Advanced Researches in Bone Marrow and Stem Cells

Advanced Researches in Bone Marrow and Stem Cells

Edited by **Rex Turner**

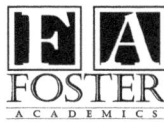

FOSTER
ACADEMICS

New Jersey

Published by Foster Academics,
61 Van Reypen Street,
Jersey City, NJ 07306, USA
www.fosteracademics.com

Advanced Researches in Bone Marrow and Stem Cells
Edited by Rex Turner

International Standard Book Number: 978-1-63242-454-9 (Hardback)

Printed in the United States of America.

Contents

Preface

Bone marrow located in the heads of long bones can be termed as a manufacturing center of red blood cells and lymphocytes as it produces billions of cells per day depending upon the requirement of the body. Bone marrow transplant is regarded as one of the most popular methods for treating blood cancer. Stem cells are generally found in embryos. These cells have a remarkable tendency to transform themselves into different body cells with the help of stem cell engineering techniques. Due to their regenerative potential they have the capability to treat diseases like heart problems, diabetes, etc. This book presents the complex subjects of bone marrow and stem cell research in the most comprehensible and easy to understand language. It attempts to understand the multiple branches that fall under the discipline of bone marrow and stem cells, and how such concepts have practical applications. The various studies that are constantly contributing towards the evolution of these fields are examined in detail. It will help the readers in keeping pace with the rapid changes in this field.

This book has been the outcome of endless efforts put in by authors and researchers on various issues and topics within the field. The book is a comprehensive collection of significant researches that are addressed in a variety of chapters. It will surely enhance the knowledge of the field among readers across the globe.

It gives us an immense pleasure to thank our researchers and authors for their efforts to submit their piece of writing before the deadlines. Finally in the end, I would like to thank my family and colleagues who have been a great source of inspiration and support.

Editor

1

Human Leukocyte Antigen Profiles of Latin American Populations: Differential Admixture and Its Potential Impact on Hematopoietic Stem Cell Transplantation

Esteban Arrieta-Bolaños,[1,2,3] **J. Alejandro Madrigal,**[1,2] **and Bronwen E. Shaw**[1,4]

[1] Clinical Research Group, The Anthony Nolan Research Institute, Royal Free & University College Medical School, London NW3 2QG, UK
[2] University College London Cancer Institute, London WC1E 6DD, UK
[3] Centro de Investigaciones en Hematología y Trastornos Afines (CIHATA), Universidad de Costa Rica, 11501-2060 San José, Costa Rica
[4] Haemato-Oncology Research Unit, Division of Molecular Pathology, The Institute of Cancer Research, London SM2 5NG, UK

Correspondence should be addressed to Esteban Arrieta-Bolaños, esteban.arrietabolanos@ucr.ac.cr

Academic Editor: Colette Raffoux

The outcome of hematopoietic stem cell transplantation (HSCT) is shaped by both clinical and genetic factors that determine its success. Genetic factors including human leukocyte antigen (HLA) and non-HLA genetic variants are believed to influence the risk of potentially fatal complications after the transplant. Moreover, ethnicity has been proposed as a factor modifying the risk of graft-versus-host disease. The populations of Latin America are a complex array of different admixture processes with varying degrees of ancestral population proportions that came in different migration waves. This complexity makes the study of genetic risks in this region complicated unless the extent of this variation is thoroughly characterized. In this study we compared the HLA-A and HLA-B allele group profiles for 31 Latin American populations and 61 ancestral populations from Iberia, Italy, Sub-Saharan Africa, and America. Results from population genetics comparisons show a wide variation in the HLA profiles from the Latin American populations that correlate with different admixture proportions. Populations in Latin America seem to be organized in at least three groups with (1) strong Amerindian admixture, (2) strong Caucasian component, and (3) a Caucasian-African gradient. These results imply that genetic risk assessment for HSCT in Latin America has to be adapted for different population subgroups rather than as a pan-Hispanic/Latino analysis.

1. Introduction

Hematopoietic stem cell transplantation (HSCT) is a curative therapy used for the treatment of malignant and nonmalignant hematologic diseases, congenital immune deficiencies, solid tumors, and metabolic diseases [1]. Its outcome is shaped not only by clinical factors [2], but also by the genetics of the patient-donor pair [3]. Apart from the normal compatibility defined by the human leukocyte antigen (HLA) system [4, 5], variation in several genetic systems is thought to have an impact on the complications experienced by patients that undergo this procedure [6].

Graft-versus-host disease (GVHD) is a major complication affecting the success of the transplant and the survival of the patients. Despite the fact that most transplants are performed with high levels of compatibility in terms of HLA, a significant proportion of these transplants is affected by GVHD. Apart from clinical factors [7], a genetic component for GVHD other than HLA has been pointed out as responsible for the occurrence of GVHD in 10/10 HLA compatible patient-donor pairs [8, 9]. Moreover, an ethnicity-driven risk of suffering GVHD after HSCT has been identified [10, 11]. However, these studies focused on "island" populations and broader populations with low admixture proportions, and further studies in admixed populations are lacking.

Latin America is a region where the most dramatic human migrations have taken place, from the early northeastern Asian bands of hunter-gatherers that conquered the last continent humanity had expanded to [12], through the 16th and 17th centuries European colonization and bringing of sub-Saharan African (SSA) slaves [13], to the latest waves of immigrants from all over the world in the last two centuries [14]. This complex population history makes present Latin American Populations (LAP) possibly the most ethnically diverse on the planet. This genetic diversity is thus likely to impact the effect of genetics on HSCT and hence it is necessary to understand it in order to be able to interpret genetic association studies in this and other medical fields.

In this study, we used population genetics tools to compare the HLA profiles of 31 LAP and 61 ancestral populations in order to characterise their diversity and classify them according to their genetic makeup.

2. Materials and Methods

2.1. Population Samples. A selection of 92 populations from Latin America, Iberia, Italy, and sub-Saharan Africa with available DNA-based typing data for HLA-A and HLA-B allele groups was made and their details are shown in Table 1. Of these, 31 LAP were defined as populations living in this region that were not classed as Amerindian. Population samples from LAP that have emigrated to the USA and Spain were also included in the analyses.

The remaining 61 populations are native population samples from the three ancestral regions that have contributed majorly to the Latin American gene pool: Amerindians (22 populations), Caucasians from Europe (Iberians and Italians, 19 populations), and SSA (20 populations). In the Caucasian population group, a sample of Italians was selected to complement the Iberian populations in view of the important immigration from this country into some LAP. In total, the population array included 384,446 chromosomes. HLA frequency data was extracted from journal articles and/or the Allele Frequencies database website [15]. The approximate geographic location for the LAP is shown in Figure 1.

2.2. Database Construction. A database containing the frequencies for 47 HLA-A and HLA-B allele groups from the 92 populations that were selected was built. When the available data were at high resolution, the data were reduced to two-digit allele groups. The database was constructed on the Multi-Variate Statistical Package (MVSP, Kovach Computing Services, Anglesey, Wales) and was independently checked for accuracy.

2.3. Population Comparisons. The HLA-A and HLA-B profiles of the 92 populations were analysed by clustering analysis and Principal Coordinates Analysis (PCO), both based on Euclidean distances. The clustering analysis was performed dually and dendrograms were generated for both analyses. The clustering method was based on minimum variance of squared Euclidean distances with a randomized input order. The Eigenanalysis for the PCO was performed at an accuracy of 1E-7 and axes were extracted according to Kaiser's rule [66].

Additionally, three ancestry-specific HLA allele groups were compared between population subgroups in order to illustrate the relative contribution of each ancestral population across LAP.

3. Results

3.1. Clustering Analysis. A dendrogram based on squared Euclidean distances was generated by the comparison of 47 HLA-A and HLA-B allele group frequencies present in the 61 ancestral populations and the 31 LAP. The results for this analysis are shown in Figure 2(a). The first split is between the Amerindian cluster and the Caucasians and SSA, which is consistent with higher differentiation of these populations. The next split is between the SSA and the Caucasian and most of the LAP.

A closer look at the clusters shows that there is a correlation between the geographic location of the ancestral populations and the branching within the clusters. Within the Amerindian cluster, 4 groups form a South American lowland group, a South American Andean group, a Central American group, and a more distinct North American-Alaskan group. A similar correlation is seen within the SSA cluster: western Africans split from the southern, eastern and central African populations. Some of the LAP cluster with the Amerindians, such as the Peruvian mestizos from Arequipa, or with the SSA, as the Cuban Mulattos and the Afro-Brazilians from Paraná. However, 90% of the LAP cluster within a distinct group which includes the Iberians and Italians.

The LAP-Iberian+Italian cluster splits further in distinct subgroups. Most of the Spanish populations, and minority populations from Spain, cluster in their own groups. Also, there is a broad group that clusters all of the remaining Brazilian and Cuban populations, and another one that clusters the Portuguese, Italian, and Argentinians from La Plata, the region of Cuyo, and Buenos Aires. Finally, the last cluster includes the admixed populations from Mexico, Colombia, Venezuela, Costa Rica, as well as the South American immigrants to Madrid and the Mexican and pan-Hispanic samples from the United States.

A dual-clustering method was applied to the dataset in order to identify the groups of alleles that are most variable between the populations. The results from this analysis are shown in Figure 2(b). Clusters of signature ancestry markers can be identified, such as frequent Amerindian input allele groups (HLA-A*68, -B*15, -A*31, -B*48, -B*40, and -B*39), frequent Iberian and Italian Caucasian markers (HLA-A*03, -A*29, -B*07, -B*44, -A*01, and-B*51), and frequent alleles that are evidence of SSA genetic input (HLA-A*30, -A*23, -B*53, -B*58, -B*45, and -B*42).

3.2. Principal Coordinates Analysis. The results from the PCO are shown in Figure 3. Firstly, the ancestral populations (Figure 3(a)) show a clear location. The first PC correlates with the Amerindian-non-amerindian split seen in the cluster analysis, whereas the second split (SSA-Caucasians) correlates with the second PC. Amerindian populations show

TABLE 1: Summary and details of the populations included in the analyses.

Code	Population	Size ($2n$)	Reference
Amerindians			
ArgCh	Argentinian Chiriguano	108	[15]
ArgET	Argentinian Eastern Toba	270	[16, 17]
ArgRT	Argentinian Toba from Rosario	172	[15]
BolA	Bolivian Aymara	204	[18]
BolQ	Bolivian Quechua	160	[19]
BraT	Brazilian Terena	120	[20]
GuaM	Guatemalan Maya	264	[21]
MexChT	Mexican Tarahumara from Chihuahua	88	[22]
MexMT	Mexican Tarasco from Michoacán	260	[23]
MexOMx	Mexican Mixe from Oaxaca	110	[24]
MexOMxt	Mexican Mixtec from Oaxaca	206	[24]
MexOZ	Mexican Zapotec from Oaxaca	180	[24]
MexTH	Mexican Teenek from Huasteca region	110	[25]
ParGua	Paraguayan Guaraní	80	[26]
PerLC	Peruvian Lama	166	[15]
PerTU	Peruvian Uro	210	[27]
VenPMB	Venezuelan Bari	110	[28]
VenSPY	Venezuelan Yucpa	146	[29]
USAYN	Alaska Yupik Natives	504	[30]
USAAI	Arizona Gila River Indian	984	[31]
USAPi	Arizona Pima	200	[28]
USSDS	South Dakota Lakota Sioux	604	[32]
LAP			
ArgBA	Argentinians from Buenos Aires	2,432	[15]
ArgCY	Argentinians from Cuyo Region	840	[15]
ArgLP	Argentinians from La Plata	200	[15]
Bra	Brazilians	216	[28]
BraBH	Brazilians from Belo Horizonte	190	[33, 34]
BraMG	Brazilians from Minas Gerais	2,000	[15]
BraPAB	Afro-Brazilians from Paraná	154	[35]
BraPCaf	Brazilian Cafuzo from Paraná	638	[35]
BraPCau	Brazilian Caucasian from Paraná	5,550	[35]
BraPMul	Brazilian Mulatto from Paraná	372	[35]
BraPS	Brazilians from Pernambuco State	202	[36]
BraSP	Brazilians from Sao Paulo	478	[15]
CCVP	Costa Ricans from the Central Valley	364	[37]
ChilS	Chileans from Santiago	140	[15]
Col	Colombians	1,122	[38]
ColMed	Colombians from Medellin	1,852	[39]
CubMx	Cubans (mixed)	378	[40]
CubMu	Cuban Mulattos	84	[33, 34]
CubWh	Cuban Whites	140	[33, 34]
MadAm	Latin American immigrants in Madrid	346	[41]
MexGM	Mexicans from Guadalajara	206	[42]
MexCM	Mexicans from Mexico City	242	[43]
MexSM	Mexicans from Sinaloa	112	[43]
MexPM	Mexicans from Puebla	198	[43]
ParM	Paraguayans	100	[44]

TABLE 1: Continued.

Code	Population	Size (2n)	Reference
PerA	Peruvians from Arequipa	336	[45]
USHis	US Hispanics	468	[15]
USHis2	US Hispanics	3,998	[46]
USHisO	US Hispanics	3,160	[47]
USMex	US Mexicans	1,106	[48]
VenCVM	Venezuelans from Caracas, Valencia, and Maracaibo	192	[15]
Iberians and Italians			
BasA	Basques from Arratia Valley	166	[49]
BasG	Basques from Guipuskoa	200	[50]
C&L	Castilians	3,880	[51]
CatG	Catalonians from Girona	176	[50]
And	Spanish from Andalucía	198	[15]
AndG	Spanish Gypsy from Andalucía	198	[15]
Ibi	Spanish from Ibiza	176	[52]
Maj	Majorcans	814	[52]
MajJD	Majorcans of Jewish descent	206	[52]
Min	Minorcans	188	[52]
Mur	Murcians	346	[53]
NCab	North Cabuernigo	190	[49]
NCant	North Cantabrians	166	[49]
PasV	Spanish from Pas Valley	176	[49]
AzoTI	Azoreans from Terceira Island	260	[15]
Ita	Italians	318,622	[54]
PorC	Portuguese from central Portugal	1,124	[15]
PorP	Portuguese from Porto	15,874	[15]
PorF	Portuguese from Faro	2,484	[15]
SSA			
CamBa	Cameroon Bamileke	154	[55]
CamBe	Cameroon Beti	348	[55]
CamYa	Cameroon Yaounde	184	[56]
CapVNW	Cape Verdeans from NW island	124	[57]
CapVSE	Cape Verdeans from SE island	124	[57]
CAFMP	Pygmy from the Central African Republic	72	[58]
GuiB	Guineans	130	[57]
Ken	Kenyans	288	[28]
KenL	Kenyans-Luo	530	[59]
KenN	Kenyans-Nandi	480	[59]
MalB	Mali Bandiagara	276	[59]
Moz	Mozambicans	500	[60]
Rwa	Rwandans	560	[61]
STIF	Sao Tome Islanders (Forro)	132	[62]
SenNM	Senegalese (Madenka)	330	[63]
SAB	Black South Africans	400	[64]
Sud	Sudanese	400	[15]
UgaK	Ugandan from Kampala	350	[65]
ZamL	Zambians from Lusaka	88	[59]
ZimHS	Zimbabwe Harare Shona	460	[28]
Total	92	384,446	

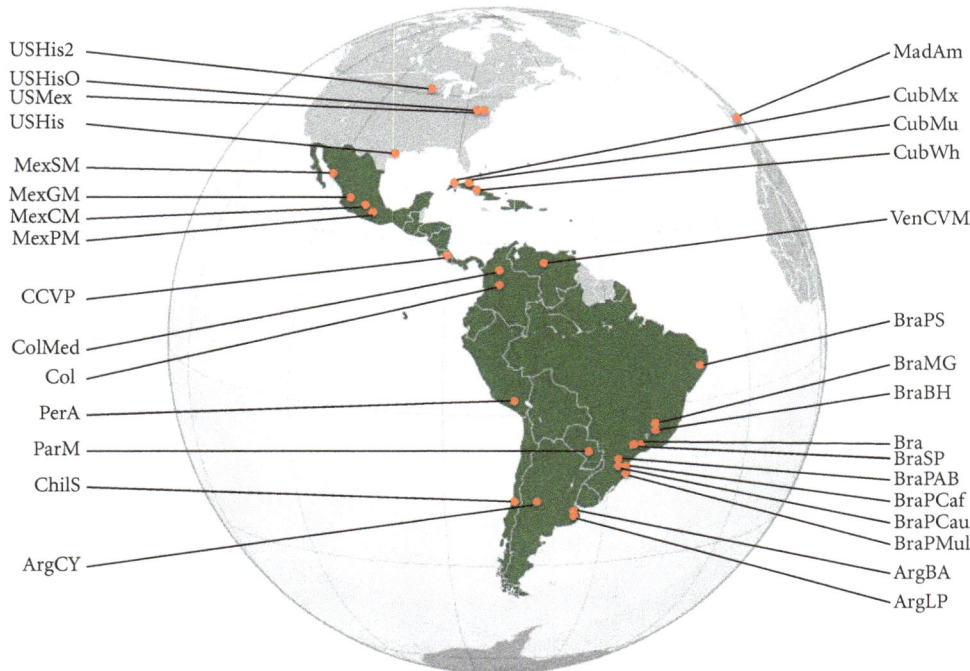

FIGURE 1: Map showing the approximate location of the LAP included in the study.

a much more dispersed array and higher distances from the Caucasians and the SSA, which is in accordance with their genetic history being shaped by the colonization of the last continent after the out-of-Africa migrations and successive bottlenecks in this process [67]. Interestingly, SSA that have been in closer genetic and geographic contact with the Caucasians, such as the Sudanese and the Cape Verdeans, are closer to these populations, whereas the southernmost Africans lie on the upper left extreme of the PCO map. Likewise, the North American Amerindians tend to be closer to the Alaskan Natives, who have been shown to be genetically different from the Amerindians of more southern regions [30].

When the LAP are included in the analysis (Figure 3(b)), the results show that LAP are located on a wide arch that connects the three ancestral populations. This arch stretches from the Peruvian mestizos from Arequipa, which appear deep into the Amerindian region, to the Afro-Brazilians from Paraná, which lie on the periphery of the SSA cluster. In between these populations there is a spectrum of locations for the remaining LAP. It is clear that there are two major regions: one that includes the LAP that lie between the Iberian and Italian populations and the Amerindian region and the others, which lie between the Caucasians and the SSA populations. Moreover, the first group seems to be divided in two subregions: one that clusters populations that lie closely to the Caucasian group (from the Argentinians from Buenos Aires to the Hispanic samples from the US), and the other (from the Mexican population from the US up to the Peruvians from Arequipa) which is dragged more intensely towards the Amerindians. The SSA component in these populations seems to be reduced, although not absent

(see below). On the other hand, the populations that lie between the Caucasians and the SSA samples also cluster closely to the Iberians and Italians, but show a gradient towards the SSA cluster. This group is composed mainly by Brazilian and Cuban populations.

A few populations seem to cluster closely enough to the ancestral populations to be considered part of those clusters. This is the case of the Cuban Mulattos and the Afro-Brazilians from Paraná, the Cuban Whites, the Brazilian Caucasians from Paraná, and the Peruvians of Arequipa. In turn, it must be noted that a population classified as Amerindian, the Argentinian Toba from the city of Rosario, show significant Caucasian admixture and, consequently, lie closer to the admixed Mexicans than the Peruvians do.

3.3. Specific Ancestry Markers. To further illustrate the differential admixture patters present in LAP based on their HLA profile, 3 allele groups which are present in one of the ancestral populations and absent or nearly absent in the other two (HLA-A*25, -B*42, and -B*48) were selected in order to evaluate their frequency among the LAP groups (Figure 4). As seen in Figure 4(a), HLA-A*25, a common allele group in western Europe and virtually absent in Amerindian and SSA populations, is present more frequently in the admixed populations with strong Caucasian component (i.e., those that lie closest to the Caucasians on the Caucasian-Amerindian axis of the PCO). Interestingly, some of the ancestral populations classified as Amerindian show evidence of Caucasian admixture as demonstrated by the presence of HLA-A*25 alleles in their gene pool.

Figure 4(b) shows the frequency of the SSA allele group HLA-B*42 in the 3 LAP subgroups. It is evident that these

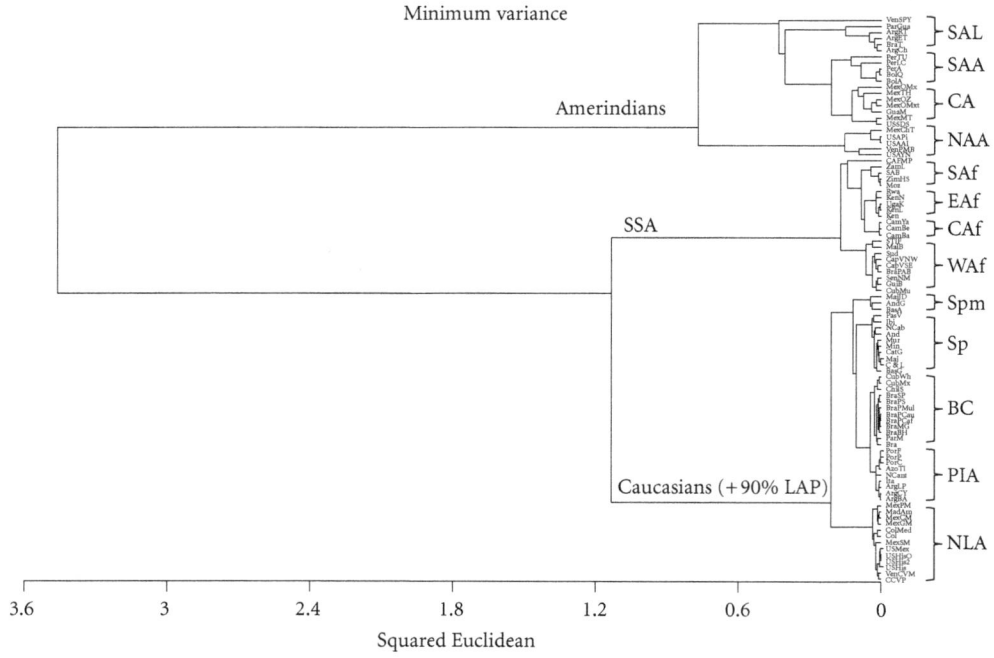

(a)

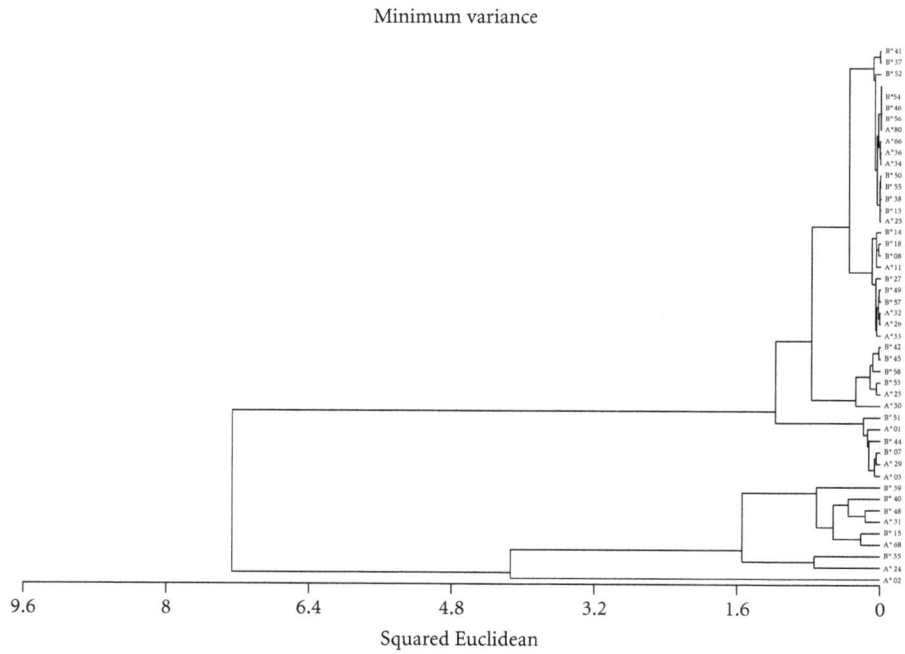

(b)

FIGURE 2: Cluster analysis based on 47 HLA-A and HLA-B allele group frequencies among 31 LAP and 61 ancestral populations. (a) Dendrogram showing the clustering of the 92 populations. (b) Dendrogram showing the dual-clustering of HLA allele groups in the dataset. SSA: Sub-Saharan Africans; SAL: South American Lowlanders; SAA: South American Andeans; CA: Central Americans; NAA: North Americans and Alaskans; SAf: Southern Africans; EAf, Eastern Africans; CAf: Central Africans; WAf: Western Africans; Spm: Spanish minorities; Sp: Spanish; BC: Brazilians and Cubans; PIA: Portuguese, Italians, and Argentinians; NLA: Northern Latin Americans.

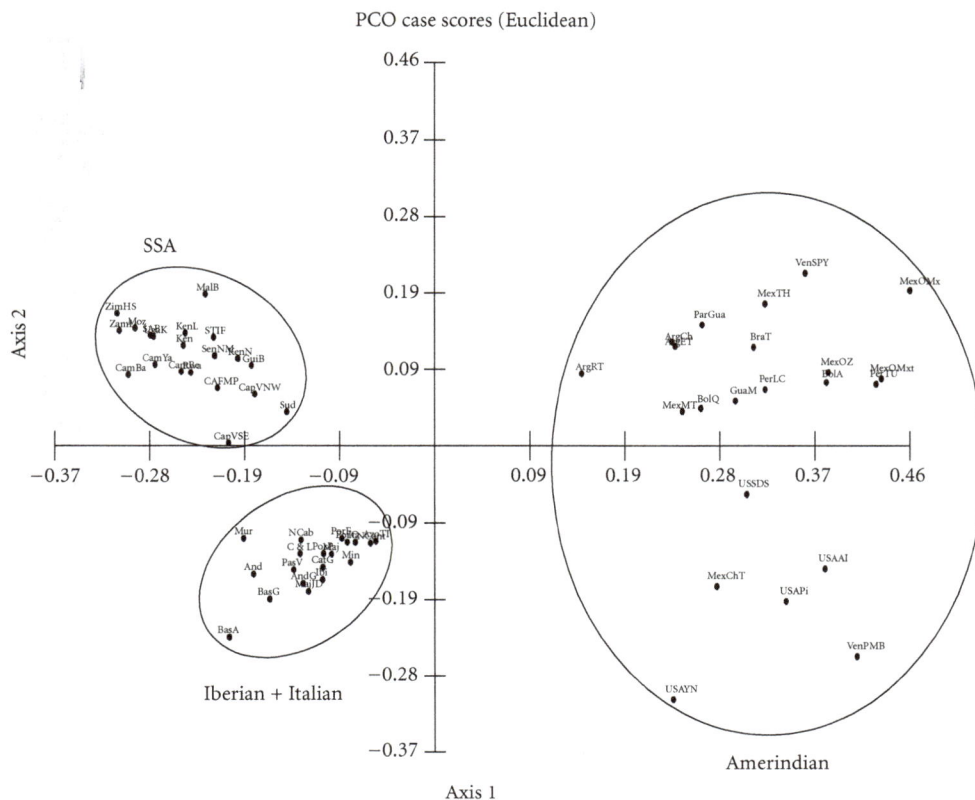

(a)

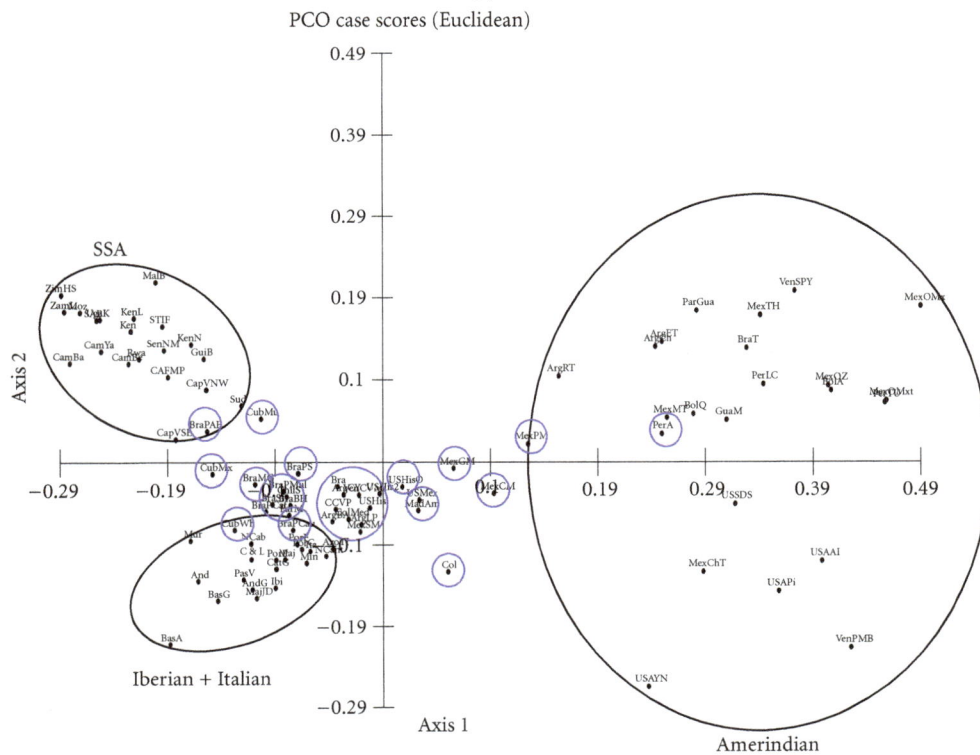

(b)

FIGURE 3: Principal coordinates analysis (PCO) based on the frequencies of 47 HLA-A and HLA-B allele groups in 31 LAP and 61 ancestral populations. (a) PCO map of the first 2 principal components (57.7% cumulative variance) for 61 ancestral populations from sub-Saharan Africa (SSA), America, and Europe. (b) PCO map showing the first 2 principal components (56.7% cumulative variance) for 31 LAP (blue) and 61 ancestral populations.

(a)

(b)

(c)

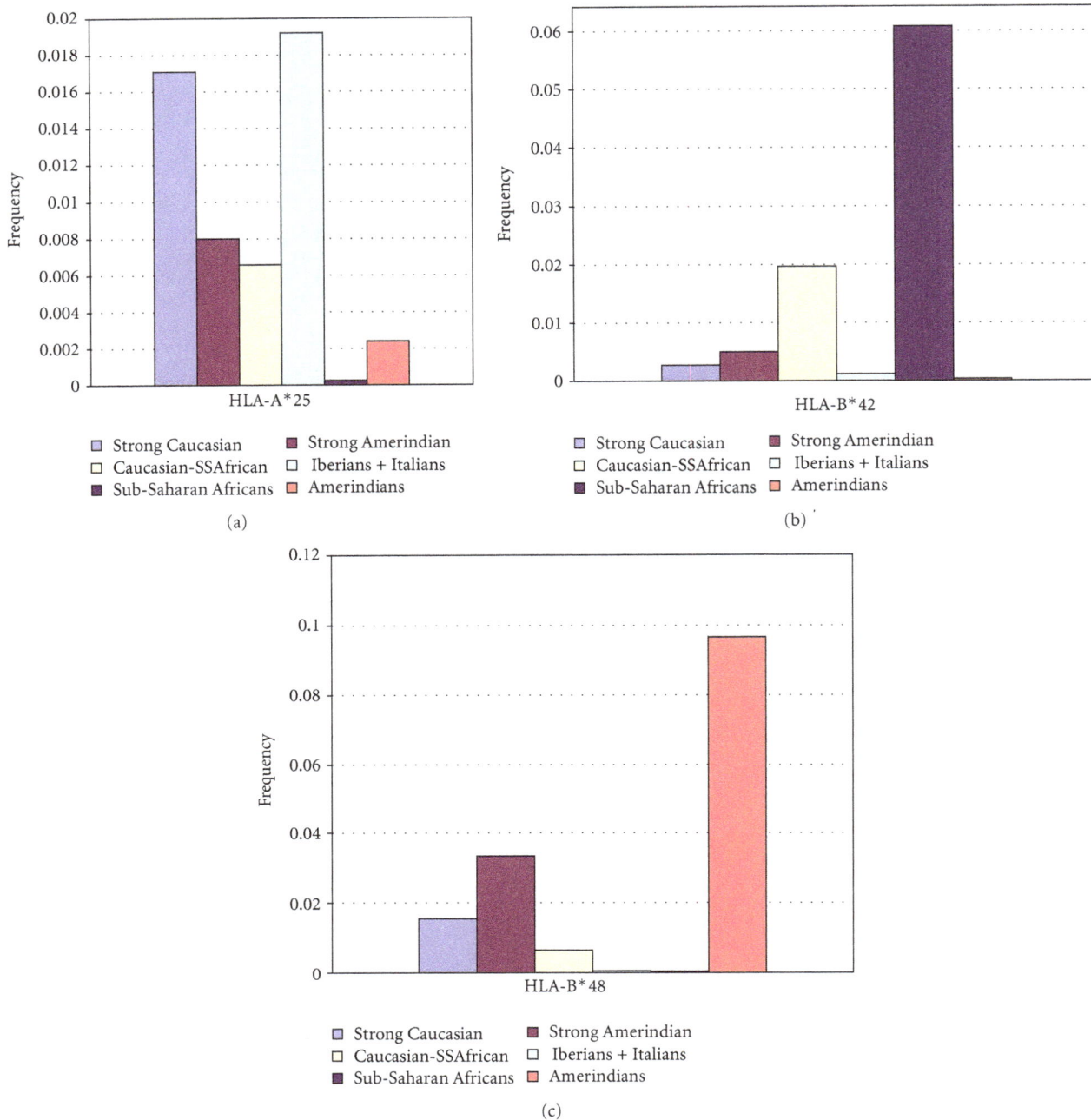

FIGURE 4: Frequency of ethnic-specific HLA allele groups among three subgroups of LAP and the ancestral populations. (a) Frequency of HLA-A*25 allele group as a Caucasian marker. (b) Frequency of HLA-B*42 allele group as a Sub-Saharan African (SSA) marker. (c) Frequency of HLA-B*48 as an Amerindian marker.

alleles are much more frequent in these populations (mainly, Brazilian and Cuban) than in the rest. However, HLA-B*42 alleles are not absent from other LAP, which may have lower levels of SSA admixture.

Finally, Figure 4(c) shows the average frequency of HLA-B*48 alleles. This group, common in Amerindians and nearly absent from SSA and Iberian and Italian populations, is more strongly represented in the populations that form the bridge between the Amerindian and Caucasian regions in the PCO.

4. Discussion

The results obtained after comparing 47 HLA-A and HLA-B allele groups among the LAP and their ancestral populations show that there is widespread variation between the genetic profiles of these admixed or exported populations. In the cluster analysis it is clear that most LAP have substantial Caucasian components, with the exception of some populations such as the Peruvians from Arequipa or the Afro-Brazilians from Paraná. This is in agreement with the uneven process of population replacement and the collapse of many Native American groups that took place throughout the continent.

However, PCO analysis showed that most LAP sit on a wide admixture arch that approaches the ancestral clusters. A few populations fall very close to or in the ancestral clusters, but most are scattered in intermediate regions. Interestingly, population samples that are likely to be a mixture of several LAP, such as those of the USA Hispanic immigrants and the Ibero-American expatriates in Madrid, sit in the center of the distribution. In fact, the heterogeneity of the Hispanic population in the US has been described using other markers [68, 69], showing differential admixture patterns between areas that have received mostly Mexican immigration and those that are predominantly colonized by Caribbean islanders from Cuba and Puerto Rico. In agreement with this, US Mexicans lie slightly closer to the Amerindian side on the PCO and locate between the Mexican populations from the center and the sample from the northern state of Sinaloa. This further illustrates the heterogeneity of the Mexican populations, where a stronger Caucasian component is preserved in the north of the country [43], while the US Mexicans are likely to be a combination of northern and southern Mexican populations.

The stronger Caucasian component in some LAP can be attributed to recent European migration [14], such as that of urban populations from Argentina and some Brazilian populations, or to relatively stronger Caucasian proportions generated at colonial times in areas where Amerindian populations were low at the time of the arrival of Europeans, which is thought to be the case of the Costa Rican Central Valley and the Colombians from Medellin [70, 71].

On the Caucasian-SSA axis of admixture, several Brazilian and Cuban populations can be found. It seems that for these populations, Amerindian admixture is very low or absent. This has been noted by others [72] and it is argued that a dual admixture model is more likely to describe the patterns seen in these populations as opposed to a triple admixture model identified for other LAP. Although not included in our analysis because of the lack of molecular HLA data, serological HLA data from Panama [73] and Puerto Rico [74] suggest that these populations are likely to join this group, whereas the data from Uruguay suggest that its major population would cluster with the strong Caucasian component group [75].

Our study is limited by both the availability of population data and the need to use HLA allele group data for comparison as opposed to high-resolution allele frequencies or haplotype frequencies. It is likely that an analysis of high-resolution frequencies would give finer results, but it would seriously diminish the number of populations that can be included in the analysis. However, the use of 47 allele groups from the most polymorphic genes in the human genome gives robustness to the analysis.

The effect of ethnicity on complications after HSCT has been suspected for many years [76, 77] but some studies have not shown such association [78]. Hence, there is growing interest in unraveling the genetic-ethnic component of GVHD in HLA-compatible HSCT. Currently, there is a project within the International Histocompatibility Working Group that aims at analyzing the risk of GVHD after HSCT in unrelated donor pairs according to the ethnic origin of both patients and donors, based on previous findings in sibling transplantations in isolated and general populations of certain countries [10]. Preliminary results in a cohort of unrelated transplants showed that Hispanic pairs have high risks of mortality and acute GVHD (grades III-IV) only second to African American pairs. Moreover, Hispanic-Hispanic pairs had the highest risk of relapse [79]. Both analyses were carried out having Asian/Pacific (mostly Japanese) ethnically matched pairs as the reference group. These findings suggest that ethnic heterogeneity in the Hispanic population may be playing a role on the risk of complications after HSCT, and the complexity of the admixture patterns illustrated in this study and others is likely to account for much of this variation. Also, ethnicity has been associated with other complications after HSCT such as chronic GVHD [80]. Moreover, an increased risk of complications has been reported specifically for Hispanic groups in North America when compared to other ethnicities in terms of survival [81] and treatment failure [82].

It is likely that the evidence for differential outcome in different ethnic groups could be explained, at least in part, by differences in allele frequencies in genes that are relevant to the immune response and that show variable interethnic polymorphism, such as the cytokine genes [83]. Moreover, polymorphisms in other genes such as those that intervene in drug metabolism or drug targets may play a role in the way patients from different ethnicities respond to treatment in HSCT, especially in admixed populations [84, 85].

LAP show widespread variation in their genetic profiles, and this complicates genetic association studies made in these populations. There is noticeable variation not only between regions and countries, but also between areas of the same country [43, 86]. Furthermore, the presence of minority populations of different ethnic composition adds to the complexity of population stratification in Latin America. Additionally, many populations remain to be studied. If an ethnic component is to be used as one prognostic factor affecting the risk of complications after HSCT, the application of this concept in Latin American populations will have to take into account the great diversity found among the different populations derived from this region and the different population subgroups generated by different admixture histories. Consequently, there is need of a more detailed understanding of the genetic profiles of the LAP, in order to be able to accurately stratify genetic risk in HSCT.

It is also important that a better definition of individual ancestry in LAP is reached in view of the evident limitations of both self-reported [87] and researcher-assigned ethnicities [41, 88]. To this purpose, the use of a more objective assignment based on ancestry markers [69] is likely to increase the accuracy of the information derived from these studies. Hopefully, a finer characterization of the risk of complications after HSCT in LAP will help foresee these complications and increase the access and success of transplantation in these populations.

Acknowledgments

This work was supported by grants from the University of Costa Rica and the Costa Rican National Council for Scientific and Technologic Research (CONICIT).

References

[1] P. Ljungman, M. Bregni, M. Brune et al., "Allogeneic and autologous transplantation for haematological diseases, solid tumours and immune disorders: current practice in Europe 2009," *Bone Marrow Transplantation*, vol. 45, no. 2, pp. 219–234, 2010.

[2] C. Anasetti, "What are the most important donor and recipient factors affecting the outcome of related and unrelated allogeneic transplantation?" *Best Practice and Research: Clinical Haematology*, vol. 21, no. 4, pp. 691–697, 2008.

[3] A. M. Dickinson, "Risk assessment in haematopoietic stem cell transplantation: pre-transplant patient and donor factors: non-HLA genetics," *Best Practice and Research: Clinical Haematology*, vol. 20, no. 2, pp. 189–207, 2007.

[4] S. J. Lee, J. Klein, M. Haagenson et al., "High-resolution donor-recipient HLA matching contributes to the success of unrelated donor marrow transplantation," *Blood*, vol. 110, no. 13, pp. 4576–4583, 2007.

[5] B. E. Shaw, R. Arguello, C. A. Garcia-Sepulveda, and J. A. Madrigal, "The impact of HLA genotyping on survival following unrelated donor haematopoietic stem cell transplantation: review," *British Journal of Haematology*, vol. 150, no. 3, pp. 251–258, 2010.

[6] A. M. Dickinson, "Non-HLA genetics and predicting outcome in HSCT," *International Journal of Immunogenetics*, vol. 35, no. 4-5, pp. 375–380, 2008.

[7] M. Jagasia, M. Arora, M. E. Flowers et al., "Risk factors for acute GVHD and survival after hematopoietic cell transplantation," *Blood*, vol. 119, no. 1, pp. 296–307, 2012.

[8] C. Baron, R. Somogyi, L. D. Greller et al., "Prediction of Graft-versus-host disease in humans by donor gene-expression profiling," *PLoS Medicine*, vol. 4, no. 1, article e23, 2007.

[9] A. M. Dickinson and E. Holler, "Polymorphisms of cytokine and innate immunity genes and GVHD," *Best Practice and Research: Clinical Haematology*, vol. 21, no. 2, pp. 149–164, 2008.

[10] H. Oh, F. R. Loberiza, M. J. Zhang et al., "Comparison of graft-versus-host-disease and survival after HLA-identical sibling bone marrow transplantation in ethnic populations," *Blood*, vol. 105, no. 4, pp. 1408–1416, 2005.

[11] S. Morishima, S. Ogawa, A. Matsubara et al., "Impact of highly conserved HLA haplotype on acute graft-versus-host disease," *Blood*, vol. 115, no. 23, pp. 4664–4670, 2010.

[12] N. Ray, D. Wegmann, N. J. R. Fagundes, S. Wang, A. Ruiz-Linares, and L. Excoffier, "A statistical evaluation of models for the initial settlement of the american continent emphasizes the importance of gene flow with Asia," *Molecular Biology and Evolution*, vol. 27, no. 2, pp. 337–345, 2010.

[13] N. Brucato, O. Cassar, L. Tonasso et al., "The imprint of the Slave Trade in an African American population: mitochondrial DNA, Y chromosome and HTLV-1 analysis in the Noir Marron of French Guiana," *BMC Evolutionary Biology*, vol. 10, article 314, 2010.

[14] M. L. Catelli, V. Alvarez-Iglesias, A. Gomez-Carballa et al., "The impact of modern migrations on present-day multi-ethnic Argentina as recorded on the mitochondrial DNA genome," *BMC Genetics*, vol. 12, article 77, 2011.

[15] F. F. Gonzalez-Galarza, S. Christmas, D. Middleton, and A. R. Jones, "Allele frequency net: a database and online repository for immune gene frequencies in worldwide populations," *Nucleic Acids Research*, vol. 39, no. 1, pp. D913–D919, 2011.

[16] M. Cerna, M. Falco, H. Friedman et al., "Differences in HLA class II alleles of isolated South American Indian populations from Brazil and Argentina," *Human Immunology*, vol. 37, no. 4, pp. 213–220, 1993.

[17] M. A. Fernández-Viña, A. M. Lázaro, C. Y. Marcos et al., "Dissimilar evolution of B-locus versus A-locus and class II loci of the HLA region in South American Indian tribes," *Tissue Antigens*, vol. 50, no. 3, pp. 233–250, 1997.

[18] A. Arnaiz-Villena, N. Siles, J. Moscoso et al., "Origin of Aymaras from Bolivia and their relationship with other Amerindians according to HLA genes," *Tissue Antigens*, vol. 65, no. 4, pp. 379–390, 2005.

[19] J. Martinez-Laso, N. Siles, J. Moscoso et al., "Origin of Bolivian Quechua Amerindians: their relationship with other American Indians and Asians according to HLA genes," *European Journal of Medical Genetics*, vol. 49, no. 2, pp. 169–185, 2006.

[20] A. M. Lázaro, M. E. Moraes, C. Y. Marcos, J. R. Moraes, M. A. Fernández-Viña, and P. Stastny, "Evolution of HLA-class I compared to HLA-class II polymorphism in Terena, a South-American Indian tribe," *Human Immunology*, vol. 60, no. 11, pp. 1138–1149, 1999.

[21] E. Gómez-Casado, J. Martínez-Laso, J. Moscoso et al., "Origin of Mayans according to HLA genes and the uniqueness of Amerindians," *Tissue Antigens*, vol. 61, no. 6, pp. 425–436, 2003.

[22] J. E. García-Ortiz, L. Sandoval-Ramírez, H. Rangel-Villalobos et al., "High-resolution molecular characterization of the HLA class I and class II in the Tarahumara Amerindian population," *Tissue Antigens*, vol. 68, no. 2, pp. 135–146, 2006.

[23] F. Loeza, G. Vargas-Alarcón, F. Andrade et al., "Distribution of class I and class III MHC antigens in the Tarasco Amerindians," *Human Immunology*, vol. 63, no. 2, pp. 143–148, 2002.

[24] J. A. Hollenbach, G. Thomson, K. Cao et al., "HLA diversity, differentiation, and haplotype evolution in mesoamerican natives," *Human Immunology*, vol. 62, no. 4, pp. 378–390, 2001.

[25] G. Vargas-Alarcón, G. Hernández-Pacheco, J. Zuñiga et al., "Distribution of HLA-B alleles in Mexican Amerindian populations," *Immunogenetics*, vol. 54, no. 11, pp. 756–760, 2003.

[26] O. Benitez, M. Busson, D. Charron, and P. Loiseau, "HLA polymorphism in a Guarani-Indian population from Paraguay and its usefulness for the Hispano-Indian admixture study in Paraguay," *International Journal of Immunogenetics*, vol. 38, no. 1, pp. 7–11, 2011.

[27] A. Arnaiz-Villena, V. Gonzalez-Alcos, J. I. Serrano-Vela et al., "HLA genes in Uros from Titikaka Lake, Peru: origin and relationship with other Amerindians and worldwide populations," *International Journal of Immunogenetics*, vol. 36, no. 3, pp. 159–167, 2009.

[28] S. Mack, Y. Tsai, A. Sanchez-Mazas, and H. A. Erlich, "Anthropology/ human genetic diversity population reports," in *Proceedings of the 13th International Histocompatibility*

Workshop and Conference on Immunobiology of the Human Genetic Diversity Population Reports, IHWG Press, Seattle, Wash, USA, 2007.

[29] Z. Layrisse, Y. Guedez, E. Domínguez et al., "Extended HLA haplotypes in a Carib Amerindian population: the Yucpa of the Perija Range," *Human Immunology*, vol. 62, no. 9, pp. 992–1000, 2001.

[30] M. S. Leffell, M. D. Fallin, H. A. Erlich et al., "HLA antigens, alleles and haplotypes among the Yup'ik Alaska natives: report of the ASHI Minority Workshops, part II," *Human Immunology*, vol. 63, no. 7, pp. 614–625, 2002.

[31] R. Williams, Y. F. Chen, R. Endres et al., "Molecular variation at the HLA-A, B, C, DRB1, DQA1, and DQB1 loci in full heritage American Indians in Arizona: private haplotypes and their evolution," *Tissue Antigens*, vol. 74, no. 6, pp. 520–533, 2009.

[32] M. S. Leffell, M. D. Fallin, W. H. Hildebrand, J. W. Cavett, B. A. Iglehart, and A. A. Zachary, "HLA alleles and haplotypes among the lakota sioux: report of the ASHI minority workshops, part III," *Human Immunology*, vol. 65, no. 1, pp. 78–89, 2004.

[33] D. Middleton, F. Williams, A. Meenagh et al., "Analysis of the distribution of HLA-A alleles in populations from five continents," *Human Immunology*, vol. 61, no. 10, pp. 1048–1052, 2000.

[34] F. Williams, A. Meenagh, C. Darke et al., "Analysis of the distribution of HLA-B alleles in populations from five continents," *Human Immunology*, vol. 62, no. 6, pp. 645–650, 2001.

[35] T. M. Ruiz, S. M. C. M. Da Costa, F. Ribas, P. R. Luz, S. S. Lima, and M. Da Graça Bicalho, "Human leukocyte antigen allelic groups and haplotypes in a Brazilian sample of volunteer donors for bone marrow transplant in Curitiba, Paraná, Brazil," *Transplantation Proceedings*, vol. 37, no. 5, pp. 2293–2296, 2005.

[36] P. Nigam, E. Dellalibera, L. Maurício-da-Silva, E. A. Donadi, and R. S. Silva, "Polymorphism of HLA class I genes in the Brazilian population from the Northeastern State of Pernambuco corroborates anthropological evidence of its origin," *Tissue Antigens*, vol. 64, no. 2, pp. 204–209, 2004.

[37] E. Arrieta-Bolaños, H. Maldonado-Torres, O. Dimitriu et al., "HLA-A, -B, -C, -DQB1, and -DRB1,3,4,5 allele and haplotype frequencies in the Costa Rica Central Valley Population and its relationship to worldwide populations," *Human Immunology*, vol. 72, no. 1, pp. 80–86, 2011.

[38] Y. R. Arias-Murillo, M. A. Castro-Jiménez, M. F. Ríos-Espinosa, J. J. López-Rivera, S. J. Echeverry-Coral, and O. Martínez-Nieto, "Analysis of HLA-A, HLA-B, HLA-DRB1 allelic, genotypic, and haplotypic frequencies in Colombian population," *Colombia Medica*, vol. 41, no. 4, pp. 336–343, 2010.

[39] L. M. Rodríguez, M. C. Giraldo, N. García et al., "Human leucocyte antigen gene (HLA-A, HLA-B, HLA-DRB1) frequencies in deceased organ donor," *Biomedica*, vol. 27, no. 4, pp. 537–547, 2007.

[40] B. Sierra, R. Alegre, A. B. Pérez et al., "HLA-A, -B, -C, and -DRB1 allele frequencies in Cuban individuals with antecedents of dengue 2 disease: advantages of the Cuban population for HLA studies of dengue virus infection," *Human Immunology*, vol. 68, no. 6, pp. 531–540, 2007.

[41] C. Parga-Lozano, D. Rey-Medrano, P. Gomez-Prieto et al., "HLA genes in Amerindian immigrants to Madrid (Spain): epidemiology and a virtual transplantation waiting list: amerindians in Madrid (Spain)," *Molecular Biology Reports*, vol. 38, no. 4, pp. 2263–2271, 2011.

[42] C. A. Leal, F. Mendoza-Carrera, F. Rivas, S. Rodriguez-Reynoso, and E. Portilla-De Buen, "HLA-A and HLA-B allele frequencies in a mestizo population from Guadalajara, Mexico, determined by sequence-based typing," *Tissue Antigens*, vol. 66, no. 6, pp. 666–673, 2005.

[43] R. Barquera, J. Zúñiga, R. Hernández-Díaz et al., "HLA class I and class II haplotypes in admixed families from several regions of Mexico," *Molecular Immunology*, vol. 45, no. 4, pp. 1171–1178, 2008.

[44] O. Benitez, C. Dehay, C. Raffoux, and J. Colombani, "Métissage hispano-indien en Amérique du Sud: essai de compréhension grâce à l'analyse sanguine du système HLA au Paraguay," *Hématologie*, vol. 1, no. 5, pp. 437–439, 1995.

[45] R. De Pablo, Y. Beraún, A. Nieto et al., "HLA class I and class II allele distribution in the Peruvian population," *Tissue Antigens*, vol. 56, no. 6, pp. 507–514, 2000.

[46] M. Maiers, L. Gragert, and W. Klitz, "High-resolution HLA alleles and haplotypes in the United States population," *Human Immunology*, vol. 68, no. 9, pp. 779–788, 2007.

[47] M. S. Leffell, W. S. Cherikh, G. Land, and A. A. Zachary, "Improved definition of human leukocyte antigen frequencies among minorities and applicability to estimates of transplant compatibility," *Transplantation*, vol. 83, no. 7, pp. 964–972, 2007.

[48] W. Klitz, L. Gragert, M. Maiers et al., "Four-locus high-resolution HLA typing in a sample of Mexican Americans," *Tissue Antigens*, vol. 74, no. 6, pp. 508–513, 2009.

[49] P. Sanchez-Velasco, E. Gomez-Casado, J. Martinez-Laso et al., "HLA alleles in isolated populations from north Spain: origin of the basques and the ancient Iberians," *Tissue Antigens*, vol. 61, no. 5, pp. 384–392, 2003.

[50] D. Comas, E. Mateu, F. Calafell et al., "HLA class I and class II DNA typing and the origin of Basques," *Tissue Antigens*, vol. 51, no. 1, pp. 30–40, 1998.

[51] M. Alcoceba, L. Mari'n, A. Balanzategui, M. E. Sarasquete et al., "Frequency of HLA-A, -B and -DRB1 specificities and haplotypic associations in the population of Castilla y Leon (northwest-central Spain)," *Tissue Antigens*, vol. 78, no. 4, pp. 249–255, 2011.

[52] C. Crespí, J. Milà, N. Martínez-Pomar et al., "HLA polymorphism in a Majorcan population of Jewish descent: comparison with Majorca, Minorca, Ibiza (Balearic Islands) and other Jewish communities," *Tissue Antigens*, vol. 60, no. 4, pp. 282–291, 2002.

[53] M. Muro, L. Marín, A. Torío et al., "HLA polymorphism in the Murcia population (Spain): in the cradle of the archaeologic Iberians," *Human Immunology*, vol. 62, no. 9, pp. 910–921, 2001.

[54] S. Rendine, I. Borelli, M. Barbanti, N. Sacchi, S. Roggero, and E. S. Curtoni, "HLA polymorphisms in Italian bone marrow donors: a regional analysis," *Tissue Antigens*, vol. 52, no. 2, pp. 135–146, 1998.

[55] J. N. Torimiro, J. K. Carr, N. D. Wolfe et al., "HLA class I diversity among rural rainforest inhabitants in Cameroon: identification of A*2612-B*4407 haplotype," *Tissue Antigens*, vol. 67, no. 1, pp. 30–37, 2006.

[56] J. M. Ellis, S. J. Mack, R. F. Leke, I. Quakyi, A. H. Johnson, and C. K. Hurley, "Diversity is demonstrated in class I HLA-A and HLA-B alleles in Cameroon, Africa: description of HLA-A*03012, *2612, *3006 and HLA-B*1403, *4016, *4703," *Tissue Antigens*, vol. 56, no. 4, pp. 291–302, 2000.

[57] H. Spínola, J. Bruges-Armas, D. Middleton, and A. Brehm, "HLA polymorphisms in Cabo Verde and Guiné-Bissau inferred from sequence-based typing," *Human Immunology*, vol. 66, no. 10, pp. 1082–1092, 2005.

[58] J. Bruges Armas, G. Destro-Bisol, A. López-Vazquez et al., "HLA class I variation in the West African Pygmies and their genetic relationship with other African populations," *Tissue Antigens*, vol. 62, no. 3, pp. 233–242, 2003.

[59] K. Cao, A. M. Moormann, K. E. Lyke et al., "Differentiation between African populations is evidenced by the diversity of alleles and haplotypes of HLA class I loci," *Tissue Antigens*, vol. 63, no. 4, pp. 293–325, 2004.

[60] A. A. A. Assane, G. M. Fabricio-Silva, J. Cardoso-Oliveira et al., "Human leukocyte antigen-A, -B, and -DRB1 allele and haplotype frequencies in the Mozambican population: a blood donor-based population study," *Human Immunology*, vol. 71, no. 10, pp. 1027–1032, 2010.

[61] J. Tang, E. Naik, C. Costello et al., "Characteristics of HLA class I and class II polymorphisms in Rwandan women," *Experimental and Clinical Immunogenetics*, vol. 17, no. 4, pp. 185–198, 2000.

[62] N. Saldanha, C. Spínola, M. R. Santos et al., "HLA polymorphisms in Forros and Angolares from Sao Tome Island (West Africa): evidence for the population origin," *Journal of Genetic Genealogy*, vol. 5, no. 2, pp. 76–85, 2009.

[63] A. Sanchez-Mazas, Q. G. Steiner, C. Grundschober, and J. M. Tiercy, "The molecular determination of HLA-Cw alleles, in the Mandenka (West Africa) reveals a close genetic relationship between Africans and Europeans," *Tissue Antigens*, vol. 56, no. 4, pp. 303–312, 2000.

[64] M. Paximadis, T. Y. Mathebula, N. L. Gentle et al., "Human leukocyte antigen class I, (A, B, C) and II, (DRB1) diversity in the black and Caucasian South African population," *Human Immunology*, vol. 73, no. 1, pp. 80–92, 2012.

[65] G. H. Kijak, A. M. Walsh, R. N. Koehler et al., "HLA class i allele and haplotype diversity in Ugandans supports the presence of a major east African genetic cluster," *Tissue Antigens*, vol. 73, no. 3, pp. 262–269, 2009.

[66] H. Kaiser, "The application of electronic computers to factor analysis," *Educational and Psychological Measurement*, vol. 20, pp. 141–151, 1960.

[67] S. L. Bonatto and F. M. Salzano, "Diversity and age of the four major mtDNA haplogroups, and their implications for the peopling of the New World," *American Journal of Human Genetics*, vol. 61, no. 6, pp. 1413–1423, 1997.

[68] B. Bertoni, B. Budowle, M. Sans, S. A. Barton, and R. Chakraborty, "Admixture in Hispanics: distribution of ancestral population contributions in the continental United States," *Human Biology*, vol. 75, no. 1, pp. 1–11, 2003.

[69] R. Kosoy, R. Nassir, C. Tian et al., "Ancestry informative marker sets for determining continental origin and admixture proportions in common populations in America," *Human Mutation*, vol. 30, no. 1, pp. 69–78, 2009.

[70] S. Wang, N. Ray, W. Rojas et al., "Geographic patterns of genome admixture in Latin American Mestizos," *PLoS Genetics*, vol. 4, no. 3, Article ID e1000037, 2008.

[71] L. G. Carvajal-Carmona, R. Ophoff, S. Service et al., "Genetic demography of Antioquia (Colombia) and the Central Valley of Costa Rica," *Human Genetics*, vol. 112, no. 5-6, pp. 534–541, 2003.

[72] A. Cintado, O. Companioni, M. Nazabal et al., "Admixture estimates for the population of Havana City," *Annals of Human Biology*, vol. 36, no. 3, pp. 350–360, 2009.

[73] A. A. Vernaza-Kwiers, I. J. de Gómez, M. Díaz-Isaacs, C. J. Cuero, E. Pérez Guardia, and M. Moreno Saavedra, "Gene frequency and haplotypes of the HLA system in the Panamanian population," *Revista Médica de Panamá*, vol. 20, no. 3, pp. 116–123, 1995.

[74] E. A. Santiago-Delpín, S. De Echegaray, F. Rivera-Cruz, and A. Rodríguez-Trinidad, "The histocompatibility profile of the Puerto Rican population," *Transplantation Proceedings*, vol. 34, no. 8, pp. 3075–3078, 2002.

[75] I. Alvarez, M. Bengochea, R. Toledo, E. Carretto, and P. C. Hidalgo, "HLA class I antigen and HLA-A, -B, and -C haplotype frequencies in Uruguayans," *Human Biology*, vol. 78, no. 4, pp. 513–525, 2006.

[76] S. J. Easaw, D. E. Lake, M. Beer, K. Seiter, E. J. Feldman, and T. Ahmed, "Graft-versus-host disease. Possible higher risk for African American patients," *Cancer*, vol. 78, no. 7, pp. 1492–1497, 1996.

[77] K. S. Baker, S. M. Davies, N. S. Majhail et al., "Race and socioeconomic status influence outcomes of unrelated donor hematopoietic cell transplantation," *Biology of Blood and Marrow Transplantation*, vol. 15, no. 12, pp. 1543–1554, 2009.

[78] P. N. Hari, N. S. Majhail, M. J. Zhang et al., "Race and outcomes of autologous hematopoietic cell transplantation for multiple myeloma," *Biology of Blood and Marrow Transplantation*, vol. 16, no. 3, pp. 395–402, 2010.

[79] Y. Morishima, "Impact of donor-recipient ethnicity on risk of acute graft-versus-host disease, leukemia relapse and survival in hematopoietic stem cell transplantation from HLA-compatible unrelated donors," in *Proceedings of the 51st ASH Annual Meeting and Exposition, A Report From the International Histocompatibility Workshop Group*, New Orleans, Miss, USA, 2009.

[80] M. Remberger, J. Aschan, B. Lönnqvist et al., "An ethnic role for chronic, but not acute, graft-versus-host disease after HLA-identical sibling stem cell transplantation," *European Journal of Haematology*, vol. 66, no. 1, pp. 50–56, 2001.

[81] D. S. Serna, S. J. Lee, M. J. Zhang et al., "Trends in survival rates after allogeneic hematopoietic stem-cell transplantation for acute and chronic leukemia by ethnicity in the United States and Canada," *Journal of Clinical Oncology*, vol. 21, no. 20, pp. 3754–3760, 2003.

[82] K. S. Baker, F. R. Loberiza, H. Yu et al., "Outcome of ethnic minorities with acute or chronic leukemia treated with hematopoietic stem-cell transplantation in the United States," *Journal of Clinical Oncology*, vol. 23, no. 28, pp. 7032–7042, 2005.

[83] S. C. Hoffmann, E. M. Stanley, E. D. Cox et al., "Ethnicity greatly influences cytokine gene polymorphism distribution," *American Journal of Transplantation*, vol. 2, no. 6, pp. 560–567, 2002.

[84] G. Suarez-Kurtz, J. P. Genro, M. O. de et al., "Global pharmacogenomics: impact of population diversity on the distribution of polymorphisms in the CYP2C cluster among Brazilians," *Pharmacogenomics Journal*, vol. 12, no. 3, pp. 267–276, 2012.

[85] G. Suarez-Kurtz and S. D. J. Pena, "Pharmacogenomics in the Americas: the impact of genetic admixture," *Current Drug Targets*, vol. 7, no. 12, pp. 1649–1658, 2006.

[86] B. Morera, R. Barrantes, and R. Marin-Rojas, "Gene admixture in the Costa Rican population," *Annals of Human Genetics*, vol. 67, no. 1, pp. 71–80, 2003.

[87] T. C. Lins, R. G. Vieira, B. S. Abreu et al., "Genetic heterogeneity of self-reported ancestry groups in an admixed Brazilian population," *Journal of Epidemiology*, vol. 21, no. 4, pp. 240–245, 2011.

[88] K. Hunley and M. Healy, "The impact of founder effects, gene flow, and European admixture on native American genetic diversity," *American Journal of Physical Anthropology*, vol. 146, no. 4, pp. 530–538, 2011.

2

New Rising Infection: Human Herpesvirus 6 Is Frequent in Myeloma Patients Undergoing Autologous Stem Cell Transplantation after Induction Therapy with Bortezomib

Netanel Horowitz,[1] Ilana Oren,[2,3] Noa Lavi,[1] Tsila Zuckerman,[1,3] Noam Benyamini,[1] Zipi Kra-Oz,[4] Viki Held,[1] and Irit Avivi[1,3]

[1] Department of Hematology and Bone Marrow Transplantation, Rambam Health Care Campus, P.O. Box 9602, Haifa 31096, Israel
[2] Unit of Infectious Diseases, Rambam Health Care Campus, P.O. Box 9602, Haifa 31096, Israel
[3] Bruce Rappaport Faculty of Medicine, Technion – Israel Institute of Technology, P.O. Box 9602, Haifa 31096, Israel
[4] Virology Laboratory, Rambam Health Care Campus, P.O. Box 9602, Haifa 31096, Israel

Correspondence should be addressed to Irit Avivi, irit_avivi@hotmail.com

Academic Editor: Catherine Bollard

Herpesvirus 6 (HHV-6) infection is a common complication during immunosuppression. Its significance for multiple myeloma (MM) patients undergoing autologous stem cell transplantation (ASCT) after treatment with novel agents affecting immune system remains undetermined. Data on 62 consecutive MM patients receiving bortezomib-dexamethasone (VD) ($n = 41$; 66%) or thalidomide-dexamethasone (TD) ($n = 21$, 34%) induction, together with melphalan $200 \, mg/m^2$ autograft between 01.2005 and 09.2010, were reviewed. HHV-6 reactivation was diagnosed in patients experiencing postengraftment unexplained fever (PEUF) in the presence of any level of HHHV-6 DNA in blood. There were no statistically significant differences in patient characteristics between the groups, excluding dexamethasone dosage, which was significantly higher in patients receiving TD. Eight patients in TD and 18 in VD cohorts underwent viral screening for PEUF. HHV-6 reactivation was diagnosed in 10 patients of the entire series (16%), accounting for 35% of those screened; its incidence was 19.5% ($n = 8$) in the VD group versus 9.5% ($n = 2$) in the TD group. All patients recovered without sequelae. In conclusion, HHV-6 reactivation is relatively common after ASCT, accounting for at least a third of PEUF episodes. Further studies are warranted to investigate whether bortezomib has an impact on HHV-6 reactivation development.

1. Introduction

Human herpesvirus 6 (HHV-6) is highly prevalent in humans, infecting almost all children during their early childhood [1–4]. Similar to other herpesviruses, it tends to remain dormant in the host tissues, but may reactivate in the presence of immune suppression, resulting in a febrile illness, often accompanied with skin eruption, encephalitis, or pneumonia [5–11]. Immune dysfunction, existing following allogeneic stem cell transplantation (Allo SCT), induced by either immunosuppressive drugs or the development of graft-versus-host disease (GvHD) appears to result in a significant risk of HHV-6 reactivation [12], approaching 33–48% [13–16].

Unlike Allo SCT, autologous stem cell transplantation (ASCT), being associated with mild transient immunodeficiency, has been traditionally considered a less probable cause of HHV-6 reactivation. However, studies exploring this risk in heterogeneous groups of autografted patients reported a similarly high risk for HHV-6 infection [16], suggesting the malignancy itself, and/or the treatment applied preautograft, to contribute to transplant-associated immune impairment.

Induction therapy for myeloma has changed dramatically over the last few years and the traditional VAD (vincristine, doxorubicin, dexamethasone) has been substituted with thalidomide, bortezomib, and lenalidomide-based regimens

[17, 18]. Apart from their well-recognized tumoricidal activity, these novel agents are known to modulate myeloma cell microenvironment and the immune system. Lenalidomide and thalidomide act as immunomodulatory drugs, inducing activation of cytotoxic T lymphocytes, and natural killer (NK) cells [19, 20], whereas bortezomib-based induction has been recently suggested to cause a transient decrease in CD8 and NK cell counts [21] and function, selective depletion of TH_1 cells [22] and dendritic cell (DC) dysfunction [23, 24].

This leads to an increased incidence of herpes Zoster infection in patients receiving bortezomib, which is reported to approach 13% [25].

The incidence of HHV-6 infection has not yet been studied in a large homogenous group of autografted MM patients. Furthermore, a potential adverse effect of pretransplant administration of novel biological agents on transplant-related HHV-6 infection has not been explored.

The current study was designed to assess the incidence, clinical significance, and risk factors for HHV-6 reactivation in a large cohort of myeloma patients, consecutively treated with novel agents and ASCT.

2. Patients and Methods

The study was approved by the Institutional Review Board (IRB) of the Rambam Health Care Campus (approval no. 0380-11RMBG).

The departmental transplant database was searched for all myeloma patients, aged 18 years or older, who underwent autologous stem cell transplantation after receiving a thalidomide or bortezomib-based therapy, completed within less than 2 months to prior transplant. Patients who received VT or TD as their second line pretransplant therapy were not included, unless they completed first therapeutic regimen, at least 6 months prior to the initiation of TD/VD. Patients receiving a second ASCT, performed in a tandem setting or at disease progression, were not included in this study. Data on induction therapy and transplant-related complications (particularly, infectious, neurological, and respiratory) were obtained from original computerized medical files.

2.1. Treatment Protocols for Multiple Myeloma. Pretransplant treatment protocols included in the current study were VD (intravenous bortezomib 1.3 mg/m² on days 1, 4, 8, 11, and dexamethasone 40 mg on the days of bortezomib administration) and TD (p.o. thalidomide 100–200 mg daily, administered together with dexamethasone).

The transplant conditioning regimen was melphalan 200 mg/m², administered over 1 day. All transplanted patients received anti-herpes-zoster prophylaxis with acyclovir 200 mg four times per day, started on day +1 after transplant and continuing up to 90 days.

2.2. Virology Screening Protocol. According to the department protocol, patients with persistent fever (temperature >38°C for ≥3 days), occurring after neutrophil engraftment (>500) or beyond day 16 after transplant, in whom detailed investigation for a causative pathogen (multiple blood cultures, polymerase chain reaction (PCR) for aspergillus,

serologic test for galactomannan, and chest CT scan) failed to detect bacterial or fungal infective cause, underwent a molecular investigation for viral infection, including PCR tests of peripheral blood (PB) for cytomegalovirus (CMV), Epstein-Barr virus (EBV), adenovirus, and HHV-6. Patients exhibiting lower or upper respiratory symptoms were also screened for respiratory viruses, using PCRs for influenza (A, B, H1N1), parainfluenza viruses types 1, 2, 3, RSV, and adenovirus, examined in respiratory secretions. Notably, criteria for performing virology screen remained unchanged during the study period.

PCR for HHV-6 was repeated only if patient's symptoms (including fever) had not resolved within one week from HHV-6 diagnosis.

2.3. Diagnosis of HHV-6 Reactivation. Diagnosis of HHV-6 reactivation was made in the presence of any level of HHV-6 DNA in blood [12] and otherwise unexplained fever after ruling out other infectious pathogens, as detailed above. High-level HHV-6 reactivation was defined as >1000 HHV-6 DNA copies/Ml plasma [12]. HHV-6 disease was diagnosed in the presence of HHV-6 related complications such as encephalitis or pneumonia [12].

Notably, the PCR test, described below, was shown to be highly sensitive (100%) and highly specific, with no false positive events, attributed to concurrent bacterial and viral infections [26].

2.4. DNA Extraction. DNA was extracted from patient's whole blood samples (200 μL per sample), using the Magna Pure LC apparatus and Magna Pure LC total Nucleic Acid Isolation Kit Reagents (Roche Diagnostics, Germany). For manual extraction the QIAamp DNA blood mini kit was used, according to the manufacturer's instructions (QIAgen LTd., Crawly, England, UK). Up to the year 2008, HHV-6 DNA was detected using nested PCR (nPCR), which was then replaced with TaqMan real time PCR.

2.5. Nested PCR. DNA was amplified by conventional nested PCR [27], in which the primers were designed to target the HHV-6 13R gene (the outer forward: 5′ AAG-CTT-GCA-CAA-TGC-CAA-AAA-AAC-AG-3′; Outer reverse: 5′ CTC-GAG-TAT-GCC-GAG-ACC-CCT-AAT-C-3′; Inner forward: 5′ TCC-ATT-ATT-TTG-GCC-GCA-TTC-GT-3; the Inner reverse: 5′ TGT-TAG-GAT-ATA-CCG-ATG-TGC-GT-3′). These primers present a genomic region showing high homology (95%) between HHV-6 A and B subtypes.

nPCR reaction was performed in 25 μL volume using ReddyMix PCR master mix (Thermo scientific, UK). Five microliters (μL) of the extracted DNA were added to the first PCR reaction and 2 μL of the first round product were added to the nested reaction. Amplification was performed by 30 cycles of denaturation at 95°C for 60 seconds, annealing at 55°C for 60 seconds, and elongation at 72°C for 90 seconds. PCR products were detected by electrophoresis in 2% agarose gel stained with ethidium bromide.

2.6. TaqMan Real Time PCR. The primers and probe were targeted—U6 gene. (Forward primer: 5′ AAAATTTCT-CACGCCGGTATTC 3′; reverse primer: 5′ CCTGCAGAC-CGTTCGTCAA 3′; probe—6-FAM-TCGGTCGACTGC-CCGCTACCA-BHQ). PCR reaction was performed in a total volume of 25 μL containing Absolute Blue QPCR mix (Thermo scientific UK) in the presence of 5 μL target DNA, 300 nM of each primer, and 200 nM of the probe. PCR was performed on the Corbet Research platform under the following conditions: 15 min at 95°C, and 45 cycles of 15 seconds at 95°C and 60 seconds at 60°C. For quantitative results analysis, a standard curve was constructed using quantified HHV-6 DNA (Advanced Biotechnology Industry). The results were reported as the number of HHV-6 genome copies per 1 mL of blood. The lowest detection level of the test is 250 genomic copies per milliliter.

3. Statistical Analysis

Analysis was performed using SPSS 18.0 software. As data were not normally distributed according to Kolmogorov-Smirnov test, quantitative variables were analyzed by Mann-Whitney U test. Categorical variables were analyzed by Fisher Exact test. $P < 0.05$ was considered significant.

4. Results

4.1. Characteristics of the Entire Patient Series. Sixty-two consecutive patients, 21 (33%) who received pretransplant TD and 41 (66%) who had VD, were analyzed. The median age at SCT for the whole series was 56.5 years (35–67 years). Characteristics of the patient group as a whole and depending on pretransplant induction regimen are presented in Table 1. No statistically significant differences were revealed in the characteristics of patients treated with VD versus TD, except for a longer time from diagnosis to SCT and a higher cumulative dose of steroids in those treated with TD (10 versus 8 months, $P = 0.024$, and 1000 versus 640 mg, $P = 0.024$, Table 1).

4.2. Characteristics of Patients Selected for Viral Screening. Twenty-six patients, 8 treated with TD and 18 treated with VD (P = n.s.), who exhibited postengraftment unexplained fever, underwent molecular blood tests for viral infections (Figure 1). Characteristics of patients selected for viral screening after treatment with TD ($n = 8$) versus VD (18) are shown in Table 2. There were no statistically significant differences between these 2 cohorts apart from a higher steroid dosage in patients receiving TD (880 mg versus 640 mg, $P = 0.022$).

4.3. Incidence of HHV-6 Reactivation and Characteristics of Infected Patients. HHV-6 reactivation was revealed in ten patients (median age 57 years; range 49–67 years), within 14 to 26 days after transplant (median 17 days).

The incidence of reactivation in the whole cohort approached 16%: 19.5% (8/41) in the VD cohort, compared to 9.5% (2/21) in the TD group (P = n.s.). While a similar proportion of patients underwent screening in both treatment groups (43% of VDs versus 38% of TDs), the

incidence of HHV-6 reactivation in the screened "VD subjects" approached 44% (8/18) versus 25% (2/8) in their "TD" counterparts (P = n.s.) (Figure 1).

Notably, the cumulative steroid dose in patients diagnosed with HHV-6 reactivation was higher than recorded in screened HHV-6 negative subjects (880 mg versus 640 mg, $P = 0.038$) and was remarkably elevated, approaching 1230 mg, in those diagnosed with high-level HHV-6 reactivation ($n = 3$).

All patients diagnosed with reactivation of HHV-6 presented with high, unexplained fever.

Causes for fever in patients undergoing a virology screen, in whom HHV-6 was found to be negative, were considered as Hickman-related infection (resolving shortly after removal of Hickman catheter, $n = 7$), drug-related (resolving immediately after drug cessation; $n = 1$), or undetermined ($n = 8$), with no significant differences in distribution of these causes among patients treated with TD versus VD.

Six of the 10 patients (60%) diagnosed with HHV-6 reactivation, were actually defined as having an HHV-6 disease, presenting with asymptomatic respiratory involvement, detected by chest CT scans, which demonstrated non-specific lung infiltrations. Notably, 3 of these 6 patients had a high level of HHV-6 reactivation.

None of the patients diagnosed with HHV-6 reactivation developed delirium or any other clinically significant neurological manifestations, and none of the patients had a skin rash.

The median time for neutrophil and platelet engraftment was similar for patients diagnosed with HHV6 infection versus the "negative" screened cohort, approaching 12 versus 14 days and 14 versus 15 days, respectively.

As expected, all patients were severely lymphopenic at the time of reactivation (absolute lymphocyte count < 500/μL). However, the median pretransplant lymphocyte count in patients diagnosed with HHV-6 reactivation did not statistically differ from that measured in the rest screened subjects (1045/μL versus 730/μL, resp.; $P = 0.24$).

Infection-related symptoms self-resolved within one week after diagnosis in 9 patients, none of whom developed a concurrent opportunistic infection.

One patient, experiencing prolonged fever (>1 week) since diagnosis of high-level HHV-6 reactivation (120,000 copies/μL), underwent a repeated PCR test, still showing a significant number of viral copies (100,000 copies/μL). PCR test for CMV was also positive, which is compatible with a concurrent CMV reactivation. Therefore, the patient was eventually treated with intravenous gancyclovir, resulting in resolution of clinical symptoms within 4 days. Three additional patients who experienced a spontaneous resolution of fever within less than one week but reported on a remarkable exhaustion, underwent a repeated PCR test (performed upon physician discretion), showing a low HHV-6 level in two (day 13 and 17, resp.), and clearance of HHV-6 in the third individual (day 14).

A long-term evaluation, performed within a median followup of 494 days (range 14–2437) after autograft showed that 49 patients were alive, including 10 of the HHV-6 positive subjects (100%), 5 of the HHV-6 negative screened

TABLE 1: Clinical characteristics of the group as a whole ($n = 62$).

	Whole group ($n = 62$)	VD cohort ($n = 41$)	TD cohort ($n = 21$)	P
Sex (male)	36 (58%)	25 (61%)	11 (52%)	n.s.
Median age, years (range)	56.5 (35–67)	58 (35–67)	56 (45–64)	n.s.
Median time from diagnosis to SCT, months (range)	9 (4–60)	8 (4–36)	10 (7–60)	0.024
Median accumulative steroid dosage, mg (range)	800 (320–4320)	640 (320–3680)	1000 (320–4320)	0.024

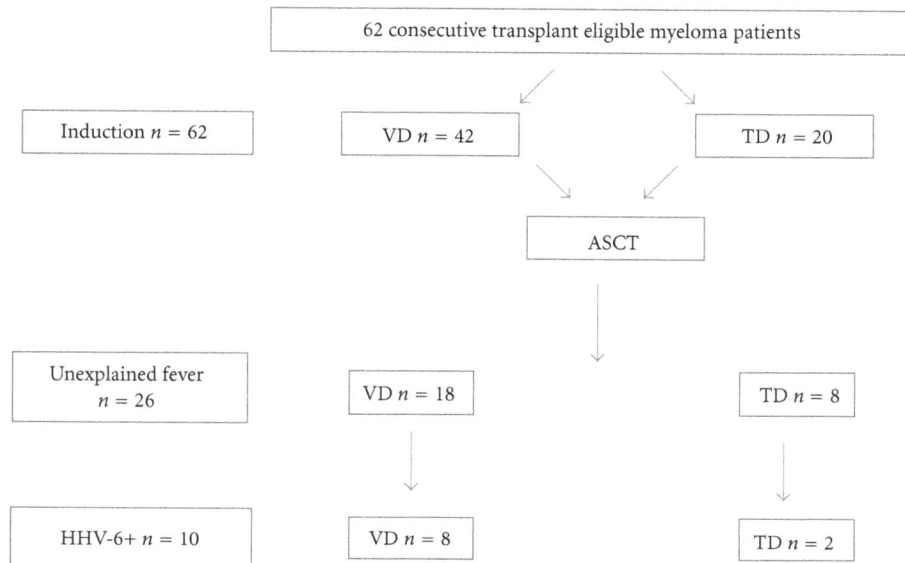

FIGURE 1: Cohort diagram.

subjects (31%), and 8 of the nonscreened subjects (25%). None of the patients in the entire cohort had clinically significant long-term neurological sequels.

4.4. Risk Factors for HHV-6 Infection. Univariate analysis of patients undergoing virology screen due to an unexplained fever following engraftment, found the exposure to a higher steroid dose to be the only statistically significant factor for HHV-6 infection (Table 3). Accumulative steroid dose in infected subjects approached 880 mg versus 640 mg in their "negative-screened" counterparts ($P = 0.038$). The incidence of HHV-6 infection appeared to be higher in subjects receiving VD versus TD (45% versus 25%), though the difference was not statistically significant. Notably, patients treated with VD received a statistically significantly lower dose of steroids (640 mg) relative to those treated with TD (880 mg) (Table 2).

5. Discussion

The prevalence and significance of HHV-6 reactivation in patients undergoing ASCT have not been fully elucidated [16, 28, 29], which could be related either to a low incidence of this complication or poor reporting attributed to limited clinical significance. The largest series ever published, prospectively evaluating HHV-6 infection in autografted patients, observed a 47% risk for HHV-6 infection [16]. This

study included 21 MM patients managed in the prenovel agent era, when treatment was based on chemotherapy rather than biological agents (e.g., thalidomide and bortezomib), which affected the immune microenvironment in addition to their direct antimalignant activity [30]. The relatively mild immunosuppression associated with ASCT might become more profound in patients whose pretransplant treatment already resulted in immunodeficiency.

Bortezomib has been reported to induce T-cell inactivation [22], leading to an increased incidence of herpes zoster in patients treated with bortezomib-containing regimens [25, 31]. Interestingly, patients receiving thalidomide do not experience such risk, despite being exposed to equal doses of steroids. The expanding use of bortezomib for pretransplant induction therapy raised the question whether this novel agent also increases the risk of post-transplant HHV-6 reactivation.

The current retrospective study explored the incidence and clinical significance of HHV-6 reactivation in 62 consecutive MM patients undergoing ASCT, after receiving induction therapy with either thalidomide or bortezomib. Notably, there were no statistically significant differences in characteristics of patients receiving VD versus TD, apart from a higher cumulative steroid dose in those receiving thalidomide. Twenty-six (42%) patients, 18 in the VD cohort (44%) and 8 in the TD group (38%), experienced a post-engraftment "unexplained" fever, hence, underwent a PCR

TABLE 2: Clinical characteristics of screened patients ($n = 26$) dependent on induction therapy.

	VD ($n = 18$)	TD ($n = 8$)	P
Sex (male)	9 (50%)	4 (50%)	
Median age, years (range)	55 (35–67)	54 (45–63)	n.s.
Disease status	CR; 2 PR: 1 VGPR: 9 Unknown: 6	PR: 5 VGPR: 2 Unknown: 1	
Median time from diagnosis to SCT, months (range)	7 (5–28)	9.5 (7–24)	n.s.
Median accumulative steroid dosage, mg (range)	640 (480–3680)	880 (320–4320)	0.022

TABLE 3: Risk factors for HHV6 reactivation after autologous SCT*.

	HHV-6 positive ($n = 10$)		HHV-6 negative ($n = 16$)		P
Age	57 (49–67)		53 (35–63)		n.s.
Male	7 (70%)		6 (37.5%)		n.s.
Female	3 (30%)		10 (62.5%)		n.s.
Median time from diagnosis to SCT, months (range)	8.5 (6–28)		7 (5–19)		n.s.
Induction regimen*	VD	TD	VD	TD	
	8 (44%)	2 (25%)	10 (54%)	8 (75%)	n.s.
Median accumulative steroid dosage, mg (range)	880 (640–1600)		640 (320–4320)		0.038
Pretransplant lymphocyte count (cells/μL)	1045		730		0.24

* Calculation represents the proportion of HHV-6 infection in screened patients that were treated with the same induction regimen (VD or TD, resp.).

virology screen. Ten patients (16.5%) were diagnosed with HHV-6 reactivation. This incidence appears to be lower than previously reported in autografted patients [16], reflecting either the lack of large homogenous historical series reliably estimating the incidence of HHV-6 reactivation in transplanted myeloma patients, or the retrospective nature of our study which selected patients for viral screen based on their symptoms. Thus, reporting was limited to clinically significant cases only, while missing asymptomatic infected subjects, those presenting with delayed engraftment as their sole complication (a presentation which is relatively rare), or those in whom fever resolved in less than 3 days.

As mentioned earlier, previous studies looked at heterogeneous groups of autographed patients treated in the prenovel agent era; hence, their data are barely comparable with ours [16, 29].

All the ten patients diagnosed with HHV-6 reactivation, presented with high unexplained fever, in the absence of other opportunistic infections, except for one subject, who had concurrent reactivation of CMV, a phenomenon recently described by Zerr et al. [12]. Respiratory involvement, though clinically insignificant, was detected in 6 subjects, whereas none had clinical evidence of neurological involvement, emphasizing the relatively innocent course of HHV-6 reactivation in this population. These findings are in line with the low PCR level observed in most our patients, which was less than reported in the allograft setting [12]. Nonetheless, HHV-6 reactivation may result in a more aggressive course, characterized with a higher frequency of

neurological complications [12, 32], and concurrent opportunistic infections, reflecting the deeper immunosuppressive milieu induced in the allogeneic setting and potentially resulting even in long-term neurological complications [12, 32].

However, the conclusion regarding the relatively innocent course of HHV-6 reactivation in autografted MM patients, previously treated with biological agents affecting immune function, should be considered with caution, given the retrospective nature of the study, the small number of evaluated patients, and the relatively short-term followup after transplant, which may interfere with proper evaluation of long-term infection-related sequels.

Nevertheless, despite the mild clinical course of HHV-6 in this setting, HHV-6 reactivation appeared to be responsible for a significant number of "post-engraftment unexplained febrile episodes," emphasizing the significance of searching for this pathogen as a potential cause for fever.

Eight patients in the VD group and 2 in the TD cohort, accounting for 19.5% of the VD versus 9.5% of the TD series, developed HHV-6 reactivation. In a similar vein, the incidence of HHV-6 in tested VDs was higher than in tested TDs (44% versus 25%), despite screening a comparable proportion of patients in both treatment groups (44% in the VD versus 36% in the TD, P = n.s.). This difference, though not statistically significant due to the low number of patients analyzed, may suggest VD to be a risk factor for post-transplant HHV-6 reactivation.

Treatment with bortezomib has been reported to be uniquely associated with an increased risk for varicella-zoster virus (VZV) infection [25]. The VZV incidence in VD-treated patients approached 13%, compared with 5% in their dexamethasone-treated counterparts ($P = 0.0002$) [25]. The mechanism of VZV reactivation has not yet been fully clarified. VZV-specific T cells appear to be necessary for suppressing VZV reactivation and preventing the VZV development [21, 33, 34]. Several studies suggested that bortezomib alters the number and function of specific lymphocyte subsets [21, 35]. Furthermore, it has been demonstrated that bortezomib impairs dendritic cell viability and function [23, 24], augmenting T-cell dysfunction. It is plausible that bortezomib also alters the function and/or interactions of key immune cells required for the suppression of HHV-6.

Consistent with our results, exposure to steroids was reported to significantly increase the risk for herpetic diseases, particularly herpes zoster [36], inducing a marked immunosuppression which allows herpes reactivation. Indeed, a high level of HHV-6 reactivation was associated with a higher accumulative steroid dose.

It is noteworthy that the low incidence of HHV-6 reactivation observed in patients receiving thalidomide may reflect induction of immunomodulation, rather than immunodeficiency [37].

6. Conclusion

The current study, investigating the incidence and clinical significance of HHV6 reactivation in a large cohort of homogenous transplanted MM patients, suggests HHV-6 is a significant cause of unexplained post-engraftment fever. Although the infection is almost always self-resolving, its detection could exclude the necessity for additional investigations and help in the management of such patients. The findings may suggest bortezomib is a potential risk factor of HHV-6 reactivation development, emphasizing the need for further large prospective studies to confirm this observation.

Conflict of Interests

Neither author has any conflict of interests.

Authors' Contribution

N. Horowitz and I. Oren contributed equally to this work.

References

[1] K. Takahashi, S. Sonoda, K. Higashi et al., "Predominant CD4 T-lymphocyte tropism of human herpesvirus 6-related virus," *Journal of Virology*, vol. 63, no. 7, pp. 3161–3163, 1989.

[2] R. W. Cone, M. L. W. Huang, R. Ashley, and L. Corey, "Human herpesvirus 6 DNA in peripheral blood cells and saliva from immunocompetent individuals," *Journal of Clinical Microbiology*, vol. 31, no. 5, pp. 1262–1267, 1993.

[3] N. Singh and D. R. Carrigan, "Human herpesvirus-6 in transplantation: an emerging pathogen," *Annals of Internal Medicine*, vol. 124, no. 12, pp. 1065–1071, 1996.

[4] D. K. Braun, G. Dominguez, and P. E. Pellett, "Human herpesvirus 6," *Clinical Microbiology Reviews*, vol. 10, no. 3, pp. 521–567, 1997.

[5] G. Campadelli-Fiume, P. Mirandola, and L. Menotti, "Human herpesvirus 6: an emerging pathogen," *Emerging Infectious Diseases*, vol. 5, no. 3, pp. 353–366, 1999.

[6] J. D. Fox, M. Briggs, P. A. Ward, and R. S. Tedder, "Human herpesvirus 6 in salivary glands," *Lancet*, vol. 336, no. 8715, pp. 590–593, 1990.

[7] R. F. Jarrett, D. A. Clark, S. F. Josephs, and D. E. Onions, "Detection of human herpesvirus-6 DNA in peripheral blood and saliva," *Journal of Medical Virology*, vol. 32, no. 1, pp. 73–76, 1990.

[8] P. K. Chan, H. K. Ng, M. Hui, and A. F. Cheng, "Prevalence and distribution of human herpesvirus 6 variants A and B in adult human brain," *Journal of Medical Virology*, vol. 64, no. 1, pp. 42–46, 2001.

[9] D. Donati, N. Akhyani, A. Fogdell-Hahn et al., "Detection of human herpesvirus-6 in mesial temporal lobe epilepsy surgical brain resections," *Neurology*, vol. 61, no. 10, pp. 1405–1411, 2003.

[10] K. Kondo, T. Kondo, T. Okuno, M. Takahashi, and K. Ymanishi, "Latent human herpesvirus 6 infection of human monocytes/macrophages," *Journal of General Virology*, vol. 72, no. 6, pp. 1401–1408, 1991.

[11] M. Luppi, P. Barozzi, C. Morris et al., "Human herpesvirus 6 latently infects early bone marrow progenitors in vivo," *Journal of Virology*, vol. 73, no. 1, pp. 754–759, 1999.

[12] D. M. Zerr, M. Boeckh, and C. Delaney, "HHV-6 reactivation and associated sequelae after hematopoietic cell transplantation," *Biology of Blood and Marrow Transplantation*, vol. 18, no. 11, pp. 1700–1708, 2012.

[13] M. P. Kadakia, "Human herpesvirus 6 infection and associated pathogenesis following bone marrow transplantation," *Leukemia and Lymphoma*, vol. 31, no. 3-4, pp. 251–266, 1998.

[14] H. G. Prentice, E. Gluckman, R. L. Powles et al., "Impact of long-term acyclovir on cytomegalovirus infection and survival after allogeneic bone marrow transplantation," *Lancet*, vol. 343, no. 8900, pp. 749–753, 1994.

[15] H. Glucksberg, R. Storb, and A. Fefer, "Clinical manifestations of graft versus host disease in human recipients of marrow from HL A matched sibling donors," *Transplantation*, vol. 18, no. 4, pp. 295–304, 1974.

[16] B. M. Imbert-Marcille, X. W. Tang, D. Lepelletier et al., "Human herpesvirus 6 infection after autologous or allogeneic stem cell transplantation: a single-center prospective longitudinal study of 92 patients," *Clinical Infectious Diseases*, vol. 31, no. 4, pp. 881–886, 2000.

[17] A. Palumbo and K. Anderson, "Multiple myeloma," *New England Journal of Medicine*, vol. 364, no. 11, pp. 1046–1060, 2011.

[18] S. V. Rajkumar, "Multiple myeloma: 2012 update on diagnosis, risk-stratification, and management," *American Journal of Hematology*, vol. 87, no. 1, pp. 78–88, 2012.

[19] F. Davies and R. Baz, "Lenalidomide mode of action: linking bench and clinical findings," *Blood Reviews*, vol. 24, no. 1, supplement, pp. S13–S19, 2010.

[20] D. S. Ritchie, H. Quach, K. Fielding, and P. Neeson, "Drug-mediated and cellular immunotherapy in multiple myeloma," *Immunotherapy*, vol. 2, no. 2, pp. 243–255, 2010.

[21] G. L. Uy, S. Peles, N. M. Fisher, M. H. Tomasson, J. F. DiPersio, and R. Vij, "Bortezomib prior to autologous transplant in multiple myeloma: effects on mobilization, engraftment, and

markers of immune function," *Biology of Blood and Marrow Transplantation*, vol. 12, supplement 1, article 116a, 2006.

[22] B. Blanco, J. A. Pérez-Simón, L. I. Sánchez-Abarca et al., "Bortezomib induces selective depletion of alloreactive T lymphocytes and decreases the production of Th1 cytokines," *Blood*, vol. 107, no. 9, pp. 3575–3583, 2006.

[23] A. Nencioni, A. Garuti, K. Schwarzenberg et al., "Proteasome inhibitor-induced apoptosis in human monocyte-derived dendritic cells," *European Journal of Immunology*, vol. 36, no. 3, pp. 681–689, 2006.

[24] A. Nencioni, K. Schwarzenberg, K. M. Brauer et al., "Proteasome inhibitor bortezomib modulates TLR4-induced dendritic cell activation," *Blood*, vol. 108, no. 2, pp. 551–558, 2006.

[25] A. Chanan-Khan, P. Sonneveld, M. W. Schuster et al., "Analysis of herpes zoster events among bortezomib-treated patients in the phase III APEX study," *Journal of Clinical Oncology*, vol. 26, no. 29, pp. 4784–4790, 2008.

[26] N. P. Tavakoli, S. Nattanmai, R. Hull et al., "Detection and typing of human herpesvirus 6 by molecular methods in specimens from patients diagnosed with encephalitis or meningitis," *Journal of Clinical Microbiology*, vol. 45, no. 12, pp. 3972–3978, 2007.

[27] A. J. Wakefield, J. D. Fox, A. M. Sawyerr et al., "Detection of herpesvirus DNA in the large intestine of patients with ulcerative colitis and Crohn's disease using the nested polymerase chain reaction," *Journal of Medical Virology*, vol. 38, no. 3, pp. 183–190, 1992.

[28] M. P. Kadakia, W. B. Rybka, J. A. Stewart et al., "Human herpesvirus 6: infection and disease following autologous and allogeneic bone marrow transplantation," *Blood*, vol. 87, no. 12, pp. 5341–5354, 1996.

[29] H. Miyoshi, K. Tanaka-Taya, J. Hara et al., "Inverse relationship between human herpesvirus-6 and -7 detection after allogeneic and autologous stem cell transplantation," *Bone Marrow Transplantation*, vol. 27, no. 10, pp. 1065–1070, 2001.

[30] S. V. Rajkumar, "Multiple myeloma: 2011 update on diagnosis, risk-stratification, and management," *American Journal of Hematology*, vol. 86, no. 1, pp. 57–65, 2011.

[31] S. J. Kim, K. Kim, B. S. Kim et al., "Bortezomib and the increased incidence of herpes zoster in patients with multiple myeloma," *Clinical Lymphoma and Myeloma*, vol. 8, no. 4, pp. 237–240, 2008.

[32] D. M. Zerr, J. R. Fann, D. Breiger et al., "HHV-6 reactivation and its effect on delirium and cognitive functioning in hematopoietic cell transplantation recipients," *Blood*, vol. 117, no. 19, pp. 5243–5249, 2011.

[33] J. I. Cohen, P. A. Brunell, S. E. Straus, and P. R. Krause, "Recent advances in varicella-zoster virus infection," *Annals of Internal Medicine*, vol. 130, no. 11, pp. 922–932, 1999.

[34] P. Schütt, D. Brandhorst, W. Stellberg et al., "Immune parameters in multiple myeloma patients: influence of treatment and correlation with opportunistic infections," *Leukemia and Lymphoma*, vol. 47, no. 8, pp. 1570–1582, 2006.

[35] G. Mele, S. Pinna, A. Quarta, M. Brocca, M. R. Coppi, and G. Quarta, "Increased incidence of Herpes Zoster in relapsed multiple myeloma patients receiving bortezomib: single institution experience," *Haematologica*, vol. 90, supplement 2, pp. 432a–433a, 2005.

[36] H. S. Lee, J. Y. Park, S. H. Shin et al., "Herpesviridae viral infections after chemotherapy without antiviral prophylaxis in patients with malignant lymphoma: incidence and risk factors," *American Journal of Clinical Oncology*, vol. 35, pp. 146–150, 2011.

[37] T. M. Tohnya and W. D. Figg, "Immunomodulation of multiple myeloma," *Cancer Biology and Therapy*, vol. 3, no. 11, pp. 1060–1061, 2004.

3

Occurrence and Impact of Minor Histocompatibility Antigens' Disparities on Outcomes of Hematopoietic Stem Cell Transplantation from HLA-Matched Sibling Donors

Monika Dzierzak-Mietla,[1] M. Markiewicz,[1] Urszula Siekiera,[2] Sylwia Mizia,[3] Anna Koclega,[1] Patrycja Zielinska,[1] Malgorzata Sobczyk-Kruszelnicka,[1] and Slawomira Kyrcz-Krzemien[1]

[1] Department of Hematology and Bone Marrow Transplantation, Medical University of Silesia, Dabrowskiego 25, 40-032 Katowice, Poland
[2] HLA and Immunogenetics Laboratory, Regional Blood Center, Raciborska 15, 40-074 Katowice, Poland
[3] Lower Silesian Center for Cellular Transplantation with National Bone Marrow Donor Registry, Grabiszynska 105, 53-439 Wroclaw, Poland

Correspondence should be addressed to Monika Dzierzak-Mietla, monajka13@o2.pl

Academic Editor: Bronwen Shaw

We have examined the alleles of eleven minor histocompatibility antigens (MiHAs) and investigated the occurrence of immunogenic MiHA disparities in 62 recipients of allogeneic hematopoietic cell transplantation (allo-HCT) with myeloablative conditioning performed between 2000 and 2008 and in their HLA-matched sibling donors. Immunogenic MiHA mismatches were detected in 42 donor-recipient pairs: in 29% MiHA was mismatched in HVG direction, in another 29% in GVH direction; bidirectional MiHA disparity was detected in 10% and no MiHA mismatches in 32%. Patients with GVH-directed HY mismatches had lower both overall survival and disease-free survival at 3 years than patients with compatible HY; also higher incidence of both severe acute GvHD and extensive chronic GVHD was observed in patients with GVH-directed HY mismatch. On contrary, GVH-directed mismatches of autosomally encoded MiHAs had no negative effect on overall survival. Results of our study help to understand why posttransplant courses of allo-HCT from siblings may vary despite the complete high-resolution HLA matching of a donor and a recipient.

1. Introduction

The allogeneic hematopoietic cell transplantation (allo-HCT) still remains a curative treatment of many severe diseases, especially hematooncological malignancies. The successful donor search is one of the most important factors deciding about the feasibility of transplantation. It starts with search among the patient's siblings as the HLA-matched sibling donor is regarded as the optimal one. The odds ratio for HLA compatibility in siblings is 1:4. The probability of having a matched sibling donor by a particular patient is determined by the formula $1 - (0.75)^n$, where n equals the number of siblings. Despite the improved matching of donor-recipient pairs that was possible after the implementation of high-resolution methods of molecular HLA typing, the better outcomes of transplantations are still limited by high number of complications: graft versus host disease (GVHD), engraftment problems (lack or loss of engraftment), and relapse [1]. The long-term survival after allo-HCT is being estimated in the range of 40–70%. Failures are mainly due to infectious complications and GVHD (30–40% each), organ toxicity of chemotherapy (20%), and relapse (20–30%) [2].

HLA matching remains the most important factor influencing both donor selection and transplantation outcomes. However, research of the human genome revealed that polymorphism of nucleotides in genes that are non-HLA related (e.g., NOD2/CARD15 or genes encoding cytokines: TNF-alpha, IL-10, IL-6, interferon gamma, IL-1, and TGF-beta) may also determine the individual immunological phenotype of donor-recipient pairs, thus influencing GVHD, infections, and overall survival [3]. Minor histocompatibility antigens (MiHAs) belong to immunogenetic non-HLA related factors encoded by polymorphic genes, which may differ between the recipient and the donor and thus they may have impact on transplant outcomes.

The impact of antigens independent from Major Histocompatibility complex on transplantation results was first observed by Counce et al. in 1950s [4]. They explored graft rejection in inbred mice, which had undergone the transplantation of skin cells and neoplasmatic cells. Genes which were not associated with MHC responsible for slower course of rejection were called weak histocompatibility genes [4, 5]. The first hypothesis concerning potential impact of MiHA on the outcome of BMT (bone marrow transplantation) was based on a case of a female recipient (with severe aplastic anemia) who received a transplant from her brother. Graft rejection after BMT was diagnosed and reactivity of cytotoxic T cells isolated from peripheral blood of recipient was directed to antigens present on donor's cells which were not associated with HLA [6].

Minor histocompatibility antigens are polymorphic peptides consisting of 9–12 amino acids. After binding to the antigen recognition site of either class I or class II HLA molecules present on a cell surface MiHAs can be recognized by T-lymphocytes. Thus the occurrence of MiHA depends on the presence of specific HLA antigens, which is called the MHC restriction. MiHAs are encoded by either autosomal chromosomes or by Y-chromosome [7–9]. Disparities of MiHA may result from polymorphism of amino acids, gene deletions [10], or from several intracellular mechanisms [11]. MiHA disparity may originate from a single or several amino-acid substitution in the part of MiHA peptide recognized by TCR (T-cell receptor), like in the case of HY and HA-1. Amino-acid polymorphism may be present in the region of MiHA that binds to HLA molecule, causing different expressions of peptide-HLA complex in the donor than in the recipient. Polymorphism may also pertain proteins responsible for intracellular processing of peptides, what leads to the presence or absence of peptides (e.g., HA-2 or HA-8) on cell's surface [12], or phosphoproteins (e.g., SP-110, MiHA discovered in 2006 by Warren et al.) [13].

Most MiHA possess only one immunogenic allele, which is sufficient to induce MiHA immunogenicity [12]. Up to date 18 autosomal and 10 Y-chromosome encoded MiHAs have been identified; those tested in our study are presented in Tables 1 and 2.

There are two patterns of MiHAs' tissue distribution: restricted and broad. Autosomal HA-3, HA-8, and most of MiHAs encoded by Y-chromosome are present in most tissues, including those crucial for GVHD: skin, intestines, and liver [11, 12]. Most of autosomal and 2 MiHAs encoded by Y-chromosome (B8/HY and B52/HY) appear only in hematologic cells including leukemic cells, dendritic cells, NK, and multiple myeloma cells [40]. Thanks to their restricted distribution all of them may be potentially exploited in immunotherapy. The other type of MiHAs' tissue distribution is their appearance on epithelial neoplasmatic cells, for example, HA-1 and ACC-1/ACC-2 [41, 42], although in normal conditions they are restricted only to hematopoietic cells and are not present on epithelial cells.

Detection of MiHA bases most often on genomic typing with PCR-SSP method. The assessment of detected immunogenic disparities is simplified by the online availability of Leiden University Medical Center's dbMinor database [43]. Disparities of immunogenic MiHA alleles between the donor and the recipient may trigger GVHD and HVG reactions, which may lead to graft rejection or to GVH/GVL reaction [44–46]. T-lymphocytes directed against recipient specific MiHAs were detected in patients with GVHD [47]. In the group of 92 recipients of allo-HCT from unrelated donors, a higher incidence of chronic GVHD was observed in those with HY disparity [48]. Many clinical trials confirm that disparities of autosomally encoded MiHAs (like HA-1, HA-2, and HA-8) may increase the incidence of GVHD [15, 17, 22], while others did not confirm such dependence [49]. Female recipients after transplantation from male donors may experience graft failure due to HVG reaction against HY antigens resulting in a worse survival [3]. MiHA present on recipient's neoplasmatic cells (HA-1, HA-2, HA-8, HB-1, and HY) may constitute the target of cytotoxic CD8+ T-lymphocytes crucial for GVL reaction [12, 50], leading to the decrease of relapse rate [51]. Use of cytotoxic T-lymphocytes recognizing selectively only MiHA present on neoplasmatic cells enables the separation of GVL effect from GVHD [52]. Such MiHAs can be used both in vivo for the production of vaccines enhancing GVL reaction and in vitro as a load to antigen presenting cells stimulating reactivity of cytotoxic T-cells [53]. HA-1 and HA-2 are the most intensively explored MiHAs in immunotherapy [12, 52–54].

The aim of this study was to determine MiHA alleles and genotypes enabling to detect their immunogenic disparities in sibling donor-recipient pairs and to explore their influence on the results of allo-HCT.

2. Material and Methods

2.1. Patients and Donors. 62 patients: 34 women and 28 men of median age 38 (range 14–59) years, who received allo-HCT from siblings in the Department of Hematology and Bone Marrow Transplantation, Medical University of Silesia, Katowice, Poland, in years 2000–2008, entered the study. The indication for transplantation was acute myeloid leukemia (45 pts), acute lymphoblastic leukemia (14 pts), chronic myeloid leukemia in chronic phase, myelodysplastic syndrome, and resistant non-Hodgkin's lymphoma (1 pt each). Donors were 30 women and 32 men of median age 35 (range 14–60) years. Median followup was 3 (0.04–10) years.

2.2. Transplantation Procedure. Conditioning treatment was myeloablative (CyTBI: cyclophosphamide + total body irradiation in 12 pts, BuCy: busulfan + cyclophosphamide in

TABLE 1: Autosomally encoded MiHA.

MiHA	Restriction	Identification	Clinical trials	Protein	Tissue distribution	Presence on cells
HA-1	HLA-A*02	Den Haan et al. 1998 [14]	Goulmy et al. 1996 [15] Tseng et al. 1999 [16] Gallardo et al. 2001 [17]	HA-1	Restricted	Hematopoietic cells Bronchial carcinomas Cervix carcinoma Breast carcinoma Prostate carcinoma
HA-1/B60	HLA-B*60	Mommaas et al. 2002 [18]	—	HA-1	Restricted	Hematopoietic cells
HA-2	HLA-A*02	Den Haan et al. 1995 [19]	Goulmy et al. 1996 [15]	Myosin 1G	Restricted	Hematopoietic cells
HA-3	HLA-A*01	Spierings et al. 2003 [20]	Tseng et al. 1999 [16]	Lymphoid blast crisis oncogene	Broad	Hematopoietic cells Keratinocytes Fibroblasts PTECs HUVECs Melanocytes
HA-8	HLA-A*02	Brickner et al. 2001 [21]	Akatsuka et al. 2003 [22] Pérez-García et al. 2005 [23]	KIAA0020	Broad	Hematopoietic cells Fibroblasts
HB-1[H/Y]	HLA-B*44	Dolstra et al. 1999 [24]	—	Unknown	Restricted	B cell ALL, EBV-BLCLs
ACC-1	HLA-A*24	Akatsuka et al. 2003 [25]	Nishida et al. 2004 [26]	BCL2A1	Restricted	Hematopoietic cells
ACC-2	HLA-B*44	Akatsuka et al. 2003 [25]	—	BCL2A1	Restricted	Hematopoietic cells
SP110 (HwA-9)	HLA-A*03	Warren et al. 2006 [13]	—	SP110 intranuclear protein	Restricted	Hematopoietic cells IFN—gamma inducible
PANE1 (HwA-10)	HLA-A*03	Brickner et al. 2006 [27]	—	PANE1	Restricted	Lymphoid cells
UGT2B17/A29	HLA-A*29	Murata et al. 2003 [28]	—	UGT2B17	Restricted	Dendritic cells, B-cells, EBV-BLCLs
UGT2B17/B44	HLA-B*44	Terrakura et al. 2007 [29]	—	UGT2B17	Restricted	Dendritic cells, B-cells, EBV-BLCLs

33 pts), reduced intensity (TreoFlu: treosulfan + fludarabine in 2 pts, TreoCy: treosulfan + cyclophosphamide in 2 pts), or nonmyeloablative (BuFlu: busulfan + fludarabine in 2 pts). Cumulative doses of drugs used in conditioning were busulfan 16 or 8 mg/kg p.o., cyclophosphamide 120 mg/kg i.v., treosulfan 42 g/m^2 i.v., fludarabine 150 mg/m^2 i.v. TBI dose was 12 Gy. Bone marrow was the source of hematopoietic cells in 40 patients, G-CSF-stimulated peripheral blood in 10 and both (harvest of insufficient number of CD34+ cells from the bone marrow followed by peripheral collection) in 12 patients. Details of transplanted cells are presented in Table 3. Standard GVHD prophylaxis consisted of cyclosporine A in initial dose 3 mg/kg i.v. starting from day −1 with dose adjusted to its serum level and shifted to oral administration about day +20, methotrexate 15 mg/m^2 i.v. on day +1 and 10 mg/m^2 i.v. on days +3 and +6. Methylprednisolone at dose 2 mg/kg i.v. was the first line therapy of aGVHD symptoms. The criteria defined by Glucksberg were used for the grading of aGVHD; the diagnosis and severity of cGVHD were determined according to NIH (National Institutes of Health) criteria established in 2005 [55].

2.3. Methods. DNA of patients and siblings was isolated from peripheral blood in the Biomolecular Laboratory of the Department of Hematology and BMT, Medical University of Silesia. Alleles of 11 autosomal and Y-chromosome encoded MiHAs were analyzed with PCR-SSP method for each donor-recipient pair in the Immunogenetics and HLA Laboratory of the Regional Blood Center in Katowice with the use of Dynal AllSet+ Minor Histocompatibility Antigen Typing Kit, according to a methodology recommended by Leiden University Medical Center. Products obtained in PCR-SSP reaction were analyzed on agarose gel and each detected allele encoding MiHA was translated into a specific letter code. dbMinor database of LUMC was used to determine the number, direction, and tissue distribution of MiHA mismatches on the base of MiHA alleles and HLA antigens

TABLE 2: Y-chromosome encoded MiHA.

MiHA	Restriction	Identification	Clinical trials	Protein	Tissue distribution	Presence on cells
A1/HY	HLA-A*01	Pierce et al. 1999 [30]	—	USP9Y	Broad	Hematopoietic cells, fibroblasts
A2/HY	HLA-A*02	Meadows et al. 1997 [31]	Goulmy et al. 1996 [15]	SMCY	Broad	Hematopoietic cells, fibroblasts
A33/HY	HLA-A*33	Torikai et al. 2004 [32]	—	TMSB4Y	Broad	Hematopoietic cells
B7/HY	HLA-B*07	Wang et al. 1995 [33]	—	KDMSD	Broad	Hematopoietic cells
B8/HY	HLA-B*08	Warren et al. 2000 [34]	—	UTY	Restricted	Hematopoietic cells
B52/HY	HLA-B*52	Ivanov et al. 2005 [35]	—	RPS4Y1	Restricted	Leukocytes, PHA blasts, EBV-BLCLs, B cells, breast carcinoma, hepatocellular carcinoma, colon adenocarcinoma, AML, ALL multiple myeloma
B60/HY	HLA-B*60	Vogt et al. 2000 [36]	—	UTY	Broad	Hematopoietic cells, fibroblasts
DRB1*1501/HY	HLA-DRB1*15	Zorn et al. 2004 [37]	—	DDX3Y (DBY)	Broad	Hematopoietic cells, fibroblasts
DRB3*0301/HY	HLA-DRB3*0301	Spierings et al.2003 [38]	—	RPS4Y1	Broad	Hematopoietic cells, fibroblasts
DQ5/HY	HLA-DQB1*05	Vogt et al. 2002 [39]	—	DDX3Y (DBY)	Broad	Hematopoietic cells, fibroblasts

Abbreviations: HUVE: human umbilical vein epithelium, PTE: proximal tubular epithelium, EBV-BLCL: Epstein Barr virus transformed B-lymphoblastoid cell lines, and PHA: phytohemagglutinine.
Data in Tables 1 and 2 are based on dbMinor database and materials presented during Minor Histocompatibility Workshop 2005, Leiden University Medical Center; Eric Spierings: minor H antigens: targets for tumor therapy—lecture at the conference "Immunogenetics in hematology and stem cell transplantation", Wroclaw 09.02.2006 and [8].

of respective donor-recipient pairs. The study has been approved by the responsible Ethical Committee of Medical University of Silesia.

2.4. Statistical Methods. Median, minimal, and maximum values were used to show numeric parameters of donor-recipient groups. Statistical analysis of MiHA mismatches' impact on transplantation outcomes was conducted in accordance to recommendation of EBMT [56]. MiHA mismatches were grouped according to mismatch direction (GVH or HVG), tissue distribution (restricted or broad), and the way of coding (autosomal or by Y-chromosome) in search for their influence on transplant results. Analysed endpoints included overall survival (OS), disease-free survival (DFS), aGVHD, and limited and extensive cGVHD. Kaplan-Meier method was used to estimate the probability of impact of MiHA mismatches on overall survival and disease-free survival. Results were presented as percent ±95% confidence interval (CI). The cumulative incidence method was used

to evaluate the probability of relapse and GVHD (acute or chronic) in order to account events which may influence the outcome as a competing risk. Results were presented also in percent ±95% CI. Results with significance level $P < 0.05$ were considered statistically significant.

3. Results

3.1. Occurrence of Alleles and Genotypes and Their Mismatches. Immunogenic MiHA mismatches were detected in 42 (68%) donor-recipient pairs; 20 (32%) pairs had no mismatched MiHAs. Unidirectional HVG-directed disparities were observed in 18 (29%) pairs (in 9 pairs MiHA mismatches were encoded by Y-chromosome, in 8 pairs autosomally, and in 1 pair both autosomally and by Y-chromosome) and GVH-directed MiHA disparities were observed in another 18 (29%) pairs (in 9 pairs MiHA mismatches were Y-chromosome encoded, in 7 pairs autosomally, and in 2 pairs both autosomally and Y-chromosome

TABLE 3: Patients characteristics ($n = 62$).

	Median (range)	Quartiles
Age (years)		
Donor	35 (14–60)	26–49
Recipient	38 (14–59)	28–47
Time from diagnosis to allo-HCT (years)	0.62 (0.24–12.91)	0.5–1.12
	n	%
Sex		
Donor		
Male	32	51.6
Female	30	48.4
Recipient		
Male	28	45.2
Female	34	54.8
Donor/recipient		
Male/male	16	25.8
Female/female	18	29
Male/female	16	25.8
Female/male	12	19.4
Compatibility of ABO blood groups		
Compatible	36	58.1
Minor incompatibility	8	12.9
Major incompatibility	14	22.5
Minor and major incompatibility	4	6.5
Diagnosis		
AML	45	72.5
ALL	14	22.5
CML	1	1.61
MDS	1	1.61
NHL	1	1.61
Regimen		
TBI + cyclophosphamide	12	19.35
Chemotherapy		
Busulfan + cyclophosphamide	33	53.2
Treosulfan + fludarabine	13	20.96
Busulfan + fludarabine	2	3.22
Treosulfan + cyclophosphamide	2	3.22
Source of hematopoietic cells		
Bone marrow	40	64.5
Peripheral blood	10	16.1
Bone marrow and peripheral blood	12	19.4
	Median (range)	Quartiles
Number of transplanted cells		
Nucleated cells (NC) $\times 10e8$/kg	3.51 (0.12–72.15)	2.34–5.84
CD34(+) $\times 10e6$/kg	2.77 (0.95–10.50)	1.68–4.19
CD3(+) $\times 10e7$/kg	3.84 (0.20–46.90)	2.71–18.01
Time range of allo-HCT	01.2000–12.2008	

TABLE 4: The occurrence of MiHA mismatches in GVH and HVG direction in 62 related donor-recipient pairs.

Immunogenic MiHA mismatches	In GVH direction	
	Present	Absent
In HVG direction		
Present	10% (6 pairs)	29% (18 pairs)
Absent	29% (18 pairs)	32% (20 pairs)

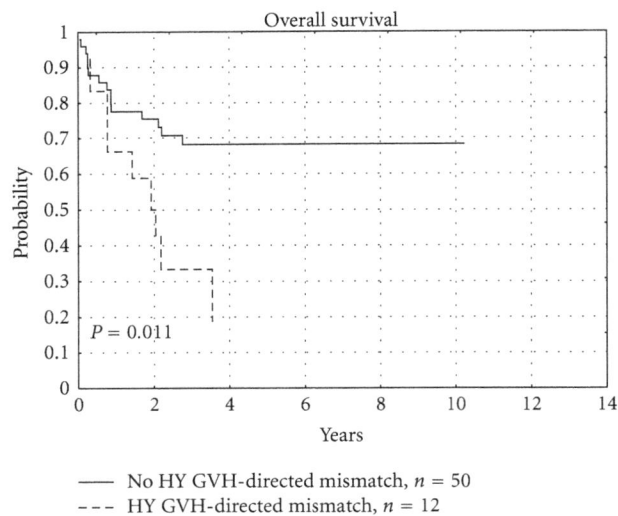

FIGURE 1: Influence of Y-chromosome encoded GVH-directed MiHA mismatch on overall survival.

encoded). In 6 (10%) pairs bi-directional (both HVG and GVH in the same donor-recipient pairs) MiHA mismatches were observed. The direction of MiHA mismatches is presented in Table 4 and the distribution of 11 MiHA alleles and genotypes in 62 related donor-recipient pairs is presented in Tables 5 and 6.

3.2. Impact of Immunogenic MiHA Mismatches on Allo-HCT Outcomes.
Analysis of overall survival showed unfavorable impact of GVH-directed Y-chromosome encoded MiHA mismatches ($P = 0.011$), as presented in Figure 1 and Table 7, and favorable trend in case of GVH-directed autosomal MiHA disparities ($P = 0.045$), as presented in Figure 2 and Table 7.

GVH-directed mismatches of Y-chromosome encoded MiHA influenced unfavorable the disease free-survival ($P = 0.05$), as shown in Figure 3 and Table 7.

Serious (grade III or IV) acute GVHD was observed in 24 patients and it was influenced by Y-chromosome encoded GVH-directed MiHA mismatches ($P = 0.037$), which is presented in Figure 4 and Table 7.

The tissue distribution of GVH- or HVG-directed MiHA mismatches did not influence the incidence of aGVHD, neither grades I-IV, nor II-IV. Higher probability of extensive chronic GVHD was observed when Y-chromosome encoded GVH-directed MiHA mismatches were present ($P = 0.017$, as shown in Figure 5 and Table 7).

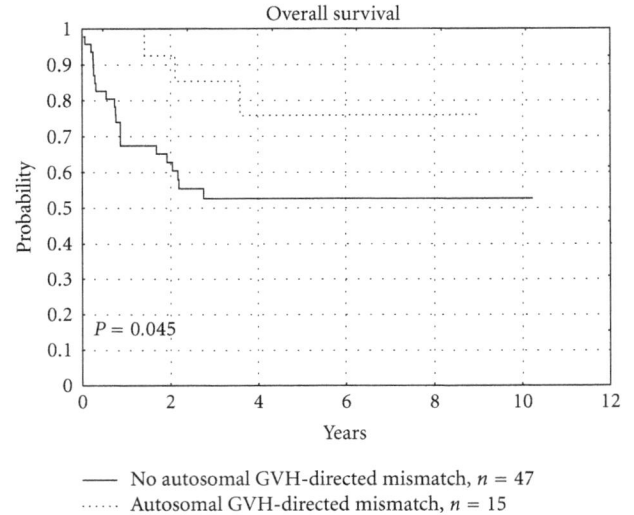

FIGURE 2: Influence of autosomal GVH-directed MiHA mismatch on overall survival.

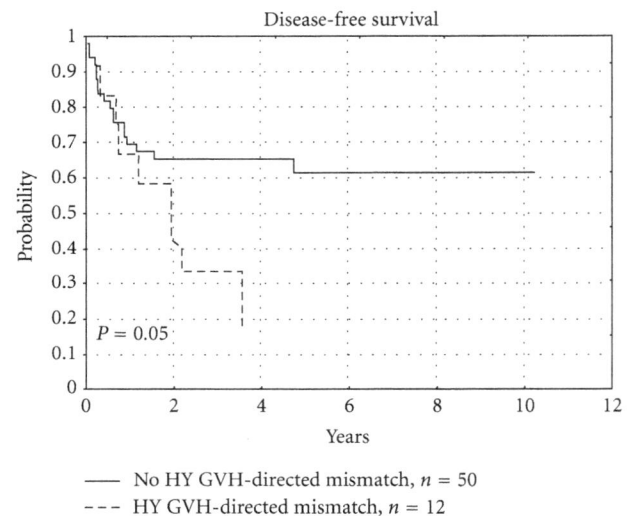

FIGURE 3: Influence of Y-chromosome encoded GVH-directed MiHA mismatch on disease-free survival.

The relapse following allo-HCT was observed in 15(24.2%) patients. Lower risk of relapse was observed in patients with HVG-directed MiHA mismatches: both autosomal (0.28(0.18–0.44) versus 0(0-0), $P = 0.032$) and with "restricted" pattern of tissue distribution (0.29(0.18–0.45) versus 0(0-0), $P = 0.028$). These data are presented in Table 7.

4. Discussion

Minor histocompatibility antigens belong to genetic factors which may vary between the donor and the recipient despite identical HLA and thus they may influence allo-HCT results. Knowledge of MiHA alleles and genotypes

TABLE 5: Distribution of 11 MiHA alleles in 62 related donor-recipient pairs.

MiHA	Allele	Recipient	Donor
HA-1	H	38.5%	41.8%
	R	61.5%	58.2%
HA-2	V	78.7%	73.0%
	M	21.3%	27.0%
HA-3	T	68.0%	70.5%
	M	32.0%	29.5%
HA-8	R	45.9%	45.9%
	P	54.1%	54.1%
HB-1	H	62.3%	64.8%
	Y	37.7%	35.2%
ACC-1	Y	23.0%	20.5%
	C	77.0%	79.5%
ACC-2	D	20.5%	19.7%
	G	79.5%	80.3%
SP110 (HwA9)	R	58.2%	58.2%
	G	41.8%	41.8%
PANE1 (HwA10)	R	67.2%	68.9%
	*	32.8%	31.1%
UGT2B17	+	86.9%	90.2%
	−	13.1%	9.8%
HY	+	50.8%	54.1%
	−	49.2%	45.9%

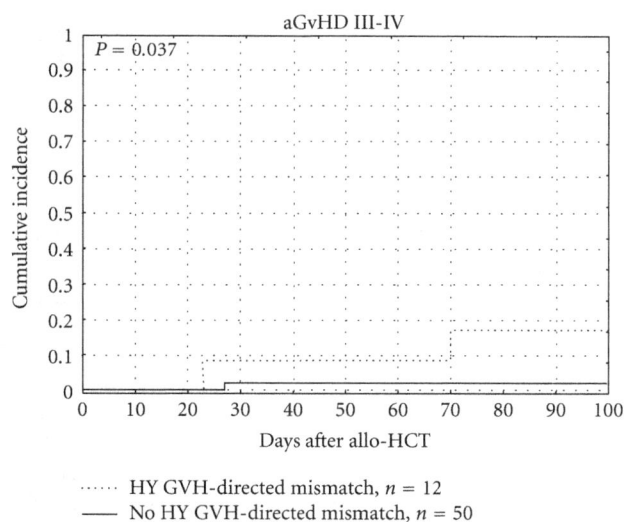

FIGURE 4: Influence of Y-chromosome encoded GVH-directed MiHA mismatches on serious aGVHD.

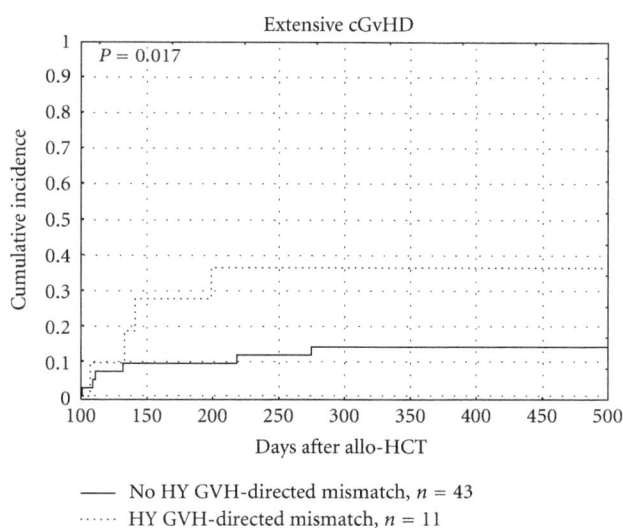

FIGURE 5: Influence of Y-chromosome encoded GVH-directed MiHA mismatches on extensive cGVHD.

enables to detect their disparities, which could be helpful not only in optimal matching of a donor/recipient pair and in understanding transplant results, but also it may create a chance to the use of MiHA in immunotherapy aiming to improve patients' survival [52–54]. The largest meta-analysis of MiHA distribution was performed by Spierings et al. who described the results of a multicenter trial of 10 MiHA

distribution in 5 different ethnic groups worldwide. The study revealed significant differences in the frequency of MiHA alleles in dependence of geographical location, with UGT2B17 being the most variable MiHA [57]. Two MiHA trials have been performed in Polish population till now: in the first one HA-1 was analyzed in a group of 30 sibling pairs [58], another trial concerned the group of 92 unrelated pairs

TABLE 6: Distribution of MiHA genotypes' frequencies in 62 related donor-recipient pairs.

MiHA	Genotype	Recipient	Donor
	HH	13.1%	16.4%
HA-1	HR	50.8%	50.8%
	RR	36.1%	32.8%
	VV	59.0%	50.8%
HA-2	VM	39.3%	44.3%
	MM	1.6%	4.9%
	TT	44.3%	47.5%
HA-3	TM	47.5%	45.9%
	MM	8.2%	6.6%
	RR	27.9%	27.9%
HA-8	RP	36.1%	36.1%
	PP	36.1%	36.1%
	HH	34.4%	36.1%
HB-1	HY	55.7%	57.4%
	YY	9.8%	6.6%
	YY	4.9%	1.6%
ACC-1	YC	36.1%	37.7%
	CC	59.0%	60.7%
	DD	3.3%	0.0%
ACC-2	DG	34.4%	39.3%
	GG	62.3%	60.7%
	RR	27.9%	31.1%
SP110 (HwA9)	RG	60.7%	54.1%
	GG	11.5%	14.8%
	RR	42.6%	42.6%
PANE1 (HwA10)	R*	49.2%	52.5%
	**	8.2%	4.9%

++ or +− genotypes' frequencies of UGT2B17 and HY are equal to the frequency of alleles + and their −− genotypes' frequencies are equal to the frequency of alleles − presented in Table 5.

[12]. In our current study alleles and genotypes of 11 MiHAs have been estimated in 62 sibling donor-recipient pairs. Basing on our results and several other studies estimating the occurrence of specific MiHA mismatches in allo-HCT [59, 60], HA-1 can be regarded as a candidate target for immunotherapeutic applications.

We have observed the unfavorable impact of GVH-directed mismatches of Y-chromosome encoded MiHAs on OS ($P = 0.011$) and DFS ($P = 0.05$). Y-chromosome encoded MiHA represents MiHA with "broad" tissue distribution. Attack of donor's T-lymphocytes on recipients' tissues precipitated by HY mismatch could explain the increased occurrence of severe forms of acute and chronic GVHD, leading to earlier deaths of recipients. In our study recipients of allo-HCT from siblings did not receive antithymocyte globulin, what probably influenced the worse course, including the fatal course of their GVHD. We have shown that GVH-directed mismatches of HY correlate significantly with serious (III or IV) aGVHD and extensive cGVHD. These results correspond to the reported influence of sex difference on transplant outcomes, especially in the case of female donor to male recipient (FDMR) transplants [61, 62]. Oppositely, Markiewicz et al. in

a study of 92 unrelated donor-recipient pairs found that HY mismatches in GVH direction influenced more favorable GVL effect than unfavorable GVHD, what resulted in the increased DFS ($P = 0.05$) [12, 63]. The probable explanation of this difference in MiHAs impact on OS and DFS between related and unrelated allo-HCT may be the use of stronger standard immunosuppressive prophylaxis including pretransplant antithymocyte globulin in unrelated allo-HCT setting. Increased incidence of serious acute and extensive chronic GVHD associated with mismatches of Y-chromosome encoded MiHAs, leading to a worse overall survival, may justify the administration of anti-thymocyte globuline before allo-HCT from sibling female donor to male recipient. Such approach could probably reduce the risk of GVHD originating from GVH-directed HY mismatch.

The analysis of GVH-directed mismatches of autosomal MiHAs, oppositely to HY, showed favorable trend to increase the OS, which was 76% in a mismatched versus 53% in a compatible groups at a 4-year posttransplant. Unlike GVH-directed HY disparities, those of autosomal MiHAs did not increase the occurrence of serious GVHD in our study, which contributed to the better survival. There are reports

TABLE 7: Influence of MiHA mismatches on allo-HCT outcomes.

Analyzed outcome	Analyzed MiHA	Direction of mismatch	Presence of mismatch	n	Probability (95% CI)	P
Overall survival	Autosomal	GVH	Yes	15	2 yrs: 0.9286 (0.5278–0.9892)	0.045
					4 yrs: 0.7619 (0.3481–0.9130)	
			No	47	2 yrs: 0.6046 (0.4329–0.7243)	
					4 yrs: 0.5265 (0.3511–0.6545)	
	HY	GVH	Yes	12	2 years: 0.4167 (0.0590–0.6384)	0.011
					3 years: 0.3333 (0.0054–0.5532)	
			No	50	2 years: 0.7546 (0.5986–0.8500)	
					3 years: 0.6822 (0.5152–0.7916)	
Disease-free survival	HY	GVH	Yes	12	2 years: 0.4167 (0.0590–0.6384)	0.050
					3 years: 0.3333 (0.0054–0.5532)	
			No	50	2 years: 0.6526 (0.4896–0.7635)	
					3 years: 0.6526 (0.4896–0.7635)	
Serious aGVHD	HY	GVH	Yes	12	0.1667 (0.0470–0.5906)	0.037
			No	50	0.0200 (0.0029–0.1392)	
Extensive cGVHD	HY	GVH	Yes	11	0.3636 (0.1664–0.7947)	0.017
			No	43	0.1395 (0.0664–0.2931)	
Relapse	Autosomal	HVG	Yes	12	0 (0–0)	0.032
			No	50	0.2836 (0.1818–0.4423)	
	Restricted	HVG	Yes	13	0 (0–0)	0.028
			No	49	0.2879 (0.1849–0.4482)	

describing the role of autosomal MiHAs in GVHD: for example, higher risk of aGVHD in the case of autosomal HA-1 incompatibility was reported in Tunisian group of 60 sibling donor-recipient pairs [64]. Others described increased incidence of cGVHD in the case of mismatched autosomal MiHAs localized on hematopoietic cells: HA-1, HA-2, and HA-8 [15, 16, 23, 65]. There are also reports that report no impact of autosomal MiHAs on GVHD [49, 66].

One could expect that disparities of MiHAs with broad tissue distribution present in the host should precipitate the posttransplant reaction of donor's lymphocytes and induce the GVHD. Unexpectedly, the tissue distribution of neither GVH- nor HVG-directed MiHA mismatches did not influence the incidence of GVHD.

Much lower probability of relapse following allo-HCT was observed by us in patients with HVG-, but not with GVH-directed MiHA mismatches. This finding, although intriguing, needs further confirmation as we do not find a reasonable explanation for this result. Japanese group found that GVH-directed HA-1 mismatches were associated with lower risk of relapse [51]. Similarly, experience of Polish group studying MiHAs in unrelated allo-HCT showed seldom episodes of relapse occurring when GVH-directed HY mismatches were present [63].

Results of our study help to explain why posttransplant courses of allo-HCT from siblings may vary despite complete high-resolution HLA-match and why cells interactions between the donor and the recipient may lead to serious complications.

5. Conclusions

GVH-directed HY mismatch significantly increased the occurrence of serious acute GVHD and extensive chronic GVHD and finally caused decreased overall survival. GVH-directed mismatches of autosomally encoded MiHAs had no negative effect on overall survival, which in fact was even longer. Findings of our study help to explain why the occurrence of immunological complications and in consequence final results of allo-HCT from high-resolution HLA-matched sibling donors are variable.

Conflict of Interests

The authors report having no conflict of interests.

References

[1] H. Greinix, "Introduction," in Graft -Versus-Host Disease, H. T. Greinix, Ed., pp. 14–15, Unimed Verlag AG, 2008.
[2] A. Szczeklik et al., "Internal Medicine State of the art in 2011," in Practical Medicine, A. Szczeklik, Ed., chapter 6K3, pp. 1683–1690, 2011.
[3] B. E. Shaw and A. Madrigal, "Immunogenetics of allogeneic HSCT," in Haematopoietic Stem Cell Transplantation, ESH-EBMT Handbook, J. Apperley, E. Carreras, E. Gluckman, and T. Masszi, Eds., pp. 74–89, 2012.
[4] S. Counce, P. Smith, R. Barth, and G. D. Snell, "Strong and weak histocompatibility gene differences in mice and their role in the rejection of homografts of tumors and skin," Annals of Surgery, vol. 144, no. 2, pp. 198–204, 1956.
[5] G. D. Snell, "Methods for study of histocompatibility genes and isoantigens," Methods in Medical Research, vol. 10, pp. 1–7, 1964.
[6] E. Goulmy, "Minor histocompatibility antigens: from transplantation problems to therapy of cancer," Human Immunology, vol. 67, no. 6, pp. 433–438, 2006.
[7] E. Simpson, D. Roopenian, and E. Goulmy, "Much ado about minor histocompatibility antigens," Immunology Today, vol. 19, no. 3, pp. 108–112, 1998.
[8] E. Spierings and E. Goulmy, "Expanding the immunotherapeutic potential of minor histocompatibility antigens," Journal of Clinical Investigation, vol. 115, no. 12, pp. 3397–3400, 2005.
[9] E. Spierings, B. Wieles, and E. Goulmy, "Minor histocompatibility antigens—big in tumour therapy," Trends in Immunology, vol. 25, no. 2, pp. 56–60, 2004.
[10] B. Mommaas, The human minor histcompatibility antigen HA-1: its processing, presentation and recognition [Ph.D. thesis], Leiden University, 2006.
[11] J. H. F. Falkenburg, L. van de Corput, E. W. A. Marijt, and R. Willemze, "Minor histocompatibility antigens in human stem cell transplantation," Experimental Hematology, vol. 31, no. 9, pp. 743–751, 2003.
[12] M. Markiewicz, Influence of donor selection and occurrence and impact of minor histocompatibility antigens' mismatches on results of hematopoietic cells transplantations from HLA-matched unrelated donors [Habilitation thesis], Medical University of Silesia, 2007, Habilitation thesis number 14/2007.
[13] E. H. Warren, N. J. Vigneron, M. A. Gavin et al., "An antigen produced by splicing of noncontiguous peptides in the reverse order," Science, vol. 313, no. 5792, pp. 1444–1447, 2006.
[14] J. M. M. den Haan, L. M. Meadows, W. Wang et al., "The minor histocompatibility antigen HA-1: a diallelic gene with a single amino acid polymorphism," Science, vol. 279, no. 5353, pp. 1054–1057, 1998.
[15] E. Goulmy, R. Schipper, J. Pool et al., "Mismatches of minor histocompatibility antigens between HLA-identical donors and recipients and the development of graft-versus-host disease after bone marrow transplantation," The New England Journal of Medicine, vol. 334, no. 5, pp. 281–285, 1996.
[16] L. H. Tseng, M. T. Lin, J. A. Hansen et al., "Correlation between disparity for the minor histocompatibility antigen HA-1 and the development of acute graft-versus-host disease after allogeneic marrow transplantation," Blood, vol. 94, no. 8, pp. 2911–2914, 1999.
[17] D. Gallardo, J. I. Aróstegui, A. Balas et al., "Disparity for the minor histocompatibility antigen HA-1 is associated with an increased risk of acute graft-versus-host disease (GvHD) but it does not affect chronic GvHD incidence, disease-free survival or overall survival after allogeneic human leucocyte antigen-identical sibling donor transplantation," British Journal of Haematology, vol. 114, no. 4, pp. 931–936, 2001.
[18] B. Mommaas, J. Kamp, J. W. Drijfhout et al., "Identification of a novel HLA-B60-restricted T cell epitope of the minor histocompatibility antigen HA-1 locus," Journal of Immunology, vol. 169, no. 6, pp. 3131–3136, 2002.
[19] J. M. M. den Haan, N. E. Sherman, E. Blokland et al., "Identification of a graft versus host disease-associated human minor histocompatibility antigen," Science, vol. 268, no. 5216, pp. 1476–1480, 1995.
[20] E. Spierings, A. G. Brickner, J. A. Caldwell et al., "The minor histocompatibility antigen HA-3 arises from differential

proteasome-mediated cleavage of the lymphoid blast crisis (Lbc) oncoprotein," *Blood*, vol. 102, no. 2, pp. 621–629, 2003.

[21] A. G. Brickner, E. H. Warren, J. A. Caldwell et al., "The immunogenicity of a new human minor histocompatibility antigen results from differential antigen processing," *Journal of Experimental Medicine*, vol. 193, no. 2, pp. 195–206, 2001.

[22] Y. Akatsuka, E. H. Warren, T. A. Gooley et al., "Disparity for a newly identified minor histocompatibility antigen, HA-8, correlates with acute graft-versus-host disease after haematopoietic stem cell transplantation from an HLA-identical sibling," *British Journal of Haematology*, vol. 123, no. 4, pp. 671–675, 2003.

[23] A. Pérez-García, R. de la Cámara, A. Torres, M. González, A. Jiménez, and D. Gallardo, "Minor histocompatibility antigen HA-8 mismatch and clinical outcome after hla-identical sibling donor allogeneic stem cell transplantation," *Haematologica*, vol. 90, no. 12, pp. 1723–1724, 2005.

[24] H. Dolstra, H. Fredrix, F. Maas et al., "A human minor histocompatibility antigen specific for B cell acute lymphoblastic leukemia," *Journal of Experimental Medicine*, vol. 189, no. 2, pp. 301–308, 1999.

[25] Y. Akatsuka, T. Nishida, E. Kondo et al., "Identification of a polymorphic gene, BCL2A1, encoding two novel hematopoietic lineage-specific minor histocompatibility antigens," *Journal of Experimental Medicine*, vol. 197, no. 11, pp. 1489–1500, 2003.

[26] T. Nishida, Y. Akatsuka, Y. Morishima et al., "Clinical relevance of a newly identified HLA-A24-restricted minor histocompatibility antigen epitope derived from BCL2A1, ACC-1, in patients receiving HLA genotypically matched unrelated bone marrow transplant," *British Journal of Haematology*, vol. 124, no. 5, pp. 629–635, 2004.

[27] A. G. Brickner, A. M. Evans, J. K. Mito et al., "The PANE1 gene encodes a novel human minor histocompatibility antigen that is selectively expressed in B-lymphoid cells and B-CLL," *Blood*, vol. 107, no. 9, pp. 3779–3786, 2006.

[28] M. Murata, E. H. Warren, and S. R. Riddell, "A human minor histocompatibility antigen resulting from differential expression due to a gene deletion," *Journal of Experimental Medicine*, vol. 197, no. 10, pp. 1279–1289, 2003.

[29] S. Terakura, M. Murata, E. H. Warren et al., "A single minor histocompatibility antigen encoded by UGT2B17 and presented by human leukocyte antigen-A*2902 and -B*4403," *Transplantation*, vol. 83, no. 9, pp. 1242–1248, 2007.

[30] R. A. Pierce, E. D. Field, J. M. M. den Haan et al., "Cutting edge: the HLA-A*0101-restricted HY minor histocompatibility antigen originates from DFFRY and contains a cysteinylated cysteine residue as identified by a novel mass spectrometric technique," *Journal of Immunology*, vol. 163, no. 12, pp. 6360–6364, 1999.

[31] L. Meadows, W. Wang, J. M. M. den Haan et al., "The HLA-A*0201-restricted H-Y antigen contains a posttranslationally modified cysteine that significantly affects T cell recognition," *Immunity*, vol. 6, no. 3, pp. 273–281, 1997.

[32] H. Torikai, Y. Akatsuka, M. Miyazaki et al., "A novel HLA-A*3303-restricted minor histocompatibility antigen encoded by an unconventional open reading frame of human TMSB4Y gene," *Journal of Immunology*, vol. 173, no. 11, pp. 7046–7054, 2004.

[33] W. Wang, L. R. Meadows, J. M. M. den Haan et al., "Human H-Y: a male-specific histocompatibility antigen derived from the SMCY protein," *Science*, vol. 269, no. 5230, pp. 1588–1590, 1995.

[34] E. H. Warren, M. A. Gavin, E. Simpson et al., "The human UTY gene encodes a novel HLA-B8-restricted H-Y antigen," *Journal of Immunology*, vol. 164, no. 5, pp. 2807–2814, 2000.

[35] R. Ivanov, T. Aarts, S. Hol et al., "Identification of a 40S ribosomal protein S4-derived H-Y epitope able to elicit a lymphoblast-specific cytotoxic T lymphocyte response," *Clinical Cancer Research*, vol. 11, no. 5, pp. 1694–1703, 2005.

[36] M. H. J. Vogt, E. Goulmy, F. M. Kloosterboer et al., "UTY gene codes for an HLA-B60-restricted human male-specific minor histocompatibility antigen involved in stem cell graft rejection: characterization of the critical polymorphic amino acid residues for T-cell recognition," *Blood*, vol. 96, no. 9, pp. 3126–3132, 2000.

[37] E. Zorn, D. B. Miklos, B. H. Floyd et al., "Minor histocompatibility antigen DBY elicits a coordinated B and T cell response after allogeneic stem cell transplantation," *Journal of Experimental Medicine*, vol. 199, no. 8, pp. 1133–1142, 2004.

[38] E. Spierings, C. J. Vermeulen, M. H. Vogt et al., "Identification of HLA class II-restricted H-Y-specific T-helper epitope evoking CD4+ T-helper cells in H-Y-mismatched transplantation," *The Lancet*, vol. 362, no. 9384, pp. 610–615, 2003.

[39] M. H. J. Vogt, J. W. van den Muijsenberg, E. Goulmy et al., "The DBY gene codes for an HLA-DQ5-restricted human male-specific minor histocompatibility antigen involved in graft-versus-host disease," *Blood*, vol. 99, no. 8, pp. 3027–3032, 2002.

[40] http://www.lumc.nl/dbminor.

[41] C. A. Klein, M. Wilke, J. Pool et al., "The hematopoietic system-specific minor histocompatibility antigen HA-1 shows aberrant expression in epithelial cancer cells," *Journal of Experimental Medicine*, vol. 196, no. 3, pp. 359–368, 2002.

[42] N. Fujii, A. Hiraki, K. Ikeda et al., "Expression of minor histocompatibility antigen, HA-1, in solid tumor cells," *Transplantation*, vol. 73, no. 7, pp. 1137–1141, 2002.

[43] E. Spierings, J. Drabbels, M. Hendriks et al., "A uniform genomic minor histocompatibility antigen typing methodology and database designed to facilitate clinical applications," *PLoS ONE*, vol. 1, no. 1, article e42, 2006.

[44] E. Simpson, D. Scott, E. James et al., "Minor H antigens: genes and peptides," *European Journal of Immunogenetics*, vol. 28, no. 5, pp. 505–513, 2001.

[45] R. Laylor, L. Cannella, E. Simpson, and F. Dazzi, "Minor histocompatibility antigens and stem cell transplantation," *Vox Sanguinis*, vol. 87, supplement 2, pp. S11–S14, 2004.

[46] R. Spaapen and T. Mutis, "Targeting haematopoietic-specific minor histocompatibility antigens to distinguish graft-versus-tumour effects from graft-versus-host disease," *Best Practice and Research*, vol. 21, no. 3, pp. 543–557, 2008.

[47] M. Stern, R. Brand, T. de Witte et al., "Female-versus-male alloreactivity as a model for minor histocompatibility antigens in hematopoietic stem cell transplantation," *American Journal of Transplantation*, vol. 8, no. 10, pp. 2149–2157, 2008.

[48] M. Markiewicz, U. Siekiera, M. Dzierzak-Mietla, P. Zielinska, and S. Kyrcz-Krzemien, "The impact of H-Y mismatches on results of HLA-matched unrelated allogeneic hematopoietic stem cell transplantation," *Transplantation Proceedings*, vol. 42, no. 8, pp. 3297–3300, 2010.

[49] M. T. Lin, T. Gooley, J. A. Hansen et al., "Absence of statistically significant correlation between disparity for the minor histocompatibility antigen HA-1 and outcome after allogeneic hematopoietic cell transplantation," *Blood*, vol. 98, no. 10, pp. 3172–3173, 2001.

[50] J. H. F. Falkenburg, H. M. Goselink, D. van der Harst et al., "Growth inhibition of clonogenic leukemic precursor

cells by minor histocompatibility antigen-specific cytotoxic T lymphocytes," *Journal of Experimental Medicine*, vol. 174, no. 1, pp. 27–33, 1991.

[51] T. Katagiri, S. Shiobara, S. Nakao et al., "Mismatch of minor histocompatibility antigen contributes to a graft-versus-leukemia effect rather than to acute GVHD, resulting in long-term survival after HLA-identical stem cell transplantation in Japan," *Bone Marrow Transplantation*, vol. 38, no. 10, pp. 681–686, 2006.

[52] J. H. F. Falkenburg and R. Willemze, "Minor histocompatibility antigens as targets of cellular immunotherapy in leukaemia," *Best Practice and Research*, vol. 17, no. 3, pp. 415–425, 2004.

[53] I. Jedema and J. H. F. Falkenburg, "Immunotherapy post-transplant," in *Haematopoietic Stem Cell Transplantation, ESH-EBMT Handbook*, J. Apperley, E. Carreras, E. Gluckman, and T. Masszi, Eds., pp. 288–301, 6th edition, 2012.

[54] A. Dickinson, "Biomarkers in acute and chronic GVHD," in *Graft -Versus-Host Disease*, H. T. Greinix, Ed., pp. 17–31, Unimed Verlag AG, 2008.

[55] J. Apperley, J. E, and T. Masszi, "Graft-versus-host disease," in *Haematopoietic Stem Cell Transplantation, ESH-EBMT Handbook*, J. Apperley, E. Carreras, E. Gluckman, and T. Masszi, Eds., pp. 216–233, 6th edition, 2012.

[56] R. M. Szydlo, "The Statistical evaluation of HSCT data," in *Haematopoietic Stem Cell Transplantation, ESH-EBMT Handbook*, J. Apperley, E. Carreras, E. Gluckman, and T. Masszi, Eds., pp. 612–628, 6th edition, 2012.

[57] E. Spierings, M. Hendriks, L. Absi et al., "Phenotype frequencies of autosomal minor histocompatibility antigens display significant differences among populations," *PLoS Genetics*, vol. 3, no. 6, article e103, 2007.

[58] U. Siekiera and J. Janusz, "Human minor histocompatibility antigens (mHag) in HLA-ABC, DR, DQ matched sib-pairs," *Transfusion Clinique et Biologique*, vol. 8, supplement 1, pp. 163s–164s, 2001.

[59] H. Y. Lio, J. L. Tang, J. Wu, S. J. Wu, C. Y. Lin, and Y. C. Yang, "Minor histocompatibility antigen HA-1 and HA-2 polymorphisms in Taiwan: frequency and application in hematopoietic stem cell transplantation," *Clinical Chemistry and Laboratory Medicine*, vol. 48, no. 9, pp. 1287–1293, 2010.

[60] H. Jung, C. S. Ki, J. W. Kim, and E. S. Kang, "Frequencies of 10 autosomal minor histocompatibility antigens in Korean population and estimated disparities in unrelated hematopoietic stem cell transplantation," *Tissue Antigens*, vol. 79, no. 1, pp. 42–49, 2012.

[61] S. S. B. Randolph, T. A. Gooley, E. H. Warren, F. R. Appelbaum, and S. R. Riddell, "Female donors contribute to a selective graft-versus-leukemia effect in male recipients of HLA-matched, related hematopoietic stem cell transplants," *Blood*, vol. 103, no. 1, pp. 347–352, 2004.

[62] T. Mutis, G. Gillespie, E. Schrama, J. H. F. Falkenburg, P. Moss, and E. Goulmy, "Tetrameric HLA class I-minor histocompatibility antigen peptide complexes demonstrate minor histocompatibility antigen-specific cytotoxic T lymphocytes in patients with graft-versus-host disease," *Nature Medicine*, vol. 5, no. 7, pp. 839–842, 1999.

[63] M. Markiewicz, U. Siekiera, A. Karolczyk et al., "Immunogenic disparities of 11 minor histocompatibility antigens (mHAs) in HLA-matched unrelated allogeneic hematopoietic SCT," *Bone Marrow Transplantation*, vol. 43, no. 4, pp. 293–300, 2009.

[64] M. H. Sellami, L. Torjemane, A. E. de Arias et al., "Does minor histocompatibility antigen HA-1 disparity affect the occurrence of graft-versus-host disease in tunisian recipients

of hematopoietic stem cells?" *Clinics*, vol. 65, no. 11, pp. 1099–1103, 2010.

[65] G. Socié, P. Loiseau, R. Tamouza et al., "Both genetic and clinical factors predict the development of graft-versus-host disease after allogeneic hematopoietic stem cell transplantation," *Transplantation*, vol. 72, no. 4, pp. 699–706, 2001.

[66] B. D. Tait, R. Maddison, J. McCluskey et al., "Clinical relevance of the minor histocompatibility antigen HA-1 in allogeneic bone marrow transplantation between HLA identical siblings," *Transplantation Proceedings*, vol. 33, no. 1-2, pp. 1760–1761, 2001.

4

Role of Killer Immunoglobulin-Like Receptor and Ligand Matching in Donor Selection

Meral Beksaç[1,2] and Klara Dalva[3]

[1] Department of Hematology, Ankara University Unrelated Donor Registry and Cord Blood Bank, Ankara, Turkey
[2] Ankara Tip Fakultesi Hematoloji Bilim Dali, Cebeci Yerleskesi, Dikimevi, 06620 Ankara, Turkey
[3] HLA Typing Laboratories, Department of Hematology, Ankara University School of Medicine, İbni Sina Hospital, Sihhiye, 06100 Ankara, Turkey

Correspondence should be addressed to Meral Beksaç, meral.beksac@medicine.ankara.edu.tr

Academic Editor: Andrzej Lange

Despite all efforts to improve HLA typing and immunosuppression, it is still impossible to prevent severe graft versus host disease (GVHD) which can be fatal. GVHD is not always associated with graft versus malignancy and can prevent stem cell transplantation from reaching its goals. Overall T-cell alloreactivity is not the sole mechanism modulating the immune defense. Innate immune system has its own antigens, ligands, and mediators. The bridge between HLA and natural killer (NK) cell-mediated reactions is becoming better understood in the context of stem cell transplantation. Killer immunoglobulin-like receptors (KIRs) constitute a wide range of alleles/antigens segregated independently from the HLA alleles and classified into two major haplotypes which imprints the person's ability to suppress or to amplify T-cell alloreactivity. This paper will summarize the impact of both activating and inhibitory KIRs and their ligands on stem cell transplantation outcome. The ultimate goal is to develop algorithms based on KIR profiles to select donors with maximum antileukemic and minimum antihost effects.

1. Introduction

Allogeneic hematopoietic stem cell transplantation is a curative approach. Removal of residual malignant cells and relapse prevention by an intensive conditioning regimen and reinstitution of a successful posttransplant anticancer immune response are the essential benefits of this treatment modality. The current donor-recipient matching criteria involve multiple factors but the only immunological barrier taken into consideration is the human leukocyte antigen system (HLA). However, an important factor affecting the success is the function of natural killer (NK) cells which are closely controlled by KIRs that interact with specific HLA class I ligands. KIR genes are encoded within 100–200 kb region of the leukocyte receptor complex (LRC) located on chromosome 19 (19q13.4) and segregated independently from the HLA genes. Most of HLA identical donor-recipient matched pairs are actually KIR mismatched. Innate system involves natural killer cells which through binding to their

ligands can inhibit or activate the anticancer or antidonor reactivity arising from HLA recognition. The KIR genes belong to the most polymorphic structures between all surface receptors, second only to MHC, and are the key regulators of NK cells. Since these receptors are located on natural killer cells, they are called killer immunoglobulin-like receptors (KIRs). KIRs may exert inhibitory or activating functions through iKIR and aKIRs. There are nine iKIR and six aKIR receptors. The number of Ig-like domains on their extracellular region and the length of the cytoplasmic tail of the KIR proteins define the acronym for each KIR gene. Most of them have 2 Ig-like domains D1, D2 or D0, D2 (KIR2D), and the others have 3 domains D0, D1, and D2 (KIR3D). Receptor families with a long tail, "L" KIRs, are mostly inhibitory (e.g., KIR2DL, KIR3DL); whereas short tail ones, "S" KIRs, are mostly activating (e.g., KIR2DS, KIR3DS) with an exception, KIR2DL4, which has a potential for activating or inhibitory function. Some but not all of natural killer receptor ligands have been defined. Some are HLA class I molecules including HLA-A (A3, A11) for KIR3DL2, HLA-B (Bw4) for KIR3DL1, HLA-C^{Lys80}, C^{Asn80}, for KIR2DL1 and KIR2DL2/3, respectively, and HLA-G for KIR2DL4 antigen subgroups. The HLA-C ligands are grouped according to their residue on position 80. The acronym of group 1 HLA-C is C1 or C^{Lys80} (HLA*C 01, 03, 07, 08, 12, 13, 14, and 16 and B*4601, B*7301) and group 2 HLA-C is C2 or C^{Asn80} (HLA*C 02, 04, 05, 06, 15, 17, and 18) [1, 2].

KIR diversity among people may originate from three reasons: allelic variations, the level of expression on the cell surface, and the haplotypic variability. Based on population studies KIR alleles are organized into two broad haplotypes: haplotype A and B. Haplotype A constitutes of 7 KIR genes, 6 inhibitory KIRs including the 4 framework genes plus the only activating gene KIR2DS4. Haplotype B is characterized by the presence of 1–5 activating KIR genes beside the increased number of genes with a greater variability, generated from recombinations of a centromeric and a telomeric cluster. Homozygosity of Haplotype A versus B defines an individual's ability to amplify or suppress immune reactions. Since NK cells can recognize donor antigens from tumor antigens, at least normal NK cell reactivity is essential for a graft versus leukemia effect in the absence of graft versus host reaction. However, to complicate the events further, even in the presence of activating KIR genes, these reactions can be silenced leading to abolition of activity.

Many investigators have evaluated the role of KIR receptor polymorphisms, KIR receptor-ligand matching on transplant outcome. The variation among studies in regard to donor or stem cell types, conditioning regimens, use of T-cell depletion has demonstrated a complex picture. To complicate analysis even further, factors that increase relapse or GVHD rates, such as disease activity at transplantation or gender matching, are not always similar between these studies. It is hypothesized that KIR-ligand mismatching is prerequisite for NK alloreactivity and, thus HLA mismatched transplants exert the best models for studying innate immune system activities [1, 2].

Previous reviews have grouped these NK alloreactivity studies in four models:

(1) KIR-ligand incompatibility, or ligand-ligand model (Ruggeri et al.);

(2) receptor-ligand model (Leung et al.);

(3) KIR gene-gene (receptor-receptor or haplotype) model (initially described by Nantes group, actually is similar to the Stanford model) (Gagne et al., Parham et al., and McQueen et al.);

(4) missing ligand model (retrospective model actually similar to the receptor-ligand model but neither the donor KIR nor HLA is considered for donor selection).

In summary, except for the fourth model which is a retrospective evaluation, the other models are based on biological matching principles and are being used for donor selection [1–5].

In this paper, these reports will be categorized and summarized according to stem cell source, donor matching, and conditioning regimens (Tables 1 and 2). It is an attempt towards a guide for use of KIR allele-ligand matching in donor selection.

2. KIR Matching in Haploidentical Stem Cell Transplants

Although NK cells activity against malignant cell were known for a long time, it was only in late 90s that the impact of KIR-ligands on allogeneic transplant was investigated. Haploidentical transplants have been an ideal model to investigate these effects. Following the initial reports by Valiante and Parham, the Perugia group and later additional groups investigated the impact of donor-ligand matching status after T cell depleted haploidentical transplantation for AML [3, 6–8]. In the presence of KIR-ligand mismatch between donor-recipient pairs, improved engraftment and a decrease in relapse rates were observed [1–3]. These effects were restricted to patients transplanted only in CR. However, subsequent studies were not able to confirm these results, directing investigators to analyze additional parameters. Recently, a study on haploidentical transplants with a posttransplant cyclophosphamide infusion have confirmed the role of haplotype B to have a GVL effect and prolongation of survival similar to the results obtained between siblings or matched unrelated subjects [7]. Multiple factors such as high T-cell content of the graft, suboptimal dose of T-cell depletion and HLA_mismatch level may effect NK-cell reconstitution and mask KIR effects [2]. A recent publication supports the following statement: T-cell alloreactivity overrides NK-mediated responses and optimal immunosuppression liberates NK-cell effects against leukemia. In other words, if extensive T-cell depletion such as CD34+ selection is performed, such as the setting of haploidentical transplantation, KIR-ligand mismatching benefits become visible [2, 3, 6–8].

3. KIR Gene-Gene Matching in Sibling Identical Stem Cell Transplants

As seen in Tables 1 and 2, Hsu, McQueen, Verheyden, Kim, Dalva, and Stringaris published reports analyzing the impact of KIRs utilizing KIR genotype, KIR haplotype, or telomeric KIR haplotype matching models [5, 10–14]. Four of these studies showed a beneficial effect of the B haplotype,which contains more activating KIRs, on both survival and relapse. These results are in accordance with results observed following haploidentical transplants by Ruggeri et al. [3] and Symons et al. [7]. It is important to note that both of the inconsistent studies include in vivo T depletion which might have unleashed NK-cell alloreactivities. However even the results from these two studies are not similar.

4. KIR Matching in Unrelated Myeloablative Stem Cell Transplants among Adults

Donor KIR3DS1, which is an activating KIR and is part of the haplotype B, is observed among 33% of donors. Transplants

TABLE 1: Characteristics of studies analyzing KIRs or KIR ligands.

Reference	n	Stem cell source	T-cell depletion	Donor type	HLA match	Diagnose
Ruggeri et al. 2002 [3]	92	PB	All	Related	Haploidentical	Various
Bishara et al. 2004 [6]	62	PB	Not all	Related	Haploidentical	Various
Symons et al. 2010 [7]	86	BM	None	Related	Haploidentical	Various
Weisdorf et al. 2012 [8]	24	PB	All	Related	Haploidentical	Myeloid
Cook et al. 2004 [9]	220	?	?	Related	HLA match	Lymphoid, myeloid
Hsu et al. 2005 [10]	178	BM	All	Sibling	HLA match	Various
Dalva et al. 2006 [11]	84	PB/BM	None	Sibling	HLA match	Various
McQueen et al. 2007 [5]	202	PB (89%)/BM	None	Sibling	HLA match	Various
Kim et al. 2007 [12]	53	BM/PB	None	Sibling	HLA match	Myeloid
Giebel et al. 2009 [13]	100	PB/BM	All	Sibling/unrelated	HLA match (81%)	Various
Stringaris et al. 2010 [14]	246	PB/BM	All	Sibling	HLA match	Myeloid
Davies et al. 2002 [15]	175	BM	34%	Unrelated	HLA mismatch	Various
Giebel et al. 2003 [16]	130	BM (96%)	81%	Unrelated	HLA match (47%)	Various
Bornhäuser et al. 2004 [17]	118	BM/PB	All	Unrelated	HLA match (46%)	Myeloid
Schaffer et al. 2004 [18]	190	BM/PB	All	Unrelated	HLA match (49%)	Various
Beelen et al. 2005 [19]	374	BM/PB	None	Unrelated (60%)	HLA match (63%)	CML (63 %)
De Santis et al.2005 [20]	104	BM/PB	14% (BM)	Unrelated	HLA mismatch	Various
Kröger et al. 2005 [21]	73	PB (63%)/BM	All	Unrelated	HLA match (86%)	Myeloma
Farag et al. 2006 [22]	1571	BM	None	Unrelated	HLA match (64%)	Various
Miller et al. 2007 [23]	1770	PB/BM	None	Unrelated	HLA match	Various
Yabe et al. 2008 [24]	1489	BM	All	Unrelated	HLA match	Various
Cooley 2009 [25]	448	?	None	Unrelated	HLA match (47%)	Myeloid
Cooley et al. 2010 [26]	1086	?	None	Unrelated	HLA match (50%)	Myeloid, lymphoid
Gagne et al. 2009 [4]	264	BM	None	Unrelated	HLA match (62 %)	Various
Venstrom et al. 2010 [27]	1087	BM (97%)	19%	Unrelated	HLA match (62%)	Myeloid, lymphoid
Brunstein et al. 2009 [28]	257	CB	32%	Unrelated	HLA mismatch (92%)	Various
Willemze et al. 2009 [29]	218	CB	81%	Unrelated	HLA mismatch	Various

BM: bone marrow, PB: peripheral blood, CB: cord blood, and CML: chronic myeloid leukemia.

performed with stem cells from donors positive for 3DS1 led to a decrease in grade II-IV GVHD and TRM without increasing relapse rate. This effect was amplified among subjects who were homozygous for this phenotype [27]. These authors have also reported a similar GVHD protection effect of Bw4 that was amplified in the presence of 3DS1. The overall effect of haplotype B on GVHD was dependent on 3DS1 and the other aKIR, 2DS2. These aKIRs are in strong linkage disequilibrium. Thus it was concluded that donor KIR 3DS1 and Bw4 expression, additively protects recipients from GVHD and TRM, without hampering the GvL effect.

5. KIR Matching in Unrelated Cord Blood Transplants

Similar to haploidentical transplants, cord blood transplants also utilize highly mismatched donors allowing a prominent GVHD effect that can be investigated under the context of KIR matching [28, 29]. So far, there are two major reports with opposing results. As seen in Tables 1 and 2, the type of conditioning regimens, in vivo T depletion, and number of cord blood units were different between these studies leading to a detrimental effect of KIRs following reduced

intensity conditioning regimen. Based on existing data, it is not possible to establish criteria for cord blood selection. There is certainly need for prospective studies analyzing the effect of KIRs and KIR-ligand matching in both GVH or HVG directions.

6. KIR Matching for Donor Selection

Finally, the first attempts of donor selection criteria based on KIR genotyping have been proposed: the studies by Cooley et al. demonstrated protection against relapse and survival benefit when donors with certain KIR B genotypes are used for T-cell replete unrelated donor HCT for AML suggesting KIR genotyping to be incorporated into unrelated donor selection algorithm [25, 26]. This finding is supported by data from sibling transplants, with the exception of data from Stanford and us, reporting an increase in relapse associated with haplotype B [5, 11, 12, 14]. On the contrary, Stringaris et al., also based on data from sibling transplants, have reported a positive effect of haplotype B on survival. Through three groups including us, we were able to show the presence of activating KIRs to augment graft versus host/leukemia immunity whereas the inhibitory KIRs cause

TABLE 2: Impact of KIR or KIR ligand matching on transplant outcome.

Reference	Overall survival	aGVHD	Graft failure	Relapse
Ruggeri et al. 2002 [3]	Better (missing KIR ligand)	Decrease (missing KIR ligand)	Decrease (missing KIR ligand)	Decrease (missing KIR ligand)
Bishara et al. 2004 [6]	Better (KIR match, GVH direction)	increase (donor aKIR)	No effect	No effect
Symons et al. 2010 [7]	Better (iKIR mm, D: haplotype B)	No effect	—	Decrease (iKIRmm; haplotype B: D/R: +/−) myeloid, lymphoid
Weisdorf et al. 2012 [8]	No effect	No effect	—	No effect (KIR increase ligand mm)
Cook et al. 2004 [9]	Unknown (haplotype A: CMV reactivation)	Unknown	—	Unknown
Hsu et al. 2005 [10]	Better (missing iKIR ligand)	No effect	—	Decrease (AML, MDS, and missing iKIR ligand)
Dalva et al. 2006 [11]	Better (aKIR m)	Decrease (iKIR m)	—	Decrease (aKIR m) Increase (D: haplotype B)
McQueen et al. 2007 [5]	Worse (donor but not recipient has haplotype B)	Increase (donor but not recipient has haplotype B, also Bw4)	—	Increase (haplotype B D/R: +/−) Decrease (D: 3DL1/3DL2; R: A3/11or Bw4+)
Kim et al. 2007 [12]	Better (D: aKIR)	Increase (D: aKIR: 2DS2-4)	—	Decrease (D: aKIR)
Giebel et al. 2009 [13]	Decrease (aKIR mm and group C2+)	Increase (aKIR mm)	—	Increase (aKIR mm)
Stringaris et al. 2010 [14]	Better (D: haplotype B)	Unknown	—	Decrease (D: aKIR or haplotype B) AML
Davies et al. 2002 [15]	Worse (missing KIR ligand) myeloid	No effect	No effect	No effect
Giebel et al. 2003 [16]	Better (KIR ligand mm)	No effect	Increase (KIR ligand match)	Decrease (KIR ligand mm) myeloid
Bornhäuser et al. 2004 [17]	No effect	No effect	—	Increase (KIR ligand mm)
Schaffer et al. 2004 [18]	Worse (increase infections)	No effect	—	No effect
Beelen et al. 2005 [19]	No effect	No effect	Increase (KIR ligand mm)	Decrease (KIR ligand mm)
De Santis et al. 2005 [20]	Worse (KIR epitope mm)	Increase (NK epitope mm)	Worse (NK epitope mm)	—
Kröger et al. 2005 [21]	No effect	Not significant	—	Decrease (KIR ligand mm)
Farag et al. 2006 [22]	No effect	No effect	No effect	No effect
Miller et al. 2007 [23]	—	Increase (KIR ligand mm)	—	Decrease (both KIR ligand and HLA mm)
Yabeet al. 2008 [24]	Worse (KIR ligand mm)	Increase (KIR ligand mm; D:2DS2)	—	No effect
Cooley et al. 2009 and 2010 [25, 26]	Better (D: haplotype B)	No effect	No effect	Decrease (D: haplotype B) AML but not ALL
Gagne 2009 [4]	No effect (D: haplotype B); Decrease (HLA identical, KIR3DL1: D+R− D: KIR3DL1+/3DS1+ R: Bw4+)	Increase (HLA I: 2DL5 mm HLA nonI: 2DS1mm) Decrease (HLA I: 2DS3 mm, D: haplotype B)	—	No effect (D: haplotype B) Increase (D: 3DL1+/3DS1+ R: Bw4−) Decrease (D: 3DL1+/3DS1+ R: Bw4+)
Venstrom et al. 2010 [27]	Better (D: KIR3DS1)	Decrease (D: KIR3DS1)	—	No effect (D: 3DS1)
Brunstein et al. 2009 [28]	Worse (only with RIC)	Increase (KIR ligand mm)(RIC)	—	Decrease (KIR ligand mm) (RIC)
Willemze et al. 2009 [29]	Better (KIR ligand mm)	Decrease	—	Decrease (KIR ligand mm)

M: match, mm: mismatch, RIC: reduced intensity conditioning, D/R: donor/recipient, HLA I: HLA identical, and HLA nonI: HLA nonidentical.

immune tolerance. This effect is observed frequently, if not exclusively, among patients with myeloid disorders [11, 12, 14]. In spite of all inconsistencies and contradictory results which are usually arising from the lack of simultaneous evaluation of donor and recipient KIR status; disease or conditioning regimen type related heterogeneity between studies, Leung was able to propose a donor selection Algorithm [2] as follows.

(I) More Than One HLA-Matched Donor Available (Sibling, Unrelated, or Cord Blood)

Selection of donor with receptor-ligand mismatch in KIR.

Selection of donor with "B" haplotype in KIR.

No need to consider KIR-ligand mismatch (as KIR-ligands always match if HLA matches).

(II) HLA-Matched Donor Not Available; T Cells Not Depleted (Related and Unrelated)

Selection of donor with the least degree of HLA mismatch.

Selection of donor with receptor-ligand mismatch in KIR.

Selection of donor with "B" haplotype in KIR.

Avoid donor with KIR-ligand mismatch.

(III) HLA-Matched Donor Not Available; T Cells Depleted or Single-Unit Cord Blood Transplant

Selection of donor with receptor-ligand mismatch in KIR.

Selection of donor with "B" haplotype in KIR.

Selection of donor with KIR-ligand mismatch.

7. Conclusion

It appears that different KIR parameters are valid for each donor-recipient pair based on the degree of HLA matching, T-cell depletion intensity, and the type of leukemia. The protective or opposite effects of haplotype B among unrelated or sibling transplants is a perfect example for inconsistent results. Thus the algorithm presented by Leung is open to further discussion.

References

[1] P. Parham, "MHC class I molecules and KIRS in human history, health and survival," *Nature Reviews Immunology*, vol. 5, no. 3, pp. 201–214, 2005.

[2] W. Leung, "Use of NK cell activity in cure by transplant," *British Journal of Haematology*, vol. 155, no. 1, pp. 14–29, 2011.

[3] L. Ruggeri, M. Capanni, E. Urbani et al., "Effectiveness of donor natural killer cell aloreactivity in mismatched

hematopoietic transplants," *Science*, vol. 295, no. 5562, pp. 2097–2100, 2002.

[4] K. Gagne, M. Bussson, J. D. Bignon et al., "Donor KIR3DL1/3DS1 gene and recipient Bw4 KIR ligand as prognostic markers for outcome in unrelated hematopoietic stem cell transplantation," *Biology of Blood and Marrow Transplantation*, vol. 15, no. 11, pp. 1366–1375, 2009.

[5] K. L. McQueen, K. M. Dorighi, L. A. Guethlein, R. Wong, B. Sanjanwala, and P. Parham, "Donor-recipient combinations of group A and B KIR haplotypes and HLA class I ligand affect the outcome of HLA-matched, sibling donor hematopoietic cell transplantation," *Human Immunology*, vol. 68, no. 5, pp. 309–323, 2007.

[6] A. Bishara, D. de Santis, C. C. Witt et al., "The beneficial role of inhibitory KIR genes of HLA class I NK epitopes in haploidentically mismatched stem cell allografts may be masked by residual donor-alloreactive T cells causing GVHD," *Tissue Antigens*, vol. 63, no. 3, pp. 204–211, 2004.

[7] H. J. Symons, M. S. Leffell, N. D. Rossiter, M. Zahurak, R. J. Jones, and E. J. Fuchs, "Improved survival with inhibitory killer immunoglobulin receptor (KIR) gene mismatches and KIR haplotype B donors after nonmyeloablative, HLA-haploidentical bone marrow transplantation," *Biology of Blood and Marrow Transplantation*, vol. 16, no. 4, pp. 533–542, 2010.

[8] D. Weisdorf, S. Cooley, S. Devine et al., "T cell-depleted partial matched unrelated donor transplant for advanced myeloid malignancy: KIR ligand mismatch and outcome," *Biology of Blood and Marrow Transplantation*, vol. 18, no. 6, pp. 937–943, 2012.

[9] M. Cook, D. Briggs, C. Craddock et al., "Donor KIR genotype has a major influence on the rate of cytomegalovirus reactivation following T-cell replete stem cell transplantation," *Blood*, vol. 107, no. 3, pp. 1230–1232, 2006.

[10] K. C. Hsu, C. A. Keever-Taylor, A. Wilton et al., "Improved outcome in HLA-identical sibling hematopoietic stem-cell transplantation for acute myelogenous leukemia predicted by KIR and HLA genotypes," *Blood*, vol. 105, no. 12, pp. 4878–4884, 2005.

[11] K. Dalva, F. Gungor, E. Soydan Akcaglayan, and M. Beksac, "Two independent effects of immunoglobulin-like receptor (KIR) allele matching between siblings: inhibitory KIR, (IKIR) mismatches are associated with graft versus host disease (GVHD) while activatory KIR matches, (AKIR) and CGVHD are associated with graft versus leukemia (GVL)," *Blood*, vol. 108, supplement 1, Article ID 2912a, 2006.

[12] H. J. Kim, Y. Choi, W. S. Min et al., "The activating killer cell immunoglobulin-like receptors as important determinants of acute graft-versus host disease in hematopoietic stem cell transplantation for acute myelogenous leukemia," *Transplantation*, vol. 84, no. 9, pp. 1082–1091, 2007.

[13] S. Giebel, I. Nowak, J. Dziaczkowska et al., "Activating killer immunoglobulin-like receptor incompatibilities enhance graft-versus-host disease and affect survival after allogeneic hematopoietic stem cell transplantation," *European Journal of Haematology*, vol. 83, no. 4, pp. 343–356, 2009.

[14] K. Stringaris, S. Adams, M. Uribe et al., "Donor KIR genes 2DL5A, 2DS1 and 3DS1 are associated with a reduced rate of leukemia relapse after HLA-identical sibling stem cell transplantation for acute myeloid leukemia but not other hematologic malignancies," *Biology of Blood and Marrow Transplantation*, vol. 16, no. 9, pp. 1257–1264, 2010.

[15] S. M. Davies, L. Ruggieri, T. DeFor et al., "Evaluation of KIR ligand incompatibility in mismatched unrelated donor

hematopoietic transplants," *Blood*, vol. 100, no. 10, pp. 3825–3827, 2002.

[16] S. Giebel, F. Locatelli, T. Lamparelli et al., "Survival advantage with KIR ligand incompatibility in hematopoietic stem cell transplantation from unrelated donors," *Blood*, vol. 102, no. 3, pp. 814–819, 2003.

[17] M. Bornhäuser, R. Schwerdtfeger, H. Martin, K. H. Frank, C. Theuser, and G. Ehninger, "Role of KIR ligand incompatibility in hematopoietic stem cell transplantation using unrelated donors," *Blood*, vol. 103, no. 7, pp. 2860–2861, 2004.

[18] M. Schaffer, K. J. Malmberg, O. Ringdén, H. G. Ljunggren, and M. Remberger, "Increased infection-related mortality in KIR-ligand-mismatched unrelated allogeneic hematopoietic stem-cell transplantation," *Transplantation*, vol. 78, no. 7, pp. 1081–1085, 2004.

[19] D. W. Beelen, H. D. Ottinger, S. Ferencik et al., "Genotypic inhibitory killer immunoglobulin-like receptor ligand incompatibility enhances the long-term antileukemic effect of unmodified allogeneic hematopoietic stem cell transplantation in patients with myeloid leukemias," *Blood*, vol. 105, no. 6, pp. 2594–2600, 2005.

[20] D. de Santis, A. Bishara, C. S. Witt et al., "Natural killer cell HLA-C epitopes and killer cell immunoglobulin-like receptors both influence outcome of mismatched unrelated donor bone marrow transplants," *Tissue Antigens*, vol. 65, no. 6, pp. 519–528, 2005.

[21] N. Kröger, B. Shaw, S. Iacobelli et al., "Comparison between antithymocyte globulin and alemtuzumab and the possible impact of KIR-ligand mismatch after dose-reduced conditioning and unrelated stem cell transplantation in patients with multiple myeloma," *British Journal of Haematology*, vol. 129, no. 5, pp. 631–643, 2005.

[22] S. S. Farag, A. Bacigalupo, M. Eapen et al., "The effect of KIR ligand incompatibility on the outcome of unrelated donor transplantation: a report from the center for international blood and marrow transplant research, the European blood and marrow transplant registry, and the Dutch registry," *Biology of Blood and Marrow Transplantation*, vol. 12, no. 8, pp. 876–884, 2006.

[23] J. S. Miller, S. Cooley, P. Parham et al., "Missing KIR ligands are associated with less relapse and increased graft-versus-host disease (GVHD) following unrelated donor allogeneic HCT," *Blood*, vol. 109, no. 11, pp. 5058–5061, 2007.

[24] T. Yabe, K. Matsuo, K. Hirayasu et al., "Donor killer immunoglobulin-like receptor (KIR) genotype-patient cognate KIR ligand combination and antithymocyte globulin preadministration are critical factors in outcome of HLA-C-KIR ligand-mismatched T cell-replete unrelated bone marrow transplantation," *Biology of Blood and Marrow Transplantation*, vol. 14, no. 1, pp. 75–87, 2008.

[25] S. Cooley, E. Trachtenberg, T. L. Bergemann et al., "Donors with group B KIR haplotypes improve relapse-free survival after unrelated hematopoietic cell transplantation for acute myelogenous leukemia," *Blood*, vol. 113, no. 3, pp. 726–732, 2009.

[26] S. Cooley, D. J. Weisdorf, L. A. Guethlein et al., "Donor selection for natural killer cell receptor genes leads to superior survival after unrelated transplantation for acute myelogenous leukemia," *Blood*, vol. 116, no. 14, pp. 2411–2419, 2010.

[27] J. M. Venstrom, T. A. Gooley, S. Spellman et al., "Donor activating KIR3DS1 is associated with decreased acute GVHD in unrelated allogeneic hematopoietic stem cell transplantation," *Blood*, vol. 115, no. 15, pp. 3162–3165, 2010.

[28] C. G. Brunstein, J. E. Wagner, D. J. Weisdorf et al., "Negative effect of KIR alloreactivity in recipients of umbilical cord blood transplant depends on transplantation conditioning intensity," *Blood*, vol. 113, no. 22, pp. 5628–5634, 2009.

[29] R. Willemze, C. A. Rodrigues, M. Labopin et al., "KIR-ligand incompatibility in the graft-versus-host direction improves outcomes after umbilical cord blood transplantation for acute leukemia," *Leukemia*, vol. 23, no. 3, pp. 492–500, 2009.

5

CMV Serostatus of Donor-Recipient Pairs Influences the Risk of CMV Infection/Reactivation in HSCT Patients

Emilia Jaskula,[1] Jolanta Bochenska,[2] Edyta Kocwin,[2]
Agnieszka Tarnowska,[2] and Andrzej Lange[1, 2]

[1] Department of Clinical Immunology, L. Hirszfeld Institute of Immunology and Experimental Therapy, Polish Academy of Sciences, 12 Rudolfa Weigla Street, 53-114 Wroclaw, Poland
[2] Lower Silesian Center for Cellular Transplantation, National Bone Marrow Donor Registry, Grabiszyńska 105, 53-439 Wroclaw, Poland

Correspondence should be addressed to Andrzej Lange, lange@iitd.pan.wroc.pl

Academic Editor: Bronwen Shaw

CMV donor/recipient serostatus was analyzed in 200 patients allografted in our institution from unrelated (122 patients) donors and 78 sibling donors in the years 2002–2011 in relation to posttransplant complications. On a group basis independently of the CMV serostatus of donor-recipient pairs sibling transplantations and those from unrelated donors that matched 10/10 at allele level had a similar rate of CMV reactivation (17/78 versus 19/71, P = ns). The rate of CMV reactivation/infection was higher in patients grafted from donors accepted at the lower level of matching than 10/10 (18/38 versus 36/149, P = 0.008). The incidence of aGvHD followed frequencies of CMV reactivation in the tested groups, being 40/156 and 25/44 in patients grafted from sibling or unrelated donors that 10/10 matched and in those grafted from donors taht HLA mismatched, respectively (P = 0.001). Regarding the rate of reactivation in both groups seropositive patients receiving a transplant from seronegative donors had more frequently CMV reactivation as compared to those with another donor-recipient matching CMV serostatus constellation (22/43 versus 32/143, P = 0 < 0.001). Multivariate analysis revealed that seropositivity of recipients with concomitant seronegativity of donors plays an independent role in the CMV reactivation/infection (OR = 2.669, P = 0.037; OR = 5.322, P = 0.078; OR = 23.034, P = 0.023 for optimally matched and mismatched patients and the whole group of patients, resp.).

1. Introduction

Donor-recipient matching for unrelated hematopoietic stem cell transplantation (HSCT) in addition to human leukocyte antigens (HLA) includes CMV serostatus of the donor and recipient to facilitate the decision [1, 2].

In the clinical practice the presence of CMV IgM antibodies is suggestive of the active infection/reactivation and the presence of IgG antibodies indicates prior infection and shows CMV immunological competence of individuals [3–5]. Unfortunately, it is very suggestive that IgG CMV antibody positive individuals harbor CMV in a latent form and their blood products are infective for CMV incompetent recipients [6]. In the present era of specific anti-CMV chemotherapy the significant impact of pretransplant donor seropositivity on the patient outcome is controversial—reviewed in the Boeckh and Nichols paper [7]. However, recipient CMV serostatus still remains an important risk factor of the patient outcome [8, 9].

HSCT involving pairs in which both donor and recipient lack CMV IgG antibodies is associated with a lower transplant mortality [10]. In the latter situation we are dealing with a donor-recipient pair in which probably neither donor nor recipient has CMV in a latent form. On the other hand, positivity of both donor and recipient should also favor the HSCT outcome—both donors and recipients likely have CMV in a latent form but the immune system of the donor should have a memory of CMV infection, which facilitates the immune response to CMV posttransplant. However, Ljungman et al. [11] in the megafile analysis

TABLE 1: Patient characteristics.

Number of patients	200
Age	
(median, range), yrs	34, 1–60
Adults > 16 yrs	174
Children ≤ 16 yrs	26
Recipient gender	
Female	91
Male	109
Donor gender	
Female	83
Male	116
Donor	
Sibling	78
Unrelated HLA matched (10/10 at the allele level),	78
Mismatched, at the allele or low resolution levels up to two mismatches	44
Transplant material	
Bone marrow (BM)	28
Peripheral blood progenitor cells (PBPC)	172
Diagnosis	
Hematological malignancies (HM)	175
Chronic myeloid leukemia (CML)	24
Chronic lymphocytic leukemia (CLL)	5
Acute myeloid leukemia (AML)	67
Acute lymphocytic leukemia (ALL)	39
Other HM	40
Anemias and immunodeficiencies	24
Osteopetrosis	1
Conditioning regimen	
Myeloablative	105
Reduced intensity conditioning (RIC)	95
Acute GvHD, grades	
0	114
I	21
II	26
III	16
IV	23
Chronic GvHD	
Extensive	38
Limited	33
EBV ≥ 100 DNA copies/10^5 cells	45/187
CMV ≥ 100 DNA copies/10^5 cells	54/187
HHV6 ≥ 100 DNA copies/10^5 cells	34/187
Polyoma (JC/BK)	19/33
CMV IgG serostatus	
Recipients	
CMV IgG negative	32
CMV IgG positive	168

TABLE 1: Continued.

Donors	
CMV IgG negative	66
CMV IgG positive	132
Recipient/donor CMV serostatus	
Recipient CMV IgG (+)/donor CMV IgG (+)	118
Recipient CMV IgG (−)/donor CMV IgG (−)	18
Recipient CMV IgG (+)/donor CMV IgG (−)	48
Recipient CMV IgG (−)/donor CMV IgG (+)	14

showed that the latter important observation seems to be valid only for the unrelated donor transplantation setting.

To add new information to the still disputable association between the CMV donor/recipient serostatus with the outcome of transplantation the present study was undertaken.

2. Materials and Methods

Two hundred patients (F/M: 91/109; 26 and 174 patients were below and above 16 years of age, resp.) allografted from unrelated donors (122 patients), and 78 from sibling (SIB) donors in our institution in the years 2002–2011 were studied. One hundred and seventy-five suffered from hematological malignancies acute myeloid leukemia (AML; $n = 67$), chronic myeloid leukemia (CML; $n = 24$), acute lymphocytic leukemia (ALL; $n = 39$), other lymphoproliferative disorders ($n = 23$), myeloproliferative diseases ($n = 10$), and myelodysplastic syndromes ($n = 12$). The others were transplanted because of anemias (10 patients) and immunodeficiencies (14 patients) and osteopetrosis ($n = 1$).

One hundred and five and 95 patients received myeloablative (based on busulfan and cyclophosphamide) and reduced intensity conditioning (reduced busulfan dose or melphalan plus fludarabine and antithymocyte globulin (ATG)), respectively. Unrelated donor transplanted patients and those on reduced intensity conditioning received ATG (10 to 12.5 mg/kg b.w. cumulative dose, 125 patients) or alemtuzumab (90 mg as a dose, 38 patients) as a part of the conditioning regimen. All patients were on cyclosporin A with a dose adjusted to the blood CsA trough a level to 200 ng/L. CMV serostatus, age, gender, underlying disease, donor source, and HLA match as well as conditioning regimen (reduced or myeloablative) are given in Table 1.

The patients were routinely followed for clinical outcome in one-week intervals until 30 days posttransplant, then monthly until one year post-transplant and as well as when clinical symptoms were suggestive of CMV, EBV, or HHV6 reactivation or any other serious post-transplant complications including relapse or GvHD. Out of 200 patients studied viral CMV, EBV and HHV6 DNA copies in blood were determined in 187 recipients transplanted after the year 2003.

The Zeus Scientific, Inc. (NJ, USA), IgG and IgM ELISA test system was used for qualitative detection of CMV-specific antibodies in donors' and recipients' plasma. The ELISA kit was used according to the manufacturer's instructions. Briefly, microtiter plates, precoated with inactivated

TABLE 2: Univariate analysis of risk factors for aGvHD and CMV reactivation/infection event(s) in patients post-alloHSCT.

Variable	aGvHD		P value	CMV absence	CMV presence	P value
	≤grade I	>grade I		Infection/reactivation until 1 year post-HSCT		
Donor/recipient HLA match						
Matched	116	40	P < 0.001	113	36	P = 0.008
Mismatched at the allele or low resolution levels up to two mismatches	**19**	**25**		**20**	**18**	
Source of HSCT						
PBPC	**111**	**61**	P = 0.029	112	48	P = 0.496
BM	24	4		21	6	
Type of donor						
SIB	65	13	P < 0.001	61	17	P = 0.074
MUD	**70**	**52**		72	37	
Conditioning regimen						
RIC	67	28	P = 0.450	60	30	P = 0.202
Myeloablative	68	37		73	24	
Donor CMV IgG						
CMV IgG−	**38**	**28**	P = 0.036	**36**	**23**	P = 0.055
CMV IgG+	96	36		96	31	
Recipient CMV IgG						
CMV IgG−	19	13	P = 0.307	24	4	P = 0.073
CMV IgG+	116	52		**109**	**50**	
Donor-recipient IgG CMV serology						
R−/D−	10	8		15	1	
R+/D−	28	20	P = 0.159	**21**	**22**	P < 0.001
R−/D+	9	5		9	3	
R+/D+	87	31		87	28	
R−/D−, R+/D−, R−/D+ , R+/D+	106	44	P = 0.115	111	32	P < 0.001
R+/D−	28	20		**21**	**22**	
Donor/recipient gender						
Male to male, female to female, and male to female	105	54	P = 0.572	105	44	P = 0.841
Female to male	29	11		28	10	
Donor gender						
Male	76	40	P = 0.543	75	32	P = 0.747
Female	58	25		58	22	
Recipient gender						
Male	76	33	P = 0.544	71	27	P = 0.747
Female	59	32		62	27	
Recipient age						
≤16	17	9	P = 0.824	20	2	P = 0.042
>16	118	56		**113**	**52**	
CMV infection/reactivation event within 1 year post-HSCT						
CMV−	97	36	P = 0.025			
CMV+	**30**	**24**				

Table 2: Continued.

Variable	aGvHD		P value	CMV absence	CMV presence	P value
	≤grade I	>grade I		Infection/reactivation until 1 year post-HSCT		
aGvHD						
aGvHD ≤ grade I				97	30	**P = 0.025**
aGvHD > grade I				**36**	**24**	
EBV infection/reactivation event within 1 year post HSCT						
EBV−	100	42	P = 0.204	104	38	P = 0.263
EBV+	27	18		29	16	
HHV6 infection/reactivation event within 1 year post HSCT						
HHV6−	103	50	P = 0.835	110	43	P = 0.677
HHV6+	24	10		23	11	

PBPC: peripheral blood progenitor cells; BM: bone marrow; R: recipient; D: donor; "−": negative; "+": positive; ATG: antithymocyte globulin; SIB: HLA-identical siblings; MUD: unrelated donors; RIC: reduced intensity conditioning.

Table 3: Multivariate analysis of risk factors for aGvHD (grade > I).

Variable	Coefficient	P value	Odds ratio	95% CI
CMV infection/reactivation event within 1 year post HSCT	0.5473	0.1362	1.7286	0.8415 to 3.5509
CMV IgG in donor serum	0.0290	0.9411	1.0295	0.4762 to 2.2254
Donor-recipient HLA mismatch	**0.8591**	**0.0421**	**2.3611**	**1.0310 to 5.4072**
Unrelated donor	**0.9520**	**0.0355**	**2.5909**	**1.0669 to 6.2921**
BM as a source of cells	−0.6177	0.3090	0.5392	0.1640 to 1.7723

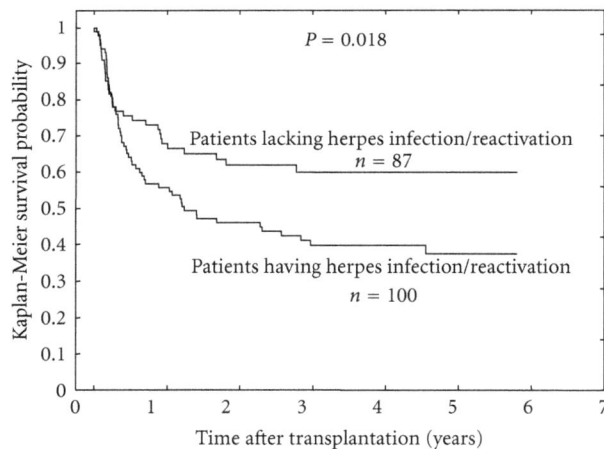

Figure 1: Overall survival in the groups of patients having and lacking *herpes* virus (CMV and/or EBV and/or HHV6) reactivations/infections.

CMV antigen, were incubated with the recipient or donor plasma. Bound IgG or IgM was detected with peroxidase labeled anti-IgG and anti-IgM antibodies by the addition of the color substrate and reading by spectrometry. Results were interpreted as seropositive or seronegative as per the manufacturer's instructions.

DNA was extracted from peripheral blood (QiAmp Blood Kit; Qiagen, Hilden, Germany) according to the manufacturer's instructions. The numbers of CMV, EBV, and HHV6 DNA copies in peripheral blood cells were determined using real-time PCR and Light Cycler II (Roche, Mannheim, Germany). The sequences of the PCR primers and the probe were selected from the *BALF5* region of EBV, the *US17* region of CMV, and the *U67* region of HHV6. PCRs were performed as described by Jaskula et al. [12].

2.1. Statistical Analysis. Statistical analysis was performed using the CSS Statistica for Windows (version 10.0) software (Stat-Soft Inc., Tulsa, OK). Univariate analyses were performed by the Fisher exact test. Logistic regression was used for the multivariate analysis, and a log-rank test to analyze the survival probability. Differences between samples were considered to be significant when $P < 0.05$ and those between 0.05 and 0.1 were indicative of a trend.

3. Results and Discussion

The presence of >100 CMV, EBV, and HHV6 DNA copies per 10^5 blood cells (clinically significant [12, 13]) was detected in 29%, 24%, and 18% of patients, respectively. Sixty out of 100 patients having during the observation period one or more reactivation events of one or more examined herpes viruses died. The mortality rate was lower in the group of patients lacking reactivations/infections (32 out of 87 patients), which resulted in a better five-year survival (59% versus 37%, $P = 0.018$, Figure 1).

TABLE 4: Multivariate analysis of risk factors for CMV reactivation/infection.

Variable	Coefficient	P value	Odds ratio	95% CI
Recipient CMV IgG seronegativity	−0.0761	0.9224	0.9267	0.2000 to 4.2929
Donor/recipient HLA mismatch	**1.2525**	**0.0155**	**3.4992**	**1.2695 to 9.6446**
R CMV IgG+/D CMV IgG−	**3.1370**	**0.0227**	**23.0340**	**1.5491 to 342.4999**
Unrelated donor	0.0021	0.9965	1.0021	0.3904 to 2.5722
aGvHD > 1	0.5363	0.1755	1.7096	0.7870 to 3.7141
Recipient age > 16 years	**2.2890**	**0.0072**	**9.8650**	**1.8606 to 52.3036**

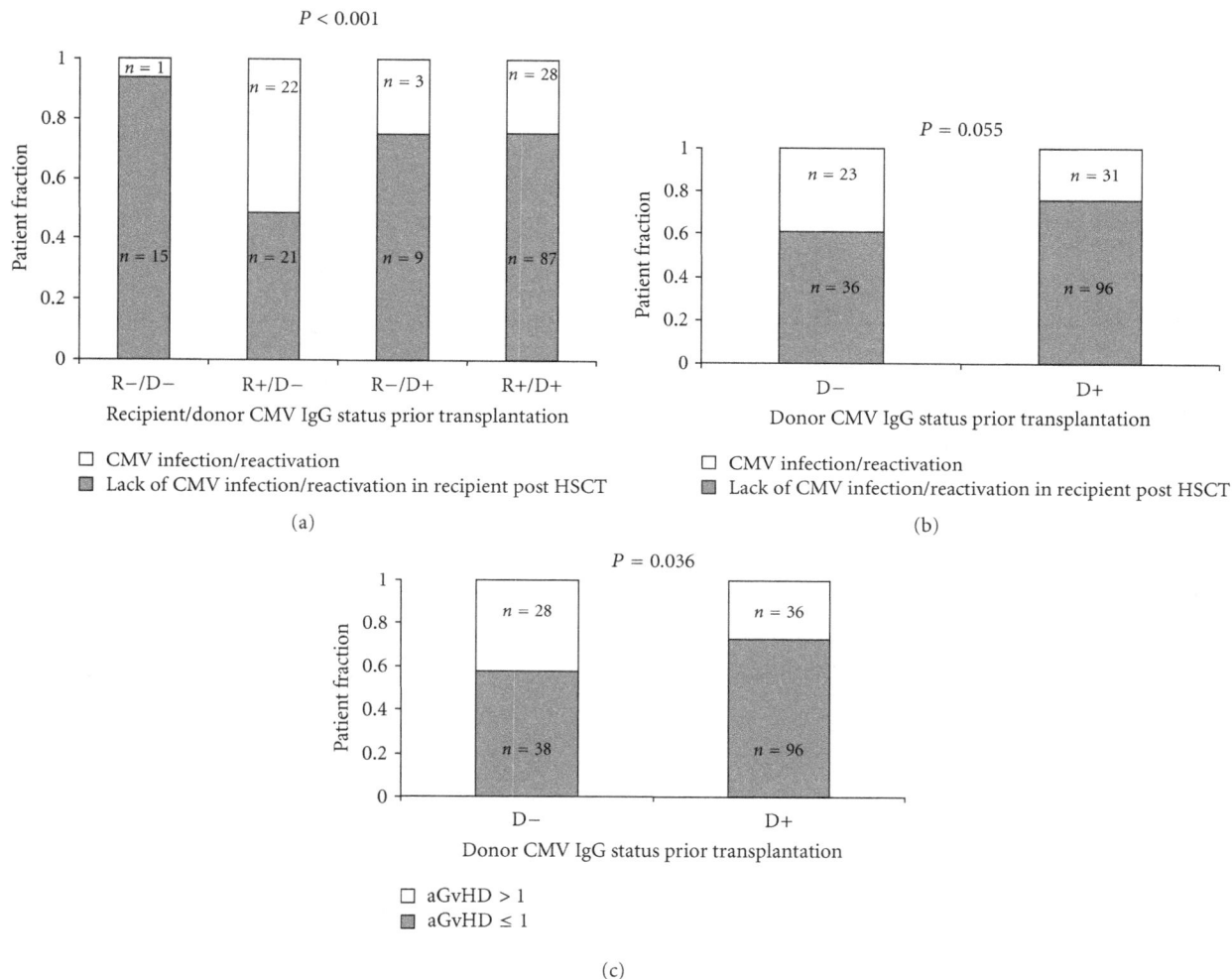

(a)

(b)

(c)

FIGURE 2: CMV reactivation/infection with respect to donor/recipient CMV serology (a) and donor CMV IgG status independently of the serostatus of recipients (b). Acute GvHD in patients transplanted from CMV IgG negative and CMV IgG positive donors (c) (R: recipient, D: donor, "+": CMV IgG positive, and "−": CMV IgG negative).

Patients receiving transplantation from the CMV IgG seronegative donors tended to suffer more frequently from CMV infection/reactivation after HSCT as compared to those grafted from CMV seropositive donors (23/59 versus 31/127, $P = 0.055$, Figure 2(b)). This association was valid for seropositive and seronegative recipients. However, the highest risk of CMV reactivation was when seropositive recipients were transplanted from the seronegative donors (22/43 versus 32/143, $P < 0.001$ Figure 2(a)). In contrast,

CMV negative serostatus of both the donor and the recipient was associated with the lowest rate of the CMV reactivation (1 out of 16 patients) as compared to other recipient (R)/donor (D) CMV IgG serostatus relations, being 22/43 versus 28/115 versus 3/12, ($P < 0.001$) for R+/D−, R+/D+, and R−/D+, resp. (Figure 2(a)). We also found that aGvHD (grade > I) was more frequently seen in patients receiving grafts from IgG negative donors (28/66 versus 36/132, $P = 0.036$, Figure 2(c)). However, donor

TABLE 5: Univariate analysis of risk factors for CMV reactivation/infection event(s) in group of SIB and MUD HLA match patients and in group of MUD HLA mismatch patients.

Variable	Optimally matched group (SIB+ 10/10 HLA matched) of patients			MUD HLA mismatched group of patients		
	CMV absence	CMV presence	P value	CMV absence	CMV presence	P value
	Infection/reactivation until 1 year post HSCT			Infection/reactivation until 1 year post HSCT		
Source of HSCT						
PBPC	95	30	1.000	17	18	0.232
BM	18	6		3	0	
Conditioning regimen						
Absence of ATG and Campath	33	5				
ATG	60	22	0.167	19	14	0.170
Campath	20	9		1	4	
RIC	**53**	**23**	**0.087**	7	7	1.000
Myeloablative	60	13		13	11	
Donor CMV IgG						
CMV IgG−	26	12	0.273	10	11	0.532
CMV IgG+	86	24		10	7	
Recipient CMV IgG						
CMV IgG−	18	2	0.160	6	2	0.238
CMV IgG+	95	34		14	16	
Donor-recipient IgG CMV serology						
R−/D−	**10**	**0**		5	1	
R−/D+	8	2	**0.032**	1	1	**0.18**
R+/D−	**16**	**12**		5	10	
R+/D+	78	22		9	6	
R−/D−, R−/D+, R+/D+	96	24	**0.015**	15	8	**0.096**
R+/D−	**16**	**12**		5	10	
Donor/recipient gender						
Male to male, female to female, and male to female	67	23	0.698	13	14	0.485
Female to male	46	13		7	4	
Donor gender						
Male	67	23	0.569	8	9	0.746
Female	46	13		12	9	
Recipient gender						
Male	59	21	0.698	12	6	0.112
Female	54	15		8	12	
Recipient age						
≤16	11	1	0.290	9	1	**0.009**
>16	102	35		**11**	**17**	
aGvHD						
aGvHD ≤ grade I	88	23	0.123	9	7	0.752
aGvHD > grade I	25	13		11	11	

serostatus did not affect the survival of HSCT recipients (Figure 3).

In addition to the factors associated with the serostatus of donors and recipients, a lack of optimal donor/recipient HLA matching was associated with a higher risk of grade > I aGvHD (25/44 versus 40/156, $P < 0.001$) and with a higher rate of CMV reactivation/infection (18/38 versus 36/149, $P = 0.008$). CMV reactivation was also more frequently

TABLE 6: Multivariate analysis of risk factors for CMV infection/reactivation in group of SIB and MUD HLA match patients and in group of MUD HLA mismatch patients.

Variable	Optimally matched group (SIB+ 10/10 HLA matched) of patients				MUD HLA mismatched group of patients			
	Coefficient	P value	Odds ratio	95% CI	Coefficient	P value	Odds ratio	95% CI
aGvHD > 1	0.7265	0.1015	2.0679	0.8667 to 4.9336	0.0185	0.9816	1.0187	0.2113 to 4.9106
Recipient CMV IgG seronegativity	0.9058	0.2601	2.474	0.5113 to 11.9711	0.5751	0.6126	1.7773	0.1918 to 16.4703
R CMV IgG+/D CMV IgG−	**0.9819**	**0.0374**	**2.6695**	**1.0587 to 6.7314**	1.6719	0.0776	5.3222	0.8313 to 34.0733
RIC conditioning regimen	−0.5655	0.1745	0.5681	0.2511 to 1.2849	0.30101	0.7333	1.3513	0.2391 to 7.6375
Recipient age > 16 years	1.2945	0.2318	3.6492	0.4371 to 30.4624	**3.1026**	**0.0148**	**22.256**	**1.8360 to 269.7835**

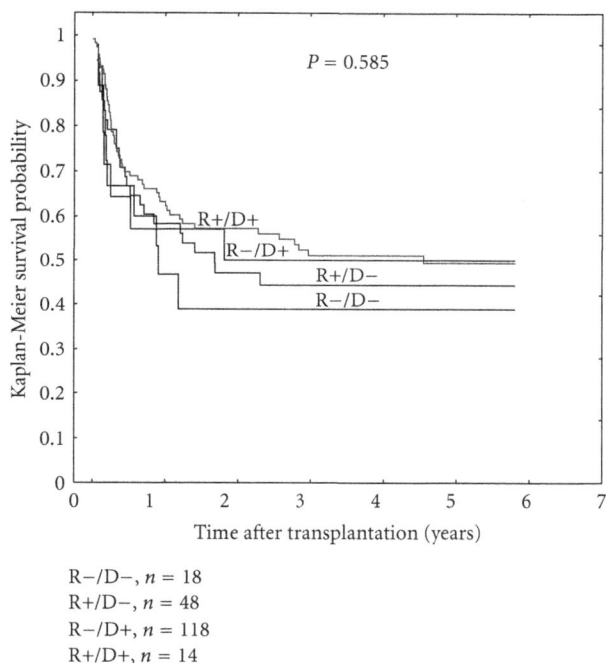

FIGURE 3: Survival of HSCT patients in the groups stratified according to CMV donor-recipient serostatus constellation (R: recipient, D: donor, "+": CMV IgG positive, and "−": CMV IgG negative).

R−/D−, n = 18
R+/D−, n = 48
R−/D+, n = 118
R+/D+, n = 14

seen in patients who were over 16 years old at the time of transplantation (52/165 versus 2/22, P = 0.042, Table 2) and in those having CMV IgG antibodies before transplantation (50/159 versus 4/28, P = 0.073, Table 2).

Multivariate analysis devoted to the evaluation of the risk factors of aGvHD showed that unrelated donor (OR = 2.591, P = 0.036) transplantation and HLA mismatch (OR = 2.361, P = 0.042) appeared as independent and significant factors associated with aGvHD grade > I (Table 3). In spite of the univariate results multivariate analysis did not confirm the role of CMV reactivation and donor serology as independent factors associated with aGvHD (Table 3).

The next statistical approach was to validate factors associated with CMV reactivation. For that also a multivariate analysis was calculated employing factors as follows: recipient IgG serology, donor-recipient HLA mismatch, transplantation recipient in CMV IgG positive/donor CMV IgG negative serology, type of donors, recipient age, and aGvHD. Among the above factors donor-recipient HLA mismatch (OR = 3.499, P = 0.016), recipient CMV IgG positive/donor CMV IgG negative serology status constellation (OR = 23.030, P = 0.023), and recipient age over 16 years (OR = 9.865, P = 0.007) were found to be significant risk factors of CMV reactivation (Table 4).

To further analyze the significance of CMV serology as a risk factor of CMV reactivation similar to that above, analysis was performed for groups consisting of SIB and MUD 10/10 matched and MUD not optimally matched (Tables 5 and 6). On a group basis independently of the CMV serostatus of donor-recipient pairs, sibling transplantations and those from unrelated donors matched 10/10 at allele level had a similar rate of CMV reactivation (17/78 versus 19/71, P = ns). Notably, the rate of CMV reactivation was higher in patients grafted from donors accepted at the lower level of matching than 10/10 (18/38 versus 36/149, P = 0.008). Also when we considered separately the optimal match group (SIB + MUD) the highest risk of CMV reactivation was observed when donors were negative but recipients were positive (12/28 versus 24/120, P = 0.015). In MUD HLA mismatched recipients a tendency to the association seropositivity of recipients with concomitant seronegativity of donors with the CMV reactivation/infection was observed (10/15 versus 8/23, P = 0.096). Notably in the MUD HLA mismatch group recipient age >16 years was a risk factor for CMV reactivation (17/28 versus 1/10, P = 0.009, Table 5). There were no significant associations between aGvHD and variables considered in this paper in the optimally matched group (SIB + 10/10 HLA matched) and in the MUD HLA mismatched group of patients.

Multivariate analysis results of patients optimally matched and separately those not optimally matched were similar and revealed that among factors analyzed for the risk of CMV reactivation seropositivity of recipients with concomitant seronegativity of donors plays an independent role (OR = 2.670, $P = 0.037$) for optimally matched and as tendency in HLA mismatched patients (OR = 5.322, $P = 0.078$, Table 6).

4. Conclusions

The information provided in the present paper shows that IgG negativity in donors favors the outcome of HSCT only when recipients are also CMV IgG negative. The worst is when donor IgG CMV negativity is confronting IgG CMV positivity in recipients. This confirms the importance of CMV IgG positivity likely associated with the immune competence of donors [3–5], which is of a special value in seropositive patients, very likely having CMV in a latent form [6]. Therefore, when recipients are IgG CMV positive the immune competence of donors is required to reduce the risk of CMV reactivation. This observation can be used as one of the factors that should be considered during donor selections for an optimal post-HSCT outcome.

Acknowledgment

This work was supported by Grant N R13 0082 06 from the Polish Ministry of Science and Higher Education.

References

[1] P. Ljungman, "Risk assessment in haematopoietic stem cell transplantation: viral status," *Best Practice and Research*, vol. 20, no. 2, pp. 209–217, 2007.

[2] International Standards for Cellular Therapy Product Collection, *Processing, and Administration*, chapter 6, FACT-JACIE Standards, 4th edition, 2008.

[3] J. W. Gratama, J. W. J. Van Esser, C. H. J. Lamers et al., "Tetramer-based quantification of cytomegalovirus (CMV)-specific CD8+ T lymphocytes in T-cell-depleted stem cell grafts and after transplantation may identify patients at risk for progressive CMV infection," *Blood*, vol. 98, no. 5, pp. 1358–1364, 2001.

[4] H. T. Maeker and V. C. Maino, "Analyzing T-cell responses to cytomegalovirus by cytokine flow cytometry," *Human Immunology*, vol. 65, no. 5, pp. 493–499, 2004.

[5] M. Sester, B. C. Gärtner, U. Sester, M. Girndt, N. Mueller-Lantzsch, and H. Köhler, "Is the cytomegalovirus serologic status always accurate? A comparative analysis of humoral and cellular immunity," *Transplantation*, vol. 76, no. 8, pp. 1229–1230, 2003.

[6] J. D. Roback, "CMV and blood transfusions," *Reviews in Medical Virology*, vol. 12, no. 4, pp. 211–219, 2002.

[7] M. Boeckh and W. G. Nichols, "The impact of cytomegalovirus serostatus of donor and recipient before hematopoietic stem cell transplantation in the era of antiviral prophylaxis and preemptive therapy," *Blood*, vol. 103, no. 6, pp. 2003–2008, 2004.

[8] W. G. Nichols, L. Corey, T. Gooley, C. Davis, and M. Boeckh, "High risk of death due to bacterial and fungal infection among cytomegalovirus (CMV)-seronegative recipients of stem cell transplants from seropositive donors: evidence for indirect effects of primary CMV infection," *Journal of Infectious Diseases*, vol. 185, no. 3, pp. 273–282, 2002.

[9] P. B. McGlave, X. O. Shu, W. Wen et al., "Unrelated donor marrow transplantation for chronic myelogenous leukemia: 9 years' experience of the National Marrow Donor Program," *Blood*, vol. 95, no. 7, pp. 2219–2225, 2000.

[10] P. Ljungman, K. Larsson, G. Kumlien et al., "Leukocyte depleted, unscreened blood products give a low risk for CMV infection and disease in CMV seronegative allogeneic stem cell transplant recipients with seronegative stem cell donors," *Scandinavian Journal of Infectious Diseases*, vol. 34, no. 5, pp. 347–350, 2002.

[11] P. Ljungman, R. Brand, H. Einsele, F. Frassoni, D. Niederwieser, and C. Cordonnier, "Donor CMV serologic status and outcome of CMV-seropositive recipients after unrelated donor stem cell transplantation: an EBMT megafile analysis," *Blood*, vol. 102, no. 13, pp. 4255–4260, 2003.

[12] E. Jaskula, D. Dlubek, D. Duda, K. Bogunia-Kubik, A. Mlynarczewska, and A. Lange, "Interferon gamma 13-CA-repeat homozygous genotype and a low proportion of CD4+ lymphocytes are independent risk factors for cytomegalovirus reactivation with a high number of copies in hematopoietic stem cell transplantation recipients," *Biology of Blood and Marrow Transplantation*, vol. 15, no. 10, pp. 1296–1305, 2009.

[13] E. Jaskula, D. Dlubek, M. Sedzimirska, D. Duda, A. Tarnowska, and A. Lange, "Reactivations of cytomegalovirus, human herpes virus 6, and Epstein-Barr virus differ with respect to risk factors and clinical outcome after hematopoietic stem cell transplantation," *Transplantation Proceedings*, vol. 42, no. 8, pp. 3273–3276, 2010.

6

Computer Algorithms in the Search for Unrelated Stem Cell Donors

David Steiner

Department of Cybernetics, Czech Technical University in Prague, Karlovo Náměstí 13, 121 35 Prague 2, Czech Republic

Correspondence should be addressed to David Steiner, david.steiner@fel.cvut.cz

Academic Editor: Colette Raffoux

Hematopoietic stem cell transplantation (HSCT) is a medical procedure in the field of hematology and oncology, most often performed for patients with certain cancers of the blood or bone marrow. A lot of patients have no suitable HLA-matched donor within their family, so physicians must activate a "donor search process" by interacting with national and international donor registries who will search their databases for adult unrelated donors or cord blood units (CBU). Information and communication technologies play a key role in the donor search process in donor registries both nationally and internationaly. One of the major challenges for donor registry computer systems is the development of a reliable search algorithm. This work discusses the top-down design of such algorithms and current practice. Based on our experience with systems used by several stem cell donor registries, we highlight typical pitfalls in the implementation of an algorithm and underlying data structure.

1. Introduction

Hematopoietic stem cell transplantation (HSCT) [1] (commonly referred to as bone marrow transplantation) is a medical procedure in the field of hematology and oncology, most often performed for patients with certain cancers of the blood or bone marrow. HSCT is the treatment of choice for people with hematopoietic malignancies, bone marrow failure, and certain types of cancer (e.g., lymphoma) which results in a compromised immune system. The most important factor in the successful outcome of HSCT is that the patient and donor are matched for the Human Leukocyte Antigens (HLA). The level of the matching required varies with the source of stem cells used for HSCT.

A lot of patients have no suitable HLA-matched donor within their family, so physicians must activate a "donor search process" by interacting with national and international donor registries who will search their databases for adult unrelated donors (AUD) or cord blood units (CBU).

Information and communication technologies play a key role in the donor search process in donor registries both nationally and internationally. One of the major challenges for donor registry computer systems is the development of a reliable search algorithm. This work discusses the top-down design of such algorithms and current practice. Based on our experience with systems used by several stem cell donor registries, we will highlight typical pitfalls in the implementation of an algorithm and underlying data structure.

2. Search Algorithm

The purpose of the donor search algorithm is to find and present a selected list of potential donors and/or CBUs, in which those most likely to be an optimal stem cell source for the patient are sorted to the top of the list [2]. Selection and sorting criteria are based on HLA compatibility and may also take into consideration secondary preference criteria, such as CMV antibody status, gender, and age.

Basic requirements for the search system used by stem cell donor registries are as follow.

(i) *Deterministic*: behavior that ensures the same results with the same input. This means, the algorithm has to reproduce exact decisions at every step.

(ii) *Clear ranking order*: results.

(iii) *Exhaustive*: all donors available for transplant in the source database should be included in the search algorithm. Exceptions must be clearly indicated to the end-user. For example, some algorithms exclude donors that are typed only at HLA-A and HLA-B.

(iv) *Scalable*: the system should be able to handle databases of varying size and type.

(v) *Fast*: search algorithms are also used in user-interactive systems, so the results should be received in seconds.

(vi) *Configurable*: search coordinator must be able to define patient-donor HLA match criteria and secondary preference criteria (CMV status, gender, and age).

(vii) *Consistently matched*: The data presented should be uniformly matched as a set for a given instance of a patient search. Different primary algorithms or matching criteria shall not be used within a single patient search.

The search algorithm is usually implemented as the key component of the stem cell donor registry software system. It has several inputs and a single output (see Figure 1). The following input data are essential.

(i) Patient's data: HLA type (minimum HLA-A, HLA-B, and HLA-DRB1 typing).

(ii) Patient's match criteria (position and number of allowable mismatches).

(iii) Database of adult unrelated (AUD) and cord blood units (CBUs) (optional).

(iv) HLA nomenclature code lists.

(v) Allele and haplotype frequencies (optional, depending on type of the algorithm).

The algorithm itself usually follows the following step.

(a) *Preprocessing*: fast preselection of donors based on predetermined internal indices.

(b) *Processing*: comparison of every (preselected) donor with the patient, calculation of match grades, matching probabilities, and filtering.

(c) *Postprocessing*: linking corresponding donor/CBU details.

The search output, which returns a sorted list of potential donors and CBUs can be presented either in the user interface, on a printed report, or transmitted to other systems (EMDIS). The presentation output may be calculated within the search engine software. For example, it is common practice to highlight patient-donor HLA mismatches as well as match grade and matching probability this may require additional data extraction from internal information calculated during the execution of the algorithm.

2.1. Patient's Data. Patient's HLA typing data must correspond to the valid HLA nomenclature and WMDA guidelines [3] and should be typed at the highest possible resolution, that is, at least intermediate resolution. Some

algorithms may return unexpected search results, if low-resolution HLA typing data is provided.

Example 1. B*35:76 has no mapping to "Unambiguous Serology" [4], but is mapped to "Possible Serology" B35 and B22. B22 is the broad HLA code with splits B54, B55, and B56. Therefore, a patient carrying B*35: XX is a potential match with a donor carrying B56. Such a result is likely to be confusing for healthcare professionals. This problem would not appear if the patient was typed at higher resolution (the B*35:76 allele is excluded). An alternative solution would be to apply an exceptions or filter by application of additional criteria, for example, matching probabilities with threshold (it is very unlikely that B*35: XX will become B*35:76).

2.2. Patient's Match Criteria. Some algorithms have hard-coded or fixed match criteria, but more sophisticated search algorithms allow users to define matching preferences for each individual search. EMDIS Matching Preferences [5] define the following criteria.

(i) Counting method for mismatches: count graft-versus-host (GvH) mismatches only or host-versus-graft (HvG) mismatches only.

(ii) Maximum number of antigen/allele mismatches for adult donors.

(iii) Maximum number of antigen/allele mismatches for CBUs.

(iv) Maximum number of antigen/allele mismatches at loci A/A*, B/B*, Cw/C*, DR/DRB1*, DQ/DQB1*.

(v) Additional sorting criteria like age of the donor, gender matching, and CMV matching.

2.3. Database of Donors and Cord Blood Units (CBUs). Database of unrelated stem cell donors and CBUs should correspond to the following requirements [6].

(i) *Current*: the data used by the algorithm should be up to date.

(ii) *Detailed*: the data presented should contain all relevant fields to the determination of match. The set of data elements should be consistent amongst the registry community.

(iii) *Integrated*: the data presented should be considered as a set and should be available to the matching party as part of a singular search event.

(iv) *Recognizable*: the data presented should uniquely reference individual sources using the identifier that is directly associated with the donor/CBU or would appear on any biological samples associated with the product.

(v) *Comprehensive*: the data presented should represent a consolidated view of the inventory. Uniform depth of access to all donors is needed.

Good implementation of the donor database is essential for acceptable performance of the search algorithm. Not all

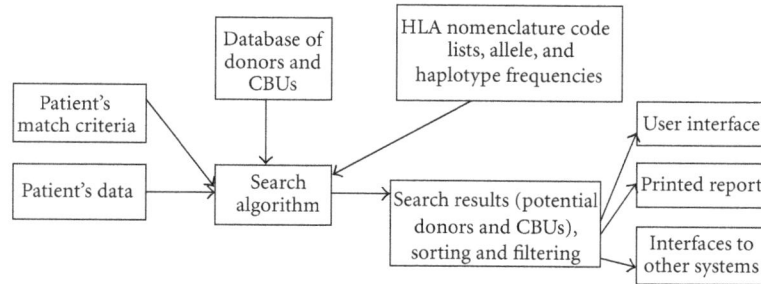

FIGURE 1: Basic concept of the donor search algorithm.

database structures of HLA applications are suitable as the data source for the algorithm.

Many small to middle size registry are colocated in a single centre with the HLA typing laboratory and there is a need for data integration of these two departments. It may seem that the registry system stores and manages the HLA typing results in the same way as the HLA laboratory information management system (LIMS), and some registries have implemented such data storage. It is a mistake to use these in search algorithms. The main differences between registry database and HLA LIMS database are as follow.

(i) The registry system needs fast access to the most current and comprehensive HLA typing results, which does not always mean the last test typing. This may be combination of multiple tests performed in the past by multiple typing techniques. The registry system always needs access to the full set of all loci that should be stored at one place, while the HLA lab system order includes only requested tests and loci, so HLA typing results of an individual may be spread in multiple typing orders.

(ii) When the HLA lab supervisor approves the order results, it cannot be changed in the lab system. However, the registry system has to keep historical HLA typing results up to date according to the latest HLA nomenclature, so it needs to update them (deleted and renamed alleles, new HLA nomenclature).

Database of donors/CBUs can simply be organized in a single relational database table. Even this may be problematic. A logical database approach is to organize HLA code-lists in separated tables (multiple-allele codes, alleles, antigens, and their relations) and define master-detail relationship between donor data and HLA codes. These systems have been implemented in some registries. The storage of donor record is using only primary keys of HLA codes (as foreign keys). The disadvantage of the master-detail storage is that the retrieval of donor's HLA typing is inefficient. Often the solution for data retrieval in such a structure is cumbersome, because the database system has to join data (database natural join) from tens of tables or do tens of joins of the same table. The advantage is easy manipulation of the properties of HLA codes or even the renaming of HLA allele codes. But such operations are much less common, compared to data retrieval.

2.4. HLA Nomenclature Code Lists. In all cases, the algorithm has to recognize the description of HLA typing codes (e.g., multiple-allele codes) and relations between HLA codes, especially DNA to serology mapping. Some algorithms even use antigen recognition site matching, amino acid sequences, or nucleotide sequences. It is recommended that code lists and code attributes are downloaded from specialist reference websites [4, 7].

Donors have been typed by various different typing techniques and many of them are registered with HLA serological assignments. The database of donors could be preprocessed, so all interpretations and mapping of HLA codes could be saved in advance, but generally, the patient's HLA type is known only at the time of the search, so HLA nomenclature code lists are needed. Of some concern is that a minority of patients are still typed only by serologic typing techniques! This means that search algorithms must be capable of using these in the search process.

3. Preprocessing

Several variants of search algorithms are being used by stem cell donor registries. Selection of the algorithm is influenced by available resources, size of the donor database, availability of haplotype frequencies of the supported population(s), and so forth. We will discuss commonly used search algorithms.

3.1. Simple Preselection. The goal of the algorithm is to find potential donors for one patient. The phenotype of the patient is compared with all donors phenotypes in the donor registry database that are "available" for transplantation purposes (simple preselection).

> For every donor D in the database
> Count Match Grade (patient P-donor D)
> If the Match Grade is acceptable, store
> data of donor D in the list of
> potential donors of patient P.

This kind of algorithm is usually used only for small to middle sized registries. Implementation enhancements can help to improve this situation. For example, increasing current capacities of server memories allows caching of all donors in the random access memory (RAM) of the server. The advantage of this algorithm is mainly in its simplicity and simple validation process. It also has very straightforward implementation of distributed or parallel computing. The drawback is the speed and memory limitation, especially where donor database is growing.

This algorithm could be extended to multiple patient searches that might be useful, for example, for EMDIS repeat searches [5], when search results from several thousands of donors have to be generated and compared with previous results. Again, the list of all patients could be cached in the server memory with one additional loop.

> For every donor D in the database
> > For every patient P in the database
> > > Count Match Grade (patient P-donor D)
> > > If the Match Grade is acceptable, store
> > > data of donor D in the list of
> > > potential donors of patient P.

3.2. Search Determinants. Databases from Registries and cord blood banks store the HLA types in many formats depending whether typing was by serology or by DNA-based methods. Registries must take these different assignments to create a match algorithm to search for a patient. This comparison is usually facilitated by the conversion of phenotypes to "search determinants" prior to development of matching algorithms [8].

The phenotype of the patient/donor is mapped to "Search Determinants" (SD) [9, 10]. The SD is a data record, based on serological antigens, corresponding to the original HLA phenotype. For example, it might be a group of six HLA, serologic-based assignments—three pairs for HLA-A, HLA-B, and HLA-DRB1 loci. There are also a number of issues with this approach, since some alleles have multiple or no serologic specificities. Therefore, an individual can have multiple SDs. SDs are used as an index to select the set of matching phenotypes. Then, more precise match grades are counted and the list of donors is filtered.

The main application of SDs is the speeding up of the match process by using SDs as key values in conjunction with a database and a matching algorithm [11]. The main disadvantage is the need for regular checks and updates of SDs of all donors in the database; due to changes of donor data, HLA nomenclature updates and changes in the "DNA to serology" mapping. There are particular problems where there is no serological equivalent for a DNA allele.

3.3. DNA Matching Only. The National Marrow Donor Program (NMDP) in the United States has developed an algorithm [12] that does not use SDs for the initial matching step as this is done by directly comparing patient DNA type to donor DNA type. The algorithm is able to account for all serologic typing possibilities with the use of a special table called the "Serology to DNA Allele Table." This table can be generated from the "rel_dna_ser.txt" and "rel_ser_ser.txt" files from hla.alleles.org [4].

4. Processing

The key element of the processing step of the algorithm is the "match grade function" that can compare data (HLA, ethnic group) of two individuals (usually patient and donor) and return their match grade and/or matching probabilities (see Figure 2). The threshold function then filters out donors that do not match patient's match criteria.

Original versions of matching algorithms compared HLA typing only at HLA-A and HLA-B loci. DNA typing was not performed. Later generations added other loci, especially HLA-DRB1, but also HLA-C and HLA-DQB1. Today, some algorithms even use HLA-DRB3/4/5, HLA-DPB1, and other loci.

Earlier versions of matching algorithms also used only serological assignments; DNA typing either did not exist or was not taken into account. Later versions have converted DNA typing results into serological assignments or vice versa, so the algorithm has a uniform typing technique view on all donors. Current search algorithms use DNA typing results as much as possible and switch to serology comparisons only if DNA typing is not provided or if they want to refine DNA to serology mapping.

The Information Technology (IT) Working Group of the World Marrow Donor Association (WMDA) has issued two key resources that describe the correct handling of HLA data and key patient-donor matching procedures:

(i) framework for the implementation of HLA matching programs in hematopoietic stem cell donor registries and cord blood banks [2]. This paper gives a bottom-up approach to the design of search algorithms: comparison of individual HLA codes, then HLA single-locus phenotypes, and eventually HLA multilocus phenotypes;

(ii) fuidelines for use of HLA nomenclature and its validation in the data exchange among hematopoietic stem cell donor registries and cord blood banks [3].

A common mistake in the design of search algorithm is the violation of the rule 2.1 of the guidelines [3]: "laboratories must assign DNA nomenclature to results obtained using DNA-based methods and serologic nomenclature to results obtained using antibody reagents." Some computer systems need to permanently store serology-derived results of DNA codes, usually because of simple DNA-serology matching. However, the mapping should be done automatically by the system and not by the user. Derived serology values must be clearly distinguished from real serology results obtained using antibody reagents. Where mapping has changed, the registry system has to know if stored serologic results should be updated or not. Moreover, some alleles are mapped to multiple serology equivalents and the system has to take this into account.

In addition to match grade, some information can be calculated. In these, the probability of HLA matching at the allele level based on local population haplotype frequencies in the underlying population can be calculated. Such prediction algorithm system has been developed and validated by the NMDP (HapLogic II) [13].

The latest, state-of-the-art versions of search algorithms (OptiMatch, HapLogic III) use these probability calculations to determine the rank order of HLA matches as the main searching and sorting criteria.

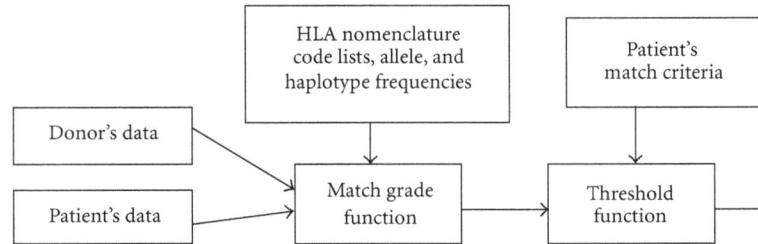

FIGURE 2: Match grade function.

5. Postprocessing

At this stage, the system retrieves corresponding donor details of all selected donors that will be displayed in the search results. If the matching probabilities are not used as the main sorting criteria, the search system can apply them at this stage (ProMatch [14], Hap-E [15] and EasyMatch [16]).

6. Probability Matching Algorithms

The search algorithms of the two largest registries in the world are based on the probability matching approach.

Using a large number of high resolution HLA types the system can estimate the probability of other less well-typed donors being matched to the patient. The system is validated by retyping these donors to obtain high resolution types/haplotypes and thereby confirming that the calculation is accurate. The limitation of this is that it may be specific to an ethnic group.

6.1. OptiMatch. OptiMatch [17] is a matching program calculating, for each donor, the probability of allelic identity to the patient. The program was developed by the German registry ZKRD. The first version (October 2006) was based on 3 locus high resolution haplotype frequencies, while the current version (June 2008) is based on 5 locus high resolution haplotype frequencies.

The web-based user interface lists potential donors with 7 probabilities: A∗ match, B∗ match, C∗ match, DRB1∗ match, DQB1∗ match, and overall probabilities of 10/10 match and 9/10 match.

6.2. HapLogic. The HapLogic program [13, 18] was developed by the NMDP registry. It works in a similar way to OptiMatch. First versions calculated probabilities of 6/6 allele matches, while the latest version III, introduced in November 2011, sorts donors based on probability of matching 10 alleles, using 5 locus high resolution haplotypes (like OptiMatch). HapLogic also uses 5 broad and 21 detailed race/ethnic groups.

The web-based user interface shows a list of potential donors with several probabilities: A∗ match, B∗ match, C∗ match, DRB1∗ match, DQB1∗ match, and overall probabilities of 10/10 match, 9/10 match, 8/10 match, 8/8 match, 7/8 match, 6/8 match, and for cord blood units also 6/6 match, 5/6 match, and 4/6 match.

7. Implementation of the Probability Matching Algorithm

If the registry wants to implement probability matching algorithm, such as OptiMatch or HapLogic, it has to successfully complete the following three steps.

(1) Design and implement the algorithm itself.

(2) Estimate haplotype frequencies of the donor (and patient) populations—these 5 locus high resolution haplotype frequencies are usually estimated from a donor registry database.

(3) Validate the search system—using retrospective data of historical searches. Usually, registry confirmatory typing requests (CTs) and their results are used.

There are two potential problems with the development of this approach: (1) unlike ZKRD and NMDP, other registries do not have sufficient donors to estimate 5 locus high resolution haplotype frequencies. Haplotype frequencies could be calculated, but their confidence is questionable. (2) Smaller registries also do not have enough high resolution HLA types (obtained at confirmatory typing, CT) for validation of the prediction algorithm. ZKRD used 9843 CTs in 2008 [17] and 22255 CTs in 2010 [19]. NMDP used about 60 000 CTs (not published). These numbers are not achievable in smaller registries.

In order to overcome these problems, the Prometheus system approximated the local population to the German (ZKRD) population, that is, by using ZKRD high resolution A∗-B∗-C∗-DRB1∗-DQB1∗ haplotype frequencies [14]. It also used high resolution HLA types from CT samples from multiple registries.

8. Validation of the Search Algorithm

All implementations of the search algorithms need to be validated before being used. The WMDA Information Technology Working Group provides validation sets of patients and donors that are used for matching trials and comparison of results with expected outcomes [2, 20]. Algorithms that do not use simple preselection approach, but use more complex preselection, have to be validated for completeness. It is important not to miss any relevant donors in the preselection [2].

Validation of the processing phase, especially the match grade function, can be done by running several automated

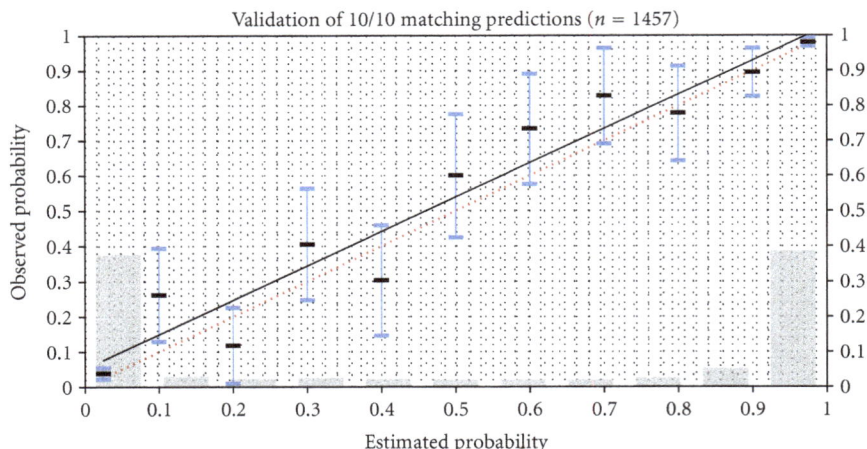

FIGURE 3: Prometheus probability matching algorithm (ProMatch): the graph shows the correlation of estimated 10/10 matching probabilities in 10% prediction intervals and corresponding observed probabilities. The population model is approximated by the German population. Blue bars show 95% confidence intervals of estimated probabilities. Grey bars show relative number of CTs in each prediction interval. Red-dotted line is the ideal correlation.

unit tests, addressing all kinds of matches and mismatches, exceptions, and rare cases. Interfaces to software source code classes, modules, or libraries are tested with a variety of input arguments to validate that the results that are returned are as expected [21].

The quality of prognostic matching algorithm and the population model used (allele and haplotype frequencies) also has to be validated. This is usually done by retrospective or prospective studies. Typically, all CTs performed by the registry that meet some criteria are used. These criteria are as the follows.

(i) Patient has been typed in high resolution.

(ii) Donor was not typed in high resolution before the CT, but has been high resolution typed at the time of CT (or later).

(iii) No discrepancy between a priori and final HLA type.

The review process retrospectively calculates the matching prognosis and compares the predicted and observed percentage of allele matches (see Figure 3).

9. Conclusions

A reliable and efficient search algorithm is the key component of the unrelated stem cell donor registry computer system. An overview of search algorithms, their design, and implementation aspects have been described. Both combinatorial and probability matching algorithms have been presented.

A top-down design approach that first lists algorithm requirements, specifies input and output parameters, and then goes deeper into details was selected. The importance of validation prior to the implementation of a new matching algorithm has been emphasized.

Conflict of Interests

The author declares no conflict of interests.

Acknowledgments

Karel Peyerl and Ann Green have provided valuable input to this paper. Yves Garcia from One Match and Matt Prestegaard from NMDP are authors of the document entitled "Unrelated Hematopoietic Stem Cell Donor Search and Facilitation Information Systems Principles" ("2012-03-15 World Match Central Glossary of Terms.docx"). The author has used their definition of terms "Consistently matched," "Current," "Detailed," "Integrated," "Recognisable," and "Comprehensive." Research described in the paper has been supported by the research Program no. MSM 6840770012 "Transdisciplinary Research in Biomedical Engineering II" of the CTU in Prague.

References

[1] Wikipedia, "Hematopoietic stem cell transplantation," http://en.wikipedia.org/wiki/Hematopoietic_stem_cell_transplantation.

[2] W. Bochtler, M. Maiers, J. N. A. Bakker et al., "World Marrow Donor Association framework for the implementation of HLA matching programs in hematopoietic stem cell donor registries and cord blood banks," *Bone Marrow Transplantation*, vol. 46, no. 3, pp. 338–343, 2011.

[3] M. Prestegaard, *Unrelated Hematopoietic Stem Cell Donor Search and Facilitation Information Systems Principles*, 2012.

[4] W. Bochtler, M. Maiers, M. Oudshoorn et al., "World Marrow Donor Association guidelines for use of HLA nomenclature and its validation in the data exchange among hematopoietic stem cell donor registries and cord blood banks," *Bone Marrow Transplantation*, vol. 39, no. 12, pp. 737–741, 2007.

[5] S. G. Marsh, "Nomenclature of HLA alleles," http://hla.alleles.org/wmda/index.html.

[6] A. Timm and H. Eberhard, "The semantics of EMDIS messages Version 1.28," 2011.

[7] NMDP, "HLA Resources - Allele Code Lists," http://bioinformatics.nmdp.org/HLA/Allele_Codes/Allele_Code_Lists/Allele_Code_Lists.aspx.

[8] E. B. I. EMBL, "IMGT/HLA Database—Search Determinants," http://www.ebi.ac.uk/imgt/hla/searchdet.html.

[9] C. K. Hurley, M. Maiers, S. G. E. Marsh, and M. Oudshoorn, "Overview of registries, HLA typing and diversity, and search algorithms," *Tissue Antigens*, vol. 69, no. 1, supplement, pp. S3–S5, 2007.

[10] C. K. Hurley, M. Setterholm, M. Lau et al., "Hematopoietic stem cell donor registry strategies for assigning search determinants and matching relationships," *Bone Marrow Transplantation*, vol. 33, no. 4, pp. 443–450, 2004.

[11] ZKRD, "IMGT/HLA Database—Search Strategies—ZKRD," http://www.ebi.ac.uk/imgt/hla/searchdet_zkrd.html.

[12] NMDP, "IMGT/HLA Database—Search Strategies—NMDP," http://www.ebi.ac.uk/imgt/hla/searchdet_nmdp.html.

[13] C. Malmberg, "Search Strategy and HapLogic: Case Studies," NMDP, http://marrow.org/News/Events/Council_Meeting/HapLogic_III_Search_Strategy_With_Answers.aspx.

[14] D. Steiner, M. Korhonen, M. Kurikova et al., "Prometheus probability matching: community technology preview," in *Proceedings of the 9th International Donor Registry Conference (IDRC '12)*, Sydney, Australia, 2012.

[15] J. Pingel, J. Hofmann, D. Baier et al., "Hap-E search: haplotype-enhanced search," in *Proceedings of the 9th International Donor Registry Conference (IDRC '12)*, Sydney, Australia, 2012.

[16] P. Gourraud, M. Balère, A. Dormoy, P. Loiseau, E. Marry, and F. Garnier, "Computer assisted search for unrelated donors using the easymatch—tool at France greffe de moelleprometheus probability matching: community technology preview," in *Proceedings of the 16th International HLA and Immunogenetics Workshop and Joint Conference*, Kings Dock, Liverpool, 2012.

[17] H. Eberhard, "Validation of the predictions of optiMatch," in *Proceedings of the 9th International Donor Registry Conference (IDRC '08)*, Berne, Switzerland, 2008.

[18] J. Dehn, "HapLogic III," NMDP, http://marrow.org/News/Events/Council_Meeting/2011_Presentations/A3_B3_Putting_HapLogic_to_Work_for_You.aspx.

[19] H.-P. Eberhard, *Schätzung von hochaufgelösten HLA-Haplotypfrequenzen deutscher Blutstammzellspender und ihre Anwendung bei der Patientenversorgung*, Institut für Transfusionsmedizin, Universität Ulm, 2010.

[20] M. Maiers, J. N. A. Bakker, W. Bochtler et al., "Information technology and the role of WMDA in promoting standards for international exchange of hematopoietic stem cell donors and products," *Bone Marrow Transplantation*, vol. 45, no. 5, pp. 839–842, 2010.

[21] Wikipedia, "Test automation," http://en.wikipedia.org/wiki/Test_automation.

7

The Role of HLA in Cord Blood Transplantation

Catherine Stavropoulos-Giokas, Amalia Dinou, and Andreas Papassavas

Hellenic Cord Blood Bank, Biomedical Research Foundation Academy of Athens (BRFAA), 4 Soranou Efessiou Street, 115 27 Athens, Greece

Correspondence should be addressed to Catherine Stavropoulos-Giokas, cstavrop@bioacademy.gr

Academic Editor: Andrzej Lange

In recent years, umbilical cord blood (CB), a rich source of hematopoietic stem cells (HSC), has been used successfully as an alternative HSC source to treat a variety of hematologic, immunologic, genetic, and oncologic disorders. CB has several advantages, including prompt availability of the transplant, decrease of graft versus host disease (GVHD) and better long-term immune recovery, resulting in a similar long-term survival. Studies have shown that some degree of HLA mismatches is acceptable. This review is intended to outline the main aspects of HLA matching in different settings (related, pediatric, adult, or double-unit HSCT), its effect on transplantation outcome and the role of HLA in donor selection.

1. Introduction

The experience of the last 20 years indicates that cord blood transplantation is a valid alternative to bone marrow (BM) and PBSC transplants. For patients suffering from malignant or nonmalignant diseases, who do not have a matched sibling donor or a matched volunteer unrelated donor, two available alternative stem cell donor sources exist: a haploidentical transplantation from a three locus mismatched family member (parents, siblings) or an unrelated cryopreserved umbilical cord blood (CB) unit from a cord blood bank [1–4]. A low rate of graft versus host disease (GVHD) in the presence of higher HLA disparity, represents the main advantage of the umbilical cord grafts, while delayed engraftment due to limited cell dose is still the major drawback [3]. Moreover, umbilical cord blood is a viable source particularly for racial and ethnic minority patients whose genetic variations are not included in unrelated volunteer donor registries [5].

The role of HLA mismatches in CBT remains unclear as most transplants have been selected on low resolution class I HLA typing and allelic level class II typing. In malignant diseases, HLA mismatching is partially overcome by increasing the cell dose [6]. Recent data on associations between HLA disparity and survival, support that there is a direct association between the number of donor-recipient HLA mismatches and the risk for GVHD, while the mismatching has a greater impact on absolute mortality differences in recipients with diseases with low risk of posttransplant recurrence [7].

The number of CB transplantations, as well as the global inventory of CB units, are growing rapidly. CB grafts, in contrast to adults unrelated donors who need 10/10 allele level matches with the patients, have a reduced risk of severe GVHD and permit a mismatched transplantation at least in one HLA locus [8, 9]. HLA matching for unrelated CBT generally focuses on three HLA loci HLA-A,-B, and -DRB1. In order to overcome limitation in cell dose, many centers perform double unit CBT (dCBT) [10].

This paper focuses on the impact of HLA-matching in CBT in different settings: related, unrelated, pediatric, adult, and double CBT; the eventual inclusion of other HLA loci in the unit selection process and the future need for high resolution typing in CBT.

2. The MHC (Major Histocompatibility Complex)

Tissue compatibility is determined by the major histocompatibility complex (MHC), also known as the HLA system in humans, a cluster of genes located on the short arm of chromosome 6, extending about 3.6 Mb, that play a fundamental role in the acceptance and rejection of transplanted tissues [11]. The MHC is the most gene-dense region of the human genome and encompasses almost 300 genes and pseudogenes, situated in three regions called the class I, class II and class III regions. About 20% of the proteins coded by the MHC have immune-related functions [12]. Immune responses against HLA incompatibility represent a major barrier to hematopoietic stem cell transplantation (HSCT) [13, 14].

The class I region encodes the classical HLA molecules HLA-A, -B and -C, the nonclassical HLA-E, -F, -G, and class I-like molecules MICA and MICB. The class II region comprises the HLA-DR region (containing the DRA, DRB1, and depending on the haplotype DRB3, DRB4, or DRB5 genes), the HLA-DP region (containing the DPA1, DPB1 genes), the HLA-DQ region (containing the DQA1, DQB1 genes), as well as genes encoding proteins involved in antigen presentation. The class III region comprises genes coding for the complement cascade, cytokines, tumor necrosis factor, lymphotoxins, and heat shock proteins [11].

HLA molecules are expressed on the surface of antigen-presenting cells, displaying peptide antigens for recognition by T-cell receptors. T-cell receptors recognize antigens only if presented in the form of peptides bound to self MHC molecules, a concept known as MHC restricted recognition.

Class I molecules are constitutively expressed at varying levels on most nucleated cells and platelets. They consist of a polymorphic transmembrane α-chain (encoded by the corresponding MHC gene) which is associated with and stabilized by a nonpolymorphic $\beta2$ microglobulin chain, coded by a gene located on chromosome 15. The class-II molecules are restricted to cells of the immune system and consist of two MHC-encoded transmembrane polymorphic glycoproteins, the α and β chain-the latter being the more polymorphic. The structure of HLA Class I and Class II molecules is similar, with most of the polymorphism located in the peptide binding groove. The HLA class I molecule peptide-binding groove can bind peptides that are 8–10 amino acids long whereas HLA class II molecules bind longer peptides (12–24 amino acids). CD4$^+$ T cells recognize antigens presented by class II HLA molecules and CD8$^+$ T cells recognize antigens presented by class I HLA molecules.

The HLA region is the most polymorphic currently known in the human genome. According to the World Health Organization Nomenclature Committee for the HLA System, at the March 2012 update [15] (http://www.ebi.ac.uk/imgt/hla/) there are 1757 HLA-A, 2338 HLA-B, and 1304 HLA-C alleles.

The set of HLA alleles inherited from one parent is referred to as a *haplotype* and is located on one chromosome, for example, the A1-B8-DR3 or the DRB1*15:01-DQB1*06:02 haplotypes. Linkage disequilibrium (LD) a hallmark for MHC, means that certain alleles occur together with a greater frequency than would be expected by chance. This is more frequently observed between closely located loci [11]. Certain haplotypes are common in particular ethnic groups. In hematopoietic cell transplantation from an unrelated donor, the probability of identifying an HLA-matched donor is higher when the patient and donor originate from the same ethnic group [16].

Because of the great polymorphism of HLA molecules, it became clear that serologic typing techniques were completely inadequate to cover all the diversities present in the HLA system. The serology-based method (microlymphocytotoxicity) is still in use for low resolution typing in many laboratories and to clarify the absence of some null alleles [17, 18]. The use of DNA-based techniques for HLA typing moved the field forward. DNA typing methods, are based on the nucleotide sequence information of the polymorphic DNA segments, using PCR technology. A number of HLA typing methods have been developed, mainly using PCR-SSP (sequence specific primers), reverse PCR-SSOP (sequence specific oligonucleotide probes), hybridization on solid support (microbead arrays), or sequence-based typing [18].

Low resolution (LR) referred to as generic typing, or 2-digit typing, corresponds to the identification of broad families of alleles (e.g., A*02) and is the equivalent of serological typing (A2). Medium resolution (MR) tissue typing techniques can define specific allele groups and subtypes. High resolution (HR) or 4-digit typing discriminates the individual alleles in each serotype (e.g., A*02:01) and resolve the tissue type to allele level, with no ambiguity [15]. The use of NMDP (http://bioinformatics.nmdp.org/HLA/hla-res-idx.html) codes can be helpful in this setting. It is recommended that selection of an unrelated donor is based on these first two sets of digits and in a second level of selection to use high resolution typing [19].

3. Related Cord Blood Transplantation

Although the primary interest in CB is an alternative unrelated donor source, CB has been used in related transplants for both malignant and nonmalignant diseases [19–21], performed almost exclusively in children. In an update of the Eurocord experience, with a median followup of 41 months after related CB transplantation for children, the survival estimate was $47 \pm 5\%$ in patients with malignancies ($n = 96$), $82 \pm 7\%$ in patients with BM failure ($n = 33$), 100% in patients with hemoglobinopathies ($n = 52$), and $70 \pm 15\%$ ($n = 10$) in patients with inborn errors of metabolism or primary immunodeficiencies [22]. By matching the Eurocord and International Bone Marrow Registry (IBMTR) [23] results of CB transplantation from HLA identical sibling donors ($n = 113$; median age, 5 years) with the results of BM transplantation (BMT) from HLA identical sibling donors ($n = 2052$; median age, 8 years), it seems that despite the lower incidence of neutrophil recovery at 1 month after CBT compared to BMT (89% versus 98%, resp.), there were no differences in 3-year survival rates (64% versus 66%, resp.), whereas incidence of grade III-IV acute GVHD and probability of chronic GVHD (3 years) were lower after CBT [24].

Related CB transplantation in patients with hemoglobinopathies, offers a probability of success comparable to that offered by BMT and is associated with a lower risk of both treatment-related mortality (TRM) and chronic GVHD, as it has been reported previously [24]. Based on this, Locatelli et al. [25], recommend collection and freezing of CB units in families in which a child is affected with genetic or hematological disease. In 2003, Reed et al. [26, 27] reported on their successful banking initiative of sibling donor CB for children with hematologic disorders, despite the challenges associated with remote-site collections. The Minesotta Group reported a case of successful CB transplantation for a patient with Fanconi anemia from unaffected HLA genotype-identical sibling selected using preimplantation genetic diagnosis [28]. The practice of preimplantation selection of HLA matched siblings for transplantation has since been established [29].

β-thalassemia is one of the most common single-gene inherited conditions in the world, with a particularly high prevalence in Mediterranean countries, including Greece. The Hellenic Cord Blood Bank, stores CB from healthy siblings of patients with β-thalassemia major. In collaboration with St Sofia Children's Hospital Stem Cell Transplant Unit, eight HLA matched units were released for transplantation and were used alone or in combination with reduced volume bone marrow from the same donor; engraftment was achieved in six out of these cases and all patients survived with 7/8 patients thalassemia-free [30].

4. Unrelated Cord Blood Transplantation in Children

The Cord Blood Transplantation Study (COBLT) [31], has reported the clinical outcomes of unrelated donor umbilical cord blood transplantation in pediatric patients with hematologic malignancies. All 193 patients had at least a 3/6 HLA match by low-resolution HLA-A, -B, and high resolution HLA-DRB1. The overall survival at 1 year was 57.3%, and grade III/IV aGVHD and cGVHD incidence was 19.5% and 20.2%, respectively. Higher TNC dose significantly improved engraftment. Retrospective high resolution (HR) HLA typing and the subsequent multivariate analysis revealed that while the level of original HLA match had no impact on the occurrence of grade II–IV or grade III-IV aGVHD, if the pair were matched for fewer than 5/6 alleles (HR) the probability of developing grade III/IV GVHD was significantly higher. Concerning overall survival, although there seemed to be a trend for survival advantage for 6/6 matched patients for both LR and HR typing the size of the cohort does not allow to draw definitive conclusions. The authors suggest selecting CB units that are at least 4 of 6 by LR typing at class I loci and HR typing at HLA-DRB1. Another concern is that even if HR matching decreases GVHD, overall survival may not be affected because of competing contributions of GVHD and graft-versus-Leukemia. Further analysis of larger series will provide more conclusive results regarding the impact of HLA matching on CBT.

On the other hand, for patients with non-malignant diseases the use of unrelated CB from HLA-mismatched unrelated donor will require a larger study, regarding engraftment, survival and GVHD.

In patients with hemoglobinopathies, the risk factors like the donor/recipient mismatching and cell dose, are probably amplified by the effect of multiple transfusion exposures, that might sensitize the recipient to donor alloantigens.

In the case of severe Sickle cell disease (SCD), the cytokine milieu of SCD, which activates the inflammation and the immune activation might also promote a host-versus-graft reaction and interfere with engraftment even after myeloablative preparation [32]. In a recent phase II (BMT CTN) study of the toxicity and efficacy of unrelated donor HSCT in children with SCD, using a reduced-intensity condition regimen, one patient had 6/6 HLA antigen matching with his donor (using low-intermediate resolution typing for HLA-A-B and high resolution for HLA-DRB1), while seven patients had 5/6 HLA antigen mismatching. The median post-thaw infused CD34+ cell dose was $1.5*10^5$/kg. All patients achieved neutrophil recovery in median 22 days. Two patients developed grade II acute GVHD, one of these chronic GVHD and died 14 months posttransplantation. According to the data a number of modifications should be done to improve the rate of engraftment after CB transplantation for severe SCD [32].

The use of CB from unrelated donors in β-thalassemia patients resulted in 77% survival in a study of 36 cases [33]. In another study investigating the feasibility of using CBT from unrelated HLA mismatched donor in 5 children with β-thalassemia major, all patients showed grade II or III acute GVHD and none developed extensive chronic GVHD. All patients were alive at a median followup of 303 days after transplantation with complete donor chimerism and transfusion independence [34].

There is a limited experience of CB transplantation in pediatric cases with idiopathic severe aplastic anemia (SAA). Information has mostly been included in registry data with very few details available [35, 36]. In a study from the Children's Hospital in San Antonio, nine children with SAA were transplanted with CB units selected from various CB banks of the USA and the choice was based on the best HLA compatibility, with at least four out of six loci matching. HLA-DRB1 compatibility between the donor and the recipient was in complete priority. At a median followup of 34 months, seven patients are alive and transfusion independent [37]. A simultaneous infusion of CD34+ haploidentical cells seems to improve CBT outcome for patients with SAA [38].

In pediatric patients with severe SCID there is a big discussion about the use either of mismatched related stem cells or unrelated cord blood for transplantation. According to a retrospective study on behalf of Eurocord and the Inborn Errors Working Party of the European Group for Blood and Marrow Transplantation, and although only 4 centers performed both techniques, the results did not differ significantly in terms of 5-years survival despite a higher incidence of chronic GVHD in CBT recipients [39]. CB transplantation has also been shown effective in metabolic diseases [19] in which time from diagnosis to definitive treatment may represent a crucial period to prevent further progression of the disease. The group at Duke University has reported outcomes in 20 children with Hurler syndrome who received condition regimen followed by infusion of unrelated 1, 2, or 3 HLA antigen mismatched CB. With a median followup of 905 days 17–20 children are alive with complete donor chimerism [40].

In a pilot study of Duke University, conducted in order to determine the safety and feasibility of intravenous administration of autologous umbilical cord blood in young children with acquired neurologic disorders, the results showed that the intravenous infusion of autologous CB is safe and feasible in young children [41].

The comparison of the results of CB and BM transplantation from unrelated donors in children is of paramount importance. It is now accepted that unrelated CB is an efficient alternative to matched unrelated BM in children and the start of a simultaneous search for BM and CB unrelated graft is supported. The final selection of unrelated donor BM versus CB should be based on the urgency of the transplant, the cell dose and HLA matching of the BM and CB unrelated donor. Moreover, CB is advantageous for children requiring urgent transplantation [9].

5. Unrelated Cord Blood Transplantation in Adults

The first unrelated cord blood transplantation was performed in 1996 and since then, more than 20.000 patients have undergone CB transplantation. In the adult setting, in a retrospective analysis of the data concerning 1525 patients with acute leukemia the results revealed that the leukemia-free survival after CBT with 4 to 6 of 6 HLA match was comparable to 7-8/8 allele-matched BMT, with grade II-IV acute and chronic GVHD and chronic GVHD lower in CBT recipients than in PBPC and BM recipients respectively. The issue of further analysis of the impact of HLA matching on transplant outcome was not addressed in this study, as for CB cell dose and not HLA matching is considered to be the limiting factor for its use: the use of a 4–6/6 match CB is considered the equivalent of a 7/8 allele matched unrelated donor when a fully matched donor is unavailable [42].

The feasibility of identifying HLA-matched donors depends on the HLA antigens of the patient and the size of the donor registries [43–45]: every patient has a mismatched donor. Intense efforts have been made to determine the "permissive" of HLA mismatches that do not increase post-transplant risks. Data for the outcomes of 1202 CB transplantations, facilitated by the New York Blood Center National Cord Blood Program, showed important differences in the small subgroups of patients with unidirectional mismatches. The graft-versus-host direction only (GVH-O) and rejection direction only (R-O) mismatches were present in 4.8% and 3.3% of the cases, respectively. According to their results, recipients of transplantation with GVH-O mismatches had neutrophil and platelet engraftment rates that were comparable to those of recipients of transplantations matched in HLA-A, -B, and -DRB1. With GVH-O mismatches, the time to engraftment was significantly faster than transplantation with R-O mismatches. In addition, patients with hematologic malignancies given GVH-O grafts had lower transplantation mortality and treatment failure compared to those with matched CB grafts [46, 47]. The practical implication is that including HLA mismatch direction in search procedures

permits easy identification of grafts with unidirectional mismatches, allowing to give priority to GVH-O and to avoid R-O grafts [47].

Since the identification of HLA-C as a classical transplantation antigen [48], donor mismatching for HLA-C has been shown to be a risk factor after myeloablative, nonmyeloablative, unrelated donor, cord blood, marrow, and peripheral blood stem cell transplantation. A retrospective study for the effect of donor-recipient HLA matching at HLA-A, -B, -C, and -DRB1 on outcomes after CBT for leukemia and myelodysplastic syndrome, underlines the importance of HLA-C matching in CB transplantation [49]. Several reports on the association between HLA matching and survival after adult unrelated donor transplantation, showed higher transplant related mortality for transplantation HLA-A, -B, and -DRB1 matched and HLA-C mismatched, or mismatched at a single HLA-A, -B, or -DRB1 locus and mismatched at HLA-C, and transplantations mismatched at a single HLA-A, -B, or -C locus and mismatched at DRB1 [50, 51]. HLA-C is an important model for understanding differential risks conferred by allele and antigen mismatches [52]. Donor recipient pairs mismatched at HLA-C are likely to be mismatched at HLA-B because of the high degree of linkage disequilibrium between these loci [53]. Studies of prognostic factors with larger series of adults given a CB transplant are still missing and any attempt to explain the different outcomes among these series is premature.

There is data analyzing the impact of administering a CB unit that shares a non inherited maternal HLA antigen (NIMA) with a mismatched HLA antigen in the recipient, for patients with hematologic malignancies treated with CB transplantation [54]. These noninherited maternal antigens may define "permissive" HLA mismatches and could be used to extend the genotypes of suitable matches for particular donors or CB units. Rocha et al., demonstrated that CB transplants matched for NIMA were associated with lower transplant related mortality and decreased relapse. A study by the CIBMTR, NMDP and Eurocord [55] found that NIMA matched CB transplantation resulted in superior survival and disease-free survival compared to equivalent NIMA mismatched transplantation. At the present time the role of NIMA matching in the engraftment in CB transplantation is not very clear and requires additional investigation.

From previous studies ABO incompatibility is not considered as a barrier to successful allogeneic HSCT, even though it can be associated with several immunohematologic complications, like delayed red blood cell engraftment, red cell aplasia, or hemolytic anemia. However, red blood cell alloimmunization was recently reported as an independent predictor of HLA alloimmunization [56, 57].

A retrospective analysis of pretransplantation sera from unrelated donor HCT recipients, showed that the presence of donor-directed, HLA specific alloantibodies was significantly associated with graft failure [58]. A recent analysis of sera from 386 myeloablative CB transplant recipients showed that the presence of donor-specific antibodies (DSA) correlated with significantly lower neutrophil recovery compared with those who lacked alloantibodies [59]. The presence of preformed DSA in double CB transplantation is predictive of higher graft failure rates and high incidence of mortality [60]. Until recently, in vitro crossmatching was used to determine compatibility between donors and recipients, and the relationship between a positive crossmatch and graft rejection in allogeneic transplantation is well established. There is strong evidence, that there is a relationship between the presence of preformed DSA and a positive crossmatch, therefore units that elicit an intense antibody response should be avoided [60, 61].

There is currently little clinical evidence suggesting an important clinical impact for HLA-DR-DQ or DP matching for CB transplantation as well as other non HLA loci like Minor Histocompatibility antigens, Killer immunoglobulin-like receptors (KIR), cytokines, chemokines, and immune response genes.

6. Double CB Transplantation

In order to overcome cell dose limitations, improve engraftment rates, and immune reconstitution, a strategy consisting of administering two partially matched CB grafts called double CBT (dCBT) has been implemented. The University of Minnesota program [62], a pioneer of double or sequential CBT using a nonmyeloblative regimen, has published impressive results. Although dCBT (like single CBT) shows delayed engraftment compared to other donor sources, the higher TRM is counterbalanced by lower relapse rate.

Avery et al. [63] examined the effect of HLA match on engraftment after dCBT. In almost all dCBT outcomes, single-unit dominance is observed. No relationship was found between CB/recipient match and unit dominance, even at the allelic (HR) level: a better HLA matched unit at high resolution was not more likely to become the dominant unit. Donor engraftment, is not influenced by the level of match (either at antigen or allelic level) between the two units administered; although high unit-unit match is associated with elevated initial engraftment it has no bearing to eventual graft failure. The authors recommend infusing two units with a cell dose in each unit adequate for engraftment, and 4/6 to 6/6 HLA matching to the recipient at antigen level at class I and allelic level at DRB1.

The influence of HLA matching on engraftment as well as other transplantation outcomes after double-unit CBT, should be readdressed in the future, when a very large number of cases will be available for study. Therefore, although double unit grafts have been widely adopted as a simple strategy to augment graft cells dose in unrelated donor CB transplantation, there is still little information to guide transplant centers in the selection of the graft.

Finally, more recently, it has been observed, that the percentage of viable CD34$^+$ cells after thaw can vary significantly according to the bank of origin, and poor viability units were unlikely to engraft [64]. Querol et al. [65], have similarly reported variable quality between units. This raises the possibility that part of the benefit of dCBT is that, by transplanting two units, we increase the chance that at least one good quality unit, with high engraftment potential, is infused. Given that unit quality is one of the most important considerations in CBT today, the field must determine how unit quality can be reliably measured and ensured, and how poor quality units are to be investigated and/or eliminated.

7. Cord Blood Unit Selection

With the number of cryopreserved CB increasing and the better understanding of the factors influencing transplant outcome (cell dose, HLA match, CD34$^+$ dose, etc.), a need has arisen for better strategies regarding unit selection. Organizations like the NMDP have published guidelines and transplant centers worldwide have established their own set of criteria regarding donor selection, adapted to the transplantation protocols they use and the type of patient they cater to.

NMDP strategy [53] for cord blood unit selection indicates that all patients should receive a cell dose of >2.5 × 10^7 NC/kg. In case of double CBT, each CB should have a cell dose of >1.5 × 10^7 NC/kg. Moreover, the patient should receive a 4/6 or better A, B, DR HLA match. For dCBT, the units should also be 4/6 or better HLA match to each other and if units have an adequate cell dose of >2.5 × 10^7 NC/kg, a 6/6 match is preferable to a 5/6 matched unit. A very important parameter, is to avoid HLA mismatches at loci in which patients have preformed HLA antibodies. It has also been suggested that if maternal typing is available, a CB with a NIMA-shared antigen should be preferred.

HLA matching for unrelated cord blood transplantation generally focuses on three loci (HLA-A,-B, -DRB1). Although selection currently is done to maximize matching at the antigen-level for HLA-A and -B, and at the allele-level for -DRB1, all three loci plus HLA-C are being typed by many centers at high-resolution. In a recent retrospective analysis from NMDP/CIBMTR and Eurocord [49], transplants mismatched at HLA-C were associated with higher transplant-related mortality compared to transplants matched at HLA-C; among transplants mismatched at two loci, mismatching at HLA-C and -DRB1 was associated with the highest risk of mortality. This study suggests that extended HLA matching may yield better outcomes after cord blood transplantation, although HLA match does not predict survival nor the predominant cord [66].

Gluckman and Rocha [9] reported a higher incident of graft-versus- host-disease (GVHD) and longer platelet recovery with both Class I and Class II mismatches. The effect of HLA mismatch is most important when the cell dose is low, and transplant centers are addressing the limitations in cell dose by combining two cord blood units for transplantation. Recent studies [67] examined the relationship between cell dose and HLA match in 1061 patients undergoing cord blood transplantation. Both cell dose and HLA match were independent predictors of transplant-related mortality. Patients receiving 6/6 matched CB unit had improved outcomes, regardless of cell dose. A 4/6 matched CB with cell dose >5.0 × 10^7 NC/kg was comparable to a 5/6 matched CB unit with cell dose 2.0–5.0 × 10^7 NC/kg. Although no consensus has yet been reached concerning intra-unit HLA match in dCBT, current practice is to maximize matching of the two units to the recipient at the antigen-level for HLA-A and -B, and at the allele-level for DRB1 with a minimum of 4/6 match [68].

8. Current Opinion in Cord Blood Banking

Since the first human CB transplant performed in 1988, CB banks (CBB) have been established worldwide for collection and cryopreservation of CB for allogeneic hematopoietic stem cells transplant [69]. CB banking includes the following phases: (1) donor recruitment, consent, and medical evaluation of the donor; (2) CB collection; short-term storage and transportation; (3) processing, testing, cryopreservation, and storage; (4) release of CB unit to transplant center; (5) quality assurance according to FACT/NETCORD standards [27].

The Netcord Foundation (http://www.netcord.org/) is a European nonprofit cooperative network of large experienced CB banks, formally established in 1998 in order to improve the quality of the grafts. The inventory of Netcord currently has more than 300.000 cryopreserved CB units ready to use, with more than 8.624 grafts shipped.

Eurocord was established in 1995 and its principal objectives were to collect data provided by CB banks and transplant centers. Eurocord (from 1988 to October 2010), has collected feedback on 6736 transplanted CB units from transplant centers in Europe and other countries. In the USA, the National Marrow Donor Program (NMDP) has established a similar CB bank network.

International search systems have been established in order to aid transplant centers to locate eligible CB and/or adult unrelated donors (AUD). These include the Bone Marrow Donors Worldwide (BMDW): a database with HLA data and other information pertaining to CB characteristics from registries and CBB worldwide, and the EMDIS (European Marrow Donor Information System) that is a network connecting 26 registries with both CB and AUD. The two systems are complementary and account for approximately 80% of the international transplant activity [70, 71].

From collection and processing through transplantation and followup, a CB quality assurance program establishes a series of controls, quality monitors, and mechanisms that ensure product uniformity, preventing errors, and promoting continuous process and improvements. This approach has elevated the fields of CB banking and transplantation to new issues in regard to quality and process control. The Netcord Foundation in cooperation with FACT (Foundation of Accreditation of Cellular Therapy) has developed standards [72] for CBB that have been adopted by the World Marrow Donor Association (WMDA) and other National and International transplant organizations.

The optimal number of CB units stored in order to provide any patient with a minimum 4/6 HLA matched unit, is not really known, but should approach 9 per 10.000 inhabitants [70]. An issue that should be addressed is the HLA haplotype content of the units stored: it should not only cover the commonest haplotypes of the population covered by the CBB, but also a variety of rare haplotypes or haplotypes characteristic of ethnic minorities. Targeted recruitment directed towards minorities is one of the measures already taken by several large CBB. Another measure, might be the use of HLA as a selection criterion by CB Banks, as volume unit or prereduction nucleated cell number, in order to store units not only with the most common HLA haplotypes but also for rare ones. The target would be to have an overrepresentation of rare haplotypes compared to the more common ones, making it easier to find a reasonable match for everyone, although the practical issues would be difficult to overcome.

9. Conclusions

The experience of last 20 years indicates that CBT is a valid alternative method for BM and PBSC transplants. The main advantage of UCB grafts is the low rate of GVHD in the presence of higher HLA disparity, while delayed engraftment is still a mayor disadvantage due to limited cell dose. The current consensus is that CB should be at least 4/6 HLA matching for HLA-A, -B at the antigen level, and HLA-DRB1 at the allelic level. The role of additional loci as well as the impact of each individual locus remains to be determined by international studies and extended meta-analysis of large numbers of cases.

Considering the additional increasing molecular understanding of most diseases, allogeneic stem cell transplantation is headed towards a next generation of transplantation procedures: the individual adaptation in terms of graft source, engineering, and post-transplant immune interventions depending on the type of disease and underlying genetic alterations of donors and patients. Furthermore, it will allow to combine the beneficial effects of several allogeneic transplantations strategies [73], such as the early haplo-mediated neutrophil recovery, the targeted antileukemia effect of NK cells (KIR mismatch) and T-cells after selected haplo-HSCT and the long term excellent T-cell recovery after CB transplantation, but also to predict, in case of a double CB transplantation, which unit will remain as the long-term graft. All this would provide a crucial advantage for patients in need of grafts with unique genetic features such as mutations in the CCR5-coreceptor rendering carriers resistant to certain types of HIV infection: taking advantage of such types of grafts would allow curing patients with hematological malignancies and co-infection with HIV [74, 75]. Cord Blood, with its immediate availability and the possibility of having genotypically well characterized units, is a prime candidate for these applications and in the future other biological markers influencing transplant outcome or providing an advantage to carriers could be added to the selection criteria used.

Much research is ongoing to investigate the potential use of UCB stem cells in regenerative medicine. Clonal lines of multipotent cells (called the multilineage progenitor cell, MLPC) have been established from full term UCB, which can expand and differentiate into cells representing all three germinal layers. Recently, it has been shown that human unrestricted somatic stem cells (USSC's) from umbilical cord blood represent pluripotent, neonatal, nonhematopoietic stem cells with the potential to differentiate into osteoblasts, chondroblasts, adipocytes, hematopoietic, and neural cells. The mesenchymal stem cells (MSC) derived from UCB or umbilical cord (Wharton's Jelly) with their differenciation potential and immune-modulatory properties are of interest in the field of cellular therapies and regenerative medecine. MSC mediated immunosuppression, after simultaneously MSC transfusion and HSCT, has been shown to contribute to faster engraftment [76] and can be used as anti-GVHD prophylaxis [77]. CB is also a convenient source of induced pluripotent stem cells [78].

As the potential uses of cord blood extend beyond HSCT, the notion of CB banking will have to be reinvented. Cellular therapies and regenerative medicine have different immunological considerations and HLA will have a role to play that will be different: that of providing individuals with well-suited therapies. In the years to come, the better understanding of the biology of CB derived stem cells, in conjunction with new technologies will provide additional tools for the realisation of both exciting new research and novel therapeutic applications.

References

[1] E. D. Thomas, C. D. Buckner, M. Banaji et al., "One hundred patients with acute leukemia treated by chemotherapy, total body irradiation, and allogenic marrow transplantation," *Blood*, vol. 49, no. 4, pp. 511–533, 1977.

[2] K. G. Blume, E. Beutler, K. J. Bross et al., "Bone-marrow ablation and allogeneic marrow transplantation in acute leukemia," *The New England Journal of Medicine*, vol. 302, pp. 1041–1046, 1980.

[3] J. E. Wagner and E. Gluckman, "Umbilical cord blood transplantation: the first 20 years," *Seminars in Hematology*, vol. 47, no. 1, pp. 3–12, 2010.

[4] J. Barrett, E. Gluckman, R. Handgretinger, and A. Madrigal, "Point-counterpoint: haploidentical family donors versus cord blood transplantation," *Biology of Blood and Marrow Transplantation*, vol. 17, supplement 1, pp. S89–S93, 2011.

[5] K. K. Ballen, J. Hicks, B. Dharan et al., "Racial and ethnic composition of volunteer cord blood donors: comparison with volunteer unrelated marrow donors," *Transfusion*, vol. 42, no. 10, pp. 1279–1284, 2002.

[6] R. Handgretinger, T. Klingebiel, P. Lang et al., "Megadose transplantation of purified peripheral blood CD34⁺ progenitor cells from HLA-mismatched parental donors in children," *Bone Marrow Transplantation*, vol. 27, no. 8, pp. 777–783, 2001.

[7] S. J. Lee, J. Klein, M. Haagenson et al., "High-resolution donor-recipient HLA matching contributes to the success of unrelated donor marrow transplantation," *Blood*, vol. 110, no. 13, pp. 4576–4583, 2007.

[8] N. Kamani, S. Spellman, C. K. Hurley et al., "State of the art review: HLA matching and outcome of unrelated donor umbilical cord blood transplants," *Biology of Blood and Marrow Transplantation*, vol. 14, no. 1, pp. 1–6, 2008.

[9] E. Gluckman and V. Rocha, "Cord blood transplantation:state of the art," *Haematologica*, vol. 94, no. 4, pp. 451–454, 2009.

[10] J. A. Gutman, S. R. Riddell, S. McGoldrick, and C. Delaney, "Double unit cord blood transplantation: who wins-and why do we care?" *Chimerism*, vol. 1, no. 1, pp. 21–22, 2010.

[11] J. Klein and A. Sato, "Advances in immunology: the HLA system," *The New England Journal of Medicine*, vol. 343, no. 11, pp. 782–786, 2000.

[12] J. Trowsdale, "HLA genomics in the third millennium," *Current Opinion in Immunology*, vol. 17, no. 5, pp. 498–504, 2005.

[13] R. I. Lechler, G. Lombardi, J. R. Batchelor, N. Reinsmoen, and F. H. Bach, "The molecular basis of alloreactivity," *Immunology Today*, vol. 11, no. 3, pp. 83–88, 1990.

[14] C. K. Hurley, M. Fernandez-Vina, W. H. Hildebrand et al., "A high degree of HLA disparity arises from limited allelic diversity: analysis of 1775 unrelated bone marrow transplant donor-recipient Pairs," *Human Immunology*, vol. 68, no. 1, pp. 30–40, 2007.

[15] S. G. Marsh, "Nomenclature for factors of the HLA system," *International Journal of Immunogenetics*, vol. 39, no. 4, pp. 370–372, 2012.

[16] J. M. Tiercy, J. Villard, and E. Roosnek, "Selection of unrelated bone marrow donors by serology, molecular typing and cellular assays," *Transplant Immunology*, vol. 10, no. 2-3, pp. 215–221, 2002.

[17] A. M. Little, S. G. E. Marsh, and J. A. Madrigal, "Current methodologies of human leukocyte antigen typing utilized for bone marrow donor selection," *Current Opinion in Hematology*, vol. 5, no. 6, pp. 419–428, 1998.

[18] P. P. J. Dunn, "Human leucocyte antigen typing: techniques and technology, a critical appraisal," *International Journal of Immunogenetics*, vol. 38, no. 6, pp. 463–473, 2011.

[19] K. K. Ballen, "New trends in umbilical cord blood transplantation," *Blood*, vol. 105, no. 10, pp. 3786–3792, 2005.

[20] J. E. Wagner, N. A. Kernan, M. Steinbuch, H. E. Broxmeyer, and E. Gluckman, "Allogeneic sibling umbilical-cord-blood transplantation in children with malignant and nonmalignant disease," *The Lancet*, vol. 346, no. 8969, pp. 214–219, 1995.

[21] J. Kurtzberg, M. Laughlin, M. L. Graham et al., "Placental blood as a source of hematopoietic stem cells for transplantation into unrelated recipients," *The New England Journal of Medicine*, vol. 335, no. 3, pp. 157–166, 1996.

[22] V. Rocha, G. Sanz, and E. Gluckman, "Umbilical cord blood transplantation," *Current Opinion in Hematology*, vol. 11, no. 6, pp. 375–385, 2004.

[23] V. Rocha, J. E. Wagner, K. A. Sobocinski et al., "Graft-versus-host disease in children who have received a cord blood or bone marrow transplant from an HLA-identical sibling," *The New England Journal of Medicine*, vol. 342, no. 25, pp. 1846–1854, 2000.

[24] Y. Cohen and A. Nagler, "Umbilical cord blood transplantation—how, when and for whom?" *Blood Reviews*, vol. 18, no. 3, pp. 167–179, 2004.

[25] F. Locatelli, V. Rocha, W. Reed et al., "Related umbilical cord blood transplantation in patients with thalassemia and sickle cell disease," *Blood*, vol. 101, no. 6, pp. 2137–2143, 2003.

[26] W. Reed, R. Smith, F. Dekovic et al., "Comprehensive banking of sibling donor cord blood for children with malignant and nonmalignant disease," *Blood*, vol. 101, no. 1, pp. 351–357, 2003.

[27] C. Stavropoulos-Giokas and A. C. Papassavas, "Cord blood banking and transplantation: a promising reality," *HAEMA*, vol. 9, no. 6, pp. 736–756, 2006.

[28] S. S. Grewal, J. P. Kahn, M. L. MacMillan, N. K. C. Ramsay, and J. E. Wagner, "Successful hematopoietic stem cell transplantation for Fanconi anemia from an unaffected HLA-genotype-identical sibling selected using preimplantation genetic diagnosis," *Blood*, vol. 103, no. 3, pp. 1147–1151, 2004.

[29] C. Basille, R. Frydman, A. E. Aly et al., "Preimplantation genetic diagnosis: state of the art," *European Journal of Obstetrics Gynecology and Reproductive Biology*, vol. 145, no. 1, pp. 9–13, 2009.

[30] E. Goussetis, E. Petrakou, M. Theodosaki et al., "Directed sibling donor cord blood banking for children with β-thalassemia major in Greece: usage rate and outcome of transplantation for HLA-matched units," *Blood Cells, Molecules, and Diseases*, vol. 44, no. 2, pp. 107–110, 2010.

[31] J. Kurtzberg, V. K. Prasad, S. L. Carter et al., "Results of the Cord Blood Transplantation Study (COBLT): clinical outcomes of unrelated donor umbilical cord blood transplantation in pediatric patients with hematologic malignancies," *Blood*, vol. 112, no. 10, pp. 4318–4327, 2008.

[32] N. R. Kamani, M. C. Walters, S. Carter et al., "Unrelated donor cord blood transplantation for children with severe sickle cell disease: results of one cohort from the phase II study from the blood and marrow transplant clinical trials network (BMT CTN)," *Biology of Blood and Marrow Transplantation*, vol. 18, no. 8, pp. 1265–1272, 2012.

[33] W. Reed, M. Walters, and B. H. Lubin, "Collection of sibling donor cord blood for children with thalassemia," *Journal of Pediatric Hematology/Oncology*, vol. 22, no. 6, pp. 602–604, 2000.

[34] T. H. Jaing, I. J. Hung, C. P. Yang, S. H. Chen, C. F. Sun, and R. Chow, "Rapid and complete donor chimerism after unrelated mismatched cord blood transplantation in 5 children with β-thalassemia major," *Biology of Blood and Marrow Transplantation*, vol. 11, no. 5, pp. 349–353, 2005.

[35] P. Rubinstein, C. Carrier, A. Scaradavou et al., "Outcomes among 562 recipients of placental-blood transplants from unrelated donors," *The New England Journal of Medicine*, vol. 339, no. 22, pp. 1565–1577, 1998.

[36] A. Yoshimi, S. Kojima, S. Taniguchi et al., "Unrelated cord blood transplantation for severe aplastic anemia," *Biology of Blood and Marrow Transplantation*, vol. 14, no. 9, pp. 1057–1063, 2008.

[37] K. W. Chan, L. McDonald, D. Lim, M. S. Grimley, G. Grayson, and D. A. Wall, "Unrelated cord blood transplantation in children with idiopathic severe aplastic anemia," *Bone Marrow Transplantation*, vol. 42, no. 9, pp. 589–595, 2008.

[38] R. Childs, "Combined CB and Haploidentical CD34+ cell transplantation improves transplant outcome for patients with treatment-refractory severe aplastic anemia," in *Proceedings of the 10th International Cord Blood Symposium*, San Francisco, Calif, USA, 2012.

[39] J. F. Fernandes, V. Rocha, M. Labopin et al., "Transplantation in patients with SCID: mismatched related stem cells or unrelated cord blood?" *Blood*, vol. 119, pp. 2949–2955, 2012.

[40] S. L. Staba, M. L. Escolar, M. Poe et al., "Cord-blood transplants from unrelated donors in patients with hurler's syndrome," *The New England Journal of Medicine*, vol. 350, no. 19, pp. 1960–1969, 2004.

[41] J. Sun, J. Allison, C. McLaughlin et al., "Differences in quality between privately and publicly banked umbilical cord blood units: a pilot study of autologous cord blood infusion in children with acquired neurologic disorders," *Transfusion*, vol. 50, no. 9, pp. 1980–1987, 2010.

[42] M. Eapen, V. Rocha, G. Sanz et al., "Effect of graft source on unrelated donor haemopoietic stem-cell transplantation in adults with acute leukaemia: a retrospective analysis," *The Lancet Oncology*, vol. 11, no. 7, pp. 653–660, 2010.

[43] M. J. Laughlin, J. Barker, B. Bambach et al., "Hematopoietic engraftment and survival in adult recipients of umbilical-cord blood from unrelated donors," *The New England Journal of Medicine*, vol. 344, no. 24, pp. 1815–1822, 2001.

[44] G. D. Long, M. Laughlin, B. Madan et al., "Unrelated umbilical cord blood transplantation in adult patients," *Biology of Blood and Marrow Transplantation*, vol. 9, no. 12, pp. 772–780, 2003.

[45] G. F. Sanz, S. Saavedra, D. Flanelles et al., "Standardized, unrelated donor cord blood transplantation in adults with hematologic malignancies," *Blood*, vol. 98, no. 8, pp. 2332–2338, 2001.

[46] M. de Lima, M. Fernandez-Vina, and E. J. Shpall, "HLA matching of CB: it's complicated," *Blood*, vol. 118, no. 14, pp. 3761–3762, 2011.

[47] C. E. Stevens, C. Carrier, C. Carpenter, D. Sung, and A. Scaradavou, "HLA mismatch direction in cord blood transplantation: impact on outcome and implications for cord blood unit selection," *Blood*, vol. 118, no. 14, pp. 3969–3978, 2011.

[48] A. Nagler, C. Brautbar, S. Slavin, and A. Bishara, "Bone marrow transplantation using unrelated and family related donors: the impact of HLA-C disparity," *Bone Marrow Transplantation*, vol. 18, no. 5, pp. 891–897, 1996.

[49] M. Eapen, J. P. Klein, G. F. Sanz et al., "Effect of donor-recipient HLA matching at HLA A, B, C, and DRB1 on outcomes after umbilical-cord blood transplantation for leukaemia and myelodysplastic syndrome: a retrospective analysis," *The Lancet Oncology*, vol. 12, no. 13, pp. 1214–1221, 2011.

[50] N. Flomenberg, L. A. Baxter-Lowe, D. Confer et al., "Impact of HLA class I and class II high-resolution matching on outcomes of unrelated donor bone marrow transplantation: HLA-C mismatching is associated with a strong adverse effect on transplantation outcome," *Blood*, vol. 104, no. 7, pp. 1923–1930, 2004.

[51] E. W. Petersdorf, C. Anasetti, P. J. Martin et al., "Limits of HLA mismatching in unrelated hematopoietic cell transplantation," *Blood*, vol. 104, no. 9, pp. 2976–2980, 2004.

[52] R. A. Bray, C. K. Hurley, N. R. Kamani et al., "National marrow donor program HLA matching guidelines for unrelated adult donor hematopoietic cell transplants," *Biology of Blood and Marrow Transplantation*, vol. 14, supplement 9, pp. 45–53, 2008.

[53] S. R. Spellman, M. Eapen, B. R. Logan et al., "A perspective on the selection of unrelated donors and cord blood units for transplantation," *Blood*, vol. 120, no. 2, pp. 259–265, 2012.

[54] J. J. Van Rood, C. E. Stevens, J. Smits, C. Carrier, C. Carpenter, and A. Scaradavou, "Reexposure of cord blood to noninherited maternal HLA antigens improves transplant outcome in hematological malignancies," *Proceedings of the National Academy of Sciences of the United States of America*, vol. 106, no. 47, pp. 19952–19957, 2009.

[55] V. Rocha, D. Purtill, M. Zhang et al., "Impact of matching at non-inherited maternal antigenson outcomes after 5/6 or 4/6 HLA mismatched unrelated cord blood transplantation for malignant haematological disease. A matched pair analysis on behalf of Eurocord, Netcord, NMDP, CIBMTR," *Bone Marrow Transplantation*, vol. 46, supplement 1, p. S2, 2011, Abstract O115.

[56] J. Kanda, T. Ichinohe, K. Matsuo et al., "Impact of ABO mismatching on the outcomes of allogeneic related and unrelated blood and marrow stem cell transplantations for hematologic malignancies: IPD-based meta-analysis of cohort studies," *Transfusion*, vol. 49, no. 4, pp. 624–635, 2009.

[57] N. Blin, R. Traineau, S. Houssin et al., "Impact of donor-recipient major ABO mismatch on allogeneic transplantation

outcome according to stem cell source," *Biology of Blood and Marrow Transplantation*, vol. 16, no. 9, pp. 1315–1323, 2010.

[58] S. Spellman, R. Bray, S. Rosen-Bronson et al., "The detection of donor-directed, HLA-specific alloantibodies in recipients of unrelated hematopoietic cell transplantation is predictive of graft failure," *Blood*, vol. 115, no. 13, pp. 2704–2708, 2010.

[59] M. Takanashi, Y. Atsuta, K. Fujiwara et al., "The impact of anti-HLA antibodies on unrelated cord blood transplantations," *Blood*, vol. 116, no. 15, pp. 2839–2846, 2010.

[60] C. Cutler, H. T. Kim, L. Sun et al., "Donor-specific anti-HLA antibodies predict outcome in double umbilical cord blood transplantation," *Blood*, vol. 118, no. 25, pp. 6691–6697, 2011.

[61] M. A. Fernandez-Vina, M. de Lima, and S. O. Ciurea, "Humoral HLA sensitization matters in CBT outcome," *Blood*, vol. 118, no. 25, pp. 6482–6484, 2011.

[62] C. G. Brunstein, J. A. Gutman, D. J. Weisdorf et al., "Allogeneic hematopoietic cell transplantation for hematologic malignancy: relative risks and benefits of double umbilical cord blood," *Blood*, vol. 116, no. 22, pp. 4693–4699, 2010.

[63] S. Avery, W. Shi, M. Lubin et al., "Influence of infused cell dose and HLA match on engraftment after double-unit cord blood allografts," *Blood*, vol. 117, no. 12, pp. 3277–3285, 2011.

[64] A. Scaradavou, K. M. Smith, R. Hawke et al., "Cord blood units with low CD34$^+$ cell viability have a low probability of engraftment after double unit transplantation," *Biology of Blood and Marrow Transplantation*, vol. 16, no. 4, pp. 500–508, 2010.

[65] S. Querol, S. G. Gomez, A. Pagliuca, M. Torrabadella, and J. A. Madrigal, "Quality rather than quantity: the cord blood bank dilemma," *Bone Marrow Transplantation*, vol. 45, no. 6, pp. 970–978, 2010.

[66] M. Delaney, C. S. Cutler, R. L. Haspel et al., "High-resolution HLA matching in double-umbilical-cord-blood reduced-intensity transplantation in adults," *Transfusion*, vol. 49, no. 5, pp. 995–1002, 2009.

[67] J. N. Barker, A. Scaradavou, and C. E. Stevens, "Combined effect of total nucleated cell dose and HLA match on transplantation outcome in 1061 cord blood recipients with hematologic malignancies," *Blood*, vol. 115, no. 9, pp. 1843–1849, 2010.

[68] C. G. Brunstein, E. J. Fuchs, S. L. Carter et al., "Alternative donor transplantation after reduced intensity conditioning: results of parallel phase 2 trials using partially HLA-mismatched related bone marrow or unrelated double umbilical cord blood grafts," *Blood*, vol. 118, no. 2, pp. 282–288, 2011.

[69] E. Gluckman, A. Ruggeri, F. Volt, R. Cunha, K. Boudjedir, and V. Rocha, "Milestones in umbilical cord blood transplantation," *British Journal of Haematology*, vol. 154, no. 4, pp. 441–447, 2011.

[70] E. Gluckman, *Choice of Donor According to HLA Typing and Stem Cell Source*, Heamatopoietic Stem Cell Transplantation, chapter 6, The EBMT Handbook, 6th edition, 2012.

[71] C. Mueller and S. Querol, *Bone Marrow Donor Registries and Cord Blood Banks*, Heamatopoietic Stem Cell Transplantation, chapter 6, The EBMT Handbook, 6th edition, 2012.

[72] NetCord and the Foundation for the Accreditation of Cellular Therapy (FACT), Ed., *NetCord-FACT International Standards For Cord Blood Collection, Processing, and Release For Administration*, 4th edition.

[73] C. Anasetti, F. Aversa, and C. G. Brunstein, "Back to the future: mismatched unrelated donor, haploidentical related donor, or unrelated umbilical cord blood transplantation?" *Biology of Blood and Marrow Transplantation*, vol. 18, supplement 1, pp. S161–S165, 2012.

[74] J. Kuball, "Towards the next generation of transplantation: HIV positive patients," in *Proceedings of the 10th International Cord Blood Symposium*, San Francisco, Calif, USA, 2012.

[75] L. D. Petz, "Cord Blood Transplants with Homozygous CCR5-Delta 32 Units as a means of providing possible cure of HIV infection," in *Proceedings of the 10th International Cord Blood Symposium*, San Francisco, Calif, USA, 2012.

[76] K. Le Blanc, I. Rasmusson, B. Sundberg et al., "Treatment of severe acute graft-versus-host disease with third party haploidentical mesenchymal stem cells," *The Lancet*, vol. 363, no. 9419, pp. 1439–1441, 2004.

[77] V. Tisato, K. Naresh, J. Girdlestone, C. Navarrete, and F. Dazzi, "Mesenchymal stem cells of cord blood origin are effective at preventing but not treating graft-versus-host disease," *Leukemia*, vol. 21, no. 9, pp. 1992–1999, 2007.

[78] A. Giorgetti, N. Montserrat, T. Aasen et al., "Generation of induced pluripotent stem cells from human cord blood using OCT4 and SOX2," *Cell Stem Cell*, vol. 5, no. 4, pp. 353–357, 2009.

8

Inhibition of Mammalian Target of Rapamycin in Human Acute Myeloid Leukemia Cells Has Diverse Effects That Depend on the Environmental *In Vitro* Stress

Anita Ryningen,[1,2] **Håkon Reikvam,**[1,2] **Ina Nepstad,**[1,2] **Kristin Paulsen Rye,**[1,2] **and Øystein Bruserud**[1,2]

[1] *Division of Hematology, Institute of Medicine, University of Bergen, N-5021 Bergen, Norway*
[2] *Department of Medicine, Haukeland University Hospital, N-5021 Bergen, Norway*

Correspondence should be addressed to Øystein Bruserud, oystein.bruserud@helse-bergen.no

Academic Editor: Guido Kobbe

Effects of the mTOR inhibitor rapamycin were characterized on *in vitro* cultured primary human acute myeloid leukemia (AML) cells and five AML cell lines. Constitutive mTOR activation seemed to be a general characteristic of primary AML cells. Increased cellular stress induced by serum deprivation increased both mTOR signaling, lysosomal acidity, and *in vitro* apoptosis, where lysosomal acidity/apoptosis were independent of increased mTOR signaling. Rapamycin had antiproliferative and proapoptotic effects only for a subset of patients. Proapoptotic effect was detected for AML cell lines only in the presence of serum. Combination of rapamycin with valproic acid, all-trans retinoic acid (ATRA), and NF-κB inhibitors showed no interference with constitutive mTOR activation and mTOR inhibitory effect of rapamycin and no additional proapoptotic effect compared to rapamycin alone. In contrast, dual inhibition of the PI3K-Akt-mTOR pathway by rapamycin plus a PI3K inhibitor induced new functional effects that did not simply reflect a summary of single drug effects. To conclude, (i) pharmacological characterization of PI3K-Akt-mTOR inhibitors requires carefully standardized experimental models, (ii) rapamycin effects differ between patients, and (iii) combined targeting of different steps in this pathway should be further investigated whereas combination of rapamycin with valproic acid, ATRA, or NF-κB inhibitors seems less promising.

1. Introduction

Acute myeloid leukemia (AML) is a heterogeneous malignancy characterized by bone marrow infiltration of immature leukemic myeloblasts, and the overall disease-free survival is only 40–50% even for the younger patients below 60–65 years of age who receive the most intensive chemotherapy [1, 2]. New therapeutic approaches are thus warranted [3], and inhibition of the phosphatidylinositol 3-kinase (PI3K)-Akt-mammalian target of rapamycin (mTOR) pathway may become a future strategy because this pathway is constitutively activated in the leukemia cells for most patients and seems important for regulation of cell proliferation, viability, and autophagy [4–8]. However, despite these observations the initial clinical studies showed an antileukemic effect

of mTOR inhibition only for a subset of patients [9]. Thus, the future development and optimal use of PI3K-Akt-mTOR inhibition as a therapeutic strategy in human AML will probably depend on a more detailed functional characterization of this pathway using standardized *in vitro* models [4–7].

2. Material and Methods

2.1. Pharmacological Agents. The first generation mTOR inhibitor rapamycin was purchased from LC Laboratories (Woburn, MA, USA). The PI3K inhibitor 3-methyladenine (3-MA) and the specific IκB-kinase/NFκB inhibitor BMS-345541 were purchased from Sigma Aldrich (St. Louis, MO,

USA). Stock solutions were dissolved in dimethylsulphoxide (DMSO), aliquoted, and stored at $-80°C$. The stock solutions were further diluted in culture medium. Pilot experiments showed that DMSO at concentrations used in the experiments did not affect AML cell proliferation. Valproic acid was from Orfiril; Destin GmbH (Hamburg, Germany) and aliquoted stock solutions in saline were stored at $-80°C$ and further diluted with culture medium. The HSP90 inhibitor 17-dimethylaminoethylamino-17-demethoxygeldanamycin (17-DMAG) was purchased from Infinity Pharmaceuticals (Cambridge, MA, US) and used at $1.0\,\mu M$.

2.2. AML Cell Cultures. The study was approved by the local Ethics Committee (University of Bergen, Norway) and patient samples collected after written informed consent. The study included primary human AML cells from unselected adult patients with peripheral blood blast counts exceeding $>7 \times 10^9/L$ and being $>80\%$ of the circulating leukocytes. The AML cell lines HL60, HEL, K562, KG1a, and CTV-1 and the acute lymphoblastic leukemia (ALL) cell lines Nalm-6 and Tanoue were purchased from Deutsche Sammlung von Mikroorganismen und Zellkulturen GmbH (GSMZ; Braunschweig, Germany). The culture medium was Stem Span (Stem Cell Technologies, Vancouver, BC, Canada) eventually supplemented with 10% heat-inactivated fetal bovine serum (FBS) [10]. Primary AML cells were isolated from the blood by density gradient separation (Lymphoprep, Axis-Shield, Oslo, Norway), contained at least 95% leukemia blasts [11, 12] and were stored in liquid nitrogen [11, 12].

2.3. Analysis of Viability, Proliferation, and Flow Cytometry

2.3.1. Viability. Leukemic cells (2×10^6 cells in 2 mL) were incubated at $37°C$ in a humidified atmosphere of 5% CO_2 in 24-well culture plates (Costar 3524; Cambridge, MA, USA) for 48 hours in StemSpan SFEM medium (referred to as StemSpan; Stem Cell Technologies; Vancouver, BC, Canada) supplemented with $100\,\mu g/mL$ of gentamicin. The fractions of viable, apoptotic, and necrotic cells were then determined by double staining of AML cells with Annexin V-fluorescein isothiocyanate and propidium iodide (PI) (Apoptest-FITC kit; NeXins Research, Kattendijke, the Netherlands) as described in detail previously [13].

2.3.2. Proliferation. AML cells 5×10^4/well were cultured in $150\,\mu L$ medium in flat-bottomed microtiter 96-well plates (Nucleon Surface, Nunc A/S, Roskilde, Denmark). Cells were cultured in medium alone or with stem cell factor (SCF), granulocyte-macrophage colony stimulating factor (GM-CSF) and FLT3 ligand (FLT3-L) (all from PeproTech Ltd.; Rocky Hill, NJ, USA). Nuclear ^3H-thymidine incorporation was assayed after seven days as described in detail previously [14].

2.3.3. Flow Cytometry. Cultured cells were washed with phosphate buffered saline (PBS) and fixed with 4% paraformaldehyde (PFA) in PBS before permeabilization with ice-cold methanol. After washing twice with PBS samples were blocked with 5% bovine serum albumin (BSA) in PBS before being incubated with primary conjugated fluorescent antibodies against phospho-S6RP (S6 ribosomal protein) and the autophagy-associated mediators LC3B and Beclin-1 (Cell Signaling Technology, Inc.; Boston, MA, USA) and ATG-3, ATG-7, ATG-10 (Biosensis; Halifax, Australia) for 1 hour. After PBS washing samples were analyzed by flow cytometry. The mean fluorescence intensity (MFI) was detected for the cells after eliminating debris and cell aggregates in a forward versus side scatter cytogram.

Lysosomal acidity was detected with LysoTracker Red DND-99 from Molecular Probes, Inc. (Eugene, OR, USA). Aliquots of the 1 mM probe stock solution were stored at $-20°C$ and diluted to a final concentration of 50 nM in growth medium. The cells were incubated with LysoTracker Red for the last 30 minutes of culture, washed with PBS, fixed with 4% paraformaldehyde (PFA) in PBS, and washed with PBS before being analyzed by flow cytometry. A cytogram based on forward versus side scatter was used to eliminate debris and cell aggregates before lysosomal acidity was analyzed.

For the cell cycle measurements PI and RNase A were purchased from Sigma-Aldrich. The cells were rapidly fixed in ice-cold 70% ethanol and incubated for at least 30 minutes at $4°C$. They were then washed once with PBS, resuspended in $800\,\mu L$ PBS + RNase A (0.1 mg/mL) + PI ($40\,\mu g/mL$) before cells were incubated in the dark at $37°C$ for 30 minutes. Samples were immediately analyzed by flow cytometry. A cytogram based on forward versus side scatter was used to eliminate aggregates, debris, and dead cells before red fluorescence in linear mode was detected on viable cells.

2.4. Statistical and Bioinformatical Approaches. All statistical analyses were performed using the Statistical Package for the Social Sciences (SPSS) version 15.0 (SPSS Inc., Chicago, IL, USA) and GraphPad Prism 5 (GraphPad Software, Inc., San Diego, CA, USA), and P values < 0.05 were regarded as statistically significant. Bioinformatical analyses were performed using the J-Express 2011 analysis suite (MolMine AS, Bergen, Norway) [15, 16]. Values were divided by the values of control culture before being transformed to logarithmic values (base 2) as described previously [16]. Unsupervised hierarchical clustering was performed with Euclidian correlation and complete linkage as distance measure.

3. Results

3.1. Primary Human AML Cells Show Constitutive mTOR-Mediated Signaling and a Wide Variation in the Expression of Proteins Involved in Autophagy. We compared the intracellular levels of the phosphorylated mTOR target S6RP and the autophagy-associated mediators LC3B, Beclin-1, ATG-3, ATG7, and ATG-10 after 4 hours of incubation in FBS-containing medium for AML cells derived from 9 patients (Figure 1). Constitutive signaling through mTOR

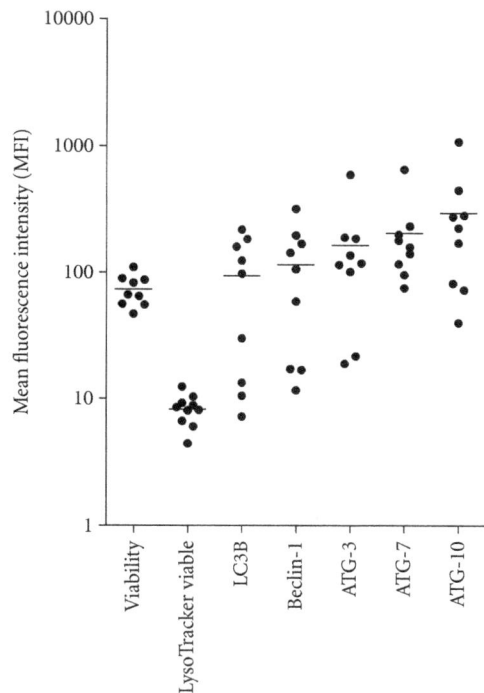

FIGURE 1: Intracellular levels of the five autophagy-involved mediators LC3B, Beclin-1, ATG3, ATG7, and ATG10 in primary human AML cells. Levels were determined by flow cytometric analysis for primary human AML cells derived from 9 unselected patients. The cells were rested in FCS-containing medium for 4 hours before the analysis. The results are presented as the mean fluorescence intensity (MFI).

was estimated as the MFI of phosphorylated S6RP (p-S6RP); this was detected for all patients but the levels showed a wide variation (MFI range 50–405). Expression of LC3B (MFI range 16.2–65.3), Beclin-1 (range 9.4–101.5), ATG-3 (range 28.5–116.3), ATG7 (range 31.2–118.5), and ATG-10 (range 9.1–105.6) also showed wide variations without any correlation with S6RP phosphorylation.

We did an unsupervised hierarchical clustering of the patients with regard to levels of autophagy-associated molecules (Figure 2). The patient clustering showed only minor differences between FBS-containing and serum-free cultures, and as would be expected from the correlation analyses (see above) the p-S6RP level clustered separately with no close association with any of the autophagy mediators. Both FBS-containing and serum-free cultures showed close associations between (i) LC3B and Beclin-1; (ii) the three ATGs, and (iii) apoptosis-regulating bcl-2, bcl-Xl and bax.

3.2. Dose-Response Effects of Rapamycin on Primary Human AML Cell Proliferation.

We investigated the effect of different rapamycin concentrations (tenfold dilution between 0.01 nM and 10^5 nM) on cytokine-dependent AML cell proliferation for 15 unselected patients. All concentrations caused a similar and statistically significant inhibition of AML cell proliferation with median proliferation varying between 68% (0.01 and 10^4 nM) and 77% (10^3 nM). Studies of

myeloma cells have also described a similar antiproliferative effect of different concentrations of rapamycin when tested over a wide concentration range [17], and previous *in vitro* studies of primary human AML cells suggest that some patients show no inhibition of mTOR activity when testing rapamycin ≤20 nM and with a maximal effect being reached at rapamycin >50 nM [18]. Based on our own dose-response experiments and these previous observations we used rapamycin 100 nM in our experiments.

3.3. Rapamycin-Induced mTOR Inhibition Does Not Reverse the Stress-Induced Increase in Lysosomal Acidity and Spontaneous Apoptosis in Primary Human AML Cells.

Even *in vitro* culture in optimal FBS-containing medium is associated with spontaneous apoptosis of primary human AML cells as well as a small but significant increase in lysosomal acidity (see Supplementary Figure 1(a) available online at doi:10.1155/2012/329061). Serum deprivation during culture is often used to increase cellular stress [19–24], and for primary AML cells such deprivation is associated both with a further increase in spontaneous apoptosis (Supplementary Figure 1(b)) and in addition increased mTOR signaling and increased lysosomal acidity (Supplementary Figures 1(c) and 1(d)) even though the intracellular levels of autophagy-(LC3B, Beclin, ATG3, ATG7, ATG10) or apoptosis-associated (bcl-2, bcl-XL, bax) molecules are not altered.

Rapamycin 100 nM significantly reduced phosphorylation of the mTOR downstream target S6RP when AML cells were cultured under serum-free conditions; this decrease was detected after only 4 hours (Figure 3; $P = 0.008$) and persisted after 24 hours ($P = 0.028$, data not shown). However, rapamycin 100 nM (24 hours cultures) had divergent effects and caused no significant alterations when comparing the overall results for cell viability, lysosomal acidity, or intracellular levels of autophagy-associated and apoptosis-regulating molecules (data not shown). Rapamycin did not affect apoptosis or lysosomal acidity for primary AML cells cultured under optimal conditions with FBS-containing medium either (data not shown) even though it decreased S6RP phosphorylation (Figure 3). These results demonstrate that the decreased viability and increased lysosomal acidity induced by serum deprivation (i.e., experimental *in vitro* stress) are not reversed by inhibition of the increased mTOR signaling. Thus, spontaneous or stress-induced *in vitro* apoptosis and mTOR signaling seem to be independent events.

As described previously the extent of spontaneous *in vitro* apoptosis shows wide variation between patients both in the presence of rapamycin 100 nM and in drug-free cultures. Furthermore, the cellular HSP70/HSP90 levels then seem important for the extent of this apoptosis [13]. We therefore investigated whether the patient heterogeneity could be reduced by adding the HSP90 inhibitor 17-DMAG 50 nM and thereby reducing the influence of variations in intracellular HSP90 levels between patients. We examined AML cells from 52 patients, but the patient heterogeneity with regard to the effect of rapamycin on cell viability persisted also in the presence of 17-DMAG. Thus, the patient

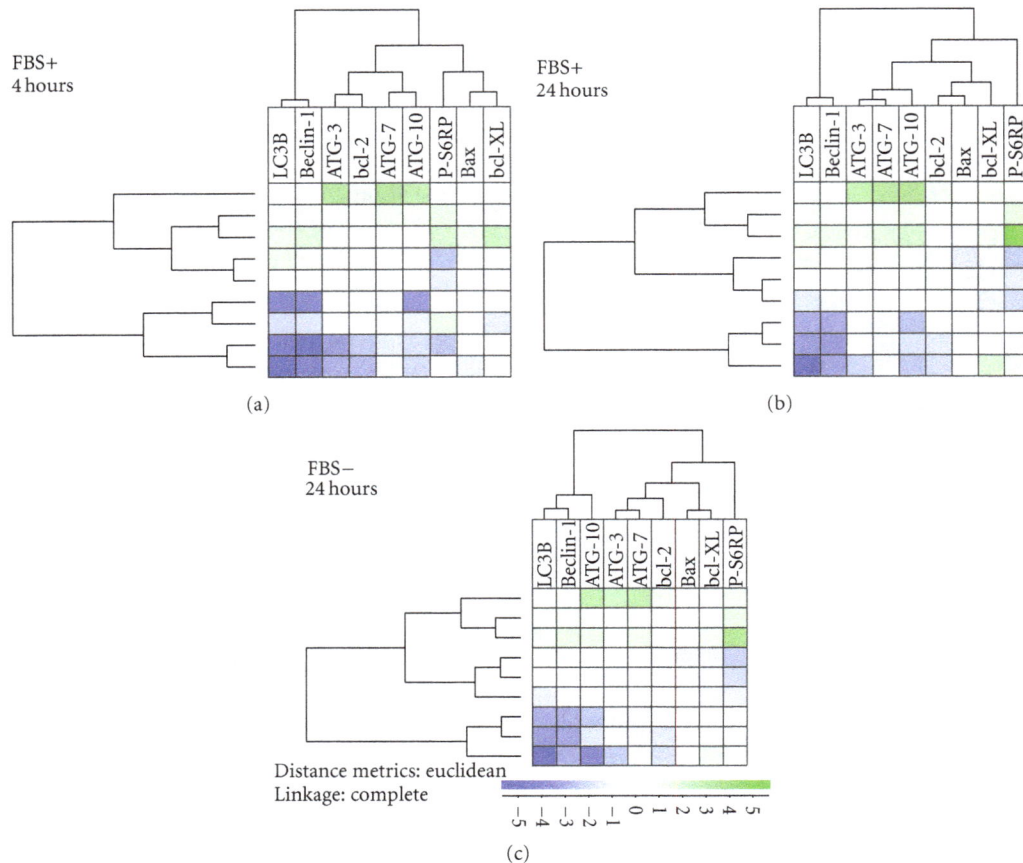

FIGURE 2: Unsupervised hierarchical cluster analysis of the intracellular levels of (i) the five autophagy-involved mediators LC3B, Beclin-1, ATG3, ATG7 and ATG10, (ii) the apoptosis regulators bcl-2, bcl-XL, and bax, and (iii) the phosphorylated form of the mTOR downstream target S6RP. The levels were determined by flow cytometry for primary human AML cells derived from 9 unselected patients. Cells were incubated in either FBS-containing or serum-free medium for 4 and 24 hours before analysis. The figure presents the results for cells incubated in FBS-containing medium for 4 (a) and 24 hours (b) and for cells incubated in serum-free medium for 24 hours (c).

heterogeneity with regard to effect of rapamycin on primary AML cell viability is not secondary to differences in HSP90 levels.

3.4. Rapamycin Has a Proapoptotic Effect on AML Cell Lines Associated with Increased Lysosomal Acidity, but This Effect Is Not Detected during Serum Deprivation. As described previously primary human AML cells show spontaneous or stress-induced *in vitro* apoptosis during *in vitro* culture, and this is seen especially during serum depletion but also for cultures supplemented with FBS. We therefore used an alternative experimental model and investigated effects of rapamycin on the viability of the five AML cell lines HL60, HEL, KG1a, CTV-1, and K562. All these cell lines proliferated when cultured in serum-free medium [13, 25], but the viability was generally lower in serum-free than FBS-containing cultures. We investigated the effect of rapamycin (100, 200, 400, 600, and 800 nM) when AML cells were cultured in medium without and with 10% inactivated FBS. For these cell lines rapamycin caused a dose-dependent reduction in AML cell viability in FBS-containing cultures. In contrast, for the serum-free cultures rapamycin even

caused a minor increase in the viability for HEL (rapamycin 100 nm, viability 63 versus 76%), HL60 (81 versus 87%), and CTV-1 cells (78 versus 89%); for higher concentrations the increased viability was also observed for K562 (600 nM, 59 versus 77% viable cells). The results for HEL and CTV-1 are presented in Supplementary Figure 2. The FBS dependency of this rapamycin-associated proapoptotic effect was reproduced for all cell lines in 4 independent experiments, the proapoptotic effect in FBS-containing cultures could be detected after 24 hours and increased gradually during the first 48 hours of culture, and the early apoptotic population remained small during culture but showed a minor increase for all except K562 (data not shown). Finally, we observed a decrease in the phosphorylation of the mTOR downstream target S6RP in all rapamycin-supplemented cultures whether FBS was added or not. To conclude, (i) AML cell lines cultured in medium alone show detectable stress-induced *in vitro* apoptosis similar to primary cells, and rapamycin then does not alter regulation of apoptosis, whereas (ii) cell lines cultured in FBS containing medium show very low stress-induced apoptosis, and under these conditions rapamycin has a proapoptotic effect.

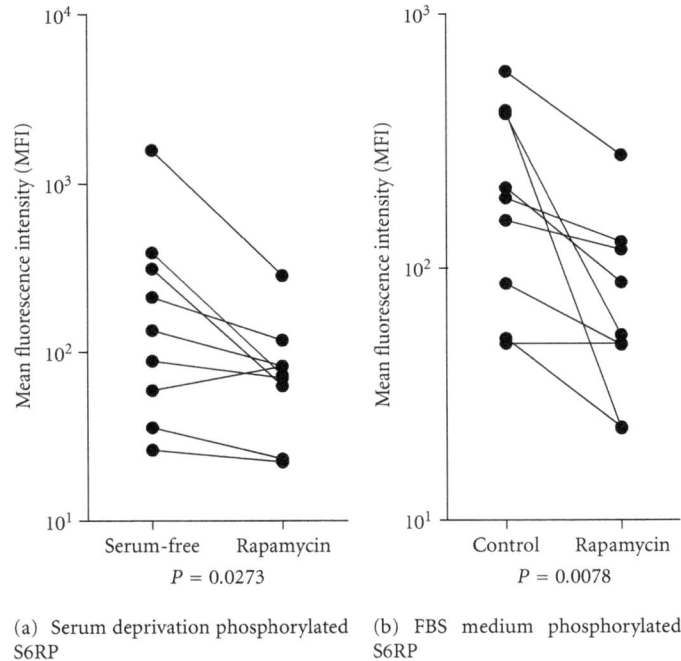

(a) Serum deprivation phosphorylated S6RP

(b) FBS medium phosphorylated S6RP

FIGURE 3: Effects of *in vitro* culture of primary human AML cells on mTOR signaling for primary human AML cells derived from unselected patients. The figure compares mTOR-mediated signaling (levels of the downstream target p-S6RP) for AML cells incubated for 24 hours in serum-free (a) or FBS-containing (b) medium alone or in the presence of rapamycin 100 nM. The results are presented as the median fluorescence intensity (MFI).

We investigated the lysosomal acidity for all AML cell lines and the ALL cell line Tanoue when cells were cultured with and without rapamycin 100 nM in serum-free and FBS-supplemented medium. The lysosomal acidity/autophagy in drug-free controls was always highest for cells cultured without FBS, and a similar difference between serum-free and FBS containing cultures was seen even in the presence of rapamycin (Supplementary Figure 3), but without any significant effect of rapamycin on autophagy (data not shown). These results were reproduced in independent experiments for all cell lines. Thus, similar to the primary cells serum deprivation of AML cell lines increased lysosomal acidity, and we did not detect any further effect of rapamycin-induced mTOR inhibition on the acidity, that is, autophagy.

3.5. Rapamycin Has a Caspase-Independent Proapoptotic Effect in AML Cell Lines. We compared cell viability in FBS-containing cultures prepared with rapamycin alone and rapamycin plus the pan-caspase inhibitor Z-VAD for three AML cell lines. For KG1a and K562 the viability was not increased by caspase inhibition. For HL60 the viability after 24 hours was 71% in control cultures, it was decreased to 33.1% by rapamycin alone, and a minor increase to 46% was seen when Z-VAD was added together with rapamycin. Thus, caspase-independent mechanisms are important for the rapamycin-induced decrease of AML cell viability, whereas bax and Bcl-2 showed only minor alteration after exposure to rapamycin and/or Z-VAD (only KG1a being examined).

3.6. Combined mTOR and PI3K Inhibition: More than a Summary of Single Drug Effects. Other inhibitors of the PI3K-Akt-mTOR pathway are now being developed, including PI3K inhibitors acting upstream to mTOR [26, 27]. These upstream inhibitors are also considered for cancer therapy [26, 27], and we therefore investigated whether combination of rapamycin with an upstream inhibitor had any additional effects compared with rapamycin alone. 3-MA is a paninhibitor of PI3K and is regarded as an inhibitor of autophagy [13]. The effects of 3-MA on KG-1a alone were decreased viability, no effect on lysosomal acidity but increased accumulation of cells in the G0/G1 phase (data not shown). When combined with rapamycin 3-MA caused an additional decrease in viability, but in contrast to the results for 3-MA alone the drug caused increased lysosomal acidity with no additional effect on the G0/G1 fraction when combined with rapamycin.

3.7. Rapamycin Combined with Valproic Acid and ATRA: Valproic Acid Alters Levels of Autophagy-Regulating Mediators in Primary Human AML Cells Whereas ATRA Has Minor Effects. Valproic acid plus ATRA is now used for AML-stabilizing palliative therapy either alone or in combination with other drugs [28, 29]. We investigated the effects of combining valproic acid and rapamycin on primary human AML cells ($n = 9$) cultured under optimal *in vitro* conditions in FBS-containing medium. Intracellular levels of ATG-3, ATG-10, and bcl-XL were significantly increased after 24 hours of exposure to the drug combination compared

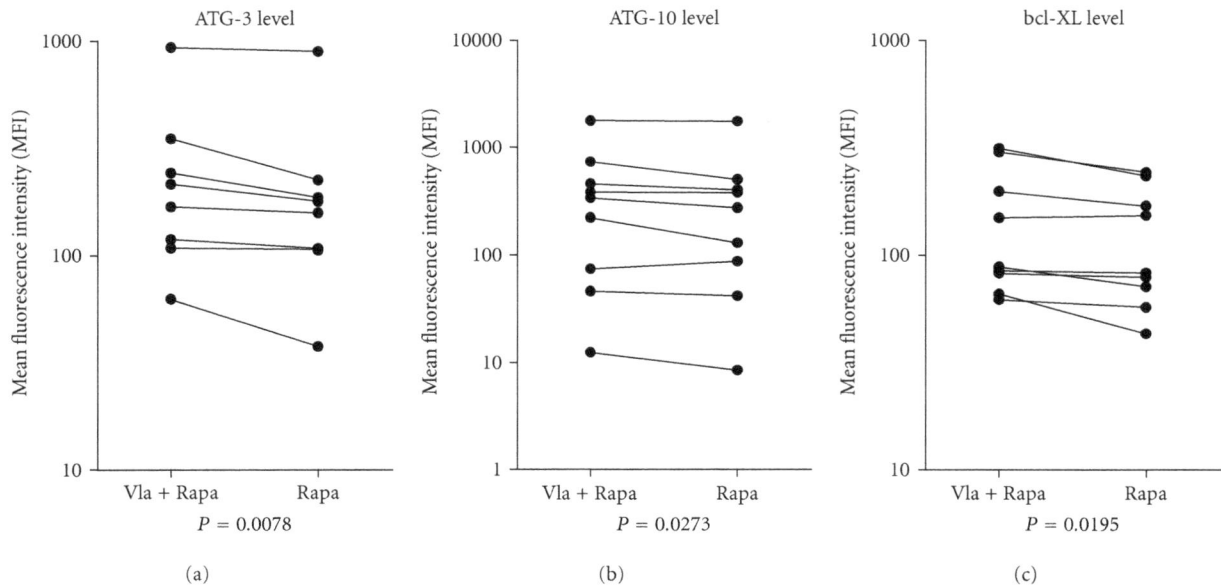

FIGURE 4: The effect of the HDAC inhibitor valproic acid on the expression ATG-3 (a), ATG-10 (b) and bcl-XL (c) when primary human on AML cells from unselected patients were cultured in serum-free medium in the presence of rapamycin 100 nM alone or in combination with valproic acid (2400 μM). The results are presented as the MFI, and the P values are given below each figure. Abbreviations: Vla, valproic acid; Rapa, rapamycin.

with rapamycin alone (Figure 4) but despite these molecular effects lysosomal acidity (i.e., autophagy) was not altered (data not shown). Valproic acid did not interfere with mTOR-mediated signaling as the phosphorylation status of S6RP in primary AML cells as well as cell lines was not altered when valproic acid was added to rapamycin. Finally, valproic acid plus rapamycin had divergent effects compared with rapamycin alone and when analyzing the overall results the combination did not significantly alter AML cell viability or intracellular levels of bcl-2 or bax (data not shown).

The effect of combining rapamycin and valproic acid on lysosomal acidity and viability was also investigated for all 5 AML cell lines, and similar to the primary cells valproic acid had (i) no or minor effects on lysosomal acidity, the only exception being HEL cells that showed increased lysosomal acidity, and (ii) minor effects on AML cell line viability (data not shown).

ATRA was also tested alone and in combination with rapamycin during 4 and 24 hours of culture for primary AML cells derived from 9 patients. The drug did not interfere with mTOR mediated signaling (i.e. S6RP phosphorylation) and had no additional effect to rapamycin alone on viability, lysosomal acidity, or intracellular protein levels of autophagy-associated (LC3B, Beclin-1, ATG-3, ATG7, ATG-10) and apoptosis-regulating intracellular mediators (bcl-2, bax, bcl-XL) (data not shown).

3.8. Rapamycin Combined with the NFκB Inhibitor BMS-345541 Increases Lysosomal Acidity.

The IκB/NFκB inhibitor BMS-345541 was tested alone and in combination with rapamycin during 4 and 24 hours of culture (AML cells from 9 patients examined), but the drug did not have any statistically significant effect on the overall results neither when tested alone nor in combination with rapamycin on the phosphorylation of the mTOR substrate S6RP, viability/apoptosis, lysosomal acidity, or intracellular protein levels of autophagy-associated (LC3B, Beclin-1, ATG-3, ATG7, ATG-10) and apoptosis-regulating intracellular mediators (bcl-2, bax, bcl-XL) (data not shown).

We investigated the effect of BMS-345541 on the KG1a AML cell line cultured in FBS-containing medium. NF-κB inhibition gradually decreased the AML cell viability during a 48-hour culture period, but the most striking effect was a considerable increase in lysosomal acidity both for viable, apoptotic, and necrotic cells (Figure 5). Furthermore, similar effects were seen when BMS-345541 was added together with rapamycin; the presence of the NF-κB inhibitor then further decreased AML cell viability and caused a gradual and strong increase in lysosomal acidity with maintenance of the rapamycin-induced accumulation of cells in the G0/1 phase during a 48-hour culture period. The increased lysosomal acidity was strongest for the small minority of dead cells but was also seen for viable cells. For viable cells cultured with FBS for 24 hours rapamycin alone increased the MFI of lysosomal acidity to 164% of the drug-free control, whereas an additional increase up to 205% was seen when BMS-345541 was added together with rapamycin. The BMS-345541-associated increase in lysosomal acidity was reproduced in three independent experiments.

To conclude, rapamycin and rapamycin plus BMS-345541 had divergent effects on the viability of primary AML cell viability, but the studies in KG1a cells suggest that decreased viability for a subset of patients is associated with increased autophagy and G0/G1 accumulation of the cells.

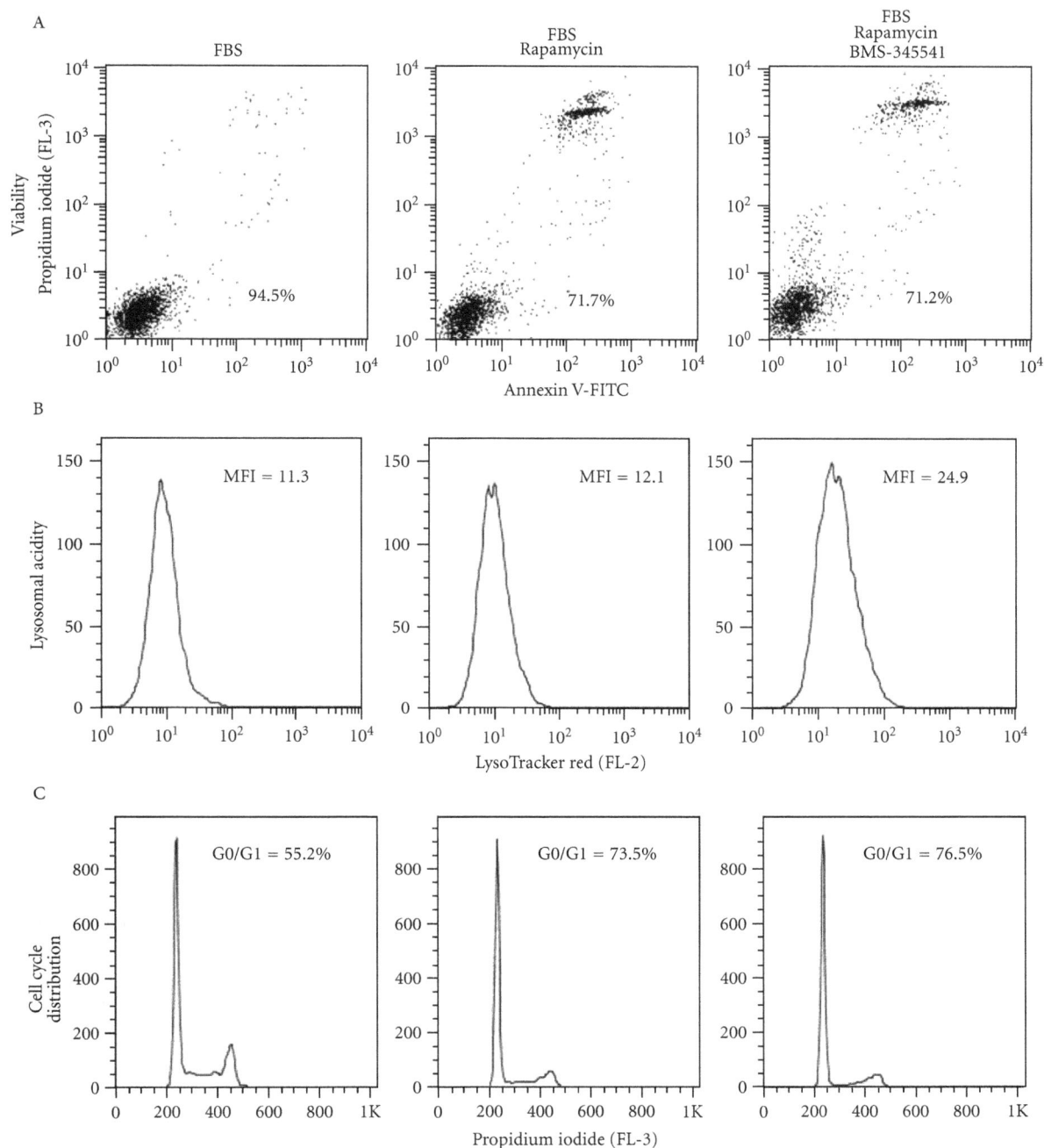

FIGURE 5: The effect of rapamycin and BMS-345541 on viability (A), lysosomal acidity (B), and cell cycle distribution (C) for the AML cell line KG1a. As is indicated at the top of the figure the AML cells were cultured for 24 hours in FBS-containing medium alone and medium supplemented with rapamycin 100 nM alone or rapamycin plus BMS-345541. The figure presents the results from flow-cytometric analyses of viability ((A) percent of viable cells is given in the diagrams), lysosomal acidity ((B) the MFI values are given in the diagrams), and cell cycle distribution ((C) percent of cells in G0/G1 phase is given in the diagrams).

4. Discussion

The median age of patients with newly diagnosed AML is 65–70 years. The majority of AML patients thus cannot receive the most intensive and potentially curative treatments for their disease [1, 2], but even for the younger patients receiving this treatment the overall disease-free survival is less than 50% [1, 2]. New therapeutic approaches are therefore considered both for combination with conventional treatment and as a basis for the development of less toxic therapeutic strategies in elderly patients [3]. Inhibition of mTOR-mediated signaling is one of these strategies [4–8], but the initial clinical experience suggests that mTOR inhibitors alone have limited antileukemic effects

[9]. Combination of mTOR inhibitors with other targeted therapies should therefore be considered, and preclinical evaluation in well-characterized experimental models will then be important.

Spontaneous or stress-induced apoptosis is seen during *in vitro* culture of primary human AML cells and is most extensive in leukemic cells with low HSP levels as well as a low bcl-2 : bax ratio [13]. Our present results show that this apoptosis is increased during serum deprivation in primary AML cells, and only experimental models using culture of AML cell lines in FBS-containing medium represent a standardized model with a minimal stress-induced apoptosis during culture [10]. The AML cell line viability was also lower during serum deprivation, that is, during experimental *in vitro* stress.

The degree of spontaneous apoptosis differed between culture conditions (serum-deprivation versus FBS-containing medium) and the type of AML cells examined (primary cells versus cell lines). The viability was highest for AML cell lines cultured in FBS-containing medium followed by cell lines cultured in serum-free medium; it was lower for primary AML cells cultured with serum, and the lowest viability was seen for primary AML cells after serum deprivation. Thus, for studies of pharmacological effects without the influence of additional stress-induced apoptosis one should investigate AML cell lines cultured in FBS-supplemented medium, whereas serum-free cultures of primary leukemic cells represent an experimental model with a relatively strong influence of environmental stress-induced proapoptotic signaling that differs between patients.

In most of our experiments we tested rapamycin at 100 nM. This concentration was chosen because mTOR signaling in primary AML cells is often inhibited by rapamycin 10–20 nM, but for exceptional patients there is a partial resistance, and concentrations exceeding 50 nM have to be used to achieve a reduction in downstream protein phosphorylation [18]. Concentrations up to 1000 nM have been used in previous *in vitro* studies [18], and another recent AML study also used rapamycin 100 nM [30]. In our dose-response experiments we observed that a plateau was reached when testing the effect of higher rapamycin concentrations (>10–20 nM) on cytokine-dependent AML cell proliferation, and a similar plateau was also observed in an experimental myeloma model [17]. The detection of a plateau suggests that no functionally important off-target effects occur when using rapamycin 100 nM. Finally, we used flow cytometric detection of the phosphorylated form of S6RP as a marker of mTOR signaling; this is a downstream mediator to mTOR, and previous AML studies using the alternative methodological approach with western blot analysis have shown that rapamycin will decrease S6RP phosphorylation [31] (Reikvam, submitted).

The intracellular levels of autophagy- and apoptosis-regulating mediators showed a considerable variation in primary AML cells, but the levels did not have a close association with spontaneous apoptosis or the effect of rapamycin. Furthermore, valproic acid altered the levels of several of these mediators but did not affect viability or autophagy when added together with rapamycin. Taken together these observations suggest that the intracellular levels of these mediators do not have any major role in our experimental model with regard to regulation of viability or lysosomal acidity.

We investigated the effects of double targeting of the PI3K-Akt-mTOR pathway by combining rapamycin and 3-MA, an upstream inhibitor of PI3K and also an inhibitor of autophagy [25]. We have previously done a detailed study of 3-MA effects on primary human AML cells showing that rapamycin and 3-MA may have additive proapoptotic and antiproliferative effects in primary human AML cells [32]. Our present results with AML cell lines showed that this double targeting caused an additive reduction of the viability had no effect on cell cycle distribution but caused an unexpected increase of lysosomal acidity consistent with increased autophagy. Based on our present results we therefore conclude that (i) inhibitors targeting different steps in the PI3K-Akt-mTOR pathway have different biological effects, and (ii) the effects of combined inhibition of different steps may induce new functional effects, and the final effects of such combinations not only represent a summary of the single drug effects. An advantage of dual targeting has also been suggested by another study [33].

The combination of valproic acid and ATRA is now tried as disease-stabilizing treatment in AML [34], and these two drugs may eventually be combined with cytotoxic agents [29]. Combination with rapamycin should also be considered because this drug shows limited toxicity, and serum level estimation is available [34]. Our present results show that valproic acid (but not ATRA) can alter the levels of autophagy-associated molecules; none of the drugs interfere with the mTOR inhibitory effect of rapamycin but they had no additional biological effects compared with rapamycin alone when comparing the overall results. Future studies should therefore focus on whether it is possible to define patient subsets that will benefit from treatment with these drug combinations.

NF-κB inhibition is also considered as a possible therapeutic strategy in AML [35]. This therapeutic approach seems to target the leukemic stem cells [35] as well as the communication with nonleukemic neighboring cells through the local cytokine network [14]. Even though BMS-345541 did not interfere with the mTOR inhibitory effect of rapamycin, the combination of rapamycin plus NFκB inhibition had divergent effects in primary AML cells compared with rapamycin alone. However, the combination caused increased apoptosis, autophagy, and G0/G1 accumulation in the KG-1a cell line, and these mechanisms may then be important for the increased antileukemic effect of this combination in certain patients.

Inhibition of the PI3K-Akt-mTOR pathway is regarded as a possible therapeutic strategy in human AML. Based on our present results we conclude that (i) future *in vitro* pharmacological characterization of PI3K-Akt-mTOR inhibitors requires carefully standardized experimental models, (ii) even though constitutive activation of this pathway and the inhibitory effect of rapamycin on this signaling seem to be a general characteristic of primary human AML cells, the final biological effects of rapamycin seem to differ between patients, and (iii) combined targeting of different steps in this pathway should be further investigated as a possible therapeutic strategy whereas combination of rapamycin with valproic acid, ATRA, or NF-κB inhibitors seems less promising.

Acknowledgments

The study received economic support from the Norwegian Cancer Society.

References

[1] H. Döhner, E. H. Estey, S. Amadori et al., "Diagnosis and management of acute myeloid leukemia in adults: recommendations from an international expert panel, on behalf of the European LeukemiaNet," *Blood*, vol. 115, no. 3, pp. 453–474, 2010.

[2] E. H. Estey, "Acute myeloid leukemia: 2012 update on diagnosis, risk stratification, and management," *American Journal of Hematology*, vol. 87, pp. 89–99, 2012.

[3] C. Stapnes, B. T. Gjertsen, H. Reikvam, and O. Bruserud, "Targeted therapy in acute myeloid leukaemia: current status and future directions," *Expert Opinion on Investigational Drugs*, vol. 18, no. 4, pp. 433–455, 2009.

[4] A. M. Martelli, C. Evangelisti, F. Chiarini, C. Grimaldi, L. Manzoli, and J. A. McCubrey, "Targeting the PI3K/AKT/mTOR signaling network in acute myelogenous leukemia," *Expert Opinion on Investigational Drugs*, vol. 18, no. 9, pp. 1333–1349, 2009.

[5] A. Fasolo and C. Sessa, "Current and future directions in mammalian target of rapamycin inhibitors development," *Expert Opinion on Investigational Drugs*, vol. 20, no. 3, pp. 381–394, 2011.

[6] S. Albert, M. Serova, C. Dreyer, M. P. Sablin, S. Faivre, and E. Raymond, "New inhibitors of the mammalian target of rapamycin signaling pathway for cancer," *Expert Opinion on Investigational Drugs*, vol. 19, no. 8, pp. 919–930, 2010.

[7] D. W. Bowles and A. Jimeno, "New phosphatidylinositol 3-kinase inhibitors for cancer," *Expert Opinion on Investigational Drugs*, vol. 20, no. 4, pp. 507–518, 2011.

[8] J. Tamburini, C. Elie, V. Bardet et al., "Constitutive phosphoinositide 3-kinase/Akt activation represents a favorable prognostic factor in de novo acute myelogenous leukemia patients," *Blood*, vol. 110, no. 3, pp. 1025–1028, 2007.

[9] K. W. L. Yee, Z. Zeng, M. Konopleva et al., "Phase I/II study of the mammalian target of rapamycin inhibitor everolimus (RAD001) in patients with relapsed or refractory hematologic malignancies," *Clinical Cancer Research*, vol. 12, no. 17, pp. 5165–5173, 2006.

[10] O. Bruserud, B. T. Gjertsen, and H. L. Von Volkman, "*In vitro* culture of human acute myelogenous leukemia (AML) cells in serum-free media: studies of native AML blasts and AML cell lines," *Journal of Hematotherapy and Stem Cell Research*, vol. 9, no. 6, pp. 923–932, 2000.

[11] O. Bruserud, "Effect of dipyridamole, theophyllamine and verapamil on spontaneous *in vitro* proliferation of myelogenous leukaemia cells," *Acta Oncologica*, vol. 31, no. 1, pp. 53–58, 1992.

[12] B. T. Gjertsen, A. M. Øyan, B. Marzolf et al., "Analysis of acute myelogenous leukemia: preparation of samples for genomic and proteomic analyses," *Journal of Hematotherapy and Stem Cell Research*, vol. 11, no. 3, pp. 469–481, 2002.

[13] A. Ryningen, E. Ersvær, A. M. Øyan et al., "Stress-induced *in vitro* apoptosis of native human acute myelogenous leukemia (AML) cells shows a wide variation between patients and is associated with low BCL-2:Bax ratio and low levels of heat shock protein 70 and 90," *Leukemia Research*, vol. 30, no. 12, pp. 1531–1540, 2006.

[14] Ø. Bruserud, A. Ryningen, A. M. Olsnes et al., "Subclassification of patients with acute myelogenous leukemia based on chemokine responsiveness and constitutive chemokine release by their leukemic cells," *Haematologica*, vol. 92, no. 3, pp. 332–341, 2007.

[15] A. K. Stavrum, K. Petersen, I. Jonassen, and B. Dysvik, "Analysis of gene-expression data using J-express," *Current Protocols in Bioinformatics*, no. 21, pp. 7.3.1–7.3.25, 2008.

[16] H. Reikvam, K. J. Hatfield, E. Ersvaer et al., "Expression profile of heat shock proteins in acute myeloid leukaemia patients reveals a distinct signature strongly associated with FLT3 mutation status—consequences and potentials for pharmacological intervention," *British Journal of Haematology*, vol. 156, pp. 468–480, 2012.

[17] L. K. Francis, Y. Alsayed, X. Leleu et al., "Combination mammalian target of rapamycin inhibitor rapamycin and HSP90 inhibitor 17-allylamino-17-demethoxygeldanamycin has synergistic activity in multiple myeloma," *Clinical Cancer Research*, vol. 12, no. 22, pp. 6826–6835, 2006.

[18] A. E. Perl, M. T. Kasner, D. Shank, S. M. Luger, and M. Carroll, "Single-cell pharmacodynamic monitoring of S6 ribosomal protein phosphorylation in AML blasts during a clinical trial combining the mTOR inhibitor sirolimus and intensive chemotherapy," *Clinical Cancer Research*, vol. 18, pp. 1716–1725, 2012.

[19] Q. Zhang, Y. J. Yang, H. Wang et al., "Autophagy activation: a novel mechanism of atorvastatin to protect mesenchymal stem cells from hypoxia and serum deprivation via AMP-activated protein kinase/mammalian target of rapamycin pathway," *Stem Cells and Development*, vol. 21, pp. 1321–1332, 2012.

[20] J. Wang, Z. Gu, P. Ni et al., "NF-kappaB P50/P65 hetero-dimer mediates differential regulation of CD166/ALCAM expression via interaction with micoRNA-9 after serum deprivation, providing evidence for a novel negative auto-regulatory loop," *Nucleic Acids Research*, vol. 39, pp. 6440–6455, 2011.

[21] Y. Ohsawa, K. Isahara, S. Kanamori et al., "An ultrastructural and immunohistochemical study of pc12 cells during apoptosis induced by serum deprivation with special reference to autophagy and lysosomal cathepsins," *Archives of Histology and Cytology*, vol. 61, no. 5, pp. 395–403, 1998.

[22] D. D. Gougoumas, I. S. Vizirianakis, I. N. Triviai, and A. S. Tsiftsoglou, "Activation of Prn-p gene and stable transfection of Prn-p cDNA in leukemia MEL and neuroblastoma N2a cells increased production of PrPC but not prevented DNA fragmentation initiated by serum deprivation," *Journal of Cellular Physiology*, vol. 211, no. 2, pp. 551–559, 2007.

[23] Y. H. Kim, M. Takahashi, E. Suzuki, and E. Niki, "Apoptosis induced by hydrogen peroxide under serum deprivation and its inhibition by antisense c-jun in F-MEL cells," *Biochemical and Biophysical Research Communications*, vol. 271, no. 3, pp. 747–752, 2000.

[24] C. J. Welsh, A. M. Sayer, L. G. Littlefield, and M. C. Cabot, "Modification of lipid acyl groups by serum deprivation does not affect phorbol ester-induced differentiation of human leukemia cells," *Cancer Letters*, vol. 16, no. 2, pp. 145–154, 1982.

[25] E. S. Bergmann-Leitner and S. I. Abrams, "Treatment of human colon carcinoma cell lines with anti-neoplastic agents enhances their lytic sensitivity to antigen-specific CD8+ cytotoxic T lymphocytes," *Cancer Immunology, Immunotherapy*, vol. 50, no. 9, pp. 445–455, 2001.

[26] J. Baselga, M. J. De Jonge, J. Rodon et al., "A first-in-human phase I study of BKM120, an oral pan-class I PI3K inhibitor, in patients (pts) with advanced solid tumors," *Journal of Clinical Oncology*, vol. 28, no. 15s, abstract 3003, 2010.

[27] A. J. Folkes, K. Ahmadi, W. K. Alderton et al., "The identification of 2-(1H-indazol-4-yl)-6-(4-methanesulfonyl-piperazin-1-ylmethyl)-4-morpholin-4-yl-thieno[3,2-d]pyrimidine (GDC-0941) as a potent, selective, orally bioavailable inhibitor of class I PI3 kinase for the treatment of cancer," *Journal of Medicinal Chemistry*, vol. 51, no. 18, pp. 5522–5532, 2008.

[28] H. Fredly, E. Ersvær, C. Stapnes, B. T. Gjertsen, and Ø. Bruserud, "The combination of conventional chemotherapy with new targeted therapy in hematologic malignancies: the safety and efficiency of low-dose cytarabine supports its combination with new therapeutic agents in early clinical trials," *Current Cancer Therapy Reviews*, vol. 5, no. 4, pp. 243–255, 2009.

[29] H. Fredly, C. Stapnes Bjørnsen, B. T. Gjertsen, and Ø. Bruserud, "Combination of the histone deacetylase inhibitor valproic acid with oral hydroxyurea or 6-mercaptopurin can be safe and effective in patients with advanced acute myeloid leukaemia—a report of five cases," *Hematology*, vol. 15, no. 5, pp. 338–343, 2010.

[30] F. Zhang, A. S. Lazorchak, D. Liu, F. Chen, and B. Su, "Inhibition of the mTORC2 and chaperone pathways to treat leukemia," *Blood*, vol. 119, pp. 6080–6088, 2012.

[31] N. Chapuis, J. Tamburini, A. S. Green et al., "Perspectives on inhibiting mTOR as a future treatment strategy for hematological malignancies," *Leukemia*, vol. 24, no. 10, pp. 1686–1699, 2010.

[32] H. Reikvam, K. Hatfield, E. Ersvaer, A. Ryningen, and Bruserud Ø, "Pharmacological targeting of the PI3K-AKT/PKB-mTOR pathway alters local angioregulation in acute myelogenous leukemia," *Haematologica*, vol. 95, no. s2, abstract 0634, 2010.

[33] A. M. Martelli, F. Chiarini, C. Evangelisti et al., "Two hits are better than one: targeting both phosphatidylinositol 3-kinase and mammalian target of rapamycin as a therapeutic strategy for acute leukemia treatment," *Oncotarget*, vol. 3, pp. 371–394, 2012.

[34] Ø. Bruserud, C. Stapnes, E. Ersvær, B. T. Gjertsen, and A. Ryningen, "Histone deacetylase inhibitors in cancer treatment: a review of the clinical toxicity and the modulation of gene expression in cancer cells," *Current Pharmaceutical Biotechnology*, vol. 8, no. 6, pp. 388–400, 2007.

[35] H. Reikvam, A. M. Olsnes, B. T. Gjertsen, E. Ersvar, and O. Bruserud, "Nuclear factor-κB signaling: a contributor in leukemogenesis and a target for pharmacological intervention in human acute myelogenous leukemia," *Critical Reviews in Oncogenesis*, vol. 15, no. 1-2, pp. 1–41, 2009.

9

Influence of Bisphosphonate Treatment on Medullary Macrophages and Osteoclasts: An Experimental Study

Natalia Daniela Escudero and Patricia Mónica Mandalunis

Histology and Embryology Department, School of Dentistry, University of Buenos Aires, Marcelo T de Alvear 2142 1° piso sector A, (C1122AAH) Ciudad Autónoma de Buenos Aires, C1122AAH Buenos Aires, Argentina

Correspondence should be addressed to Natalia Daniela Escudero, nataliaescudero5@yahoo.com.ar

Academic Editor: Helen A. Papadaki

Nitrogen-containing bisphosphonates are widely used for treating diverse bone pathologies. They are anticatabolic drugs that act on osteoclasts inhibiting bone resorption. It remains unknown whether the mechanism of action is by decreasing osteoclast number, impairing osteoclast function, or whether they continue to effectively inhibit bone resorption despite the increase in osteoclast number. There is increasing evidence that bisphosphonates also act on bone marrow cells like macrophages and monocytes. The present work sought to evaluate the dynamics of preosteoclast fusion and possible changes in medullary macrophage number in bisphosphonate-treated animals. Healthy female Wistar rats received olpadronate, alendronate, or vehicle during 5 weeks, and 5-bromo-2-deoxyuridine (BrdU) on day 7, 28, or 34 of the experiment. Histomorphometric studies were performed to study femurs and evaluate: number of nuclei per osteoclast (N.Nu/Oc); number of BrdU-positive nuclei (N.Nu BrdU+/Oc); percentage of BrdU-positive nuclei per osteoclast (%Nu.BrdU+/Oc); medullary macrophage number (mac/mm^2) and correlation between N.Nu/Oc and mac/mm^2. Results showed bisphosphonate-treated animals exhibited increased N.Nu/Oc, caused by an increase in preosteoclast fusion rate and evidenced by higher N.Nu BrdU+/Oc, and significantly decreased mac/mm^2. Considering the common origin of osteoclasts and macrophages, the increased demand for precursors of the osteoclast lineage may occur at the expense of macrophage lineage precursors.

1. Introduction

Bisphosphonates, especially nitrogen-containing bisphosphonates, are the first-choice drugs in the pharmacological treatment of osteoporosis and other less prevalent bone pathologies. It is well documented that these anticatabolic drugs exert their action by partly inhibiting bone resorption caused by osteoclasts, either by decreasing the number of osteoclasts, altering recruitment, and/or stimulating apoptosis, [1–7], after which the apoptotic remains are phagocytosed by neighboring macrophages in bone marrow microenvironment. Nevertheless, there are reports indicating that the number of osteoclasts remains unchanged in spite of the significant increase in bone volume [8, 9]. Moreover, a number of studies including our research group have observed a significant increase in the number of osteoclasts [10–18]. More recently, patients treated with alendronate were found to exhibit large osteoclasts, with peculiar morphological features, termed "giant osteoclasts", whose formation, lifespan, and potential risk to patients remain unknown [19]. Similar findings from experimental studies in animals are scarce [16, 17, 20]. In addition, it has been reported that macrophages and monocytes are affected by bisphosphonate administration and the acute phase of the adverse reaction as well as the antitumor effects could be associated with the action of bisphosphonates on these cells [21].

Furthermore, it has been posited that the alteration of macrophages may play a role in the development of ONJ [22]. Preosteoclasts and macrophages have a common precursor: monocytes. The finding of hypernucleated osteoclasts in bisphosphonate-treated patients [19, 23] and in experimental animal models [16, 17, 20], has drawn attention to the dynamics of hypernucleated osteoclast formation and to the question whether macrophages are affected due to an increase in monocyte differentiation to the osteoclastic lineage. Based on the above, the aim of the present study was to assess the effect of bisphosphonates on macrophages and osteoclasts *in vivo*.

2. Materials and Methods

2.1. Experimental Design. Twenty female Wistar rats, aged 2 months, 170 ± 10 gr body weight, were used throughout. Housing conditions included galvanized wire cages, five animals per cage, 21–$24°C$ temperature, 52–56% humidity and 12-12 hrs light-dark cycles. The Guide for the Care and Use of Laboratory Animals (NRC 1996) was observed. The animals had free access to water and food (standard rat-mouse diet, Cooperación, Argentina) containing 23% protein, 1–1.4% calcium and 0.5–0.8% phosphorous. The animals were divided into three groups: two experimental and one sham. The experimental groups were i.p. injected with 0.3 mg/kg/week of monosodic olpadronate (OPD) and alendronate (ALN) (Gador SA), respectively, during 5 weeks; the dose was adjusted to body weight weekly. The sham group received an equal dose of saline solution during the same time interval. In addition, all animals received a single i.p. dose of 100 mg/kg body weight of 5-Bromo 2-deoxyuridine (BrdU). The animals in each of the groups were assigned to one of three subsets and injected with BrdU on day 7, 28, or 34 (i.e., one month, one week, or one day prior to euthanasia, resp.) (Figure 1). Euthanasia was performed on day 35 by administering acepromazine in a dose of 0.5 mg/kg bw (Acepromacina, Holliday Laboratories), ketamine 40 mg/kg bw (Ketamina 50, Holliday Laboratories), sodium pentobarbital 50 mg/kg bw and diphenylhydantoin sodium 6 mg/kg bw (Euthanyle, Brouwer Laboratories), all administered via i.p. After euthanasia left, femurs were resected.

2.2. Immunohistochemistry. The femurs were fixed in PBS-formalin at pH 7.2 and $4°C$ for 48 hrs and then decalcified in EDTA at the same temperature and pH. They were then dehydrated in ethyl alcohol (Biopack Argentina), clarified in xylol (Biopack Argentina) and embedded in paraffin to obtain longitudinal sections of the distal epiphysis. Two histologic sections were obtained from each femur; one was processed for immunohistochemical (IHC) detection of ED1 to detect cells of the phagocytic mononuclear system (macrophages, preosteoclasts, and osteoclasts belong to the phagocytic mononuclear system, so they express ED1 in the surface of their lysosomes), and the other was processed for immunohistochemical detection of BrdU to determine the number of stained nuclei in the osteoclasts.

For IHC detection of ED1, the sections were rehydrated in ethyl alcohol and washed with PBS 0.02 M (DakoCytomaton S3024). Antigen retrieval was performed with 0.1% trypsin in tris-maleate (Sigma-Aldrich, T0303-1G) at pH 7 and $37°C$ for 10 minutes. Following antigen retrieval, the sections were washed with PBS and endogenous peroxidase was blocked with 3% hydrogen peroxide (Biopack Argentina) in PBS for 10 minutes. The sections were incubated with mouse anti-rat ED1 monoclonal antibody (MAB 1435, Chemicon

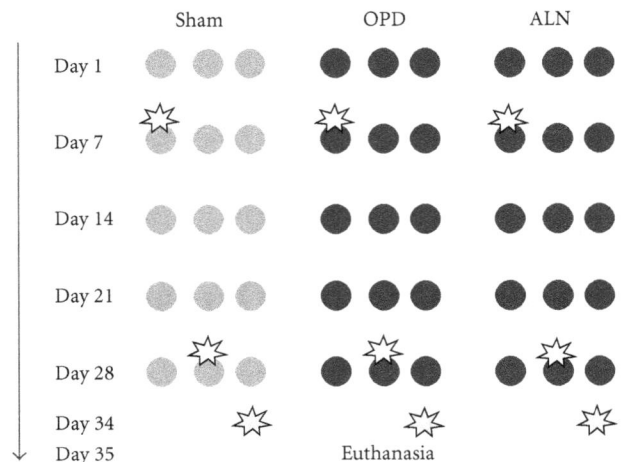

FIGURE 1: Experimental Design. Female Wistar rats were used, divided into three groups: Sham, OPD, and ALN. Each one of the groups was divided into three subgroups and the columns of circles indicate these subsets into which the animals in each group were divided. The rows show weekly administration of vehicle (light gray) or 0.3 mg/kg of the corresponding bisphosphonate olpadronate or alendronate (dark gray). The star indicates the time of administration of the single dose of BrdU, that is, days 7, 28, or 34 of the experiment. All animals were euthanized on day 35 of the experiment.

International Inc.) diluted $1:450$ in PBS in a humidity chamber at $4°C$ overnight, following the manufacturer's instructions.

For IHC detection of BrdU, the sections were dehydrated in ethanol and methanol (both Biopack Argentina). Endogenous peroxidase was then blocked with 1% hydrogen peroxide in methanol for 30 minutes. After washing with distilled water, antigen retrieval was performed by two, 3-minute cycles in 0.01 M citrate buffer in a microwave oven. Following antigen retrieval, the sections were allowed to cool to room temperature and unspecific reactions were blocked by immersion in 0.1% BSA (Sigma Aldrich) in PBS for 1 hour. The sections were incubated with the primary antibody reagent ($1:100$ in PBS with 1% BSA and 0.09% sodium azide at pH 7.6) (AM 247-5 M Biogenex) at room temperature in a humidity chamber for 30 minutes.

After incubation with the primary antibody, anti-ED1 or anti-BrdU, the sections were washed with PBS and incubated with biotinylated antibody (BioGenex) for 1 hr, washed with PBS, and incubated with streptavidin-peroxidase complex. The sections were revealed with Diaminobenzidine (DAB) for 7 to 10 minutes (SK 4100, Vector Laboratories Inc), contrasted with hematoxylin, dehydrated, and mounted with Canada balsam. All sections for ED1 IHC detection were processed simultaneously, as BrdU sections.

2.3. Histomorphometry. From each histological section stained for detection of ED1, 35 digital microphotographs at 1000X magnification were obtained using a photomicroscope (Axioskop 2, Carl Zeiss Jena, Germany), and the number of macrophages in the dyaphiseal bone marrow was determined using Image Pro Plus 6.1 computer software

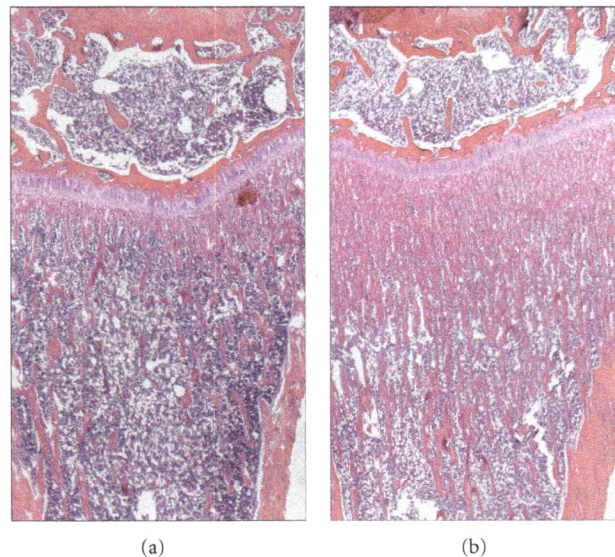

(a)   (b)

FIGURE 2: Microphotographs of hematoxylin-eosin-stained histological sections of distal tibia. Animals treated with BPs showed a larger number of subchondral trabecualae (b) compared to sham (a).

(Media Cybernetics). Mononuclear cells showing cytoplasmic expression of ED1 were diagnosed as macrophages. Diaphyseal bone marrow was used, distant from any bone surface, because mononuclear cells neighboring bone trabeculae and cortical bone could be either macropages or preosteoclasts. In addition, the distribution of ED1 in the cytoplasm of osteoclasts located near the surface of subchondral trabeculae was observed and evaluated using 1000X magnification. Cells with 2 or more nuclei, in close relation with bone surface were diagnosed as osteoclasts (preosteoclasts are mononucleated, so 2 nuclei already represents multinucleation, and only osteoclasts are multinucleated).

Histologic sections stained for BrdU detection were examined by direct observation under a light-field microscope using 1000X magnification to evaluate osteoclasts in primary and secondary spongiosa. The following parameters were studied: number of nuclei (N.Nu/Oc), mean number of BrdU-positive nuclei per osteoclast (N.Nu BrdU+/Oc), and percentage of BrdU-positive nuclei per osteoclast (%Nu. BrdU+/Oc).

The results were analyzed using one-way ANOVA or the Kruskal Wallis test accordingly, and the Bonferroni post hoc test; in order to study dependence between the number of nuclei per Oc and number of macrophages, Spearman's rank correlation was used. p values below 0.05 were considered significant.

3. Results

The effect of BPs on bone volume in tibia are illustrated in Figure 2.

Sections stained immunohistochemically for detection of ED1 corresponding to bisphosphonate-treated animals showed a decrease in the number of macrophages per mm²: sham 54.6 ± 19.6 mac/mm², OPD 21.3 ± 10 mac/mm², ALN 12.3 ± 4.1 mac/mm²; Anova $p < 0.01$ (Bonferroni test: sham versus OPD and sham versus ALN) (Figures 3 and 4).

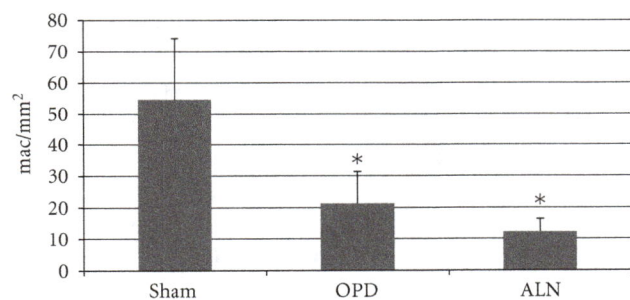

FIGURE 3: Number of macrophages in diaphyseal bone marrow. The number of macrophages, measured using IHC ED1 detection, was significantly lower in bisphosphonate-treated animals compared to sham (*: Anova $p < 0.01$ compared to sham).

Evaluation of IHC expression of ED1 by osteoclasts showed all osteoclasts were ED1-positive, regardless of the treatment and osteoclast features. Even those exhibiting morphological features compatible with apoptosis were found to be ED1-positive (Figure 5(d)). Cytoplasmic expression varied in intensity and distribution pattern in the cytoplasm, and in some cases was found in some sectors only. Sham osteoclasts showed marked vacuolization whereas osteoclasts corresponding to bisphosphonate-treated animals exhibited a more homogenous distribution pattern (Figures 5(a), 5(b) and 5(c)). Large hypernucleated osteoclasts were found in the latter groups, and though most were detached from bone trabeculae they presented some active sectors superficially associated with an erosive bone surface. The presence of osteoclasts with long cytoplasmic projections extending through tubular resorption cavities in the bone matrix was a characteristic finding (Figures 5(b) and 5(c)).

As regards BrdU, because this marker is incorporated into the cell nucleus during the S period of the cell cycle (prior to mitosis), osteoclasts of animals receiving BrdU on

(a)

(b)

(c)

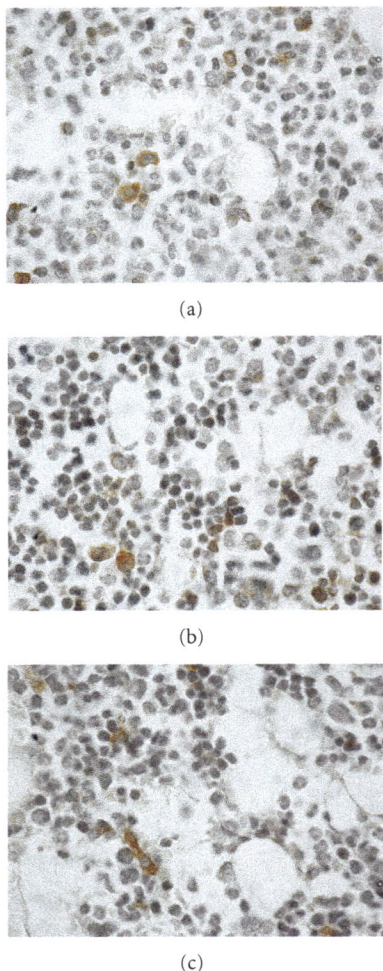

FIGURE 4: Macrophages in diaphyseal bone marrow. Micropho-tographs of histologic sections with ED1 immunohistochemical detection and hematoxylin-counterstain. Brown cells correspond to positive cells (macrophages). (a) shows a microphotograph of a sham animal, (b) an olpadronate-treated animal and (c) and alendronate-treated one. (b) and (c) show a lower number of positive cells.

day 34 (24 hr before euthanasia) exhibited intense nuclear staining (when positive). The intensity of IHC staining for BrdU in histologic sections corresponding to animals receiving BrdU on day 28 of the experiment (one week prior to euthanasia) was similar to that observed on day 34. Both administration times were useful to assess recruitment of osteoclast precursors and their differentiation into multi-nucleated osteoclasts (taking into account that osteoclasts originate from fusion of posmitotic precursors). Nuclear staining in histologic sections of animals receiving BrdU on day 7 of the experiment, which was performed mainly to observe changes in osteoclast lifespan, was not as intense as that observed in sections corresponding to animals receiving BrdU on day 28 or 34 and it is in agreement with the fact that the intensity of BrdU staining is inversely proportional to the number of mitosis of the monocytic precursor in bone marrow.

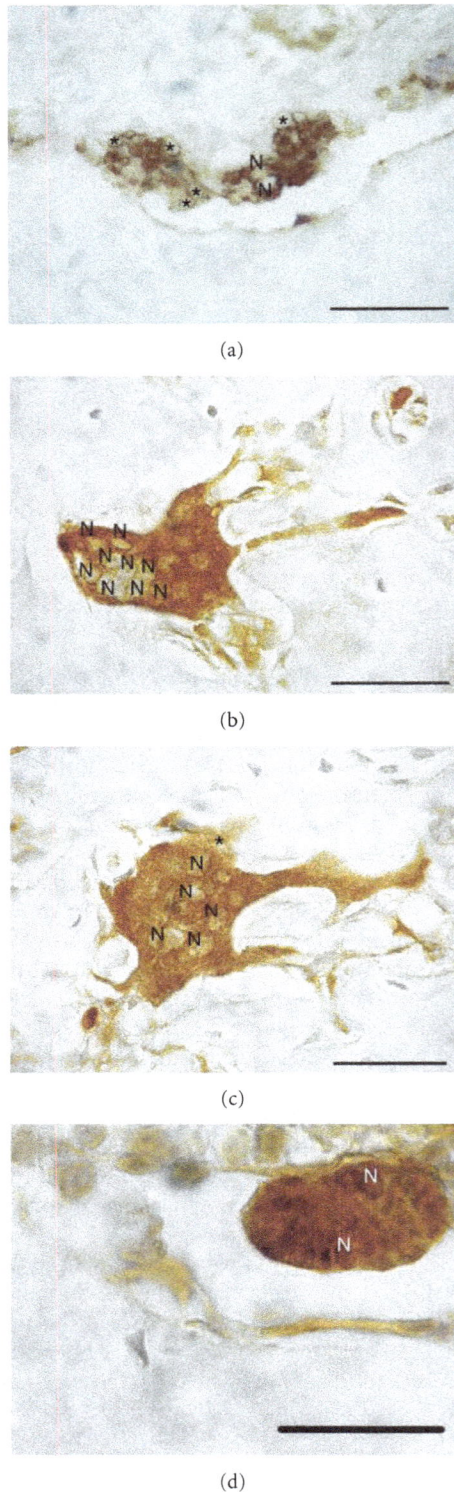

(a)

(b)

(c)

(d)

FIGURE 5: Microphotographs of osteoclasts stained for IHC detec-tion of ED1. Microphotograph (a) shows the distribution pattern of the marker in the cytoplasm of osteoclasts of sham group sections; the light areas indicate abundant vesicles (*). (b) and (c) show osteoclasts corresponding to olpadronate and alendronate-treated animals, respectively. The cytoplasm exhibits a homogenous distribution pattern of ED1. (d) shows an apoptotic osteoclast staining intensely positive for ED1. N: nucleus. The bar represents 50 microns.

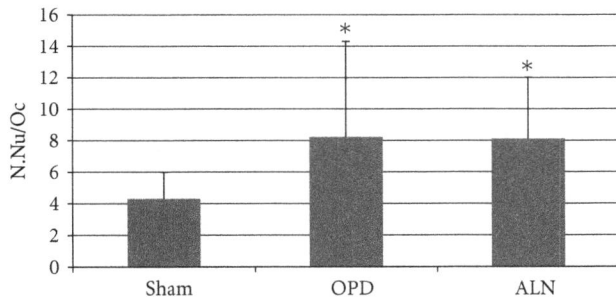

FIGURE 6: Mean number of nuclei in osteoclasts. The mean number of nuclei per osteoclast was evaluated in BrdU-detection sections, was significantly higher in bisphosphonate-treated animals compared to sham (*: Kruskal Wallis $p < 0.01$). Both positive and negative nuclei were counted to assess this parameter.

N.Nu/Oc. sham 4.3 ± 1.7 Nu/Oc, $n = 7$ animals; OPD 8.2 ± 6.1 Nu/Oc, $n = 7$ animals; ALN 8.1 ± 3.9 Nu/Oc, $n = 7$ animals, Kruskal Wallis $p < 0.01$, Bonferroni test: sham versus OPD and ALN, 825 Ocs were assessed in the three groups (Figure 6). Taking into account that number of nuclei is directly associated with osteoclast size, it follows that osteoclasts of bisphosphonate-treated animals were larger than those of sham animals.

N.Nu BrdU+/Oc. Both groups of bisphosphonate-treated animals receiving BrdU on day 7 of the experiment showed a greater number of stained nuclei as compared to shams (sham 0.38 ± 0.68 Nu+/Oc $n = 70$ Ocs, OPD 1.86 ± 2.32 Nu+/Oc $n = 75$ Ocs, ALN 1.28 ± 2.18 Nu+/Oc $n = 80$ Ocs, Kruskal Wallis $p < 0.001$, Bonferroni sham versus OPD and sham versus ALN). The same trend was observed in animals receiving BrdU on day 28 (sham 0.05 ± 0.22 Nu+/Oc $n = 40$ Ocs, OPD 0.46 ± 0.95 Nu+/Oc $n = 80$ Ocs, ALN 0.74 ± 1.42 Nu+/Oc $n = 120$ Ocs, Kruskal Wallis $p < 0.05$, Bonferroni sham versus OPD and sham versus ALN) and in the subsets receiving BrdU on day 34 (sham 0.03 ± 0.18 Nu+/Oc $n = 120$ Ocs, OPD 0.3 ± 0.82 Nu+/Oc $n = 120$ Ocs, ALN 0.46 ± 0.86 Nu+/Oc $n = 120$ Ocs, Kruskal Wallis $p < 0.001$, Bonferroni sham versus OPD and sham versus ALN) (Figures 7 and 8).

%Nu.BrdU+/Oc. A significant increase in the percentage of positive nuclei per osteoclast (Oc) was observed in all BrdU subsets of bisphosphonate-treated animals: day 7: sham $10.3 \pm 19.6\%$ $n = 70$ Ocs, OPD $30.5 \pm 31.6\%$ $n = 75$ Ocs, ALN 16.3 ± 25.6 $n = 105$ Ocs; day 28: sham $0.98 \pm 4.5\%$ $n = 40$ Ocs, OPD $7 \pm 14.2\%$ $n = 80$ Ocs, ALN: $8.3 \pm 15.3\%$ $n = 120$ Ocs; day 34: sham $0.63 \pm 3.5\%$ $n = 120$ Ocs, OPD $4.6 \pm 11.2\%$ $n = 120$ Ocs, ALN $7.4 \pm 13.5\%$ $n = 120$ Ocs, Kruskal Wallis $p < 0.05$ in all cases, Bonferroni sham versus OPD and sham versus ALN at all three BrdU administration times (Figure 9).

Correlation between the Number of Nuclei per Osteoclast and Number of Macrophages. An inverse correlation (-0.6)

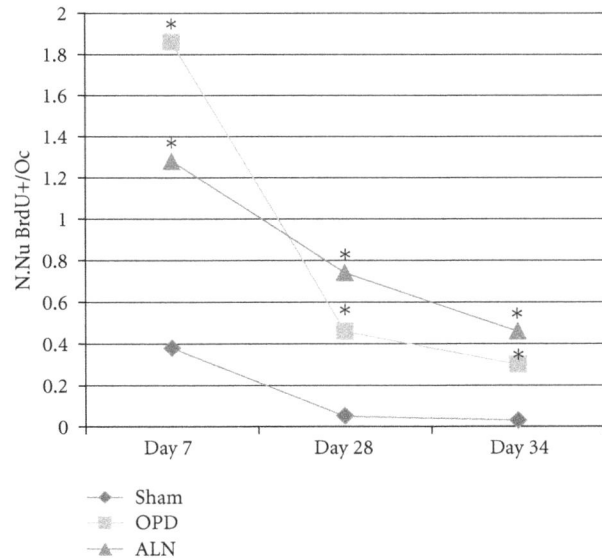

FIGURE 7: The number in BrdU-positive nuclei per osteoclast was greater in bisphosphonate-treated animals at all three BrdU administration times (*: Kruskal Wallis $p < 0.001$ for days 7 and 34, $p < 0.05$ for day 28). Standard deviations are not represented because of high dispersion, which produces lines superposition (see data on text).

was found between N.Nu/Oc and mac/mm^2 (Figure 10): as number of nuclei per osteoclasts increased in BP-treated groups, the number of macrophages decreased (Spearman's test $p < 0.05$).

4. Discussion

The results of the present work show that animals treated with both the bisphosphonates exhibited a significant decrease in the number of medullary macrophages as compared to shams. In their 1999 study on mice treated with the aminobisphosphonate AHBuBP, Nakamura et al. also observed a decrease in erythroblastic island macrophages [14]. Macrophages have multiple functions, and their decrease, therefore, can have a number of implications. One such function is the removal of apoptotic cells. In previous works in bisphosphonate-treated animals, we found an increase in the number of osteoclasts as well as an increase in the number of apoptotic osteoclasts [17]. The question thus arises whether the increase in the number of apoptotic osteoclasts observed in histologic sections is caused only by the effect of bisphosphonates on osteoclasts, or whether apoptotic debris remain in the bone microenvironment over a more prolonged period of time due to a deficiency in phagocytosis. As osteoclast size is directly associated with the number of precursors that fuse to form multinucleated osteoclasts, it can be posited that those presenting a large number of nuclei were, in turn, large osteoclasts; removal of such large osteoclasts may contribute to the inefficient clearance of debris.

Macrophages also have an immune function, and its impairment could thus be associated with the development

(a)

(b)

(c)

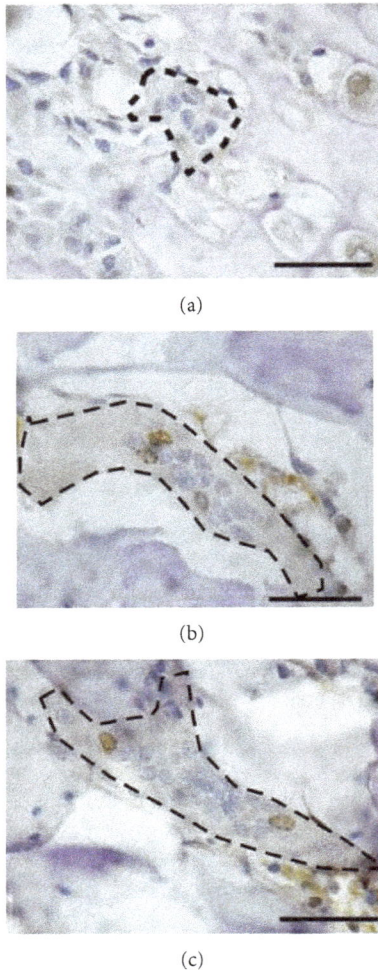

FIGURE 8: Microphotographs of osteoclasts stained immunohistochemically for BrdU. (a): dotted line: osteoclasts corresponding to the sham group showing 8 nuclei, none of which were BrdU-positive. (b): osteoclast corresponding to an olpadronate-treated animal showing at least 15 nuclear profiles, 3 of which were BrdU-positive. (c): osteoclast corresponding to an ALN-treated animal showing 2 BrdU-positive nuclei out of more than 25. The bar represents 50 microns.

FIGURE 9: Percentage of BrdU positive-nuclei per osteoclast. The percentage of BrdU-positive nuclei per osteoclast was higher in the bisphosphonate-treated groups at all three BrdU administration times (day 7, 28, or 35 of the experiment corresponding to one month, one week, and one day before euthanasia resp.) (*Kruskal Wallis $p < 0.05$ compared to sham).

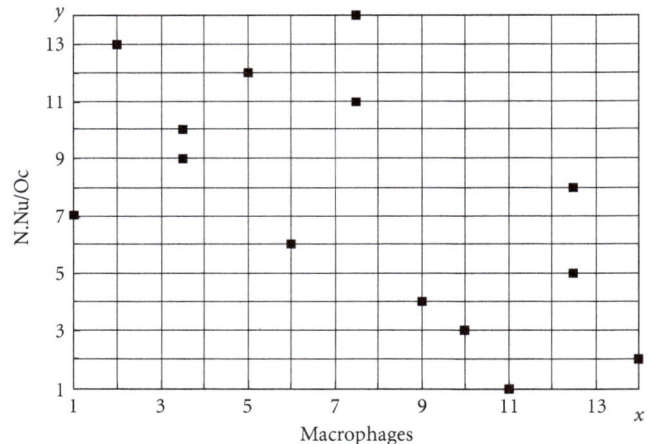

FIGURE 10: Number of nuclei per osteoclast and number of macrophages. These two variables showed a negative correlation (−0.6), as number of nuclei increased in BP-treated animals, the number of macrophages in bone marrow consequently decreased (n sham = 7, n BP-treated = 7). $p < 0.05$, Spearman's test.

of osteonecrosis of the jaw, as has been suggested previously [22, 24].

The finding of a large number of nuclei in BrdU-stained sections is in agreement with reports by other authors [19] who found "giant" osteoclasts containing a large number of nuclei and that were detached from the bone surface. Our observation of giant osteoclasts coexisting with normal-appearing osteoclasts in bisphosphonate-treated animals is also in keeping with the aforementioned report. The coexistence of osteoclasts similar in size to controls with other larger osteoclasts is shown by the greater dispersion of the data on the number of nuclei found in both bisphosphonate-treated groups. Based on the observation of stained nuclei in bisphosphonate-treated animals receiving BrdU 24 hrs before euthanasia it can be inferred that not all giant osteoclasts detached from the bone surface are inactive forms

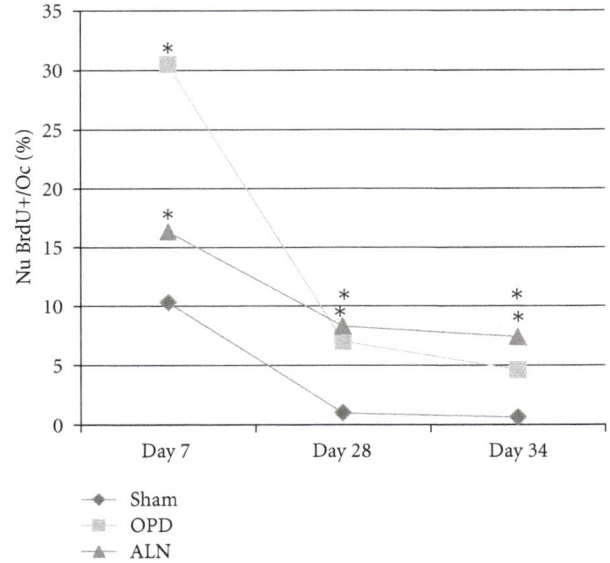

that will remain inactive from a recruitment viewpoint, but rather may be found to be actively incorporating precursors. It cannot be concluded that these osteoclasts were significantly smaller and functionally normal at some previous stage. The finding of a greater number of nuclei in osteoclasts from bisphosphonate-treated animals is in agreement with previous in vivo studies in children with osteogenesis imperfecta treated with risedronate [23] and patients with osteoporosis treated with alendronate [19]. BrdU staining resulting from BrdU administration 24 hrs and 1 week before euthanasia showed that the number and percentage of stained nuclei were higher in both bisphosphonate-treated groups. Our results are in keeping with those of other authors who used BrdU [11] and tritiated thymidine [25]; the latter are the only studies reported in the literature using nuclei staining to evaluate osteoclast recruitment. Staining with BrdU administered 1 month before euthanasia was almost undetectable; the number and percentage of stained nuclei were higher in bisphosphonate-treated than sham animals and in the subset receiving BrdU on day 7 compared to the remaining subsets of the same group. The difference between bisphosphonate-treated and sham animals may be due to an increased fusion of osteoclast precursors caused by bisphosphonates, as found in groups receiving BrdU 24 hrs and 1 week prior to euthanasia. The difference among subsets of the same group may be because renewal of hematopoietic stem cells results in a greater number of stained precursors, though intensity of staining is proportionally lower to the number of mitosis of the hematopoietic stem cell. The main aim of administering BrdU at this experimental time (1 month before euthanasia) was to observe changes in osteoclast lifespan. Such changes could be a shortening of osteoclast longevity manifesting as fewer or lack of BrdU-positive nuclei compared to shams, or a lengthening of osteoclast lifespan made apparent by more intensely stained nuclei in bisphosphonate treated animals as compared to controls. Our study could not detect changes in osteoclast lifespan. The lack of differences indicates that the lifespan of osteoclasts was less than one month, that is, the administration time used to evaluate osteoclast lifespan, and would explain why less-marked changes might not have been detected in our experimental design. The use of shorter administration times of BrdU that allow assessing less extreme changes in osteoclast lifespan may prove useful for designing future studies.

Considering that osteoclasts with 30 or more nuclei had 1 or 2 positive nuclei when BrdU was administered 24 hrs prior to euthanasia, it follows that the time course of osteoclast formation in this case could not have been less than 15 days, provided that the rate of precursor fusion remained constant. The time course of normal osteoclast formation, however, is no longer than 4 to 6 days [26]. Hence, although no changes in osteoclast lifespan were detected, it can be concluded that the time for fusion of osteoclasts with additional mononuclear progenitors is longer in bisphosphonate-treated animals. In addition, as mentioned previously, some giant osteoclasts seemed to be partially active. It remains to be clarified whether in spite of having initiated resorption, fusion of these osteoclasts with precursors continues, thus increasing in size as they continue to attempt but fail to resorb bone matrix.

As to the rate of precursor recruitment, the sharper slope observed in bisphosphonate-treated animals from day 28 to day 34 of BrdU administration depicted in Figure 5 may be associated with a higher rate of precursor fusion. The greater number of stained nuclei observed in animals receiving BrdU on day 7 as compared with the subsets of the same group (i.e., the remaining BrdU administration times) is due to mitosis of the hematopoietic stem cell.

It remains to be elucidated whether the decrease in the number of macrophages observed in the present study is due to a direct effect of bisphosphonates on these cells [21, 27] or whether monocytes, the precursors of macrophages and preosteoclasts, become committed to the osteoclast lineage at the expense of the macrophagic lineage [14] supporting our finding of negative correlation between number of nuclei and number of macrophages, also explaining the presence of hypernucleated, large osteoclasts. Further studies are necessary to determine if macrophage depletion is directly related to the increase in osteoclast number or if they are effects of bisphosphonates, independent one to another.

It is well documented that increased RANKL expression in the environment promotes differentiation of preosteoclasts to osteoclasts [28, 29]. In addition, previous findings reported by our group showed that nitrogen-containing bisphosphonates increase the number of megakaryocytes, which express RANKL, and thus might act as an additional source of RANKL in the bone microenvironment and contribute to precursor cells committing to the osteoclast lineage at the expense of the macrophagic lineage [17].

Acknowledgments

This work was supported by Grant UBACyT 20020090100210 from the University of Buenos Aires. The authors wish to thank Gador S.A. for supplying both bisphosphonates, alendronate and olpadronate, Dr. Mariel Itoiz and Dr. Miguel Pérez for kindly supplying BrdU and training us in its use, Victor Tomas CLT for performing the BrdU IHC detection, Ms. Lewicki DVM for her collaboration during the experiments, and Mariela Lacave CLT for obtaining histological sections and carrying out IHC staining for ED1.

References

[1] E. Hiroi-Furuya, T. Kameda, K. Hiura et al., "Etidronate (EHDP) inhibits osteoclastic-bone resorption, promotes apoptosis and disrupts actin rings in isolate-mature osteoclasts," *Calcified Tissue International*, vol. 64, no. 3, pp. 219–223, 1999.

[2] H. L. Benford, N. W. A. McGowan, M. H. Helfrich, M. E. Nuttall, and M. J. Rogers, "Visualization of bisphosphonate-induced caspase-3 activity in apoptotic osteoclasts in vitro," *Bone*, vol. 28, no. 5, pp. 465–473, 2001.

[3] E. R. Van Beek, C. W. G. M. Löwik, and S. E. Papapoulos, "Bisphosphonates suppress bone resorption by a direct effect on early osteoclast precursors without affecting the osteoclastogenic capacity of osteogenic cells: the role of protein geranylgeranylation in the action of nitrogencontaining bisphosphonates on osteoclast precursors," *Bone*, vol. 30, no. 1, pp. 64–70, 2002.

[4] H. Sudhoff, J. Y. Jung, J. Ebmeyer, B. T. Faddis, H. Hildmann, and R. A. Chole, "Zoledronic acid inhibits osteoclastogenesis in vitro and in a mouse model of inflammatory osteolysis," *Annals of Otology, Rhinology and Laryngology*, vol. 112, no. 9, pp. 780–786, 2003.

[5] H. B. Kwak, J. Y. Kim, K. J. Kim et al., "Risedronate directly inhibits osteoclast differentiation and inflammatory bone

loss," *Biological and Pharmaceutical Bulletin*, vol. 32, no. 7, pp. 1193–1198, 2009.

[6] L. C. Spolidorio, E. Marcantonio Jr., D. M. P. Spolidorio et al., "Alendronate therapy in cyclosporine-induced alveolar bone loss in rats," *Journal of Periodontal Research*, vol. 42, no. 5, pp. 466–473, 2007.

[7] K. E. S. Poole, S. Vedi, I. Debiram et al., "Bone structure and remodelling in stroke patients: early effects of zoledronate," *Bone*, vol. 44, no. 4, pp. 629–633, 2009.

[8] V. Breuil, F. Cosman, L. Stein et al., "Human osteoclast formation and activity in vitro: effects of alendronate," *Journal of Bone and Mineral Research*, vol. 13, no. 11, pp. 1721–1729, 1998.

[9] Y. Koshihara, S. Kodama, H. Ishibashi, Y. Azuma, T. Ohta, and S. Karube, "Reversibility of alendronate-induced contraction in human osteoclast- like cells formed from bone marrow cells in culture," *Journal of Bone and Mineral Metabolism*, vol. 17, no. 2, pp. 98–107, 1999.

[10] M. J. Marshall, A. S. Wilson, and M. W. J. Davie, "Effects of (3-amino-1-hydroxypropylidene)-1,1-bisphosphonate on mouse osteoclasts," *Journal of Bone and Mineral Research*, vol. 5, no. 9, pp. 955–962, 1990.

[11] M. J. Marshall, I. Holt, and M. W. J. Davie, "Osteo-clast recruitment in mice is stimulated by (3-amino-1- hydroxypropylidene)-1,1-bisphosphonate," *Calcified Tissue International*, vol. 52, no. 1, pp. 21–25, 1993.

[12] Y. Endo, M. Nakamura, T. Kikuchi et al., "Aminoalkylbis-phosphonates, potent inhibitors of bone resorption, induce a prolonged stimulation of histamine synthesis and increase macrophages, granulocytes, and osteoclasts *in vivo*," *Calcified Tissue International*, vol. 52, no. 3, pp. 248–254, 1993.

[13] I. Holt, M. J. Marshall, and M. W. J. Davie, "Pamidronate stimulates recruitment and decreases longevity of osteoclast nuclei in mice," *Seminars in Arthritis and Rheumatism*, vol. 23, no. 4, pp. 263–264, 1994.

[14] M. Nakamura, H. Yagi, Y. Endo, H. Kosugi, T. Ishi, and T. Itoh, "A time kinetic study of the effect of aminobisphosphonate on murine haemopoiesis," *British Journal of Haematology*, vol. 107, no. 4, pp. 779–790, 1999.

[15] E. J. Smith, A. McEvoy, D. G. Little, P. A. Baldock, J. A. Eisman, and E. M. Gardiner, "Transient retention of endochondral cartilaginous matrix with bisphosphonate treatment in a long-term rabbit model of distraction osteogenesis," *Journal of Bone and Mineral Research*, vol. 19, no. 10, pp. 1698–1705, 2004.

[16] G. Shu, K. Yamamoto, and M. Nagashima, "Differences in osteoclast formation between proximal and distal tibial osteoporosis in rats with adjuvant arthritis: inhibitory effects of bisphosphonates on osteoclasts," *Modern Rheumatology*, vol. 16, no. 6, pp. 343–349, 2006.

[17] N. D. Escudero, M. Lacave, A. M. Ubios, and P. M. Mandalu-nis, "Effect of monosodium olpadronate on osteoclasts and megakaryocytes: an *in vivo* study," *Journal of Musculoskeletal Neuronal Interactions*, vol. 9, no. 2, pp. 109–120, 2009.

[18] S. Ralte, K. Khatri, and M. Nagar, "Short-term effects of zoledronate on the histomorphology of osteoclast in young albino rats," *Annals of Anatomy*, vol. 193, no. 6, pp. 509–515, 2011.

[19] R. S. Weinstein, P. K. Roberson, and S. C. Manolagas, "Giant osteoclast formation and long-term oral bisphosphonate therapy," *The New England Journal of Medicine*, vol. 360, no. 1, pp. 53–62, 2009.

[20] Y. Bi, Y. Gao, D. Ehirchiou et al., "Bisphosphonates cause osteonecrosis of the jaw-like disease in mice," *American Journal of Pathology*, vol. 177, no. 1, pp. 280–290, 2010.

[21] A. J. Roelofs, M. Jauhiainen, H. Mönkkönen, M. J. Rogers, J. Mönkkönen, and K. Thompson, "Peripheral blood monocytes are responsible for $\gamma\delta$ T cell activation induced by zoledronic acid through accumulation of IPP/DMAPP," *British Journal of Haematology*, vol. 144, no. 2, pp. 245–250, 2009.

[22] M. Pazianas, "Osteonecrosis of the jaw and the role of macrophages," *Journal of the National Cancer Institute*, vol. 103, no. 3, pp. 232–240, 2011.

[23] M. S. Cheung, F. H. Glorieux, and F. Rauch, "Large osteoclasts in pediatric osteogenesis imperfecta patients receiving intra-venous pamidronate," *Journal of Bone and Mineral Research*, vol. 24, no. 4, pp. 669–674, 2009.

[24] E. L. Scheller, K. D. Hankenson, J. S. Reuben, and P. H. Krebsbach, "Zoledronic acid inhibits macrophage SOCS3 expression and enhances cytokine production," *Journal of Cellular Biochemistry*, vol. 112, no. 11, pp. 3364–3372, 2011.

[25] S. C. Miller, W. S. S. Jee, D. B. Kimmel, and L. Woodbury, "Ethane 1 hydroxy 1,1 diphosphonate (EHDP) effects on incorporation and accumulation of osteoclast nuclei," *Calcified Tissue International*, vol. 22, no. 3, pp. 243–252, 1977.

[26] T. Kurachi, I. Morita, T. Oki et al., "Expression on outer membranes of mannose residues, which are involved in osteoclast formation via cellular fusion events," *Journal of Biological Chemistry*, vol. 269, no. 26, pp. 17572–17576, 1994.

[27] F. P. Coxon, K. Thompson, A. J. Roelofs, F. H. Ebetino, and M. J. Rogers, "Visualizing mineral binding and uptake of bisphosphonate by osteoclasts and non-resorbing cells," *Bone*, vol. 42, no. 5, pp. 848–860, 2008.

[28] J. R. Edwards and G. R. Mundy, "Advances in osteoclast biology: old findings and new insights from mouse models," *Nature Reviews Rheumatology*, vol. 7, no. 4, pp. 235–243, 2011.

[29] M. J. Oursler, "Recent advances in understanding the mech-anisms of osteoclast precursor fusion," *Journal of Cellular Biochemistry*, vol. 110, no. 5, pp. 1058–1062, 2010.

10

Differential Expression of Matrix Metalloproteinase-2 Expression in Disseminated Tumor Cells and Micrometastasis in Bone Marrow of Patients with Nonmetastatic and Metastatic Prostate Cancer: Theoretical Considerations and Clinical Implications—An Immunocytochemical Study

Nigel P. Murray,[1,2,3] **Eduardo Reyes,**[1,4] **Pablo Tapia,**[5]
Leonardo Badínez,[6] **and Nelson Orellana**[1]

[1] Hematology, Division of Medicine, Hospital de Carabineros de Chile, Simón Bolívar 2200, Ñuñoa, 7770199 Santiago, Chile
[2] Instituto de Bio-Oncología, Avenida Salvador 95, Oficina 95, Providencia, 7500710 Santiago, Chile
[3] Circulating Tumor Cell Unit, Faculty of Medicine, Universidad Mayor, Renato Sánchez 4369, Las Condes, 7550224 Santiago, Chile
[4] Faculty of Medicine, Universidad Diego Portales, Manuel Rodriguez Sur 415, 8370179 Santiago, Chile
[5] Faculty of Medicine, Universidad Pontificia Católica de Chile, Avenida Libertador Bernardo O'Higgins 340, 8331150 Santiago, Chile
[6] Radiotherapy, Fundación Arturo López Pérez, Rancagua 899, Providencia, 7500921 Santiago, Chile

Correspondence should be addressed to Nigel P. Murray, nigelpetermurray@gmail.com

Academic Editor: Joseph H. Antin

Matrix metalloproteinase-2 (MMP-2) is important in the dissemination and invasion of tumor cells and activates angiogenesis. We present an immunocytochemical study of MMP-2 expression in circulating prostate cells (CPCs), disseminated tumor cells (DTCs), and micrometastasis (mM) in bone marrow of men with prostate cancer. *Methods and Patients.* Tumor cells were identified with anti-PSA immunocytochemistry. Positive samples underwent processing with anti-MMP-2, its expression was compared with Gleason score, concordance of expression, and metastatic and nonmetastatic disease. *Results.* 215 men participated, CPCs were detected in 62.7%, DTCs in 62.2%, and mM in 71.4% in nonmetastatic cancer; in metastatic cancer all had CPCs, DTCs, and mM detected. All CPCs and DTCs expressed MMP-2; in mM MMP-2 expression was positively associated with increasing Gleason score. MMP-2 expression in CPCs and DTCs showed concordance. In low grade tumors, mM and surrounding stromal cells were MMP-2 negative, with variable expression in high grade tumors; in metastatic disease, both mM and stromal cells were MMP-2 positive. *Conclusions.* CPCs and DTCs are different from mM, with inhibition of MMP-2 expression in mM of low grade tumors. With disease progression, MMP-2 expression increases in both mM and surrounding stromal cells, with implications for the use of bisphosphonates or MMP-2 inhibitors.

1. Introduction

With the increasing use of prostate specific antigen as a screening test to detect prostate cancer, the frequency of men presenting with metastatic disease has decreased [1, 2]. However, the death rate from prostate cancer has only slightly fallen [3], with metastatic disease being the commonest scenario leading to death. At least 85% of men with advanced disease will have bone metastasis [4, 5], with an increasing number of these patients believed to be metastasis-free at the time of initial treatment but who had occult micrometastasis. Furthermore, 30% to 50% of men with localized prostate cancer will develop biochemical failure with an increased PSA at 10 years. This is due to dissemination of cancer cells early in the disease and being not detected by conventional methods.

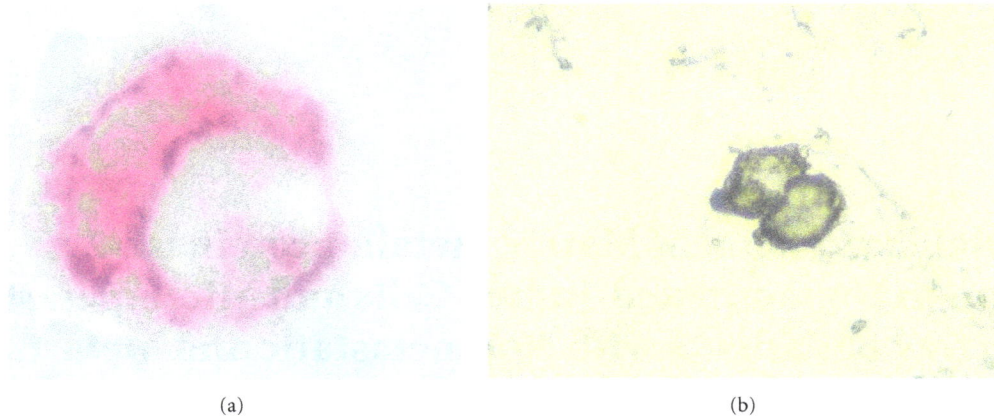

(a)   (b)

FIGURE 1: (a) PSA (+) CPC. (b) circulating leucocytes.

Cancer cells disseminate from the original cancer, first to the neurovascular structures and then to the blood [6]. From there they pass to other tissues where they may pass through (cells in transit) or adhere to the capillary endothelium and invade, forming micrometastasis. Tumor invasion is considered to be an unregulated physiological activity, with similarities between the molecular events of tumor invasion and normal processes such as angiogenesis and wound healing. One common denominator is the involvement of the matrix metalloproteinases. These are endopeptidases capable of degrading the extracellular matrix, contain zinc in their structure, and are secreted in latent form and later activated. It is postulated that they have an important role in metastasis and the liberation of growth factors [7, 8]. Matrix metalloproteinase-2 (MMP-2) is a gelatinase and its expression has been reported to be increased in prostate cancer [9–11]. There is an association between MMP-2 expression in the primary tumor and the Gleason score, pathological stage, and as an independent prognostic factor [11, 12]. In addition MMPs have been shown to be involved in the release of growth factors that enhance tumor growth and aggressiveness [13–15].

If, as the reports indicate, increased MMP-2 expression in the primary tumor is associated with a worse prognosis, one explication could be that cells expressing MMP-2 disseminate early to distant tissues, are not therefore affected by loco-regional treatments, and as a consequence are able to develop into metastasis. If this hypothesis is correct, circulating tumor cells should express MMP-2 whether they are circulating in blood or the bone marrow, and MMP-2 expression would permit the invasion of the endostium and therefore facilitate the formation of micrometastasis. The coexpression of PSA and MMP-2 in bone marrow fragments would confirm this hypothesis.

These data prompted us to investigate the expression of MMP-2 in circulating prostate cells in blood and bone marrow, and in the micrometastasis in bone marrow fragments in a population of patients with prostate cancer, after radical prostatectomy, both in patients bone scan negative and positive.

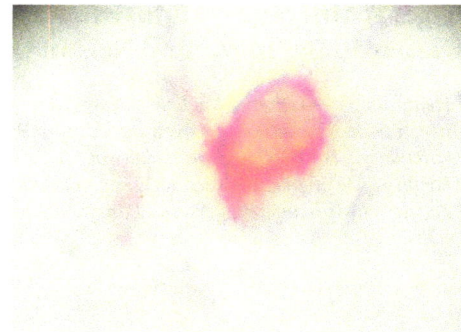

FIGURE 2: Disseminated tumor cell.

2. Methods and Patients

The transverse population included patients diagnosed with prostate cancer attending the Hospital de Carabineros de Chile and the Instituto of BioOncología, Santiago, Chile between 2008 and 2011. Patient records were used to retrieve clinical information (age, stage, Gleason score, treatment, bone scan results, and serum PSA at the time of sampling).

The following is definition of circulating prostate cells (CPCs), disseminated tumor cells (DTCs) in bone marrow aspirates, and micrometastasis (mM). The criteria of ISHAGE were used to evaluate immunostained cells [16].

(a) CPCs: secondary CPC: detected in blood after radical treatment (Figure 1(a)).

(b) DTCs: cells detected in bone marrow aspirates or bone marrow biopsy touch preparations, but not in bone marrow fragments (Figure 2).

(c) Micrometastasis: cells detected in bone marrow fragments from biopsy specimens (Figures 3(a)–3(i)).

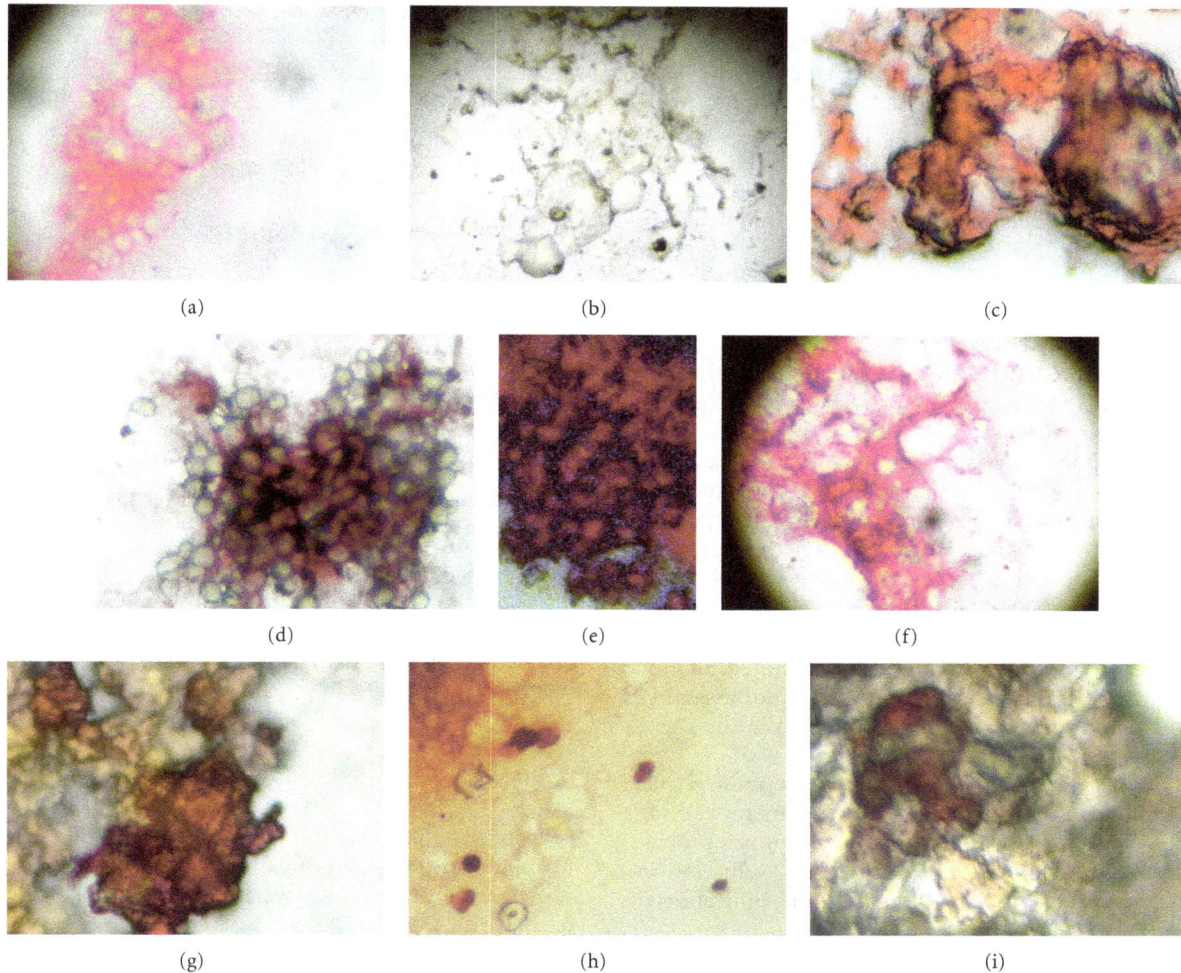

FIGURE 3: (a) Micrometastasis PSA (+). (b) Biopsy PSA (−). (c) Borders of microfragment MMP-2 (+). (d) Central pattern MMP-2 (+) stromal cells MMP-2 (+). (e) Central pattern MMP-2. (f) Microfragment MMP-2 (−), surrounding stromal cells MMP-2 (−). (g) Borders of microfragment MMP-2 (+), surrounding stromal cells MMP-2 (−). (h) Microfragment MMP-2 (−), stromal cells MMP-2 (−), DTC MMP-2 (+). (i) Borders of microfragment MMP-2 (+), some stromal cells MMP-2 (+).

2.1. Inclusion Criteria

(a) Biopsy proven prostate cancer.

(b) Written informed consent.

(c) Bone scan within three months of the sampling.

2.2. Sample Preparation.
After written informed consent bone marrow samples were obtained by an aspiration (4 mL) and a biopsy from the posterior superior iliac crest, and an 8 mL venous blood sample was taken at the same time.

2.2.1. Blood and Bone Marrow Aspiration.
4 mL aspirate sample of bone marrow and 8 mL of blood were collected into EDTA (Beckinson-Vacutainer) and processed within 30 minutes. The sample was layered onto 2 mL Histopaque 1.077 (Sigma-Aldrich) at room temperature. The mononuclear cells were obtained according to manufacturer's instructions and finally washed 3 times in phosphate buffered saline

pH 7.4 (PBS). The pellet was resuspended in $100\,\mu$L of autologous plasma and $25\,\mu$L was used to prepare each slide (silanized DAKO, USA). The slides were air-dried for 24 hours and finally fixed in a solution of 70% ethanol, 5% formaldehyde and 25% PBS for 5 minutes and then washed 3 times with PBS.

2.2.2. Biopsy.
The bone marrow biopsy sample was used to make 3 "touch-preps" using silanized slides (DAKO, USA) and fixed as previously described.

2.3. Immunocytochemistry.
Monoclonal antibodies directed against PSA clone 28A4 (Novacastro, UK) in a concentration of 2,5 μg/mL were used to detect prostate cells and identified using a detection system based on alkaline phosphatase-antialkaline phosphatase (LSAB2 DAKO, USA) with newfuchsin as the chromogen. To permit the rapid identification of positive cells there was no counter staining with Mayer's

hematoxilin. Levisamole (DAKO, USA) was used as an inhibitor of endogenous alkaline phosphatase. Positive and negative controls were processed in the same way.

Positive samples underwent a second stage of processing, using the monoclonal antibody against MMP-2 clone 1B4 (Novocastra, UK) and a system of detection based on peroxidase (LSAB2, DAKO, USA) with DAB (DAKO, USA) as the chromogen. Endogenous peroxidase was inhibited using an inhibitor (DAKO, USA) according to the manufacturer's instructions.

2.4. Definition of Expression of MMP-2. The criteria to define a cell expressing MMP-2 were that of Trudel et al. (2003) [12], con the percentage of PSA positive cells coexpressing MMP-2 grouped as 0%, 1–10%, 11–50%, and >50%, and the cells were additionally classified semiquantitatively as having 0, 1+, 2+, 3+ intensity of immunostaining (see Figure 1). A mean MMP-2 score was calculated for each sample, defined as total MMP-2 expression/N° of cells. In the samples of bone marrow biopsy touch preps the expression of MMP-2 in the surrounding non-PSA expressing cells was analyzed. The expression in these cells was noted as present or absent and the intensity of MMP-2 expression was noted. In blood and bone marrow aspirate samples this was not assessed as due to the nature of cell separation, and cells in the stained stain have no relation between each other.

Samples were analyzed at low power and photographed at a magnification of 400x using a digital camera, Samsung Digimax D73, and processed with the Digimax program for Windows 98. The immunocytochemical evaluation was performed by a single person, blinded to the clinical details using a coded system.

The patients were divided into 2 groups:

(I) postradical prostatectomy and bone scan negative, with or without biochemical failure,

(II) postradical prostatectomy bone scan positive with evidence of biochemical failure, defined as a PSA > 0.2 ng/mL in patients after radical prostatectomy.

2.5. Statistical Analysis. Descriptive statistics were used for demographic variables, expressed as mean and standard deviation in the case of continuous variables with a normal distribution. In case of an asymmetrical distribution the median and interquartile range (IQR) values were used. Noncontiguous variables were presented as frequencies. The Student's *t*-Test was used to compare continuous variables with a normal distribution, chi-squared, Kruskal-Wallis and log regression for the differences in frequency. The kappa test was used for tests of concordance.

2.6. Ethical Considerations. The study was directed with complete conformity with the principles of the declaration of Helsinki and approval of the local ethical committees.

3. Results

185 men bone scan negative and 30 men bone scan positive participated in the study. The presence of circulating prostate

TABLE 1: Demographic characteristics of the study group.

	Group 1	Group 2
Patient number (*n*)	185	30
Mean age ± SD (years) at sampling	72.2 ± 9.0	76.4 ± 8.7
Median serum PSA (IQR) (ng/mL) at sampling	1,32 (0,01–5,77)	43,81 (27,72–150)
Median Gleason score at diagnosis (IQR)	6 (5–7)	6 (5–7)
Median stage at diagnosis (IQR)	3 (2-3)	3 (2-3)
Median time from diagnosis (IQR) (years)	3 (1–7)	6 (4–9)
% (*n*) detection of prostate cells		
CPCs	62.7% (116)	100% (30)
DTCs	62.2% (115)	100% (30)
mM	71.4% (132)	100% (30)

IQR: interquartile range, CPCs: circulating prostate cells, and DTC: disseminated tumor cells.

cells in bone marrow aspirates as well as in bone marrow of prostate cancer patients was analyzed by determining PSA protein expression. CPCs were detected in 62.7%, DTCs in 62.2%, and mM in 71.4% of patients. All men bone scan positive had CPCs, DTCs, and mM detected in 100% of the cases (Table 1).

PSA protein expression in cells present in blood, bone marrow aspirate (BMA), and biopsy of cancer patients was compared with the Gleason score in patients without evidence of micrometastatic disease. There was no difference in the detection of cells in relation to age or serum PSA levels or the time from diagnosis to test time. Patients with higher Gleason scores had significantly higher stage disease. There were no differences in the frequency of detection of CPCs and DTCs with regards to Gleason score; however, the frequency of detection of mM was significantly lower in patients with Gleason 4 in comparison with higher Gleason scores (Kruskal-Wallis, $P < 0.001$) (Table 2).

PSA protein expression in cells present in blood, bone marrow aspirates (BMA), and biopsy of cancer patients with macrometastasis was compared with the Gleason score. There were no significant differences in the frequency of detection of CPCs, DTCs or mM with regard to Gleason score or relation to the serum PSA at the time of sampling (Table 3).

The expression of matrix metalloproteinase-2 (MMP-2), in patients positive for prostate cells in blood ($n = 116$), bone marrow aspirates ($n = 115$), and bone marrow biopsy ($n = 132$) of men without metastatic disease showed that MMP-2 expression was commonly limited to the edge of the bone marrow fragment (Figure 3(c)). Men with higher

TABLE 2: Demographic variables according to Gleason score.

	Gleason 4	Gleason 5 + 6	Gleason 7	Gleason 8 + 9	P = (statistical test)
No. of patients (n)	28	106	31	20	
Mean age ± SD (years)	71.1 ± 8.7	73.2 ± 9.4	70 ± 8.9	71.7 ± 6.7	NS (ANOVA)
Median serum PSA (IQR) ng/mL	1.0 (0.5–4.8)	1.68 (0.5–5.5)	0.57 (0.1–10.0)	1.68 (0.32–28.7)	NS (Kruksal-Wallis)
Median stage (IQR)	2 (1-2)[a,b,c]	3 (2-3)[a,d]	3 (2-3)[b]	3 (3-4)[c,d]	a-a < 0.001 b-b < 0.001 c-c < 0.001 d-d < 0.002 Kruksal-Wallis (significant <0.004)
Median time from diagnosis (IQR) (years)	2 (1–4)	4 (1–8)	3 (1–5)	2 (1–5)	NS (Kruksal-Wallis)
Detection prostate cells % (n)					Chi-squared Log regression
CPC	46.4% (13)	63.2 (67)	64.5 (20)	80 (16)	P = 0.0123
DTC	35.7% (10)	65.1(69)	67.7 (21)	75 (15)	P = 0.015
mM	32.1% (9)	77.4 (82)	77.4 (24)	85 (17)	P = 0.001

IQR: interquartile range, CPC: circulating prostate cell, DTC: disseminated tumor cell, mM: micrometastasis, and NS: not significant.

TABLE 3: Demographic variables according to Gleason score in men with metastatic disease.

	Gleason 4	Gleason 5 + 6	Gleason 7	Gleason 8 + 9	P = (statistical test)
No. of patients (n)	1	13	11	5	
Mean age ± SD (years)	75.1 ± 7.7	74.2 ± 8.7	75 ± 7.2	74.2 ± 6.5	NS (ANOVA)
Median serum PSA (IQR) ng/mL	26	29 (19.0–150)	31 (22–150.0)	30 (19–150)	NS (Kruksal-Wallis)
Median stage at diagnosis	3	3	3	3	NS (Kruksal-Wallis)
Median time from diagnosis (IQR) (years)	8	8 (5–11)	7 (6–9)	7 (4–9)	NS (Kruksal-Wallis)

IQR: inter-quartile range, CPC: circulating prostate cell, DTC: disseminated tumor cell mM: micrometastasis, and NS: not significant.

Gleason scores had a significantly higher frequency of MMP-2 expression in the mM (chi squared for trends, P = 0.031), and all CPCs and DTCs expressed MMP-2 (Table 4).

There was concordance in MMP-2 expression between CPCs and DTCs but not with mM for all Gleason scores in men with nonmetastatic cancer.

In men with metastatic disease MMP-2 expression was present in all CPCs and DTCs as well as mM but was expressed in all parts of the bone marrow fragment, defined as central expression (Figures 3(d) and 3(e)). There was concordance between CPCs, DTCs, and mM for all Gleason scores for the expression of MMP-2 (Table 5).

Stromal cell expression of MMP-2 was variable, and in the majority of microfragments MMP-2 negative the stromal cells were also negative (Figure 3(f)). In those microfragments with borders positive for MMP-2 the stromal cells were usually MMP-2 negative (Figure 3(g)) but in one case of Gleason 9 some of the surrounding stromal cells were MMP-2 positive (Figure 3(i)). In samples of microfragments and stromal cells MMP-2 negative, DTCs nearby were MMP-2 positive (Figure 3(h)). Stromal cells surrounding microfragments centrally expressing MMP-2 also expressed MMP-2 (Figure 3(d)) (see Table 6).

4. Discussion

MMP-2 is one of a family of enzymes that cleave a broad range of components of the extracellular matrix (ECM), basement membrane, growth factors, and cell surface receptors [17, 18]. MMPs are upregulated in cancer progression, can act as oncogenes, and promote invasion and metastasis in virtually all solid tumors [17, 18]. These enzymes play a role not only in tumor initiation and invasion but also in angiogenesis, metastasis and in releasing other tumor-promoting factors. Stromal and inflammatory cells in the primary tumor, rather than tumor cells, typically synthesize MMPs, which can then act on the stroma and regulate the tumor microenvironment as well as act on tumor cells themselves [17, 18]. A key role in this process is carried out by integrins, a widespread family of ECM-specific cell surface receptors. Integrins are major mediators of both cell-ECM interactions and transduction of matrix generated signals regulating cell proliferation, motility, and apoptosis. In human breast carcinoma cells it has been shown that alpha5-beta1 integrin promotes invasion of breast carcinoma cells by upregulating MMP-2 activity [19]. Likewise tumor cell extravasation is a critical step in metastasis, studies

TABLE 4: Frequency of MMP-2 expression in CPCs, DTCs, and mM in patients with nonmetastatic disease.

No. of patients	Gleason 4	Gleason 5 + 6	Gleason 7	Gleason 8 + 9	P = (statistical test, log regression)
Total 100% ($n = 185$)	15.1% (28)	57.3% (106)	16.8% (31)	10.8% (20)	
CPC positive 62.7% ($n = 116$)	46.4% (13)	63.2% (67)	64.5% (20)	80.0% (16)	NS
MMP-2	100% (13)	100% (67)	100% (20)	100% (16)	NS
DTC positive 62.5% ($n = 115$)	35.7% (10)	65.1% (69)	67.7% (21)	75.0% (15)	
MMP-2	100% (10)	100% (69)	100% (21)	100% (15)	NS
mM positive 71.4% ($n = 132$)	32.1% (9)	77.4% (82)	77.4% (22)	85% (17)	
MMP-2	0%[a,b,c]	14.6%[a,d] (11)	20.8%[b] (5)	41.1%[c,d] (7)	a-a < 0.002 b-b < 0.002 c-c < 0.002 d-d < 0.002 Trend chi squared $P = 0.031$

CPC: circulating prostate cell, DTC: disseminated tumor cell, mM: micrometastasis, and NS: not significant.

TABLE 5: Concordance between the expression of MMP-2 in CPCs, DTCs, and mM according to Gleason score.

Kappa: MMP-2	Gleason 4	Gleason 5 + 6	Gleason 7	Gleason 8 + 9
CPC + DTC	0.64	0.59	0.78	0.57
CPC + mM	0	0.14	0.19	0.23
DTC + mM	0	0.13	0.17	0.30

Kappa values: 0–0.2 no concordance, 0.21–0.40 low concordance, 0.41–0.60 moderate concordance, 0.61–0.8 good concordance, >0.80 excellent concordance.

TABLE 6: Expression of MMP-2 in mM and surrounding stromal cells in patients with MMP-2 expressing mM.

No. of patients	Gleason 4	Gleason 5 + 6	Gleason 7	Gleason 8 + 9	
mM positive 71.4% ($n = 132$)	32.1% (9)	77.4% (82)	77.4% (22)	85% (17)	
MMP-2 in mM	0%	14.6% (11)	20.8% (5)	41.1% (7)	Trend chi squared $P = 0.031$
MMP-2 in stromal cells	0%	0%	4.5% (1)	11.8% (2)	

show that this is an active [20, 21] and not a passive process driven by mechanical factors as first thought [22]. It is characterized by orchestrated signaling events involving adhesion molecules and cytokines, and the binding of and activation of MMP-2 promote tumor cell transmigration across the endothelial barrier and thus invade the distant tissue [23].

We believe that this is the first paper to describe the expression of MMP-2 in CPCs, DTCs, and mM. That both CPCs and DTCs express MMP-2 is consistent with the theory of the role of MMP-2 in the metastatic process of dissemination that cells expressing MMP-2 are able to penetrate the basement membrane and spread via the blood. That there is no association with the clinical parameters is in agreement with studies on prostate tissues [12], but also implies that only cells expressing the metalloproteinase have the inherent capacity to migrate.

There is a differential expression of MMP-2 in bone marrow micrometastasis, where the presence of MMP-2 detected by immunocytochemistry is in almost all cases zero in low grade cancer and suggests the inhibition of MMP-2. That the stromal microenvironment plays a critical role in determining tumor cell behavior has been shown in primary tumors [24, 25], where stromal cells increase MMP-2 expression in tumor cells. We describe, for the first time in prostate cancer, that bone marrow stromal cells produce the opposite reaction, that of inhibition of MMP-2 expression. The stromal cells surrounding the micrometastasis do not express MMP-2 in those cases where the micrometastasis is MMP-2 negative, stromal cell MMP-2 expression is variable when the micrometastasis has borders expressing MMP-2 and is stromal cell MMP-2 expression is positive when the micrometastasis has central expression of MMP-2. This might suggest that the inhibitor or inhibitors affect both stromal and tumor cell MMP-2 expression. In the case of border positive micrometastasis the variable stromal cell expression of MMP-2 may be explained by possible tumor cell factors stimulating the production of MMP-2 in both tumor and stromal cells. Thus stromal cell MMP-2 expression maybe a consequence of tumor cell activity. It has been shown that ANT2 shRNA suppresses induced migration and invasion by depletion of HER2/neu protein and, in turn, suppression of HER2/PI3 K/Akt pathway signaling and subsequent suppression of proteolytic activity by downregulating the activity of metalloproteinases [26]. Men with metastasis frequently have been treated previously with androgen blockade; androgen blockade has been shown to select prostate tumor cells which express HER-2 [27]. We suggest that it may be possible that micrometastasis from higher grade tumors or those micrometastases exposed previously to androgen blockade have a higher expression of HER-2 protein; this in turn leads to higher MMP-2 expression with increased invasion, secondary dissemination and finally angiogenesis and macrometastasis formation.

That the expression in mM is different to that in CPCs and DTCs is a supportive evidence that prostate cells detected in bone marrow aspirates are different and are not true micrometastasis [28], but represent circulating tumor cells in the bone marrow compartment. It has been shown that the bone marrow microenvironment is composed of specific niches that provide support for the proliferation and maintenance of hematopoietic stem cells [29], and interactions between the stem cells and their microenvironment regulate their maintenance, proliferation, differentiation, and migration into the blood circulation. Distinct niches have been anatomically and physiologically defined within the bone marrow [30, 31]. In the endosteal region, osteoblasts and other mesenchymal-derived stromal cells such as reticular cells, fibroblasts, and adipocytes constitute the osteoblastic niche that supports the maintenance of hematopoietic stem cells in a quiescent and undifferentiated state, by adhesion and humoral factors [32].

We propose that the expression of MMP-2 is inhibited by bone marrow stromal cells, in a process similar to that seen with hematopoietic stem cells, possibly by TIMP-2, although that other inhibitors modulate this function cannot be ruled out.

The inhibition of MMP-2 decreases the ability of the cancer to migrate from its new site, but does not inhibit proliferation directly. However, the decreased release of growth factors produced by MMP-2 and decreased initiation of angiogenesis by MMP-9 induced in part by MMP-2 [33] may limit the microfoci's growth potential. However, in high grade cancer, such as Gleason 9, tumor cells in micrometastasis continue to proliferate; as they divide and expand towards the intertrabecular surface, the inhibition by stromal cells decreases. This permits the reappearance of MMP-2 expression, as seen in the microfragment borders but not in the centre of the fragment, where MMP-2 suppression continues, which in turn allows the cell to escape and to disseminate, forming 2° CPCs.

In men with bone scan positive prostate cancer the expression of MMP-2 is throughout the bone fragment and involves the surrounding stromal tissue. These men had been previously treated with standard androgen blockade, and the overexpression of HER-2 protein caused by prior androgen blockade could increase MMP-2 expression and as a consequence MMP-2 is found throughout the microfragment (central pattern) and the surrounding stromal cells. Thus there may be two mechanisms involved in MMP-2 expression seen in the microfragments, firstly a passive phenomenon caused by cell proliferation towards the intertrabecular space resulting in decreased suppression of MMP-2 and secondly in more advanced disease, an active mechanism whereby HER-2 coexpression increases MMP-2 expression.

There is evidence for tumor-stroma crosstalk at metastatic sites; Kaminski et al. [34] described the effect of metastatic prostate cancer cell lines and nonprostatic stromal fibroblasts which are encountered by metastatic cells at most sites. For continuous growth and propagation at metastatic sites tumor cells have to induce a supportive stroma. Media conditioned by metastatic cell lines are able of inducing cultured fibroblasts to proliferate which corresponds to fibrous stroma induction *in vivo* [34]. Media conditioned by DU-145 metastatic prostate cell line can induce in fibroblasts the expression of MMP-14 mRNA, although other factors such as bFGF, PDGF, and TNF-alpha are also secreted in low amounts by DU-145 cells and they also stimulate the production of MMP-14 mRNA, possibly by activation of the Ets-1 transcription factor [35]. This crosstalk between stromal and cancer cells would explain the differences in MMP-2 expression found in the three groups of patients. Firstly the stromal cells inhibit MMP-2 expression, then with cancer progression the cancer cells induce stromal expression of MMP-2, which in turn leads to the release of other growth factors and angiogenic factors [36, 37].

This process may have important clinical implications; firstly the differential expression of MMP-2 between circulating cells and micrometastasis could explain the early dissemination of cancer cells through mechanisms mediated for MMP-2; having invaded the bone, the inhibition of MMP-2 has a direct effect of trapping the cancer cell in its new environment and through indirect processes limits its growth in terms of the size of the focus (bone scan negative), thus could explain why although bone marrow micrometastasis are frequent, local gross recurrence is more common than metastatic relapse [38], the microfoci entering a state of dormancy. In cancer cells that are proliferating in the bone marrow, for mechanical reasons, the cells grow into the intertrabecular space and as a result the inhibition of MMP-2 decreases and secondary dissemination is possible.

In patients with macrometastasis, that is, bone scan positive patients, these inhibitory mechanisms have been overcome, possibly by HER-2 overexpression, and MMP-2 expression is found throughout the bone marrow fragment; this in turn permits activation of the physiological mechanism previously mentioned, angiogenesis and growth of the secondary tumor.

Secondly, one of the mechanisms of action of the bisphosphonates is inhibiting MMP-2 through MMP-14 (MMP-MT1), if as we have shown that micrometastases do not express MMP-2. This may explain why clinical studies of bisphosphonates in prostate cancer patients have shown conflicting results in bone scan negative patients [39]. Thus inhibition of MMP-2 by BFs would decrease dissemination and infiltration of circulating cells, but would not affect the established micrometastasis. They may prevent or delay the appearance of MMP-2 expression thus delaying the formation of macrometastasis. However, in men with macrometastasis, with a positive bone scan the use of bisphosphonates may have a better therapeutic effect for the increased MMP-2 expression. Thus the role of bisphosphonates would have two different roles depending on the presence of micro- or macrometastatic disease.

Acknowledgments

The study was funded by a research grant from the Teaching Council, Hospital de Carabineros de Chile, Santiago. There was no conflict of interests. The authors would like to thank Mrs. Ana Maria Palazuelos for her help in this study.

References

[1] H. S. Evans and H. Møller, "Recent trends in prostate cancer incidence and mortality in Southeast England," *European Urology*, vol. 43, no. 4, pp. 337–341, 2003.

[2] National Cancer Institute, *Cancer Trends Progress Report: 2005 Update*, NCI, Bethesda, MD, USA, 2005.

[3] E. Oliver, D. Gunnell, and J. L. Donovan, "Comparison of trends in prostate-cancer mortality in England and Wales and the USA," *The Lancet*, vol. 355, no. 9217, pp. 1788–1789, 2000.

[4] B. I. Carlin and G. L. Andriole, "The natural history, skeletal complications, and management of bone metastases in patients with prostate carcinoma," *Cancer*, vol. 88, no. 12, pp. 2989–2994, 2000.

[5] W. F. Whitmore, "Natural history and staging of prostate cancer," *Urologic Clinics of North America*, vol. 11, no. 2, pp. 205–220, 1984.

[6] J. G. Moreno, C. M. Croce, R. Fischer et al., "Detection of hematogenous micrometastasis in patients with prostate cancer," *Cancer Research*, vol. 52, no. 21, pp. 6110–6112, 1992.

[7] A. F. Chambers and L. M. Matrisian, "Changing views of the role of matrix metalloproteinases in metastasis," *Journal of the National Cancer Institute*, vol. 89, no. 17, pp. 1260–1270, 1997.

[8] M. Stearns and M. E. Stearns, "Immunohistochemical studies of activated matrix metalioproteinase-2 (MMP-2a) expression in human prostate cancer," *Oncology Research*, vol. 8, no. 2, pp. 63–67, 1996.

[9] D. P. Wood and M. Banerjee, "Presence of circulating prostate cells in the bone marrow of patients undergoing radical prostatectomy is predictive of disease-free survival," *Journal of Clinical Oncology*, vol. 15, no. 12, pp. 3451–3457, 1997.

[10] H. Kuniyasu, P. Troncoso, D. Johnston et al., "Relative expression of type IV collagenase, E-cadherin, and vascular endothelial growth factor/vascular permeability factor in prostatectomy specimens distinguishes organ-confined from pathologically advanced prostate cancers," *Clinical Cancer Research*, vol. 6, no. 6, pp. 2295–2308, 2000.

[11] J. S. Ross, P. Kaur, C. E. Sheehan, H. A. G. Fisher, R. A. Kaufman Jr., and B. V. S. Kallakury, "Prognostic significance of matrix metalloproteinase 2 and tissue inhibitor of metalloproteinase 2 expression in prostate cancer," *Modern Pathology*, vol. 16, no. 3, pp. 198–205, 2003.

[12] D. Trudel, Y. Fradet, F. Meyer, F. Harel, and B. Têtu, "Significance of MMP-2 expression in prostate cancer: an immunohistochemical study," *Cancer Research*, vol. 63, no. 23, pp. 8511–8515, 2003.

[13] A. R. Nelson, B. Fingleton, M. L. Rothenberg, and L. M. Matrisian, "Matrix metalloproteinases: biologic activity and clinical implications," *Journal of Clinical Oncology*, vol. 18, no. 5, pp. 1135–1149, 2000.

[14] Y. A. DeClerck, S. Imren, A. M. P. Montgomery, B. M. Mueller, R. A. Reisfeld, and W. E. Laug, "Proteases and protease inhibitors in tumor progression," *Advances in Experimental Medicine and Biology*, vol. 425, pp. 89–97, 1997.

[15] A. Noël, V. Albert, K. Bajou et al., "New functions of stromal proteases and their inhibitors in tumor progression," *Surgical Oncology Clinics of North America*, vol. 10, no. 2, pp. 417–432, 2001.

[16] E. Borgen, B. Naume, J. M. Nesland et al., "Standardization of the immunocytochemical detection of cancer cells in BM and blood: I. Establishment of objective criteria for the evaluation of immunostained cells," *Cytotherapy*, vol. 1, no. 5, pp. 377–388, 1999.

[17] M. Egeblad and Z. Werb, "New functions for the matrix metalloproteinases in cancer progression," *Nature Reviews Cancer*, vol. 2, no. 3, pp. 161–174, 2002.

[18] M. D. Sternlicht and Z. Werb, "How matrix metalloproteinases regulate cell behavior," *Annual Review of Cell and Developmental Biology*, vol. 17, pp. 463–516, 2001.

[19] G. Morozevich, N. Kozlova, I. Cheglakov, N. Ushakova, and A. Berman, "Integrin $\alpha5\beta1$ controls invasion of human breast carcinoma cells by direct and indirect modulation of MMP-2 collagenase activity," *Cell Cycle*, vol. 8, no. 14, pp. 2219–2225, 2009.

[20] O. V. Glinskii, V. H. Huxley, J. R. Turk et al., "Continuous real time ex vivo epifluorescent video microscopy for the study of metastatic cancer cell interactions with microvascular endothelium," *Clinical and Experimental Metastasis*, vol. 20, no. 5, pp. 451–458, 2003.

[21] A. B. Al-Mehdi, K. Tozawa, A. B. Fisher, L. Shientag, A. Lee, and R. J. Muschel, "Intravascular origin of metastasis from the proliferation of endothelium-attached tumor cells: a new model for metastasis," *Nature Medicine*, vol. 6, no. 1, pp. 100–102, 2000.

[22] O. V. Glinskii, V. H. Huxley, G. V. Glinsky, K. J. Pienta, A. Raz, and V. V. Glinsky, "Mechanical entrapment is insufficient and intercellular adhesion is essential for metastatic cell arrest in distant organs," *Neoplasia*, vol. 7, no. 5, pp. 522–527, 2005.

[23] F. W. Orr, H. H. Wang, R. M. Lafrenie, S. Scherbarth, and D. M. Nance, "Interactions between cancer cells and the endothelium in metastasis," *The Journal of Pathology*, vol. 190, pp. 310–329, 2000.

[24] L. W. K. Chung, A. Baseman, V. Assikis, and H. E. Zhau, "Molecular insights into prostate cancer progression: the missing link of tumor microenvironment," *Journal of Urology*, vol. 173, no. 1, pp. 10–20, 2005.

[25] T. Sato, T. Sakai, Y. Noguchi, M. Takita, S. Hirakawa, and A. Ito, "Tumor-stromal cell contact promotes invasion of human uterine cervical carcinoma cells by augmenting the expression and activation of stromal matrix metalloproteinases," *Gynecologic Oncology*, vol. 92, no. 1, pp. 47–56, 2004.

[26] J. Y. Jang, Y. K. Jeon, and C. W. Kim, "Degradation of HER2/neu by ANT2 shRNA suppresses migration and invasiveness of breast cancer cells," *BMC Cancer*, vol. 10, article 391, 2010.

[27] N. P. Murray, L. V. Badinez, R. R. Dueñas, N. Orellana, and P. Tapia, "Positive HER-2 protein expression in circulating prostate cells and micro-metastasis, resistant to androgen blockage but not diethylstilbestrol," *Indian Journal of Urology*, vol. 27, no. 2, pp. 200–207, 2011.

[28] N. P. Murray, G. M. Calaf, and L. Badínez, "Presence of prostate cells in bone marrow biopsies as a sign of micrometastasis in cancer patients," *Oncology Reports*, vol. 21, no. 3, pp. 571–575, 2009.

[29] B. Heissig, Y. Ohki, Y. Sato, S. Rafii, Z. Werb, and K. Hattori, "A role for niches in hematopoietic cell development," *Hematology*, vol. 10, no. 3, pp. 247–253, 2005.

[30] I. Yaniv, J. Stein, D. L. Farkas, and N. Askenasy, "The tale of early hematopoietic cell seeding in the bone marrow niche," *Stem Cells and Development*, vol. 15, no. 1, pp. 4–16, 2006.

[31] R. N. Kaplan, B. Psaila, and D. Lyden, "Niche-to-niche migration of bone-marrow-derived cells," *Trends in Molecular Medicine*, vol. 13, no. 2, pp. 72–81, 2007.

[32] R. S. Taichman, "Blood and bone: two tissues whose fates are intertwined to create the hematopoietic stem-cell niche," *Blood*, vol. 105, no. 7, pp. 2631–2639, 2005.

[33] G. Bergers, R. Brekken, G. McMahon et al., "Matrix metalloproteinase-9 triggers the angiogenic switch during carcinogenesis," *Nature Cell Biology*, vol. 2, no. 10, pp. 737–744, 2000.

[34] A. Kaminski, J. C. Hahne, E. L. M. Haddouti, A. Florin, A. Wellmann, and N. Wernert, "Tumour-stroma interactions between metastatic prostate cancer cells and fibroblasts," *International Journal of Molecular Medicine*, vol. 18, no. 5, pp. 941–950, 2006.

[35] N. Wernert, F. Gilles, V. Fafeur et al., "Stromal expression of c-Ets1 transcription factor correlates with tumor invasion," *Cancer Research*, vol. 54, no. 21, pp. 5683–5688, 1994.

[36] B. C. Patterson and Q. A. Sang, "Angiostatin-converting enzyme activities of human matrilysin (MMP-7) and gelatinase B/type IV collagenase (MMP.9)," *Journal of Biological Chemistry*, vol. 272, no. 46, pp. 28823–28825, 1997.

[37] M. Suzuki, G. Raab, M. A. Moses, C. A. Fernandez, and M. Klagsbrun, "Matrix metalloproteinase-3 releases active heparin-binding EGF-like growth factor by cleavage at a specific juxtamembrane site," *Journal of Biological Chemistry*, vol. 272, no. 50, pp. 31730–31737, 1997.

[38] G. P. Swanson, M. A. Hussey, C. M. Tangen et al., "Predominant treatment failure in postprostatectomy patients is local: analysis of patterns of treatment failure in SWOG 8794," *Journal of Clinical Oncology*, vol. 25, no. 16, pp. 2225–2229, 2007.

[39] M. D. Mason, M. R. Sydes, J. Glaholm et al., "Oral sodium clodronate for nonmetastatic prostate cancer—results of a randomized double-blind placebo-controlled trial: medical research council PR04 (ISRCTN61384873)," *Journal of the National Cancer Institute*, vol. 99, no. 10, pp. 765–776, 2007.

11

Hematopoietic Stem and Progenitor Cells as Effectors in Innate Immunity

Jennifer L. Granick,[1] Scott I. Simon,[2] and Dori L. Borjesson[1]

[1] Department of Pathology, Microbiology, Immunology, University of California School of Veterinary Medicine, Davis, CA 95616, USA
[2] Department of Biomedical Engineering, University of California, Davis, CA 95616, USA

Correspondence should be addressed to Jennifer L. Granick, jlgranick@ucdavis.edu

Academic Editor: Meenal Mehrotra

Recent research has shed light on novel functions of hematopoietic stem and progenitor cells (HSPC). While they are critical for maintenance and replenishment of blood cells in the bone marrow, these cells are not limited to the bone marrow compartment and function beyond their role in hematopoiesis. HSPC can leave bone marrow and circulate in peripheral blood and lymph, a process often manipulated therapeutically for the purpose of transplantation. Additionally, these cells preferentially home to extramedullary sites of inflammation where they can differentiate to more mature effector cells. HSPC are susceptible to various pathogens, though they may participate in the innate immune response without being directly infected. They express pattern recognition receptors for detection of endogenous and exogenous danger-associated molecular patterns and respond not only by the formation of daughter cells but can themselves secrete powerful cytokines. This paper summarizes the functional and phenotypic characterization of HSPC, their niche within and outside of the bone marrow, and what is known regarding their role in the innate immune response.

1. Introduction

Hematopoietic stem cells (HSC) maintain and replenish all blood cell types in the bone marrow and respond to changing needs for blood cells in peripheral tissues. They give rise to multipotent (produce most blood cell subsets), oligopotent (lymphoid or myeloid restricted), and unipotent hematopoietic progenitor cells (HPC), the latter type restricted to proliferation into a single set of mature blood cells. Throughout embryonic and fetal development, there are multiple sequential sites of hematopoiesis. Though primitive HSC form nucleated red blood cells in the yolk sac, the first definitive HSC appear in the aorta-gonad-mesonephros (AGM) and expand in the fetal liver before finding their niche in the bone marrow (and spleen in rodents) [1, 2]. In adult life, hematopoietic stem and progenitor cells (HSPC) primarily reside in the bone marrow, though recent work has shown that they circulate in blood and lymph and traffic to other hematopoietic and nonhematopoietic organs during homeostasis and stress [3–6]. This roving nature of

adult HSPC should not be surprising when one considers the changing location of hematopoiesis throughout HSPC ontogeny. Additionally, extramedullary hematopoiesis is well described in the adult and typically occurs at sites of prenatal hematopoiesis [7]. Given the ability of HSPC to leave the bone marrow and circulate in the periphery, that they express pattern recognition receptors (PRR) and respond to conserved microbial and viral molecular patterns [8], it is reasonable to hypothesize that HSPC are active in innate immune and inflammatory responses outside of the bone marrow.

2. Phenotypic and Functional Definitions of Hematopoietic Stem and Progenitor Cells

In order to study the potential function of HSPC outside the bone marrow, it is essential that these cells be discriminated experimentally from leukocytes and other lineage-committed cells. HSPC can be identified by their surface marker expression, unique staining properties of vital dyes, and by specific functional assays. HSC are defined by their ability to self-renew and to produce all blood cell types, while HPC do not have self-renewal capacity and are more restricted in the mature blood cells they can produce. Investigators typically use a combination of functional and phenotypic characteristics to categorize populations of HSPC.

Fluorescence activated cell sorting (FACS) schemes can identify and enrich stem and progenitor cells in sorted populations, although more committed progenitors are also present. For example, the "KSL" scheme in mice and CD34 in humans identify a heterogenous group of cells including HSC capable of long-term repopulation of bone marrow (long-term repopulating cells or LT-HSC), short-term repopulating cells (ST-HSC), and restricted progenitor cells incapable of long-term hematopoietic reconstitution. Murine KSL cells are c-Kit$^+$, Sca-1$^+$, and negative for lineage markers of mature blood cell types [9]. The addition of the Flk-2/Flt3 receptor tyrosine kinase to the KSL markers enhances separation of ST-HSC (Flk-2$^+$) from LT-HSC (Flk-2$^-$) [10]. There is no human homolog for murine Sca-1. Instead, human HSC are identified on the basis of CD34 expression. Interestingly, more primitive HSC in mice have low or absent expression of CD34 [11]. The DNA-binding dye Hoechst 33342 can be used to identify low staining "side populations" (SP) of HSPC [12]. Hoechst staining is often combined with KSL markers to further enrich HSC numbers, so called SP^{KLS} cells. The purity of HSC in sorted SP, KSL or CD34$^+$ HSPC can be increased by using the signaling lymphocyte activation molecule (SLAM) family proteins CD150, CD244, and CD48. The presence of CD150 distinguishes HSC from HPC; multipotent progenitors are CD150$^-$CD244$^+$CD48$^-$ and more committed progenitors are CD150$^-$CD244$^+$CD48$^+$[13], though there is even variability among CD150$^+$ HSC in their ability to provide balanced repopulation of irradiated bone marrow in mice [14, 15].

There are many limitations of phenotypic markers for identification of HSC and HPC in the context of infection and inflammation. For example, Sca-1 is upregulated on hematopoietic cells other than HSC during inflammation via interferons (INF) and tumor necrosis factor (TNF) [16, 17]. LT-HSC reduce expression of c-Kit tenfold after exposure to the chemotherapeutic agent 5-fluoruracil (5-FU) [18]. In addition, 5-FU increases expression of Mac-1 (CD11b/CD18) [18], a β2-integrin used by HPC for adhesion to bone marrow stroma [19] and a marker of myeloid lineage cells. Infection with an intracellular pathogen increases CD48 expression, indicative of multipotent progenitors and proliferating cells, on CD150$^+$ KSL cells that would otherwise be termed LT-HSC [20]. Infection-induced stress may alter other stem and progenitor cell markers as well. Thus phenotypic strategies for detecting HSC and HPC in infection must be evaluated to avoid mistaken identification.

Regardless of the FACS methods used to isolate HSPC, functional assays are required to truly determine a cell's ability to self-renew and form mature cell lineages. In vitro assays generally measure HPC rather than primitive HSC, while long-term in vivo assays are a measure of LT-HSC. Colony-forming cell (CFC) assays determine the capacity of cells to form lineage-restricted colonies in a semi-solid, usually methylcellulose-based, media, but do not identify HSC, rather only HPC. The gold standard for differentiating LT-HSC from ST-HSC and progenitors is their ability to engraft in vivo into irradiated hosts and maintain multilineage hematopoiesis indefinitely and through serial transplantation into new hosts [21].

3. The HSPC Niche: The Bone Marrow and Beyond

As was first proposed by Schofield in 1978, HSC and HPC occupy different stem cell niches that determine cell behaviors, such as, self-renewal versus differentiation, quiescence versus proliferation, and inertia versus mobilization [22]. These behaviors are dictated by the microenvironment including physical and structural features, humoral, paracrine and neural signals, and metabolic factors. The HSPC niche most studied is the adult bone marrow, comprised of the osteoblastic and vascular niches. It is generally believed that a minority of HSC associate with endosteum and are quiescent, while a larger portion of HSC as well as HPC are located next to vascular endothelial cells and are cycling [13]. The cues received by HSPC in these environments provide a critical balance of quiescence, self-renewal, and differentiation that provides for adequate blood cells over a lifetime.

Though HSPC primarily reside in the bone marrow, there is increasing evidence that they may find suitable niches elsewhere in the body. Indeed, it has long been recognized that extramedullary hematopoiesis (EMH), production of hemic cells outside the bone marrow, typically occurs in sites of early blood formation, such as, the liver and spleen [7]. Many tissues, however, can accommodate hematopoiesis [23] and thus may contain the essential elements of a stem cell niche. EMH has been reported in such diverse tissues as the skin, joint, urinary bladder, peritoneum, pleura, testes, adrenal glands, and gastrointestinal tract [24–31]. Myelofibrosis, inflammation, and infection are frequent underlying causes of EMH. In cutaneous pyogenic granulomas, trauma-induced vascular lesions can contain de novo formation of erythroid and myeloid cells [26, 32]. In intestinal helminth infection, multipotent progenitors cells (MPP) are induced by IL-25 in gut-associated lymphoid tissue and give rise to monocyte/macrophages and granulocytes [33]. Pleural and pericardial EMH has been associated with sepsis as well as local infections [34]. The granulocytotropic organism *Anaplasma phagocytophilum* causes mobilization of HSPC from bone marrow and enhanced myelopoiesis in the spleen [35, 36]. Thus stress, infection, and inflammation can produce stem cell niches outside of the bone marrow, which, under specific conditions, can support HSPC proliferation and differentiation.

In the bone marrow, HSC intimately associate with osteoblasts and endothelial cells, an interaction facilitated in part by the α-chemokine CXCL12, also denoted stromal-derived factor-1 (SDF-1). SDF-1 is secreted by osteoblasts, stromal cells, and reticular endothelial cells and binds its receptor CXCR4 on the HSPC surface [37]. SDF-1 is the most important chemokine for maintaining HSPC within the marrow, but peripheral sites also produce this HSPC attracting chemokine. It is produced by Langerhans cells, endothelial cells, and pericytes in human skin during homeostasis and additionally by fibroblasts during inflammation [38]. SDF-1 is upregulated in many tissues secondary to ischemia and inflammation [39]. Ischemia induces SDF-1 expression by endothelial cells via hypoxia-inducible factor-1 [40]. Peripheral tissue hypoxia results in oxygen tensions similar to the bone marrow osteoblastic niche, and recruited macrophages can be supportive cells for EMH [41]. As in the bone marrow, SDF-1 gradients may play a role in the maintenance of HSPC in damaged or infected peripheral tissues.

There is a close association between HSC and endothelial cells that begins during embryogenesis [42] and remains throughout ontogeny [43]. Kiel et al. used SLAM family receptor expression to localize HSC within bone marrow and found that 60% of HSC in the bone marrow was associated with sinusoids compared to 14% associated with endosteum [13]. Their findings suggest that the endothelium expresses factors important for HSC maintenance and function. Indeed, endothelial cells in the bone marrow constitutively express adhesion molecules, such as, P-selectin, E-selectin, and vascular cell adhesion molecule-1 (VCAM-1) that are expressed by extramedullary endothelial cells during inflammation [44]. Bone marrow endothelium also elaborates hematopoietic cytokines during homeostasis, such as, stem cell factor (SCF), interleukin-6 (IL-6), granulocyte colony stimulating factor (G-CSF), and granulocyte-macrophage colony stimulating factor (GM-CSF), highlighting the role of the vascular niche in the regulation of HSC proliferation and differentiation [45]. Though bone marrow endothelium is unique in its constitutive expression of adhesion molecules and cytokines, endothelial cells from other organs can support HSPC function to varying degrees by secretion of soluble factors [46, 47]. Inflamed endothelial cells express adhesion molecules required for capture and transmigration of leukocytes and their precursors. Upon stimulation with inflammatory mediators, endothelial cells upregulate P- and E-selectins as well as adhesion molecules of the immunoglobulin superfamily, including ICAM-1 and VCAM-1 [48]. Hematopoietic growth factors are secreted by activated endothelial cells, fibroblasts, macrophages, and other innate immune cells. Interleukin-1 induces G-CSF and GM-CSF production by human umbilical endothelial cells in culture [49]. Lipopolysaccharide induces GM-CSF secretion by human pulmonary microvascular endothelial cells in vitro, and peri-tumoral inflammation leads to GM-CSF elaboration by pulmonary endothelial cells in vivo [50]. *Staphylococcus aureus* and its exotoxins induce cultured endothelial cells to secrete G-CSF as well as IL-6 and IL-8 [51]. Sites of tissue inflammation thus provide the critical constellation of cellular and soluble elements required for HSPC homing, retention, and function.

4. HSPC Mobilization and Homing to Sites of Inflammation

HSPC travel through peripheral blood and lymph at low number during homeostasis, but they are mobilized by inflammation, infection, stress, and injury [4, 52–54]. Disruption of the CXCR4/SDF-1 axis results in rapid release of HSPC to the periphery [35]. In response to tissue inflammation or infection, neutrophil numbers increase in the bone marrow and release proteases, such as, matrix metalloproteinase-9 (MMP-9), neutrophil elastase, and cathepsin G [55]. These proteins act upon chemotactic and adhesion factors, such as, SDF-1, CXCR4, SCF, c-Kit, and VCAM-1, to release HSPC into circulation [54]. Additionally, cleavage fragments of the fifth complement cascade protein, C5, contribute to a proteolytic environment in the bone marrow [56]. Bacterial infection upregulates G-CSF on endothelium in the bone marrow, which inhibits osteoblast SDF-1 production and liberates HSPC from the endosteal niche [51, 57, 58]. Neural inputs to the stem cell niche also regulate HSPC mobilization. The bone marrow is innervated with noradrenergic sympathetic fibers, and HSPC express receptors for the sympathetic neurotransmitter dopamine on their surface [59, 60]. G-CSF and GM-CSF can increase neuronal receptor density on HSPC, augmenting their proliferation and motility [60]. Norepinephrine, another sympathetic neurotransmitter, suppresses osteoblast function, causing SDF-1 downregulation [61]. Thus stress works to mobilize HSPC to the periphery, where they may act in concert with other innate immune effectors for resolution of inflammation.

Homing of mobilized bone marrow HSPC to injured tissue is well documented. Hypoxic tissue, injured vasculature, and thrombi-forming platelets upregulate SDF-1 via HIF-1α, thus recruiting bone marrow progenitors for tissue repair [40, 62, 63]. Cleavage fragments of the third complement component (C3) increase sensitivity of CXCR4-expressing HSPC to SDF-1 gradients in injured tissue [64]. Chemokines other than SDF-1 can also attract HSPC to inflammatory sites. Monocyte chemoattractant proteins draw CCR2-expressing LT-HSC, ST-HSC and progenitor cells to injured liver and peritoneum, where they differentiate along the myeloid and lymphoid lineages [6]. Ischemia and inflammation may alter chemokine gradients between bone marrow and sites of injury to direct homing of HSPC to areas in need.

The requirement for adhesion molecules to support HSPC homing to inflamed tissues is poorly understood. The most critical adhesion molecule for HSC maintenance in the bone marrow is VCAM-1, which binds the $\alpha_4\beta_1$ integrin very late antigen-4 (VLA-4) on the HSC surface [65–67], though the importance of this adhesion pair for HSC recruitment to nonmedullary sites is not fully defined. VLA-4 is required for HSPC entry to injured liver, whereas CD18, CD44, and PECAM-1 are not [68]. VLA-4 is also important for HSPC migration to the heart [69]. However, CD18, not VLA-4, is required for HSC homing to radiation-damaged gut [67]. Much remains to be discovered regarding the requirements for HSPC homing to infected and inflamed sites, though they are likely to include both adhesion molecules and chemokines used for BM homing as well as some that are unique to the inflamed tissue.

5. HSPC Sense Infection and Inflammation Directly and Indirectly

HSPC can sense infection and inflammation directly as well as indirectly via inflammatory cytokines produced by other cells. While HSC have been found to be resistant to infection by a variety of pathogens, including *Mycobacterium avium*, *Listeria monocytogenes*, *Salmonella enterica ser. typhimurium*, and *Yersinia enterocolitica* [70, 71], direct infection of HSC by pathogens, such as retroviruses, alters hematopoiesis [72]. However, intracellular infection is not the only situation in which HSPC can respond to pathogens. Ligation of HSPC pattern recognition receptors (PRR) can lead to proliferation, differentiation and elaboration of cytokines, growth factors, integrins, and receptors. Infection-induced INF signaling can cause HSC activation or inhibition depending on chronicity and context. Though HSC remain quiescent while committed progenitors supply mature leukocytes during equilibrium, they can respond rapidly during infection [73].

Interferons are mediators of inflammation, with type I INF (INF-α and INF-β) produced by virally infected cells and type II INF (INF-γ) produced by stimulated T cells and NK cells [73]. Toll-like receptor-3 (TLR3) recognizes viral double-stranded RNA, and injection of its ligand poly(I:C) induces type I INF, causing quiescent HSC to proliferate [74]. This response may be adaptive in viral infection but could be detrimental to maintenance of the HSC compartment with long-term exposure [74]. Although INF-γ inhibits hematopoiesis, maintaining homeostasis of effector cells during infection [73], several studies describe the opposite effect. Vaccinia virus infection expands the KSL bone marrow fraction and differentially regulates common myeloid progenitors (CMP) and common lymphoid progenitors (CLP) [75]. CLP differentiate to INF-β-producing plasmacytoid dendritic cells to combat viral infection [75]. Lymphocytic Choriomeningitis virus drives monocyte differentiation of CMP and inhibition of granulopoiesis in an INF-γ-dependent manner [76]. Acute malarial infection results in INF-γ induced c-Kit^{hi} IL-7-receptor$^+$ bone marrow progenitors with both myeloid and lymphoid potential [77]. In a model of acute human monocytic ehrlichiosis, infection-induced INF-γ drives HSC out of dormancy and expands the KSL population in the bone marrow [20]. Interferon-γ likewise steers hematopoietic progenitors towards granulocyte and monocyte differentiation [20]. HSC are similarly activated in chronic infection. Persistent infection with *Mycobacterium avium* increases proliferation of KSL/Flk2$^-$/CD34$^-$ and SP^{KLS} LT-HSC without an increase in LT-HSC number via INF-γ [70]. Instead KSL/Flk2$^+$/CD34$^+$ ST-HSC were significantly increased, suggesting compensatory proliferation of LT-HSC to supply the ST-HSC and progenitors required to meet increased peripheral leukocyte demand [70]. HSPC can sense and respond to infection indirectly via both type I and type II INF, though overstimulation of the bone marrow compartment with INF could lead to ineffective hematopoiesis and HSC exhaustion [73].

Innate immune cells can respond directly to signals of infection via PRR. PRR are signaling receptors that recognize conserved pathogen-associated molecular patterns (PAMPs) and endogenous danger-associated molecular patterns (DAMPs) to elicit immune responses. There are four main classes of PRR. These include the transmembrane toll-like receptors (TLRs) and C-type, lectin receptors (CLRs), the cytoplasmic retinoic acid-inducible gene (RIG)-I-like receptors (RLRs), and nucleotide-binding oligomerization domain or NOD-like receptors (NLRs). PRR signaling induces gene transcription leading to inflammatory responses. Recently, PRR have been identified on HSPC [8, 78–80]. Nagai et al were the first to reveal the presence of functional TLR on murine HSPC [8]. In one study, human CD34$^+$ HSPC predominantly expressed transcripts for TLR1, 2, 3, 4, and 6 [81], while others have shown that TLR4, 7, and 8 are most highly expressed [80]. Additionally, the NLR NOD2 has been identified in human HSPC [78]. The expression of PRR suggests that HSPC may be an important component of the innate immune response.

When HSPC encounter microbial pathogens there is a tendency towards myeloid rather than lymphoid differentiation. TLR ligands upregulate the myeloid transcription factors PU.1, C/EBPa, and GATA-1 on HSPC, directing lineage fate decisions [81]. The NLR NOD2 in human CD34$^+$ HSPC is activated by the bacterial peptidoglycan muramyl dipeptide (MDP) resulting in increased expression of PU.1, a transcription factor important in driving hematopoietic progenitor lineage fate [80]. NOD2-stimulated HSPC differentiate to dendritic cells and macrophages. Upon ligand binding in vitro, both TLR2 and TLR4 expressed on HSPC induce proliferation and differentiation to monocytes and dendritic cells in the absence of hematopoietic growth factors [8]. *Candida albicans* yeast and hyphae are signals through HSPC TLR2 to produce phagocytic macrophages and neutrophils in vitro [82, 83]. In an in vivo mouse model of invasive candidiasis, hematopoiesis was skewed towards granulocytes and monocytes, with a corresponding decrease in B-cell formation [83]. Thus, upon detection of PAMPs, HSPC preferentially differentiate towards mature myeloid immune cells to fight infection.

6. HSPC as Immune Effectors

Stem and progenitor cell function in peripheral sites of inflammation has only recently been reported. Circulating HSPC may act as sentinels of infection, serve as readily available precursors of mature blood leukocytes, or participate as effectors themselves. HSPC respond to and secrete chemokines, pro- and anti-inflammatory cytokines and growth factors [84, 85]. For example, human CD34$^+$ cells secrete SCF, FLT3-ligand, insulin-like growth factor-1, thrombopoietin, and transforming growth factor-β1 (TGF-β1) and TGF-β2, which have variable effects on HSC viability [84]. Conditioned media from CD34$^+$ cells was a chemoattractant and increased survival and proliferation of other CD34$^+$ cells [84]. After stimulation with *S. aureus* CD34$^+$ HSPC produced high levels of TNF, IL-6, IL-8, IL-23, and IL-10 [85]. Upon ligation of NOD2 by MDP, human CD34$^+$ cells expressed TNFα, IL-1β, and GM-CSF [78]. They also upregulated intracellular stores of α-defensins 1–3, suggesting that they may be able to directly fight bacterial infections [78]. There appears to be synergism between NOD2 and TLR signaling, as cytokine production is significantly elevated when HSPC are stimulated with NOD2 and TLR ligands together versus individually [78]. Infection indirectly stimulates HSPC to generate reparative growth factors, including TGF-β, epithelial growth factor, angiogenin, fibroblast growth factor, platelet-derived growth factor, SDF-1, and vascular endothelial growth factor [85]. CD34$^+$ human HSPC can produce Th2 cytokines, like IL-5, IL-13, IL-6, and GM-CSF, at levels up to 100-fold greater than activated mast cells [85, 86]. In a mouse model of intestinal helminth infection, c-Kit$^+$/lineage$^-$ multipotent hematopoietic progenitor cells trafficked to gut-associated lymphoid tissue where they secreted Th2 cytokines [33]. The resulting progeny provided protective immunity when transferred to mice susceptible to helminth infection. Thus HSPC can secrete inflammatory cytokines, chemokines, growth factors, and antimicrobial peptides and may participate in the response to invading pathogens.

HSPC can directly respond to infection in the periphery. The seminal work of Massberg et al. illustrated not only the roaming nature of HSPC in blood and lymph but also the ability of LPS to activate HSPC injected into the renal subcapsular space to produce myeloid and dendritic cells [3]. More recently, Kim et. al. demonstrated that lineage-negative c-Kit$^+$ HSPC traffic to *Staphylococcus aureus*-infected skin wounds and proliferate and differentiate locally to mature neutrophils [5]. This response is mediated in part by TLR2 and MyD88 [87]. Schmid et al. demonstrated that common dendritic cell progenitors in the bone marrow express TLR2, 4, and 9 and, upon activation, downregulated CXCR4 [88]. These common dendritic cell progenitors preferentially trafficked to inflamed lymph nodes and gave rise to dendritic cells [88]. HSPC act in the periphery as a source of mature effectors, providing for immediate local leukocyte needs, and as innate immune cells, elaborating inflammatory responses and mediating tissue repair.

7. Future Directions

HSPC can respond to infection and inflammation by expansion in the bone marrow, mobilization to the circulation and peripheral tissue, proliferation, differentiation, and elaboration of secreted factors. HSPC thus may fine-tune the innate immune response. It is unknown whether peripheral HSPC responses influence the outcome of inflammatory or infectious diseases. As one arm of innate defense, the roles of HSPC could be beneficial or detrimental. Indeed, HSPC may contribute to maintenance of aberrant inflammation in allergy and asthma [89]. HSPC may alter the phenotype of other immune cells. For example, HSPC may direct

a proinflammatory versus anti-inflammatory macrophage phenotype or a Th1 versus Th2 T-cell response.

In order to fully dissect HSPC function, it will be critical to understand the mechanisms for HSPC homing to infected tissue. There is evidence that the chemotactic signals and adhesion molecules used by HSPC to recruit to inflamed vessels are tissue specific. Thus it may be conceivable to prevent or augment HSPC entry into a particular organ of interest. One significant challenge in this endeavor is that HSPC share chemokine receptors and adhesion molecules with other leukocytes, thus blocking one cell type would affect others. A novel approach for more specifically manipulating HSPC trafficking is needed.

It is likely that the HSPC response to infection will depend on the pathogen, the tissue, and the infectious burden. The magnitude and type of HSPC activation during sepsis versus localized infection will likely diverge. It will be important to determine if effector cells produced de novo by HSPC at sites of inflammation are functionally distinct from leukocytes entering these sites from peripheral blood. HSPC expansion within infected tissue could be doing more than simply providing mature leukocytes, but rather they could be orchestrating the local innate immune response. Exploiting the HSPC response might provide a novel means of biological therapy in an era of increasing antibiotic-resistant infections. A deeper understanding of the mechanisms of HSPC mobilization, recruitment, and activation could provide the tools necessary to manipulate them for endogenous cell-based therapy.

8. Conclusions

Mounting evidence suggests that HSPC are not simply a source of leukocytes in the bone marrow but are active players in the innate immune response to local and systemic insults. As more studies employ population-specific phenotyping and functional verification of those populations, the identification of specific HSC and HPC effects in the response to infection will become increasingly clear. HSPC produce mature effector cells in the bone marrow upon sensing danger signals from the periphery. That HSPC can traffic to sites of inflammation outside of the bone marrow suggests that they are playing a relevant within these sites. They may combat infection on the front line by providing reconnaissance, peripheral hematopoiesis, and battling pathogens via elaboration of soluble mediators of inflammation. Further exploration of the role of HSPC in innate immunity may provide valuable tools for fighting infection.

References

[1] A. Medvinsky and E. Dzierzak, "Definitive hematopoiesis is autonomously initiated by the AGM region," *Cell*, vol. 86, no. 6, pp. 897–906, 1996.

[2] A. Medvinsky, S. Rybtsov, and S. Taoudi, "Embryonic origin of the adult hematopoietic system: advances and questions," *Development*, vol. 138, no. 6, pp. 1017–1031, 2011.

[3] S. Massberg, P. Schaerli, I. Knezevic-Maramica et al., "Immunosurveillance by hematopoietic progenitor cells trafficking through blood, lymph, and peripheral tissues," *Cell*, vol. 131, no. 5, pp. 994–1008, 2007.

[4] D. E. Wright, A. J. Wagers, A. Pathak Gulati, F. L. Johnson, and I. L. Weissman, "Physiological migration of hematopoietic stem and progenitor cells," *Science*, vol. 294, no. 5548, pp. 1933–1936, 2001.

[5] M. H. Kim, J. L. Granick, C. Kwok et al., "Neutrophil survival and c-kit+-progenitor proliferation in Staphylococcus aureus-infected skin wounds promote resolution," *Blood*, vol. 117, no. 12, pp. 3343–3352, 2011.

[6] Y. Si, C. L. Tsou, K. Croft, and I. F. Charo, "CCR2 mediates hematopoietic stem and progenitor cell trafficking to sites of inflammation in mice," *Journal of Clinical Investigation*, vol. 120, no. 4, pp. 1192–1203, 2010.

[7] J. L. Johns and M. M. Christopher, "Extramedullary hematopoiesis: a new look at the underlying stem cell niche, theories of development, and occurrence in animals," *Veterinary Pathology*, vol. 49, no. 3, pp. 508–523, 2012.

[8] Y. Nagai, K. P. Garrett, S. Ohta et al., "Toll-like receptors on hematopoietic progenitor cells stimulate innate immune system replenishment," *Immunity*, vol. 24, no. 6, pp. 801–812, 2006.

[9] S. Okada, H. Nakauchi, K. Nagayoshi, S. I. Nishikawa, Y. Miura, and T. Suda, "In vivo and in vitro stem cell function of c-kit- and Sca-1-positive murine hematopoietic cells," *Blood*, vol. 80, no. 12, pp. 3044–3050, 1992.

[10] J. L. Christensen and I. L. Weissman, "Flk-2 is a marker in hematopoietic stem cell differentiation: a simple method to isolate long-term stem cells," *Proceedings of the National Academy of Sciences of the United States of America*, vol. 98, no. 25, pp. 14541–14546, 2001.

[11] M. Osawa, K. I. Hanada, H. Hamada, and H. Nakauchi, "Long-term lymphohematopoietic reconstitution by a single CD34- low/negative hematopoietic stem cell," *Science*, vol. 273, no. 5272, pp. 242–245, 1996.

[12] M. A. Goodell, K. Brose, G. Paradis, A. S. Conner, and R. C. Mulligan, "Isolation and functional properties of murine hematopoietic stem cells that are replicating in vivo," *Journal of Experimental Medicine*, vol. 183, no. 4, pp. 1797–1806, 1996.

[13] M. J. Kiel, Ö. H. Yilmaz, T. Iwashita, O. H. Yilmaz, C. Terhorst, and S. J. Morrison, "SLAM family receptors distinguish hematopoietic stem and progenitor cells and reveal endothelial niches for stem cells," *Cell*, vol. 121, no. 7, pp. 1109–1121, 2005.

[14] I. Beerman, D. Bhattacharya, S. Zandi et al., "Functionally distinct hematopoietic stem cells modulate hematopoietic lineage potential during aging by a mechanism of clonal expansion," *Proceedings of the National Academy of Sciences of the United States of America*, vol. 107, no. 12, pp. 5465–5470, 2010.

[15] G. A. Challen, N. C. Boles, S. M. Chambers, and M. A. Goodell, "Distinct hematopoietic stem cell subtypes are differentially regulated by TGF-β1," *Cell Stem Cell*, vol. 6, no. 3, pp. 265–278, 2010.

[16] F. J. Dumont and L. Z. Coker, "Interferon-α/β enhances the expression of Ly-6 antigens on T cells in vivo and in vitro," *European Journal of Immunology*, vol. 16, no. 7, pp. 735–740, 1986.

[17] T. R. Malek, K. M. Danis, and E. K. Codias, "Tumor necrosis factor synergistically acts with IFN-γ to regulate Ly-6A/E expression in T lymphocytes, thymocytes and bone marrow cells," *Journal of Immunology*, vol. 142, no. 6, pp. 1929–1936, 1989.

[18] T. D. Randall and I. L. Weissman, "Phenotypic and functional changes induced at the clonal level in hematopoietic stem cells after 5-fluorouracil treatment," *Blood*, vol. 89, no. 10, pp. 3596–3606, 1997.

[19] D. R. Coombe, S. M. Watt, and C. R. Parish, "Mac-1 (CD11b/CD18) and CD45 mediate the adhesion of hematopoietic progenitor cells to stromal cell elements via recognition of stromal heparan sulfate," *Blood*, vol. 84, no. 3, pp. 739–752, 1994.

[20] K. C. MacNamara, K. Oduro, O. Martin et al., "Infection-induced myelopoiesis during intracellular bacterial infection is critically dependent upon IFN-γ signaling," *Journal of Immunology*, vol. 186, no. 2, pp. 1032–1043, 2011.

[21] L. E. Purton and D. T. Scadden, "Limiting factors in murine hematopoietic stem cell assays," *Cell Stem Cell*, vol. 1, no. 3, pp. 263–270, 2007.

[22] R. Schofield, "The relationship between the spleen colony-forming cell and the haemopoietic stem cell. A hypothesis," *Blood Cells*, vol. 4, no. 1-2, pp. 7–25, 1978.

[23] D. P. O'Malley, "Benign extramedullary myeloid proliferations," *Modern Pathology*, vol. 20, no. 4, pp. 405–415, 2007.

[24] M. O. Muench, J.-C. Chen, A. I. Beyer, and M. E. Fomin, "Cellular therapies supplement: the peritoneum as an ectopic site of hematopoiesis following in utero transplantation," *Transfusion*, vol. 51, supplement 4, pp. 106S–117S, 2011.

[25] T. Miyata, M. Masuzawa, K. Katsuoka, and M. Higashihara, "Cutaneous extramedullary hematopoiesis in a patient with idiopathic myelofibrosis," *Journal of Dermatology*, vol. 35, no. 7, pp. 456–461, 2008.

[26] S. M. Vega Harring, M. Niyaz, S. Okada, and M. Kudo, "Extramedullary hematopoiesis in a pyogenic granuloma: a case report and review," *Journal of Cutaneous Pathology*, vol. 31, no. 8, pp. 555–557, 2004.

[27] Y. K. Mak, C. H. Chan, C. C. So, M. K. Chan, and Y. C. Chu, "Idiopathic myelofibrosis with extramedullary haemopoiesis involving the urinary bladder in a Chinese lady," *Clinical and Laboratory Haematology*, vol. 24, no. 1, pp. 55–59, 2002.

[28] M. H. Heinicke, M. H. Zarrabi, and P. D. Gorevic, "Arthritis due to synovial involvement by extramedullary haematopoiesis in myelofibrosis with myeloid metaplasia," *Annals of the Rheumatic Diseases*, vol. 42, no. 2, pp. 196–200, 1983.

[29] T. T. Kuo, "Cutaneous extramedullary hematopoiesis presenting as leg ulcers," *Journal of the American Academy of Dermatology*, vol. 4, no. 5, pp. 592–596, 1981.

[30] D. P. Sarma, "Extramedullary hemopoiesis of the skin," *Archives of Dermatology*, vol. 117, no. 1, pp. 58–59, 1981.

[31] F. Revenga, C. Hörndler, C. Aguilar, and J. F. Paricio, "Cutaneous extramedullary hematopoiesis," *International Journal of Dermatology*, vol. 39, no. 12, pp. 957–958, 2000.

[32] C. G. Rowlands, D. Rapson, and T. Morell, "Extramedullary hematopoiesis in a Pyogenic granuloma," *American Journal of Dermatopathology*, vol. 22, no. 5, pp. 434–438, 2000.

[33] S. A. Saenz, M. C. Siracusa, J. G. Perrigoue et al., "IL25 elicits a multipotent progenitor cell population that promotes T H 2 cytokine responses," *Nature*, vol. 464, no. 7293, pp. 1362–1366, 2010.

[34] B. Vaunois, M. Breyton, D. Seigneurin, and J. Boutonnat, "Intra-serous haematopoiesis," *In Vivo*, vol. 19, no. 2, pp. 407–416, 2005.

[35] J. Johns and D. Borjesson, "Downregulation of CXCL12 signaling and altered hematopoietic stem and progenitor cell trafficking in a murine model of acute anaplasma phagocytophilum infection," *Innate Immunity*, vol. 18, no. 3, pp. 418–428, 2012.

[36] J. L. Johns, K. C. MacNamara, N. J. Walker, G. M. Winslow, and D. L. Borjesson, "Infection with Anaplasma phagocytophilum induces multilineage alterations in hematopoietic progenitor cells and peripheral blood cells," *Infection and Immunity*, vol. 77, no. 9, pp. 4070–4080, 2009.

[37] T. Sugiyama, H. Kohara, M. Noda, and T. Nagasawa, "Maintenance of the hematopoietic stem cell pool by CXCL12-CXCR4 chemokine signaling in bone marrow stromal cell niches," *Immunity*, vol. 25, no. 6, pp. 977–988, 2006.

[38] J. L. Pablos, A. Amara, A. Bouloc et al., "Stromal-cell derived factor is expressed by dendritic cells and endothelium in human skin," *American Journal of Pathology*, vol. 155, no. 5, pp. 1577–1586, 1999.

[39] I. Petit, D. Jin, and S. Rafii, "The SDF-1-CXCR4 signaling pathway: a molecular hub modulating neo-angiogenesis," *Trends in Immunology*, vol. 28, no. 7, pp. 299–307, 2007.

[40] D. J. Ceradini, A. R. Kulkarni, M. J. Callaghan et al., "Progenitor cell trafficking is regulated by hypoxic gradients through HIF-1 induction of SDF-1," *Nature Medicine*, vol. 10, no. 8, pp. 858–864, 2004.

[41] Y. Sadahira and M. Mori, "Role of the macrophage in erythropoiesis," *Pathology International*, vol. 49, no. 10, pp. 841–848, 1999.

[42] K. Choi, M. Kennedy, A. Kazarov, J. C. Papadimitriou, and G. Keller, "A common precursor for hematopoietic and endothelial cells," *Development*, vol. 125, no. 4, pp. 725–732, 1998.

[43] H. G. Kopp, S. T. Avecilla, A. T. Hooper, and S. Rafii, "The bone marrow vascular niche: home of HSC differentiation and mobilization," *Physiology*, vol. 20, no. 5, pp. 349–356, 2005.

[44] I. B. Mazo, J. C. Gutierrez-Ramos, P. S. Frenette, R. O. Hynes, D. D. Wagner, and U. H. Von Andrian, "Hematopoietic progenitor cell rolling in bone marrow microvessels: parallel contributions by endothelial selectins and vascular cell adhesion molecule 1," *Journal of Experimental Medicine*, vol. 188, no. 3, pp. 465–474, 1998.

[45] S. Rafii, F. Shapiro, R. Pettengell et al., "Human bone marrow microvascular endothelial cells support long-term proliferation and differentiation of myeloid and megakaryocytic progenitors," *Blood*, vol. 86, no. 9, pp. 3353–3363, 1995.

[46] W. Li, S. A. Johnson, W. C. Shelley, and M. C. Yoder, "Hematopoietic stem cell repopulating ability can be maintained in vitro by some primary endothelial cells," *Experimental Hematology*, vol. 32, no. 12, pp. 1226–1237, 2004.

[47] J. P. Chute, G. G. Muramoto, J. Fung, and C. Oxford, "Soluble factors elaborated by human brain endothelial cells induce the concomitant expansion of purified human BM CD34+CD38- cells and SCID-repopulating cells," *Blood*, vol. 105, no. 2, pp. 576–583, 2005.

[48] B. Walzog and P. Gaehtgens, "Adhesion molecules: the path to a new understanding of acute inflammation," *News in Physiological Sciences*, vol. 15, no. 3, pp. 107–113, 2000.

[49] K. M. Zsebo, V. N. Yuschenkoff, S. Schiffer et al., "Vascular endothelial cells and granulopoiesis: interleukin-1 stimulates release of G-CSF and GM-CSF," *Blood*, vol. 71, no. 1, pp. 99–103, 1988.

[50] J. Burg, V. Krump-Konvalinkova, F. Bittinger, and C. J. Kirkpatrick, "GM-CSF expression by human lung microvascular endothelial cells: in vitro and in vivo findings," *American Journal of Physiology-Lung Cellular and Molecular Physiology*, vol. 283, no. 2, pp. L460–L467, 2002.

[51] B. Söoderquist, J. Källman, H. Holmberg, T. Vikerfors, and E. Kihlström, "Secretion of IL-6, IL-8 and G-CSF by human endothelial cells in vitro in response to Staphylococcus aureus and staphylococcal exotoxins," *APMIS*, vol. 106, no. 12, pp. 1157–1164, 1998.

[52] W. H. Fleming, E. J. Alpern, N. Uchida, K. Ikuta, and I. L. Weissman, "Steel factor influences the distribution and activity of murine hematopoietic stem cells in vivo," *Proceedings of the National Academy of Sciences of the United States of America*, vol. 90, no. 8, pp. 3760–3764, 1993.

[53] J. W. Goodman and G. S. Hodgson, "Evidence for stem cells in the peripheral blood of mice," *Blood*, vol. 19, pp. 702–714, 1962.

[54] J. P. Lévesque, I. G. Winkler, S. R. Larsen, and J. E. Rasko, "Mobilization of bone marrow-derived progenitors," *Handbook of Experimental Pharmacology*, no. 180, pp. 3–36, 2007.

[55] J. P. Lévesque, Y. Takamatsu, S. K. Nilsson, D. N. Haylock, and P. J. Simmons, "Vascular cell adhesion molecule-1 (CD106) is cleaved by neutrophil proteases in the bone marrow following hematopoietic progenitor cell mobilization by granulocyte colony-stimulating factor," *Blood*, vol. 98, no. 5, pp. 1289–1297, 2001.

[56] A. Jalili, N. Shirvaikar, L. Marquez-Curtis et al., "Fifth complement cascade protein (C5) cleavage fragments disrupt the SDF-1/CXCR4 axis: further evidence that innate immunity orchestrates the mobilization of hematopoietic stem/progenitor cells," *Experimental Hematology*, vol. 38, no. 4, pp. 321–332, 2010.

[57] M. H. Cottler-Fox, T. Lapidot, I. Petit et al., "Stem cell mobilization," *Hematology*, pp. 419–437, 2003.

[58] C. L. Semerad, M. J. Christopher, F. Liu et al., "G-CSF potently inhibits osteoblast activity and CXCL12 mRNA expression in the bone marrow," *Blood*, vol. 106, no. 9, pp. 3020–3027, 2005.

[59] M. Artico, S. Bosco, C. Cavallotti et al., "Noradrenergic and cholinergic innervation of the bone marrow," *International journal of molecular medicine*, vol. 10, no. 1, pp. 77–80, 2002.

[60] A. Spiegel, S. Shivtiel, A. Kalinkovich et al., "Catecholaminergic neurotransmitters regulate migration and repopulation of immature human CD34+ cells through Wnt signaling," *Nature Immunology*, vol. 8, no. 10, pp. 1123–1131, 2007.

[61] Y. Katayama, M. Battista, W. M. Kao et al., "Signals from the sympathetic nervous system regulate hematopoietic stem cell egress from bone marrow," *Cell*, vol. 124, no. 2, pp. 407–421, 2006.

[62] E. Karshovska, A. Zernecke, G. Sevilmis et al., "Expression of HIF-1α in injured arteries controls SDF-1α-mediated neointima formation in apolipoprotein E-deficient mice," *Arteriosclerosis, Thrombosis, and Vascular Biology*, vol. 27, no. 12, pp. 2540–2547, 2007.

[63] S. Massberg, I. Konrad, K. Schürzinger et al., "Platelets secrete stromal cell-derived factor 1α and recruit bone marrow-derived progenitor cells to arterial thrombi in vivo," *Journal of Experimental Medicine*, vol. 203, no. 5, pp. 1221–1233, 2006.

[64] M. Z. Ratajczak, R. Reca, M. Wysoczynski, J. Yan, and J. Ratajczak, "Modulation of the SDF-1-CXCR4 axis by the third complement component (C3)—Implications for trafficking of CXCR4+ stem

cells," *Experimental Hematology*, vol. 34, no. 8, pp. 986–995, 2006.

[65] R. A. J. Oostendorp, G. Reisbach, E. Spitzer et al., "VLA-4 and VCAM-1 are the principal adhesion molecules involved in the interaction between blast colony-forming cells and bone marrow stromal cells," *British Journal of Haematology*, vol. 91, no. 2, pp. 275–284, 1995.

[66] T. Papayannopoulou and B. Nakamoto, "Peripheralization of hemopoietic progenitors in primates treated with anti-VLA4 integrin," *Proceedings of the National Academy of Sciences of the United States of America*, vol. 90, no. 20, pp. 9374–9378, 1993.

[67] D. P. J. Kavanagh and N. Kalia, "Hematopoietic stem cell homing to injured tissues," *Stem Cell Reviews and Reports*, vol. 7, no. 3, pp. 672–682, 2011.

[68] D. P. J. Kavanagh, L. E. Durant, H. A. Crosby et al., "Haematopoietic stem cell recruitment to injured murine liver sinusoids depends on $\alpha 4\beta 1$ integrin/VCAM-1 interactions," *Gut*, vol. 59, no. 1, pp. 79–87, 2010.

[69] S. Zhang, E. Shpall, J. T. Willerson, and E. T. H. Yeh, "Fusion of human hematopoietic progenitor cells and murine cardiomyocytes is mediated by $\alpha 4\beta 1$ integrin/vascular cell adhesion molecule-1 interaction," *Circulation Research*, vol. 100, no. 5, pp. 693–702, 2007.

[70] M. T. Baldridge, K. Y. King, N. C. Boles, D. C. Weksberg, and M. A. Goodell, "Quiescent haematopoietic stem cells are activated by IFN-γ in response to chronic infection," *Nature*, vol. 465, no. 7299, pp. 793–797, 2010.

[71] A. Kolb-Mäurer, M. Wilhelm, F. Weissinger, E. B. Bröcker, and W. Goebel, "Interaction of human hematopoietic stem cells with bacterial pathogens," *Blood*, vol. 100, no. 10, pp. 3703–3709, 2002.

[72] P. Banerjee, L. Crawford, E. Samuelson, and G. Feuer, "Hematopoietic stem cells and retroviral infection," *Retrovirology*, vol. 7, article no. 8, 2010.

[73] M. T. Baldridge, K. Y. King, and M. A. Goodell, "Inflammatory signals regulate hematopoietic stem cells," *Trends in Immunology*, vol. 32, no. 2, pp. 57–65, 2011.

[74] T. Sato, N. Onai, H. Yoshihara, F. Arai, T. Suda, and T. Ohteki, "Interferon regulatory factor-2 protects quiescent hematopoietic stem cells from type i interferon-dependent exhaustion," *Nature Medicine*, vol. 15, no. 6, pp. 696–700, 2009.

[75] P. Singh, Y. Yao, A. Weliver, H. E. Broxmeyer, S. C. Hong, and C. H. Chang, "Vaccinia virus infection modulates the hematopoietic cell compartments in the bone marrow," *Stem Cells*, vol. 26, no. 4, pp. 1009–1016, 2008.

[76] A. M. de Bruin, S. F. Libregts, M. Valkhof, L. Boon, I. P. Touw, and M. A. Nolte, "Ifngamma induces monopoiesis and inhibits neutrophil development during inflammation," *Blood*, vol. 119, no. 6, pp. 1543–1554, 2012.

[77] N. N. Belyaev, D. E. Brown, A. I. G. Diaz et al., "Induction of an IL7-R+ c-Kithi myelolymphoid progenitor critically dependent on IFN-γ signaling during acute malaria," *Nature Immunology*, vol. 11, no. 6, pp. 477–485, 2010.

[78] M. Sioud and Y. Fløisand, "NOD2/CARD15 on bone marrow CD34+ hematopoietic cells mediates induction of cytokines and cell differentiation," *Journal of Leukocyte Biology*, vol. 85, no. 6, pp. 939–946, 2009.

[79] N. N. Zhang, S. H. Shen, L. J. Jiang et al., "RIG-I plays a critical role in negatively regulating granulocytic proliferation," *Proceedings of the National Academy of Sciences of the United States of America*, vol. 105, no. 30, pp. 10553–10558, 2008.

[80] M. Sioud, Y. Fløisand, L. Forfang, and F. Lund-Johansen, "Signaling through toll-like receptor 7/8 induces the differentiation of human bone marrow CD34+ progenitor cells along the myeloid lineage," *Journal of Molecular Biology*, vol. 364, no. 5, pp. 945–954, 2006.

[81] K. De Luca, V. Frances-Duvert, M. J. Asensio et al., "The TLR1/2 agonist PAM3CSK4 instructs commitment of human hematopoietic stem cells to a myeloid cell fate," *Leukemia*, vol. 23, no. 11, pp. 2063–2074, 2009.

[82] A. Yanez, C. Murciano, J. E. O'Connor, D. Gozalbo, and M. L. Gil, "Candida albicans triggers proliferation and differentiation of hematopoietic stem and progenitor cells by a MyD88-dependent signaling," *Microbes and Infection*, vol. 11, no. 4, pp. 531–535, 2009.

[83] A. Yanez, A. Flores, C. Murciano, J. E. O'Connor, D. Gozalbo, and M. L. Gil, "Signalling through TLR2/MyD88 induces differentiation of murine bone marrow stem and progenitor cells to functional phagocytes in response to Candida albicans," *Cellular Microbiology*, vol. 12, no. 1, pp. 114–128, 2010.

[84] M. Majka, A. Janowska-Wieczorek, J. Ratajczak et al., "Numerous growth factors, cytokines, and chemokines are secreted by human CD34+ cells, myeloblasts, erythroblasts, and megakaryoblasts and regulate normal hematopoiesis in an autocrine/paracrine manner," *Blood*, vol. 97, no. 10, pp. 3075–3085, 2001.

[85] Z. Allakhverdi and G. Delespesse, "Hematopoietic progenitor cells are innate Th2 cytokine-producing cells," *Allergy*, vol. 67, no. 1, pp. 4–9, 2012.

[86] Z. Allakhverdi, M. R. Comeau, D. E. Smith et al., "CD34+ hemopoietic progenitor cells are potent effectors of allergic inflammation," *Journal of Allergy and Clinical Immunology*, vol. 123, no. 2, pp. 472–e1, 2009.

[87] J. L. Granick, D. L. Borjesson, and S. I. Simon, "Hematopoietic stem and progenitor cells traffic to s. Aureus-infected wounds where they proliferate and differentiate along the myeloid lineage in a myd88-dependent manner," in *Proceedings of the Annual Meeting of the Society for Leukocyte Biology*, 2011.

[88] M. A. Schmid, H. Takizawa, D. R. Baumjohann, Y. Saito, and M. G. Manz, "Bone marrow dendritic cell progenitors sense pathogens via Toll-like receptors and subsequently migrate to inflamed lymph nodes," *Blood*, vol. 118, no. 18, pp. 4829–4840, 2011.

[89] M. R. Blanchet and K. M. McNagny, "Stem cells, inflammation and allergy," *Allergy, Asthma & Clinical Immunology*, vol. 5, no. 1, p. 13, 2009.

12

The Presence of Anti-HLA Antibodies before and after Allogeneic Hematopoietic Stem Cells Transplantation from HLA-Mismatched Unrelated Donors

Anna Koclega,[1] Miroslaw Markiewicz,[1] Urszula Siekiera,[2] Alicja Dobrowolska,[2] Mizia Sylwia,[3] Monika Dzierzak-Mietla,[1] Patrycja Zielinska,[1] Malgorzata Sobczyk Kruszelnicka,[1] Andrzej Lange,[3] and Slawomira Kyrcz-Krzemien[1]

[1] Department of Hematology and BMT, Medical University of Silesia, Dabrowskiego 25, 40-032 Katowice, Poland
[2] HLA and Immunogenetics Laboratory, Regional Blood Center, Raciborska 15, 40-074 Katowice, Poland
[3] Lower Silesian Center for Cellular Transplantation with National Bone Marrow Donor Registry, Grabiszynska 105, 53-439 Wroclaw, Poland

Correspondence should be addressed to Anna Koclega, annakkoc@wp.pl

Academic Editor: Bronwen Shaw

Although anti-human leukocyte antigen antibodies (anti-HLA Abs) are important factors responsible for graft rejection in solid organ transplantation and play a role in post-transfusion complications, their role in allogeneic hematopoietic stem cell transplantation (allo-HSCT) has not been finally defined. Enormous polymorphism of HLA-genes, their immunogenicity and heterogeneity of antibodies, as well as the growing number of allo-HSCTs from partially HLA-mismatched donors, increase the probability that anti-HLA antibodies could be important factors responsible for the treatment outcomes. We have examined the incidence of anti-HLA antibodies in a group of 30 allo-HSCT recipients from HLA-mismatched unrelated donors. Anti-HLA Abs were identified in sera collected before and after allo-HSCT. We have used automated DynaChip assay utilizing microchips bearing purified class I and II HLA antigens for detection of anti-HLA Abs. We have detected anit-HLA antibodies against HLA-A, B, C, DR, DQ and DP, but no donor or recipient-specific anti-HLA Abs were detected in the studied group. The preliminary results indicate that anti-HLA antibodies are present before and after allo-HSCT in HLA-mismatched recipients.

1. Introduction

Allogeneic hematopoietic stem cell transplantation (allo-HSCT) is an effective treatment of both congenital and acquired disturbances of hematopoiesis, especially of hematological malignancies.

The selection of the optimal donor is based on high-resolution HLA typing. The MHC (Major Histocompatibility Complex) contains more than 200 genes which are situated on the short arm of chromosome 6 at 6p21.3. It is divided into three main regions: HLA class I (containing *HLA-A*, *B*, and *C* genes), class II (containing *HLA-DR*, *DQ*, and *DP* genes), and class III region. The role of HLA molecules is to present peptides to T cells (both CD4 and CD8 T cells), enabling them to recognize and eliminate "foreign" particles and also to prevent the recognition of "self" as foreign. HLA mismatches may occur at antigenic or allelic level; the first are characterized by amino acid substitutions in both peptide-binding and T-cell recognition regions, whereas the latter are characterized by amino-acid substitution in the peptide binding regions only [1].

HLA antigens are recognized by immunocompetent T cells, what may lead to graft failure, graft versus host disease (GVHD), and other posttransplant complications as well as to favorable graft versus leukemia (GVL) effect. HLA molecules bear multiple antigenic epitopes, many of which are the so-called "public" epitopes that are shared among the products of several different HLA alleles, resulting in the apparent cross-reactive groups of antigens (CREGs). These shared epitopes may be responsible for patient's sensitization to multiple HLA antigens, despite a single antigen mismatch only [2–4].

The participation of cellular arm of immunological response to HLA antigens is well known, but the role of humoral arm of immunity is also very interesting, especially when we consider the enormous polymorphism of HLA-genes, their immunogenicity and huge heterogeneity of antibodies. Antibodies are glycoproteins that belong to the superfamily of immunoglobulins [5]. The basic structural units of antibodies are two heavy chains (α, γ, ε, δ or μ) and two light chains (κ or λ). The type of a heavy chain determines the class of antibody: IgA, IgG, IgM, IgE or IgM [6]. The region of chromosome that encodes the antibody is large and contains several distinct genes. The locus containing heavy chain genes is found on chromosome 14; loci containing κ and λ light chain genes are found on chromosomes 2 and 22, respectively. The enormous diversity of antibodies allows the immune system to recognize an equally wide variety of antigens [5]. It has been known that humans produce about 10 billion different antibodies capable of binding a distinct epitope of an antigen [7]. Such a diversity of antibodies is caused by domain variability, recombination, somatic hypermutation and affinity maturation, class switching, and affinity designations [8–10]. Anti-HLA Abs may be present in healthy individuals [11, 12]. The sensitization to MHC antigens may be caused by transfusions, pregnancy, or failed previous grafts [13]. Anti-HLA Abs are more frequently detected in patients with hematological disorders due to their alloimmunization, resulting mainly from common use of transfusions [14].

The clinical significance of anti-HLA Abs is well known in the field of transfusional medicine. The presence of anti-HLA Abs in patients is one of the major causes of platelet transfusion refractoriness [15]. On the other hand, anti-HLA Abs present in blood products have been shown to be a major cause of transfusion-related acute lung injury (TRALI) [16, 17]. The role of anti-HLA Abs is also well known in solid organ transplantation—especially in kidney transplantation, because transplanted kidneys are highly susceptible to antibody-mediated injury [18, 19]. Antibodies produced before kidney transplantation (reacting with donor's HLA antigens) induce hyperacute or acute vascular rejections which frequently result in transplant failure [20, 21].

Despite the well-recognized role of antibody-mediated rejection in solid organ transplantation, the graft rejection following allo-HSCT is generally attributed to cytolitic host-versus-graft (HVG) reaction mediated by host T and NK cells, that survived the conditioning regimen [22–25]. Engraftment failure rate is approximately 4% in allo-HSCT from matched unrelated donor (MUD) and about 20% in cord blood or T-cell-depleted haploidentical transplantations [26, 27]. Antibody-mediated bone marrow failure after allogeneic bone marrow transplantation can be also caused by antibody-dependent cell-mediated cytotoxicity (ADCC), or complement-mediated cytotoxicity [28–30]. In ADCC, the cytotoxic destruction of antibody-coated target cells by host cells is triggered when an antibody bound to the surface of a cell interacts with Fc receptors on NK cells or macrophages. Preformed antibodies present at the time of hematopoietic stem cell infusion are unaffected by standard transplantation conditioning regimens, T- or B-cell immunosuppressive drugs or modulatory strategies given in the pretransplantation period [31].

Albeit the T-cell-mediated cellular immunity is the primary barrier for bone marrow allorejection in nonsensitized recipients in the animal models (mice), the humoral arm of the immune response plays a very important, previously unappreciated, role in the rejection of allogeneic stem cell transplantation in sensitized mice and in such case the rejection of a bone marrow is T-cell independent [31, 32]. Moreover, the achievement of a mixed allogeneic chimerism resulted in reverse of the sensitization in allosensitized recipients [30, 33]. Probably not only antigen-specific but also cross-reactive or broadly reactive alloantibodies may be responsible for the graft failure [32]. Spellman and Bray have demonstrated in a retrospective, case-controlled study that the prevalence of donor-specific anti-HLA antibodies was higher in a group of mismatched unrelated donor recipients who suffered graft rejection than in a control group that engrafted. Among the 37 recipients who failed to engraft 9 (24%) possessed DSAS against HLA-A, B, or DP, but only 1 (1%) recipient of 78 controls did [34]. In the study of Ciurea et al. DSAS was the single most important factor associated with graft failure and HLA-mismatches increased the occurrence of donor-specific HLA antibodies in MUD transplantation [35]. Takanashi et al. demonstrated the impact of anti-HLA antibodies on engraftment after myeloablative single unit cord blood transplantation. Patients with anti-HLA antibodies experienced slower neutrophils and platelet recovery than antibody-free patients. Although no effect of anti-HLA antibodies on GvHD grade II-IV, relapse, or TRM has been observed, the overall and event-free survival were significantly inferior in antibody-positive patients [36]. Similar observations were made after double umbilical cord blood transplantation [37].

As presented above, the influence of anti-HLA Abs, including Abs directed against mismatched antigens, on the results of allo-HSCT, especially on graft failure, has been proved in several reports. However, in patients following allo-HSCT, the series of time remote complications may occur. As antibodies appearing in the result of the earlier immunization are detected before transplantation, the question of their presence and specificity after transplant, after the myeloablative conditioning treatment, and during administration of immunosuppressive therapy is open, when the hematopoietic function is taken over by the donor's cells. The first cells to reconstitute (within the first 100 days) after the transplantation are granulocytes, monocytes, macrophages, and NK cells. In contrast, T and B lymphocytes remain severely reduced and their function is impaired from 6 months to 1 year after the transplantation [1].

Therefore, the aim of our study was to examine the presence and the specificity of anti-HLA antibodies before and following the allo-HSCT.

2. Materials and Methods

We included 30 patients who received allo-HSCT from partially HLA-mismatched unrelated donors and who agreed to participate in the study. Donors lacking full HLA compatibility with recipients were chosen when compatible donors were not available. Standard high-resolution allelic typing of HLA-A, B, C, DRB1, and DQB1, without HLA-DP, was performed. The study was carried out in the Department of Hematology and Bone Marrow Transplantation of the Medical University of Silesia in Katowice, Poland, between 2007 and 2011. The examination of patient's sera was scheduled at 4 time points: before the start of conditioning treatment and 30 days, 100 days, and 1 year after transplant.

The preparative treatment was myeloablative in 28 (93%) and reduced in 2 (7%) pts. Standard GVHD prophylaxis consisted of pretransplant antithymocyte globulin, cyclosporine A in initial dose 3 mg/kg i.v. starting from day −1 with dose adjusted to its serum level and shift to oral administration about day +20, methotrexate 15 mg/m^2 i.v. on day +1, and 10 mg/m^2 i.v. on days +3 and +6. Methylprednisolone at dose 2 mg/kg i.v. was the first line therapy of aGVHD symptoms; in few patients mycophenolate mofetil or tacrolimus was used. The source of cells was the bone marrow in 9 (30%) and peripheral blood in 21 (70%) patients.

The detailed characteristics of the study population are presented in Table 1.

Patient's sera were tested for the presence of anti-HLA Abs in the HLA and Immunogenetics Laboratory of Regional Blood Center in Katowice, Poland. Anti-HLA A, B, C, DR, DQ, and DP antibodies were detected and identified using the ELISA-based DynaChip Technology. The DynaChip HLA Antibody analysis system utilizes microchips spotted with purified HLA antigens immobilized on the surface of the glass chip. Test serum was free of aggregates and excess lipids before testing. This was achieved by centrifugation for 10 minutes at 10,000 g. The clarified supernatant was diluted with the Sample Diluent contained within the kit and then it was added to the DynaChip wells. Anti-HLA Abs present in the test serum were bound to the HLA antigens on the surface on the chip. Bound antibodies were then detected using the Antibody Detection Reagent (antihuman IgG and horseradish peroxidase complex). The assay was completed with colorimetric detection. The resulting patterns of blue-positive and clear-negative spots were recorded by the software and subsequently automatically analyzed by the DynaChip Analysis Software. The presence of at least one anti-HLA antibody was regarded as presence of anti-HLA Abs, whereas if the examined serum contained antibodies against more than 50 different HLA antigens they were regarded as "anti-HLA Abs to many specificities." Applied DynaChip HLA Antibody analysis system did not allow to measure the concentration of detected antibodies.

The study has been approved by the responsible Ethical Committee of Medical University of Silesia.

3. Results

Anti-HLA Abs were detected in 26 (86.6%) patients. Anti-HLA Abs against HLA class I, II, or both were detected in 8 (26.6%), 2 (6,6%), or 16 (53.3%) patients, respectively. In 4 (13.3%) patients they were detected before transplant only,

TABLE 1: Patients characteristics ($n = 30$).

Median age (range)	
Recipient	37 (13–57) years
Donor	36 (19–55) years
Mean time from diagnosis to allo-HSCT (range)	0.75 (0.63–10.3) years
	Number (%)
Sex	
Donor	
Male	19 (63.3%)
Female	11 (36.7%)
Recipient	
Male	16 (53.3%)
Female	14 (46.7%)
Sex matching	
Male donor, male recipient	10 (33.3%)
Female donor, female recipient	5 (16.6%)
Male donor female recipient	9 (30%)
Female donor, male recipient	6 (20%)
HLA- mismatch	
Antigen A	4 (13.3%)
Antigen C	12 (40%)
Antigen DQ	2 (6.6%)
Allele A	2 (6.6%)
Allele B	5 (16.6%)
Allele DQ	3 (10%)
Antigen B + Antigen C	1 (3.3%)
Antigen A + Allele B	1 (3.3%)
Primary indication for allo-HSCT	
Acute lymphoblastic leukemia (ALL)	6 (20%)
Acute myeloid leukemia (AML)	15 (20%)
Chronic myeloid leukemia (CML)	5 (16.6%)
Chronic lymphocytic leukemia (CLL)	1 (3.3)
Severe aplastic anemia (SAA)	2 (6.6%)
Paroxysmal nocturnal hemoglobinuria (PNH)	1 (3.35)
Preparative regimen	
Cyclophosphamide	1 (3.3%)
TBI + Cyclophosphamide	6 (20%)
TBI + Fludarabine	1 (3.3%)
Treosulfan + Fludarabine	6 (20%)
Busulfan + Cyclophosphamide	12 (40%)
Busulfan + Fludarabine	1 (3.3%)
Treosulfan + Cyclophosphamide	1 (3.3%)
Busulfan + Cyclophosphamide + Gemtuzumab Ozogamycin	1 (3.3%)
Rituximab + Alemtuzumab + Melphalan	1 (3.3%)
Immunosuppressive treatment	
Glycocorticoid	27 (90%)
Cyclosporine	30 (100%)
Mycophenolate mofetil	7 (23%)
Tacrolimus	1 (3.3%)
Source of cells	
Bone marrow	9 (30%)
Peripheral blood	21 (70%)

TABLE 2: Anti-HLA antibodies detected before and 30 days, 100 days and 1 year after allo-HSCT in 30 recipients.

No	Typing of mismatched HLA		HLA-mismatch	Detected anti-HLA Abs with regard to allo-HSCT			
	Recipient	Donor		Before	+30 days	+100 days	+1 year
1	C 0401 C 0501	C 12XX C 0501	Antigen C	Many specificities	Not tested	DR15	Not tested
2	DQB1 0202 DQB1 0302	DQB1 0202 DQB1 0301	Allele DQB1	Many specificities	Not tested	B70	Not tested
3	C 0802 C 1203	C 0802 C 0303	Antigen C	Many specificities	Not tested	Not tested	Not detected
4	C 0501 C 0702	C 0201 C 0702	Antigen C	Not detected	B65, B46, B37, C36, C10	DRB1*15, DQB1*06	Not detected
5	A 0201 A 0302	A 0201 A 0301	Allele A	Not detected	Not detected	Not tested	C14, B62, C9, A26
6	C 0401 C 1602	C 0401 C 1502	Antigen C	Not detected	Not tested	Many specificities	Not detected
7	C 0802 C 1502	C 0702 C 0702	Antigen C	Not detected	Not tested	Many specificities	Not detected
8	DQB1 0202 DQB1 0301	DQB1 0303 DQB1 0301	Antigen DQB1	Not detected	Not tested	Not detected	Not detected
9	C 0303 C 0102	C 0403 C 0102	Antigen C	Not detected	Not tested	DR13	B82, B49
10	C 0303 C 0401	C 0401 —	Antigen C	A23, A24, B27, B35, B38, B40, C0803, C0804	Not tested	B45, A66	DQ8, DR4
11	C 0303 C 0602	C 0403 C 0602	Antigen C	B75, B46, DR13, DQ3	Not tested	Not detected	Not detected
12	DQB1 0301 DQB1 0504	DQB1 0301 DQB1 0501	Allele DQB1	Not detected	Not tested	Not detected	B82, A34, DQ8, DR4
13	C 0202 C 0102	C 0202 C 0202	Antigen C	Not detected	Not tested	Not tested	B70
14	DQB1 0602 DQB1 0602	DQB1 0602 DQB1 0603	Allele DQB1	Many specificities	Many specificities	Not detected	Not detected
15	C 0102 C 0602	C 0302 C 0602	Antigen C	Not detected	C18, DRB3*, DPB1*05, DRB104, DQB1*06	Not tested	Not tested
16	A 1101 A 2601	A 24xx A 2601	Antigen A	Not detected	Not detected	Not tested	DQ2, DQ4, DQA02, DQA04
17	A 0205 A 2402	A 0201 A 2402	Allele A	DQB1*03, DRB1*04	Not tested	Not tested	Not tested
18	B 4102 B 5601 C 0401 C 1703	B 4102 B 5501 C 0301 C 1703	Antigen B, antigen C	Not detected	Not detected	Not detected	Not tested
19	A 2601 A 3201	A 0201 A 3201	Antigen A	DQ8, DR4	DQ8, DR4	Not detected	B45, A66, DR10, DR12
20	DQB1 0301 DQB1 0302	DQB1 0301 DQB1 0402	Antigen DQB1	A2, 2C A0302, B67	A2, C2, B67	A2, DR 16	Not tested
21	A 0201 A 2901	A 0205 A 2901	Allele A	B7, 7C, B60, B81, A2403, A2608, C0727, C0804	B7	B47, B63	Not tested

TABLE 2: Continued.

No	Typing of mismatched HLA		HLA-mismatch	Detected anti-HLA Abs with regard to allo-HSCT			
	Recipient	Donor		Before	+30 days	+100 days	+1 year
22	C 0501 C 1203	C 0501 —	Antigen C	Not detected	Not detected	Not detected	Not detected
23	C 0304 C 0702	— C 0702	Antigen C	A2 A0302, B2703, B3501, B3503, 4006, B4101, B45, B4604, B67, B76, B78, C0103, C0403, DR51, DR15, DQ6, DR16, DQA01 DPB39, DPB3901, DPB85, DPB8501, DQB0502	A2, A0207, A0302, B2703, B3503, B4006, B4101, B67, B76, C0403, DR51, DR15, DQ6, DR16 DPB39, DPB3901, DPB85, DPB8501, DQB0502	A2, DR51, DR16	DQ7, DQA05
24	B 3501 B 5701	B 3503 B 5701	Allele B	B42, A80, C17	Not detected	B77	Not detected
25	A 2402 A 2601	A 03xx 2601	Antigen A	Not detected	Not detected	Not detected	Not tested
26	B 3501 B 3502	B 3501 B 35xx	Allele B	C7, DQ8	Not detected	Not detected	Not detected
27	A 3001 A 3101	A 01xx —	Antigen A	DR10, DR11	B77, B38	Not detected	Not tested
28	A 2501 A 3201	A 2501 A 23xx	Antigen A	Not detected	B77, A36	Not detected	Not detected
29	B 1801 B 4402	B 1801 B 4427	Allele B	A31	Not detected	B61, C15, B35	Not tested
30	B 3503 B 3501	B 3503 B 3503	Allele B	DQ5, DQ6, DQA01	C7, DQ6, DR51, DPB39, DPB3901, DPB85, DPB8501, DQB0502,	C7, DR 51, DPB14, DPB1401, DQB0502, DQB0602, DQB0608, DR0806, DR2, DQ6, DQA01	Not tested

in 10 (33.3%) patients after transplant only, and in 12 (40%) patients both before and after transplantation. In 4 (13.3%) patients anti-HLA Abs were not detected neither before nor after allo-HSCT. Anti-HLA Abs directed against the class or antigens of mismatched HLA were detected in 4 patients before transplant and in 9 patients after transplant. In 5 patients we identified antibodies with the same specificities before and 30 days after the transplantation (as presented in Table 2, cases' numbers: 19, 20, 21, 23, and 30). Although we did not identify neither donor or recipient allele-specific anti-HLA Abs, antibodies that detected after transplant in 3 patients belonged to the same CREG (Cross-Reactive Group) as recipient's mismatched HLA antigen (as presented in

Table 2, cases' numbers: 19-10CREG, 24-5CREG, and 29-12CREG). These antibodies were detected more than 100 days after transplantation, so it is very likely that they were produced by donor cells.

The specificities of anti-HLA Abs detected before allo-HSCT and at different time-points after transplant are presented in Table 2. We have succeed only partially in consequent collecting sera at all scheduled timepoints from patients included into the study for analysis due to the fact that some patients were referred to our center for allo-HSCT from remote parts of Poland. After allo-HSCT they have moved for care to their home centers and collection of the complete set of sera from them was impossible.

4. Conclusions

Our preliminary results indicate that preformed anti-HLA Abs can be detected before and may also appear after transplant in mismatched allo-HSCT recipients. Anti-HLA Abs present in 3 patients were directed against HLA antigens which belonged to the same serological Cross Reactive Groups as the mismatched HLA antigens.

In 5 patients anti-HLA Abs directed against the same HLA antigen were detected before and after allo-HSCT what may indicate that they were not destroyed during the myeloablative conditioning treatment and standard immunosuppressive therapy. These antibodies belonged to the same serological Cross Reactive Group as the recipient's but not donor's mismatched HLA antigens, so it is possible to conclude that donor's cells may produce anti-HLA Abs against the recipients cells after allo-HSCT. Therefore, they may theoretically be responsible for induction of several immunological posttransplant complications. Antibodies detected after transplantation may also result from immunization, for example, by transfusions, as allo-HSCT recipients often require intensive supportive treatment with blood derivatives.

We believe that our observations help to better understand the immune mechanisms contributing to allogeneic sensitization which may influence allo-HSCT results. It is possible that sensitized patients who possess anti-HLA antibodies before or after the transplantation could benefit from modification of conditioning and immunosuppressive therapeutic approaches in the future.

Presented preliminary outcomes of 30 patients are based only on part of our whole study group which consists of 70 patients. The statistical analysis aimed to reveal the eventual impact of anti-HLA Abs on allo-HSCT results will be performed after completion and examination of sera taken at all scheduled timepoints from the whole group. We also consider the extension of the search for anti-HLA Abs with utilization of Luminex Labscreen method which enables to calculate the mean fluorescence intensity and thus to assess the concentration of detected antibodies.

Conflict of Interests

The authors report having no conflict of interests.

References

[1] J. Apperley, E. Carreras, E. Gluckman, and T. Masszi, *Haematopoietic Stem Cell Transplantation-The EBMT Handbook*, 6th edition, 2012.

[2] F. Legrand and J. Dausset, "Serological evidence of the existence of several antigenic determinants (or factors) on the HLA-A gene products," in *Histocompatibility Testing 1972*, J. Dausset and J. Colombani, Eds., Munksgaard, Copenhagen, Denmark, 1973.

[3] G. E. Rodey and T. C. Fuller, "Public epitopes and the antigenic structure of the HLA molecules," *Critical reviews in immunology*, vol. 7, no. 3, pp. 229–267, 1987.

[4] B. D. Schwartz, L. K. Luehrman, and G. E. Rodey, "Public antigenic determinant on a family of HLA-B molecules. Basis

[5] for cross-reactivity and a possible link with disease predisposition," *Journal of Clinical Investigation*, vol. 64, no. 4, pp. 938–947, 1979.

[5] R. A. Rhoades and R. G. Pflanzer, *Human Physiology*, Thomson Learning, Stockholm, Sweden, 4th edition, 2002.

[6] J. Charles, *Immunobiology*, Garland Publishing, New York, NY, USA, 5th edition, 2001.

[7] L. J. Fanning, A. M. Connor, and G. E. Wu, "Development of the immunoglobulin repertoire," *Clinical Immunology and Immunopathology*, vol. 79, no. 1, pp. 1–14, 1996.

[8] P. Peter, *The Immune System*, Garland Science, New York, NY, USA, 2nd edition, 2005.

[9] Y. Bergman and H. Cedar, "A stepwise epigenetic process controls immunoglobulin allelic exclusion," *Nature Reviews Immunology*, vol. 4, no. 10, pp. 753–761, 2004.

[10] M. Or-Guil, N. Wittenbrink, A. A. Weiser, and J. Schuchhardt, "Recirculation of germinal center B cells: a multilevel selection strategy for antibody maturation," *Immunological Reviews*, vol. 216, no. 1, pp. 130–141, 2007.

[11] N. El-Awar, P. I. Terasaki, A. Nguyen et al., "Epitopes of human leukocyte antigen class I antibodies found in sera of normal healthy males and cord blood," *Human Immunology*, vol. 70, no. 10, pp. 844–853, 2009.

[12] L. E. Morales-Buenrostro, P. I. Terasaki, L. A. Marino-Vázquez, J. H. Lee, N. El-Awar, and J. Alberú, "Natural human leukocyte antigen antibodies found in nonalloimmunized healthy males," *Transplantation*, vol. 86, no. 8, pp. 1111–1115, 2008.

[13] W. E. Braun, "Laboratory and clinical management of the highly sensitized organ transplant recipient," *Human Immunology*, vol. 26, no. 4, pp. 245–260, 1989.

[14] A. Idica, N. Sasaki, S. Hardy, and P. Terasaki, "Unexpected frequencies of HLA antibody specificities present in sera of multitransfused patients." *Clinical transplants*, pp. 139–159, 2006.

[15] E. Hod and J. Schwartz, "Platelet transfusion refractoriness," *British Journal of Haematology*, vol. 142, no. 3, pp. 348–360, 2008.

[16] R. A. Middelburg, D. Van Stein, E. Briët, and J. G. Van Der Bom, "The role of donor antibodies in the pathogenesis of transfusion-related acute lung injury: a systematic review," *Transfusion*, vol. 48, no. 10, pp. 2167–2176, 2008.

[17] A. Reil, B. Keller-Stanislawski, S. Günay, and J. Bux, "Specificities of leucocyte alloantibodies in transfusion-related acute lung injury and results of leucocyte antibody screening of blood donors," *Vox Sanguinis*, vol. 95, no. 4, pp. 313–317, 2008.

[18] E. R. Vasilescu, E. K. Ho, A. I. Colovai et al., "Alloantibodies and the outcome of cadaver kidney allografts," *Human Immunology*, vol. 67, no. 8, pp. 597–604, 2006.

[19] A. A. Zachary, L. E. Ratner, J. A. Graziani, D. P. Lucas, N. L. Delaney, and M. S. Leffell, "Characterization of HLA class I specific antibodies by ELISA using solubilized antigen targets: II. Clinical relevance," *Human Immunology*, vol. 62, no. 3, pp. 236–246, 2001.

[20] F. Kissmeyer-Nielsen, S. Olsen, V. P. Petersen, and O. Fjeldborg, "Hyperacute rejection of kidney allografts, associated with pre-existing humoral antibodies against donor cells." *The Lancet*, vol. 2, no. 7465, pp. 662–665, 1966.

[21] G. M. Williams, D. M. Hume, R. P. Hudson Jr, P. J. Morris, K. Kano, and F. Milgrom, "Hyperacute renal-homograft rejection in man." *New England Journal of Medicine*, vol. 279, no. 12, pp. 611–618, 1968.

[22] E. Schwartz, T. Lapidot, and D. Gozes, "Abrogation of bone marrow allograft resistance in mice by increased total body

irradiation correlates with eradication of host clonable T cells and alloreactive cytotoxic precursors," *Journal of Immunology*, vol. 138, no. 2, pp. 460–465, 1987.

[23] D. A. Vallera and B. R. Blazar, "T cell depletion for graft-versus-host disease prophylaxis: a perspective on engraftment in mice and humans," *Transplantation*, vol. 47, no. 5, pp. 751–760, 1989.

[24] K. Fleischhauer, N. A. Kernan, R. J. O'Reilly, B. Dupont, and S. Y. Yang, "Bone marrow-allograft rejection by T lymphocytes recognizing a single amino acid difference in HLA-B44," *New England Journal of Medicine*, vol. 323, no. 26, pp. 1818–1822, 1990.

[25] J. Pei, Y. Akatsuka, C. Anasetti et al., "Generation of HLA-C-specific cytotoxic T cells in association with marrow graft rejection: analysis of alloimmunity by T-cell cloning and testing of T-cell-receptor rearrangements," *Biology of Blood and Marrow Transplantation*, vol. 7, no. 7, pp. 378–383, 2001.

[26] S. M. Davies, C. Kollman, C. Anasetti et al., "Engraftment and survival after unrelated-donor bone marrow transplantation: a report from the national marrow donor program," *Blood*, vol. 96, no. 13, pp. 4096–4102, 2000.

[27] P. Rubinstein, C. Carrier, A. Scaradavou et al., "Outcomes among 562 recipients of placental-blood transplants from unrelated donors," *New England Journal of Medicine*, vol. 339, no. 22, pp. 1565–1577, 1998.

[28] C. Anasetti, K. C. Doney, and R. Storb, "Marrow transplantation for severe aplastic anemia. Long-term outcome in fifty 'untransfused' patients," *Annals of Internal Medicine*, vol. 104, no. 4, pp. 461–466, 1986.

[29] R. P. Warren, R. Storb, P. L. Weiden, P. J. Su, and E. D. Thomas, "Lymphocyte-mediated cytotoxicity and antibody-dependent cell-mediated cytotoxicity in patients with aplastic anemia: distinguishing transfusion-induced sensitization from possible immune-mediated aplastic anemia.," *Transplantation Proceedings*, vol. 13, no. 1, pp. 245–247, 1981.

[30] Y. L. Colson, M. J. Schuchert, and S. T. Ildstad, "The abrogation of allosensitization following the induction of mixed allogeneic chimerism," *Journal of Immunology*, vol. 165, no. 2, pp. 637–644, 2000.

[31] P. A. Taylor, M. J. Ehrhardt, M. M. Roforth et al., "Preformed antibody, not primed T cells, is the initial and major barrier to bone marrow engraftment in allosensitized recipients," *Blood*, vol. 109, no. 3, pp. 1307–1315, 2007.

[32] R. J. Greenwald, G. J. Freeman, and A. H. Sharpe, "The B7 family revisited," *Annual Review of Immunology*, vol. 23, pp. 515–548, 2005.

[33] A. Bartholomew, D. Sher, S. Sosler et al., "Stem cell transplantation eliminates alloantibody in a highly sensitized patient," *Transplantation*, vol. 72, no. 10, pp. 1653–1655, 2001.

[34] S. Spellman, R. Bray, S. Rosen-Bronson et al., "The detection of donor-directed, HLA-specific alloantibodies in recipients of unrelated hematopoietic cell transplantation is predictive of graft failure," *Blood*, vol. 115, no. 13, pp. 2704–2708, 2010.

[35] S. O. Ciurea, P. F. Thall, X. Wang et al., "Donor-specific anti-HLAAbs and graft failure in matched unrelated donor hematopoietic stem cell transplantation," *Blood*, vol. 118, no. 22, pp. 5957–5964, 2011.

[36] M. Takanashi, Y. Atsuta, K. Fujiwara et al., "The impact of anti-HLA antibodies on unrelated cord blood transplantations," *Blood*, vol. 116, no. 15, pp. 2839–2846, 2010.

[37] C. Cutler, H. T. Kim, L. Sun et al., "Donor-specific anti-HLA antibodies predict outcome in double umbilical cord blood transplantation," *Blood*, vol. 118, no. 25, pp. 6691–6697, 2011.

13

Hematopoietic Stem Cell Development, Niches, and Signaling Pathways

Kamonnaree Chotinantakul[1, 2] and Wilairat Leeanansaksiri[1, 2]

[1] Stem Cell Therapy and Transplantation Research Group, Suranaree University of Technology, Nakhon Ratchasima 30000, Thailand
[2] School of Microbiology, Institute of Science, Suranaree University of Technology, Nakhon Ratchasima 30000, Thailand

Correspondence should be addressed to Wilairat Leeanansaksiri, wilairat@g.sut.ac.th

Academic Editor: Amanda C. LaRue

Hematopoietic stem cells (HSCs) play a key role in hematopoietic system that functions mainly in homeostasis and immune response. HSCs transplantation has been applied for the treatment of several diseases. However, HSCs persist in the small quantity within the body, mostly in the quiescent state. Understanding the basic knowledge of HSCs is useful for stem cell biology research and therapeutic medicine development. Thus, this paper emphasizes on HSC origin, source, development, the niche, and signaling pathways which support HSC maintenance and balance between self-renewal and proliferation which will be useful for the advancement of HSC expansion and transplantation in the future.

1. Introduction

Hematopoietic stem cells (HSC) are adult stem cells that contain the potentiality in self-renew and differentiation into specialized blood cells that function in some biological activities: control homeostasis balance, immune function, and response to microorganisms and inflammation. HSCs can also differentiate into other specialized cell or so called plasticity such as adipocytes [1], cardiomyocytes [2], endothelial cells [3], fibroblasts/myofibroblasts [4], liver cells [5, 6], osteochondrocytes [7, 8], and pancreatic cells [9]. Most HSCs are in quiescent state within the niches that maintain HSC pool and will respond to the signals after the balance of blood cells or HSC pool is disturbed from either intrinsic or extrinsic stimuli.

In addition, HSCs have been studied extensively, especially, for the therapeutic purposes in the treatment of blood diseases, inherited blood disorders, and autoimmune diseases. Nonetheless, advanced development in this field needs knowledge in the biological studies as a background in performing strategy and maintaining of HSCs. Thus, HSC source, origin, niches for HSC pool, and signaling pathways, essential for the regulation of HSCs, will be discussed in this review.

2. HSCs Origin and Development

In the hematopoietic system, the discovery of HSCs has shed the light on stem cell biology studies including connection to other adult stem cells through the basic concepts of differentiation, multipotentiality, and self-renewal. In the early period of those discoveries, lethally irradiated animals were found to be rescued by spleen cells or marrow cells [17, 18]. After mouse bone marrow cells were transplanted into irradiated mice, the clonogenic mixed colony of hematopoietic cells (often composed of granulocyte/megakaryocyte and erythroid precursors) were formed within the spleen, which these colonies were then termed colony-forming unit spleen (CFU-S) [19]. Some colonies of primary CFU-S could reconstitute hematopoietic system in the secondary irradiated mice after receiving transplantation [20]. Initially, CFU-S was first proposed that it may be differentiated from HSC, but subsequently, CFU-S was demonstrated to be originated from more committed progenitor cells [21]. The discovery by Till and McCulloch embarked on a new journey toward many investigations to clarify HSC biology, functional characterization, purify, cultivation, and other stem cells research.

Duration	Source
	Gestation
	E7 Yolk sac
	E8.5–10.5 Placenta
	E10.5 AGM
	E11 Liver
	E16 Bone marrow
	Adult

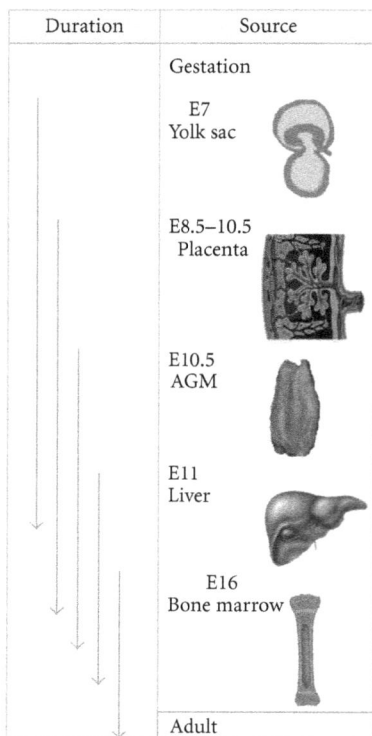

FIGURE 1: Source of blood cells during gestation through after birth. Intraembryonic yolk sac is the first site of blood cells observation at around E7.0–E7.5. The *de novo* hematopoiesis in the placenta and AGM occurs at nearly similar wave of gestation (around E8.5–E10.5) beforeit circulates into fetal liver where there is the large HSC pool during gestation. At around E16.5, the HSCs migrate and reside within the bone marrow which finally becomes the source of HSC in adult life (adapted from [10]).

Hematopoiesis and HSC development are the key role to improve efficient HSC expansion for the transplantations. Embryogenesis study has been performed to identify HSC origin and activity from various anatomical sites of several kinds of animals such as zebrafish, chicken, and mouse including human embryos model have been emerging. Initially, Moore and Metcalf showed that hematopoietic cells in the yolk sac could generate hematopoietic progenitors that restricted to only erythroid and myeloid lineages [22]. Moreover, the Runx1 (transcription factor for the onset of definitive hematopoiesis) was first identified to express at embryonic day 7.5 (E7.5) in the yolk sac, the chorionic mesoderm, and parts of allantoic mesoderm [23]. However, HSCs found in the yolk sac lacked the definitive hematopoietic stem cells which did not show long-term hematopoietic reconstitution activity in mouse embryo prior to E11.5 [24]. On the other hand, long-term repopulating HSCs (LT-HSCs) were shown to increase largely in the aorta-gonad mesonephros (AGMs) region of the mouse embryo including the serially transplantable irradiated mice, suggesting that AGM region is the first site for HSCs detection [24, 25]. Vitelline and umbilical arteries were also

endowed with hematopoietic potential [26]. The presence of HSC phenotype in the embryo was supported by the evidence that a high number of nonerythroid progenitors with high-proliferative potential was observed from which the liver rudiment has been removed [27]. A dense population of CD34+ cells adhering to the ventral side of the aortic endothelium within the embryonic compartment was shown to display a cell-surface and molecular phenotype of primitive hematopoietic progenitors (CD45+, CD34+, CD31+, CD38−, negative for lineage markers, GATA-2+, GATA-3+, c-myb+, SCL/TAL1+, c-kit+, flk-1/KDR+) [28, 29]. Moreover, the autonomously emergence of myelolymphoid lineage from progenitors was found in splanchnopleural mesoderm and derived aorta within the human embryo proper, while restricted progenitors were generated in the yolk sac [30]. Altogether, AGM region in the embryo is suggested as the source of definitive hematopoiesis as the generation occurs between E10.5 and E12.0 with the enhance activity of HSC after mid-day 11 of gestation [10, 31–33]. Even though, the main source of fetal hematopoiesis was considered in AGM including vitelline and umbilical arteries, the question is raised whether the rare population produced in those regions would be enough for the distribution into fetal liver for alternative development of enormous HSCs before the transition of hematopoiesis continues to occur in the fetal thymus and bone marrow in postnatal life. Recently, the placenta, an extraembryonic organ, has been considered as the other hematopoietic organ for *de novo* hematopoiesis [34, 35]. This may be due to the physiology of the placenta containing highly vascularized blood vessels, and cytokines and growth factors rich environment for proper microenvironment of hematopoiesis and development [36]. Additionally, privilege site within the placenta may hide the HSCs from the promoting signal into differentiation stage. However, there is no experimental evidence to support that HSCs are generated *de novo* in the extraembryonic tissues. Therefore, future works will be needed to elucidate this enigma. Summarization of the source of blood cells during gestation through adult life has been elucidated in Figure 1.

The origin of HSC in the placenta is being questioned. Understanding how theplacenta develops might be useful to define the source and the niches supporting HSC development. Mouse and human placentas are anatomically similar and its genes have analogous identity [37, 38]. The placenta is formed from trophectoderm, mesodermal tissues, chorionic mesoderm, and allantois (Figure 2) [39]. At E8.5 of mouse gestation, the allantois develops and fuses with chorionic mesoderm through its distal part generating the chorioallantoic mesenchyme in the chorionic plate and continuing to form the fetal vascular compartment of the placental labyrinth, while the proximal part becomes the umbilical cord [11].

The umbilical cord (a constitution of the fetal arteries and veins that inserted within chorionic plate of the placenta) is attached to the center of fetal surface for uteroplacenta circulation through maternal blood. Maternal blood passes through the placenta from uterine arteries to spiral arteries in the maternal decidua. Thereafter, the maternal blood percolates through the villous tree in humans (or the

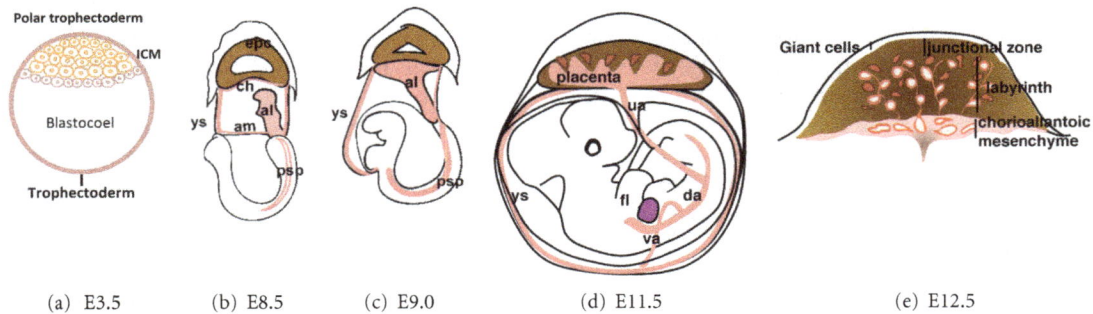

(a) E3.5　　(b) E8.5　　(c) E9.0　　(d) E11.5　　(e) E12.5

FIGURE 2: Mouse placenta development. (a) At E3.5 of early embryogenesis, blastocyst is formed, containing inner cell mass located at one side of the blastocoelic cavity and outer layer (trophectodermal epithelium) which give rise to the placenta. (b) Between E7.5–E8.25 mesodermal precursors originating from the primitive streak grow into the allantois (light grey) which then develops toward the ectoplacental cone (dark grey). (c) Chorioallantoic fusion between the allantoic and chorionic mesoderm at E8.5. After that, Chorionic villi and vasculature are formed producing and generates extensive villous branching called labyrinth. (d) At E11.5, umbilical cord is fully formed to connect the placenta with fetus where fetomaternal bloods circulate. (e) Cross-section of the placenta at E12.5 showing the chorioallantoic mesenchyme lies cover the placenta labyrinth with fetal vessels lined by fetal endothelium (dark vessels with lumen) and trophoblast lined by maternal blood spaces (grey vessels surrounded by dark trophoblasts). al, allantois; ch, chorion; am, amnion; epc, ectoplacental cone; ys, yolk sac; psp, para-aortic splanchnopleura; da, dorsal aorta; ua, umbilical artery; va, vitelline artery; fl, fetal liver (modified from [11]).

labyrinth in mice) known as chorionic villi which created and lined by fetal trophoblast cells [37, 39]. The inner core of the chorionic villi consists of allantoic mesenchyme and vasculature which is continuous with that of the umbilical cord. The chorioallantoic vasculature connects the placenta via the dorsal aorta and fetal liver through the umbilical cord vessels. These regions are localized by an equally dense network of fetal capillaries where the fetomaternal exchange occurs [37].

Because of the mesoderm layer gives rise to all blood cells, the chorionic and allantoic mesoderms are considered as the origin of HSC in the placenta. This can be explained by the observation that hematopoietic potential emerging from both tissues and has been identified with myeloerythroid potential [40]. In addition, hematopoietic cells ($CD34^+CD45^+$) collected from placental villi stroma and highly expression of $CD45^+$ cells that appear to be budding from the vasculature have been found from human placenta during midgestation [35]. Moreover, cells harvested from term human placenta vessels and tissues could generate human hematopoietic repopulation of nonobese diabetic (NOD)-SCID mice, which harbored and/or amplified in vascular labyrinth placenta niche [35]. These observations imply that the placenta is the HSC source along with umbilical cord blood. At E10.5, first HSC emerge in the dorsal aorta before the onset of heart beat where the circulation has not been formed. One study showed that in the absence of heat beat in Ncx1 (the sodium and calcium exchange pump1) knockout embryos, the HSC development was verified to initiate in the placental vasculature [41]. Additionally, multilineage hematopoietic potential could be obtained from placentas of Ncx1 knockout embryos. Thus, within the extraembryonic tissues, fetal HSCs were observed in placenta, vitelline, and umbilical arteries.

The true origin of HSC in the intraembryonic hematopoiesis remains controversial. One of the main hypotheses

is hemangioblasts or hemogenic endothelial while the alternative model is mesodermal precursors. The blood islands originated in the yolk sac are derived from mesodermal cell aggregates, which contain the ability to differentiate into both hematopoietic and endothelial cells. The common precursor by those lineages is suggested to be so called the hemangioblast [42]. Hematopoietic phenotype originated from hemogenic endothelium has been found in avian and mouse during ontogeny [43, 44]. Imaging and cell-tracking study explored that hemogenic endothelial cells could give rise to hematopoietic cells [45]. By time-lapse imaging study in single-cell mouse mesodermal cells demonstrated that it could generate endothelial sheet colonies and some colonies developed the hematopoietic morphology that upregulating the blood-specific proteins CD45, CD41, and CD11b and losing their intact morphology. Recently, this evidence has been supported by the observation on time-lapse confocal imaging from live mouse aorta showing that HSCs (Sca^+, c-kit^+, $CD41^+$) could emerge directly from ventral aortic endothelial cells [46]. Moreover, Oberlin and colleagues proved that the origin of adult bone marrow HSCs which most of them derived were from the vascular endothelial-cadherin ancestor [47]. Taken together, these studies pinpoint the evidence that definitive hematopoietic stem and progenitor cells emerge from the hemogenic endothelium at the AGM region.

3. HSC Niches

Homing of HSC from other definitive hematopoiesis to fetal bone marrow is thought to involve some signaling factors such as stromal derived factor-1 (SDF-1 or CXCL12)/chemokine C-X-C receptor 4 (CXCR4) axis [48, 49]. Soluble factors are not only mediated in fetal bone marrow but also in adult bone marrow to maintain HSC in undifferentiated state and regulate HSC in proliferative and differentiated states within the specific microenvironments termed "niche" throughout the life [12]. Stem cell niche was first proposed by Schofield [21], with the later identification in *Drosophila melanogester*'s ovary to confirm the existence of HSC niche [50]. Germline stem cells resided in the Drosophila ovary that is surrounded by differentiated somatic cells have been shown to be essential for maintaining stem cells survival and division [50]. Thus, HSC niche is the special local environments of HSCs that maintains and controls HSCs function by regulating survival, self-renewal ability, and cell fate decision. Such molecules have been identified to be associated with HSC homing to bone marrow, for example, SDF1-α, β1-integrins, metalloproteinases (MMP), and serine-threonine protein phosphatase (PP)2A [51, 52]. By using real-time imaging, it is possible to explore the localization of HSCs with their function [53]. HSCs lodge in the endosteal surface, osteoblasts, and blood vessels, particularly in trabecular regions, in the mouse calvaria. On the contrary, more mature cells reside away from the endosteum. Similarly, a study by developed *ex vivo* real-time imaging in irradiated mice show the homing and lodgment of transplantable HSCs in the endosteal region of the trabecular bone area where they respond to bone marrow damage by rapidly dividing [54].

Recently HSCs niches are suggested to be mediated in two main microenvironments within bone marrow: endosteal niche and vascular niche (Figure 3). First, endosteal niche: osteoblasts derived from mesenchymal precursors are localized in the endosteal regions which are well vascularized. The activation of osteoblastic differentiation is in part mediated by HSC-derived bone morphogenic protein-2 (BMP-2) and BMP-6 [55]. Osteoblasts are suggested as the niche due to the finding that the number of osteoblasts is increased from parathyroid hormone activation and results in an increase HSCs number *in vivo* [56]. This signal was found to be activated through Jagged1, a serrate family of Notch ligand, on osteoblasts [57]. Study by Chitteti and colleagues supports this evidence and shows that enhancing hematopoiesis promoted by osteoblast via Notch signaling not only through Jagged1 upregulation, but also Notch2, Jagged2, Delta1 and 4, Hes1 and 5, and Deltex ligands [58]. Soluble factors produced from osteoblasts function in regulating HSC quiescence, HSC pool and fate such as angiopoietin-1 (Ang-1) [59], SDF-1 (CXCL12) [60], and osteopontin [61]. Recently, osteoblasts secreted cysteine protease cathepsin X have been found to catalyze the chemokine CXCL-12, a potent chemoattractive cytokine for HSCs, and ablate the attachment of CD34$^+$ cells with the osteoblasts [62]. This result suggests the role of osteoblasts in regulate HSCs trafficking in the bone marrow.

A group of de Borros supports this hypothesis by showing that the 3D spheroid of noninduced and one week osteo-induce bone marrow stromal cell (active osteoblasts) formed an informative microenvironment that control migration, lodgment, and proliferation of HSCs [63]. Bone marrow endosteal cells, particularly, osteoblast-enriched ALCAM$^+$Sca-1$^-$ cells promoted LT-reconstitution activity of HSCs via the upregulation of genes related in homing and cell adhesion [64]. In addition, HSCs were found to adhere with spindle-shaped N-cadherin$^+$ osteoblastic (SNO) cells which are a subpopulation of osteoblasts [65]. BMP receptor type IA mutant mice have been shown to increase in the number of SNO cells that correlated to an increase in HSC number [65]. Consistently, green fluorescent protein-positive (GFP$^+$) HSCs derived from *Col2.3*-GFP$^+$ transgenic mouse were found to attach to SNO cells but not all GFP$^+$ HSCs were in contact with SNO cells showing that N-cadherin$^-$ component might be the other niche for HSCs [54]. Cumulatively, osteoblasts and SNO cells are suggested as the niche for hematopoietic stem and progenitor cells where this microenvironment termed "Endosteal niche."

Some observations have suggested that another niche, vascular niche, might involve in HSC maintenance within the bone marrow. Studies in osteoblast depletion demonstrated that there was a loss of B lymphopoiesis but not immediately loss of HSC number [66, 67] and few bone-marrow HSCs (CD150$^+$CD48$^-$CD41$^-$lineage$^-$) were localized to the endosteum [68]. Mice model defected in osteoblast function conferred no changes in LT-reconstitution function of HSCs [69]. Additionally, the loss of N-cadherin did not any effect on HSC maintenance and hematopoiesis [70]. Most HSCs in the bone marrow have been observed to reside in the sinusoid, where fenestrated endothelium persists and allows blood flow for an exchange of blood cells and small molecules. Taken together, the vascular niche is suggested as the other niche for HSC maintenance [68]. Bone-marrow endothelial cells have been proposed to play a role in HSC controlling within vascular niche. Primary CD31$^+$ microvascular endothelial cells can restore hematopoiesis in mice when they receive bone-marrow lethal doses of irradiation [71]. Study by a group of Salter shows a consistent observation that endothelial progenitor cells injected in total body irradiated mice can stimulate HSC reconstitution and hematologic recovery [72]. Furthermore, selective activation of Akt in endothelial cells produced angiocrine factors mediated in the reconstitution, expansion, and maintenance of HSCs [73]. Nonetheless, constitutively activation of Akt, a binding ligand of phosphoinositide 3 in the phospho-inositide 3-kinase pathway, impaired engraftment ability and preferable generated leukemia in mice [74]. Sinusoidal endothelial cells are essential for engraftment of hematopoietic stem and progenitor cells (HSPCs) and restoration of hematopoiesis after myeloablation [75]. Angiocrine factors, such as Notch ligands, released by endothelial cells *in vivo* contributed to the replenishment of the LT-HSC pool and resulted in reconstitution of hematopoiesis [76]. Altogether, vascular niche containing endothelial cells is suggested as the major HSC pool and maintenance conferring proliferation and differentiation selection.

Additionally, Sugiyama and colleagues demonstrated that reticular cells located around the sinusoid endothelium could produce stromal cell-derived factor 1 (SDF-1, aka CXCL12) mediated in HSC niche [77]. These cells have been named CXCL12 abundant reticular cells (CAR cells). This study showed that almost all HSCs were found in contact with CAR cells and all HSCs allocated at endosteum were also found to be in contact with CAR cells, suggesting that these cells play

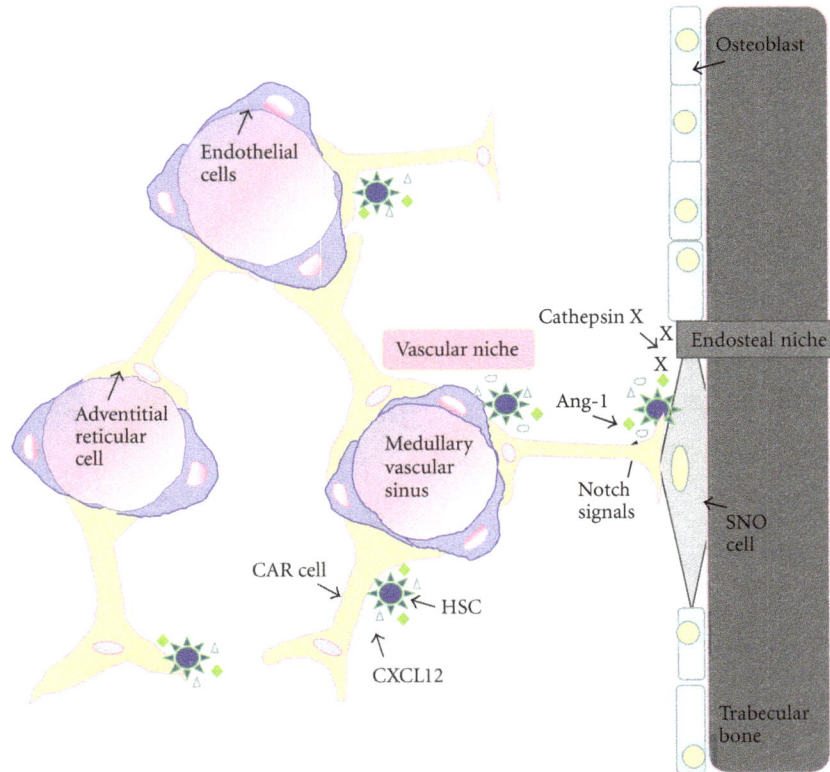

FIGURE 3: Candidate cellular niches mediated in maintenance and regulation of HSCs in bone marrow; endosteal and vascular niches. HSCs are in contact with SNO cells, bone-lining osteoblasts, within endosteal niche. Osteblasts produce several signal molecules such as Notch ligands, angiopoietin-1 (Ang-1), CXCL12, and cathepsin X mediated in control HSC pool and maintenance. Most HSCs are found in sinusoids, particularly adherence to CAR cells that surround sinusoidal endothelial cells (reticular niche). Similarly, CAR cells produce CXCL12 in association with CXCR4 signaling essentially for HSC maintenance (modified from [12]).

a crucial role in HSC niches by homing HSCs in both vascular and endosteal niches [77]. CXCL12/CXCR4 signaling is essential in maintaining the HSC pool, development of B cells and plasmacytoid dendritic cells [78–81]. Moreover, short-term ablation of CAR cells resulted in the impairment of adipogenic and osteogenic differentiation. Thus, CAR cells are suggested as the adipo-osteogenic progenitors [82]. Study in CAR cell-depleted mice demonstrated that HSCs were reduced in number and cell size, which were more quiescent and highly expressed early myeloid selector genes [82]. CAR cells were suggested to coincide with CD146$^+$ stromal progenitors that express CXCL12 and Ang-1. CD146$^+$ cells could generate osteoblast that form bone and could function as skeletal progenitor cells [83]. Taken together, CAR cells provide or generate the hematopoietic microenvironment that link to the hematopoietic regulation in both vascular and endosteal niches.

4. Hierarchy of Human Hematopoiesis

Based on the study of molecular marker expression by flow cytometry analysis has led the identification of each blood cell subpopulations in terms of their biology and potential when combined with other functional assays. As a result, schematic demonstration of hematopoietic hierarchy has been proposed (Figure 4) [13]. The origin of all blood cell in hematopoietic system is believed to be derived from HSCs that contain self-renewal capacity and give rise to multipotent progenitors (MPPs) which lose self-renewal potential but remain fully differentiate into all multilineages. MPPs further give rise to oligopotent progenitors which are common lymphoid and myeloid progenitors (CLPs and CMPs, resp.). All these oligopotent progenitors differentiate into their restricted lineage commitment: (1) CMPs advance to megakaryocyte/erythrocyte progenitors (MEPs), granulocyte/macrophage progenitors (GMPs), and dendritic cell (DC) progenitors, (2) CLPs give rise to T cell progenitors, B cell progenitors, NK cell progenitors and DC progenitors. Notably, DC progenitors (CD8α^+ DC, CD8α^- DC, and plasmacytoid DC) could be derived from both CMPs and CLPs [84–86].

Among the isolation and characterization of HSCs and progenitors, CD34 molecule is the first widely chosen for the study by several researchers. CD34 is comprised in the CD34 family of cell-surface transmembrane proteins together with podocalyxin and endoglycan [87–89]. CD34 expression on blood cells is about 0.1–4.9% in human cord blood, bone marrow, and peripheral blood [90–92]. The first candidate human HSCs was a population of cells

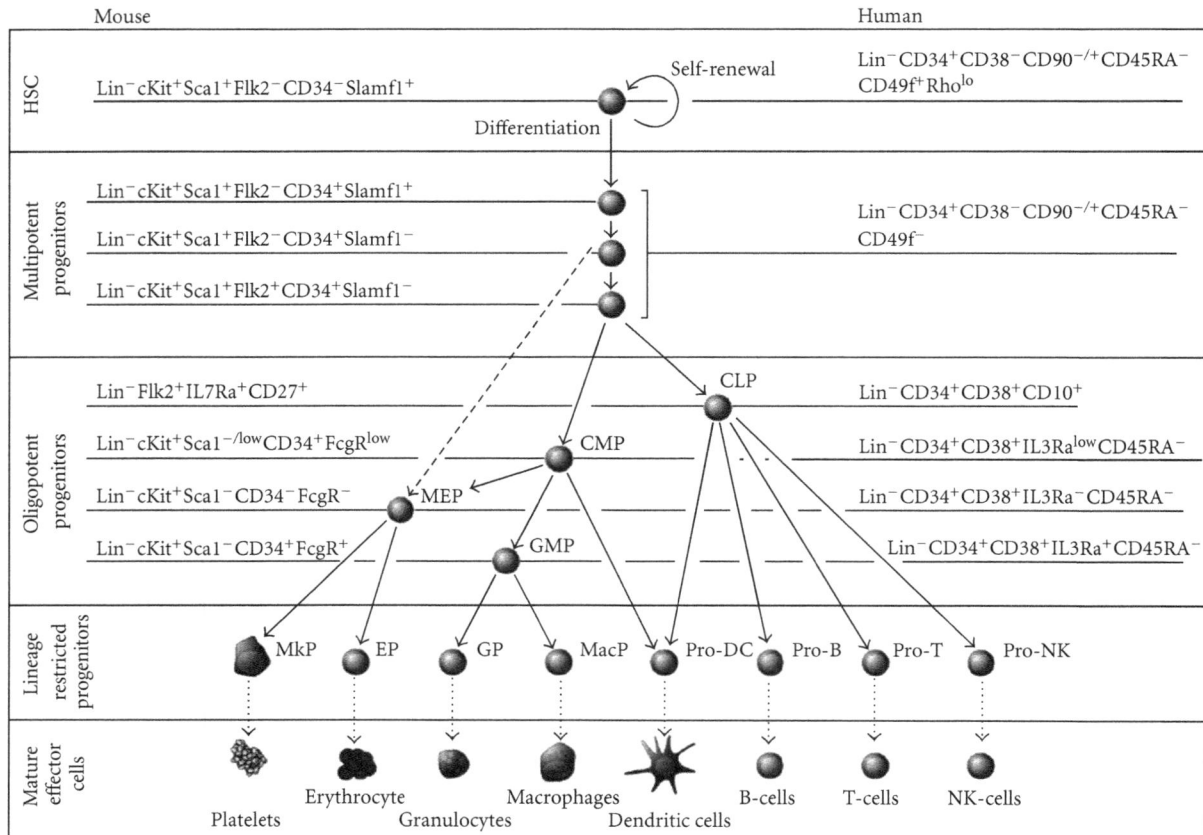

FIGURE 4: Hierarchy of hematopoiesis. The phenotypic cell surface marker of each population of mouse and human blood system is shown (modified from [13]). In the mouse hematopoiesis system, MPPs omit CMPs which directly give rise to MEPs unlink in the human system (dash line). CLP, common lymphoid progenitor; CMP, common myeloid progenitor; DC, dendritic cell; EP, erythrocyte progenitor; GMP, granulocyte/macrophage progenitor; GP, granulocyte progenitor; HSC, hematopoietic stem cell; MacP, macrophage progenitor; MEP, megakaryocyte/erythrocyte progenitor; MkP, megakaryocyte progenitor; NK, natural killer; Lin, lineage markers.

expressing $CD34^+CD90^+$(Thy-1)Lin^- which could give rise to T and B lymphocytes and myeloerythroid activities in both *in vitro* and *in vivo* human fetal thymus transplanted into SCID mice while some subset of $CD34^-$, $CD90^-$, Lin^- lacked of multipotent progenitors [93]. Further isolation of HSCs was based on the expression of CD38 [94, 95] and CD45RA [96]. This data could be concluded that $Lin^-CD34^+CD38^-CD90^+CD45RA^-$ population enriches for human HSCs and the candidate human MPP fraction of multipotency with an incomplete self-renewal capacity is enriched in $Lin^-CD34^+CD38^-CD90^-CD45RA^-$ population [97]. However, recently observation using HSC xenograft assay in NOD-SCID-IL2Rgc$^{-/-}$ (NSG) mice has shown that both $Lin^-CD34^+CD38^-CD90^-CD45RA^-$ and $Lin^-CD34^+CD38^-CD90^+CD45RA^-$ contain LT repopulating activity in secondary recipients with different frequency [98]. In addition, CD49f (integrin $\alpha6$) marker has been shown as a specific HSC marker within $Lin^-CD34^+CD38^-CD45RA^-$ population which as single-sorted HSC is highly efficient in generating long-term multilineage grafts while the loss of CD49f expression results in the absence of long-term grafts [98]. Furthermore,

Rhodamine-123 marker (efflux of the mitochondrial dye) is added to enrich for HSCs where high Rho efflux (Rho^{lo})$Lin^-CD34^+CD38^-CD90^+CD45RA^-$ can also repopulate all blood lineages in secondary recipients [98]. Taken together, these results demonstrate that human HSCs are enriched in the $Lin^-CD34^+CD38^-CD90^{+/-}CD45RA^-Rho^{lo}$ population of hematopoietic cells (Figure 4).

5. Signaling Pathways in Self-Renewal and Maintenance of HSCs

The balance that controls between self-renewal and differentiation (or cell fate decision) of HSCs in the bone marrow is mediated by several factors. There are a number of animal models promoting the concept that the niches inside bone marrow provide the maintenance and regulation of HSCs by some microenvironmental-dependent signals. Most HSCs are in quiescent state (i.e., in G0/G1 phase of the cell cycle) [99], however, when the hematopoietic cells disturbance occurs, hematopoiesis system will respond by shutting down or turning on the regulators mediated in the regulations. Several pathways have been studied in relation to that circumstance which are SDF-1 (CXCL12)/CXCR4 signaling, BMP signaling, Mpl/Thrombopoietin (TPO) signaling, Tie2/Ang-1 signaling, hedgehog and Notch signaling, as well as Wingless (Wnt) signaling.

5.1. SDF-1 (CXCL12)/CXCR4 Signaling Pathway. Stromal cell-derived factor 1 (SDF-1) is constitutively expressed in several organs including lung, liver, skin, and bone marrow [100]. SDF-1 belongs to α-chemokines that functions as chemoattractant for both committed and primitive hematopoietic progenitors and regulates embryonic development including organ homeostasis [100]. There are two main splicing forms that have been identified, SDF-1α and SDF-1β, which ubiquitously expressed with highest levels detected in liver, pancreas, and spleen [101]. Additionally, another variant form, SDF-γ, has been characterized in the nervous system [102]. Subsequently, SDF-1δ, SDF-1ε, and SDF-ϕ have been identified with highly expression in pancreases and lower levels detection in heart, kidney, liver, and spleen [103]. SDF-1 counteracts with its cognate receptor, CXCR4 that expresses widely in numerous tissues including hematopoietic and endothelial cells to stimulate the physiological processes. SDF-1/CXCR4 signaling plays a critical role during embryonic development by regulating B-cell lymphopoiesis, myelopoiesis in bone marrow and heart ventricular septum formation [104–106]. In addition, SDF-1 has been shown to be mediated in the recruitment of endothelial progenitor cells (EPCs) from the bone marrow through a CXCR4 dependent mechanism suggesting the functional role in vasculogenesis in which EPCs could form blood vessels [107]. A number of observations demonstrated that there was an increase in SDF-1 expression the ischemic sites [108, 109]. More evidence demonstrated that locally injection of SDF-1 augmented vasculogenesis and subsequently contributed to ischemic neovascularization *in vivo* by promoting EPC recruitment in ischemic tissues [110]. Recently, Liu and colleagues have shown that signal of SDF-1/CXCR4 together with CXCR7 can increase the mobilization and paracrine actions of mesenchymal stem cells (MSCs) ischemic kidneys under hypoxia condition [111]. Moreover, SDF-1/CXCR4 not only plays a role in HSC maintenance but also regulates HSC attachment within the niche. The mechanism mediated in this regulation was found to be activated through matrix metalloproteinase-9 that mediated in the releasing of soluble Kit-ligand [112]. Inactivation or deletion of CXCR4 in mice resulted in HSC pool reduction and hyperproliferation responsive to HSC defections [77, 78]. Tzeng and colleagues also confirmed the role of SDF-1 in HSC maintenance by demonstrating that a conditional SDF-1-deficient mice conferred an impairment in HSC quiescence and endosteal niche localization [113].

5.2. BMP Signaling Pathway. Bone morphogenic proteins (BMPs) are a group of growth factors that belongs to a TGF-β family member [114]. BMPs are mainly produced by osteoclasts in HSC niche [115]. During embryogenesis, BMP-4 regulates hematopoietic lineage commitment from mesodermal cell, while HSC number and function within bone marrow niche is controlled by Bmp-4 during adult life [116, 117]. Knowledge of BMP signaling and receptor related adult HSC within bone marrow has been studied in a small number and is elusive. BMP signaling impairment displayed an increase in the niche size, leading to the enhancement in the number of HSCs [65]. Differential response of HSC to soluble BMPs observed by a group of Bhatia showed that higher concentrations of BMP-2, BMP-4 and BMP-7 maintained human CB HSCs *in vitro* while at lower concentrations of BMP-4-induced proliferation and differentiation of HSCs [118].

5.3. c-Mpl/TPO Signaling Pathway. c-Mpl and its ligand, thrombopoietin (TPO), are known to regulate megakaryopoiesis [119]. c-Mpl receptor is expressed mainly on HSCs, with a lesser extent on megakaryocytic progenitors, megakaryocytes and platelets [120]. Various tissues expressing c-Mpl are mediated in hematopoiesis, including bone marrow, spleen, and fetal liver [14]. Based on the crystallographic EPO receptor study and its analogy to the TPO receptor have led to the postulation that TPO initiates the signal transduction by binding to the c-Mpl at the distal part, which in turn a homodimer of c-Mpl becomes active [15]. Consequently, Janus kinase 2 (JAK2) can phosphorylate tyrosine residues within the receptor itself which at least two tyrosine residues, Tyr625 and Tyr630, are phosphorylated on c-Mpl [15, 122], thereby stimulating the downstream cascade STATs, PI3K, the mitogen-activated protein kinases (MAPKs), and extracellular signal regulated kinases-1 and -2 (Figure 5) [123, 124]. c-Mpl/TPO signaling involved in postnatal steady-state HSC maintenance and cell-cycle progression at the endosteal surface [125, 126]. Mpl-expressed LT-HSCs were found in correlation to cell cycle quiescence and that was closely associated with TPO-producing osteoblastic cells in the bone marrow [125]. Additionally, the inhibitory adaptor protein Lnk was suggested as a negative regulator of JAK2 in HSCs following TPO stimulation, in which HSC quiescence and self-renewal controls were predominantly through Mpl [127]. Therefore, TPO/Mpl/JAK2/Lnk pathway can be concluded as a gatekeeper for HSC quiescence. Recently, TPO knock-in RAG2$^{-/-}$γc$^{-/-}$ mice has been shown to improve human engraftment in the bone marrow and maintenance of HSPCs pool by serial transplantation [128]. Taken together, TPO has an important function in maintenance and self-renewal of HSCs.

5.4. Tie2/Ang-1 Signaling. Angiopoietin-1 (Ang-1) is the ligand of Tie2, a receptor tyrosine kinase, which expresses predominantly on osteoblastic cells in endosteum [59] and in MSCs [83]. Interaction of Tie2 with its ligand, Ang-1, resulted in tightly adhesion of HSCs to the niche and become more quiescence [59]. Moreover, Ang-1 conferred the maintenance of LT-HSCs while Ang-2 did not antagonize the effects of Ang-1 on gene expression, Akt (aka protein B) phosphorylation [129].

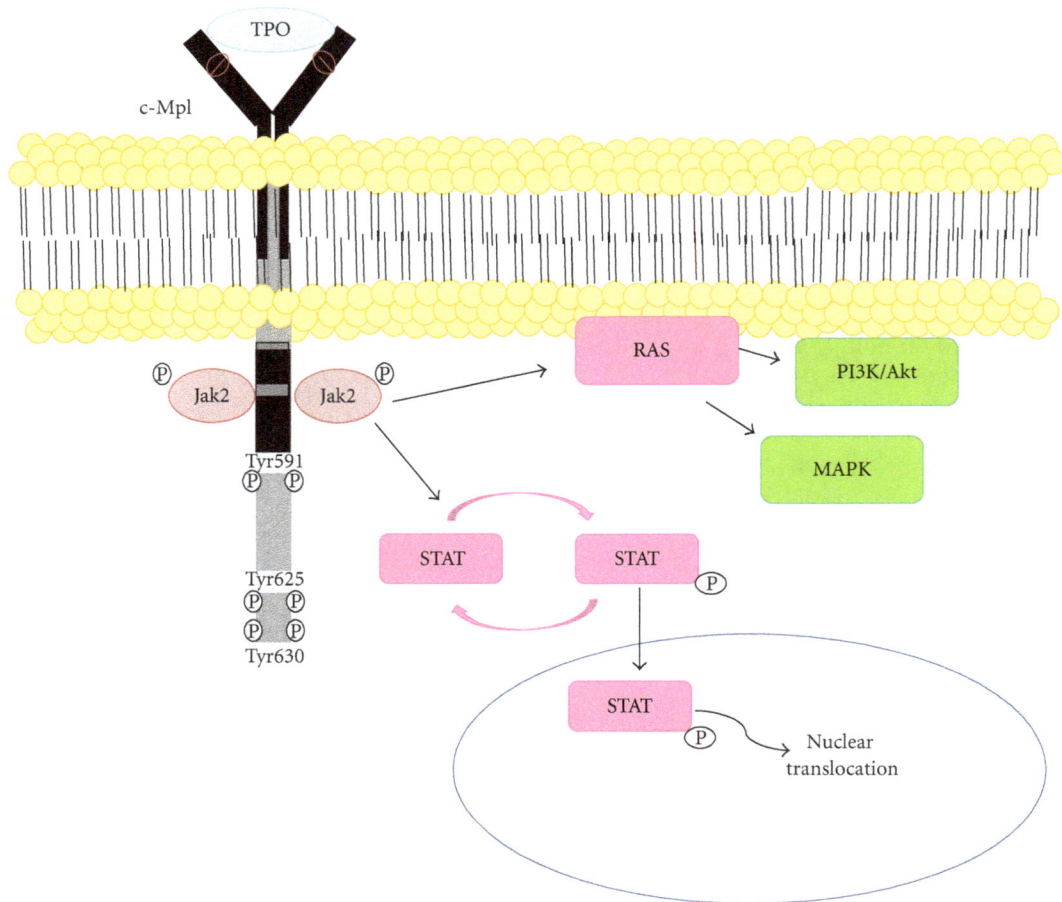

FIGURE 5: c-Mpl/TPO signaling pathway. TPO signals to its receptor, c-Mpl, and induces the downstream signaling cascades: STATs, PI3K, MAPKs, and extracellular signal regulated kinases-1 and -2 (modified from [14, 15]).

5.5. *Hedgehog Signaling Pathway.* Hedgehog (Hh) is proposed as a negative regulator of the HSC quiescence [130]. Hh ligand binds to the transmembrane receptor Patched (Ptc) and subsequently allows the signaling function of a second transmembrane protein, Smoothened (Smo), essentially for the Hh signal to be active. Trowbridge and colleagues demonstrated that constitutive activation of the Hh signaling pathway in Ptc heterozygous (Ptc-1$^{+/-}$) mice resulted in induction of cell cycling and expansion of primitive bone marrow hematopoietic cells [130]. To support this hypothesis, deletion of *Smo* in the in utero of transgenic mice was performed and the result demonstrated that there was an impaired stem cell self-renewal and the inhibition in engraftment activity of HSCs [131]. Furthermore, the common downstream positive effector of Hg signaling, Gli1, has been shown to play a critical role in normal and stress hematopoiesis [132]. Nonetheless, the discrepancies on Hg role in hematopoiesis were shown in some studies claiming that the conditional loss of *Smo* within adult HSCs is dispensable for hematopoiesis [133, 134]. These conflicts might be due to the difference of the mice model and conditional system used to impair Hg signaling.

5.6. *Notch Signaling Pathway.* Notch signaling plays a key role in several fundamental functions including proliferation, differentiation and cell fate decision [135, 136]. Four notch receptors (Notch 1–4) and five ligands (Jagged1-2 and Delta-like 1, 3, and 4) have been identified in mammals [137]. Cells expressing Notch ligands or engineered immobilized Notch ligands could maintain or enhance HSC self-renewal in the culture [138, 139]. Some investigations demonstrated that there were an impaired HSCs differentiation both *in vitro* [140, 141] and *in vivo* [139, 141] studies following interaction of Notch receptors and Notch ligands. Transcription factor act upstream of the Notch signaling cascade, Hes2, was shown to be essential in HSCs formation in zebrafish embryos when *hes2* expression was knockdown, whereas HSC formation could be rescued by the activation of Notch signal [142]. One study showed that an increase in *in vitro* maintenance of hematopoietic functions and repopulating potential on osteoblasts and Lineage⁻Sca-1⁺CD117⁺ (LSK) cells coculture was mediated by the up-regulation of Notch signal (Notch2, Jagged1 and 2, Delta1 and 4, Hes1 and 5, and Deltex) [58]. Taken together, these studies support the role of Notch signaling mediated in HSC hematopoiesis and maintenance. In the contrary, some investigations proposed that Notch signaling was not important for HSC self-renewal and maintenance [143, 144]. Inactivation of Notch1 and Jagged1 in bone marrow progenitors and bone marrow stroma, respectively, did not impair HSC maintenance and reconstitution [144]. The inhibition of Notch1–4 signaling via a developed dominant-negative Mastermind-like1 construct was transfected into LSK and demonstrated similar result of LT reconstitution in bone marrow compared to LSK control, except for T-cells [143]. Nevertheless, the study by Kim and colleague explored the important of Notch in normal hematopoiesis [145]. Mind bomb (Mib)-1, which regulates the endocytosis of Notch ligands and activation, was inactivated in mice leading to myeloproliferative disease (MPD). Surprisingly, when transplanted with wild-type bone marrow cells into the Mib1-null microenvironment, it results in a *de novo* MPD. The MPD progression was suppressed by transplantable Notch activating cells, suggesting that MPD develops from the nonhematopoietic microenvironmental cells with defective Notch signaling. Therefore, Notch signaling is indeed required for normal hematopoiesis. Santaguida and colleague developed *JunB*-decient mice which resulted in impairment of Notch and transforming growth factor-β (TGF-β) signaling, in part via the transcriptional regulation of Hes1 [146]. This study showed an increase in LT-HSCs proliferation and differentiation without impairing their self-renewal *in vivo*, suggesting that LT-HSC proliferation rate is not exclusively compelling to self-renewal activity and maintenance of HSC in the BM niches.

5.7. Wnt Signaling Pathway. Notch signaling is involved in the cross-talk with other pathways particularly Wnt signaling not only in hematopoiesis [147] but also in other cellular development [136, 148–151]. In addition, Wnt signaling pathway is mediated in the regulation of stem cell fate and maintenance of mouse ESCs and human ESCs in undifferentiated state [152, 153]. There are at least two independent pathway comprised in Wnt signaling: canonical Wnt and noncanonical Wnt signaling pathways. The canonical Wnt signal interacts with Frizzled (Fz) receptors and single-pass co-receptors LDL-receptor-related proteins 5 and 6 (LRP 5 and 6). The Fz protein contains a conserved motif, a cysteine rich domain (CRD) located on the extracellular domain that binds to multiple Wnts with a high affinity (Figure 6) [154]. Specifically, Dishevelled (DVL) is phosphorylated by casein kinase Iε (CKIε), which then binds typically to FRAT and confers the assembly between Fz to DVL (Fz-DVL complex) and LRP5/6 to AXIN and FRAT (LRP5/6-AXIN-FRAT complex) [155, 156]. After that, β-catenin is stabilized and released from phosphorylation by CKIα and GSK3β. Then, β-catenin forms the complex with T-cell factor/lymphoid enhancer binding factor (TCF/LEF) family transcription factors and also with Legless family docking proteins (BCL9 and BCL9L) associated with PYGO family coactivators for stabilization and nuclear accumulation [157–159]. Typically, the downstream effectors for transcriptional activation target genes are *FGF20, DKK1, WISP1, MYC,* and *CCND1* [160–163]. In the absence of Wnt, β-catenin is destabilized by

phosphorylation of CKIα and glycogen synthase kinase 3β (GSK 3β), which then resulted in a formation of a destruction complex facilitating by Axin (β-catenin-APC-AXIN) that is polyubiquitinated by βTRCP1 or βTRCP2 complex for the degradation by proteasome [16, 159].

In the second pathway, "noncanonical Wnt signal" exerts the independent β-catenin signaling. The Wnt subfamily members, for example, Wnt5a binds to the Frizzled receptor, stimulates downstream intracellular signaling, resulting in an increase in intracellular Ca2+, and then activates protein kinase C and calmodulin-dependent kinase [159]. The cross-talk between Notch and Wnt signaling pathways was found in the stabilizing β-catenin on bone-marrow stroma cells that promoted maintaining and self-renewal of HSCs [164]. Moreover, the induction of Jagged1 and delta-like 1 was observed in Wnt/β-catenin-activated bone-marrow stroma or in bone-marrow stroma cultured with Wnt3a-conditioned medium [164]. Mice lacking Wnt3a resulted in prenatal death [165]. Moreover, Wnt3a deficiency reduced the number of HSCs in fetal liver and impaired the repopulating activity *in vivo* [165]. However, the exact role of Wnt signaling pathway in regulation of HSCs remains a controversy. Some studies demonstrated that constitutive activation of Wnt/β-catenin in transgenic mice resulting in the multilineage differentiation block and loss of repopulating stem cell activity due to the induction of quiescent stem cells entering into cell cycle and arresting their differentiation [166, 167]. In contrast to previous works, the administration of an inhibitor of GSK-3β *in vivo* displayed the enhancement in the recovery of hematopoietic cells for neutrophil and megakaryocytic lineages as well as primitive LSK cell population together with the upregulation of *Wnt, Notch,* and *Hedgehog* genes [168].

Furthermore, inhibition of Wnt signaling in HSCs by overexpression of the paninhibitor of canonical Wnt signaling, Dickkopf1 (Dkk1), resulted in the induction of cell cycling and reduction in repopulating ability in transplanted induction mice [169]. When the inhibitor of GSK-3β, 6-bromoindirubin 3'-oxime was used to treat CB-CD34+ cells, cell cycle progression was delayed including promoted engraftment of *ex vivo*-expanded HSCs [170]. Cumulatively, these studies suggest the positive regulatory role of Wnt/β-catenin signal on the proliferative or repopulating activity of HSCs. 12/15-lipoxygenase-mediated unsaturated fatty acid metabolism has been implicated in canonical Wnt-related signaling in the maintenance of LT-HSC quiescence and number [171]. Taken together, the canonical Wnt signal is mediated in the regulation of HSC function by maintaining quiescence and balance in proliferation.

6. Concluding Remarks

HSCs have been studied extensively for HSC source, hematopoiesis, biological functions, and signaling pathways related to the maintenance and regulation of HSCs. Advance researches such as imaging system clearly provide useful information on tracking the HSC origin, pool, and transplantation outcome in the mouse models. The observation

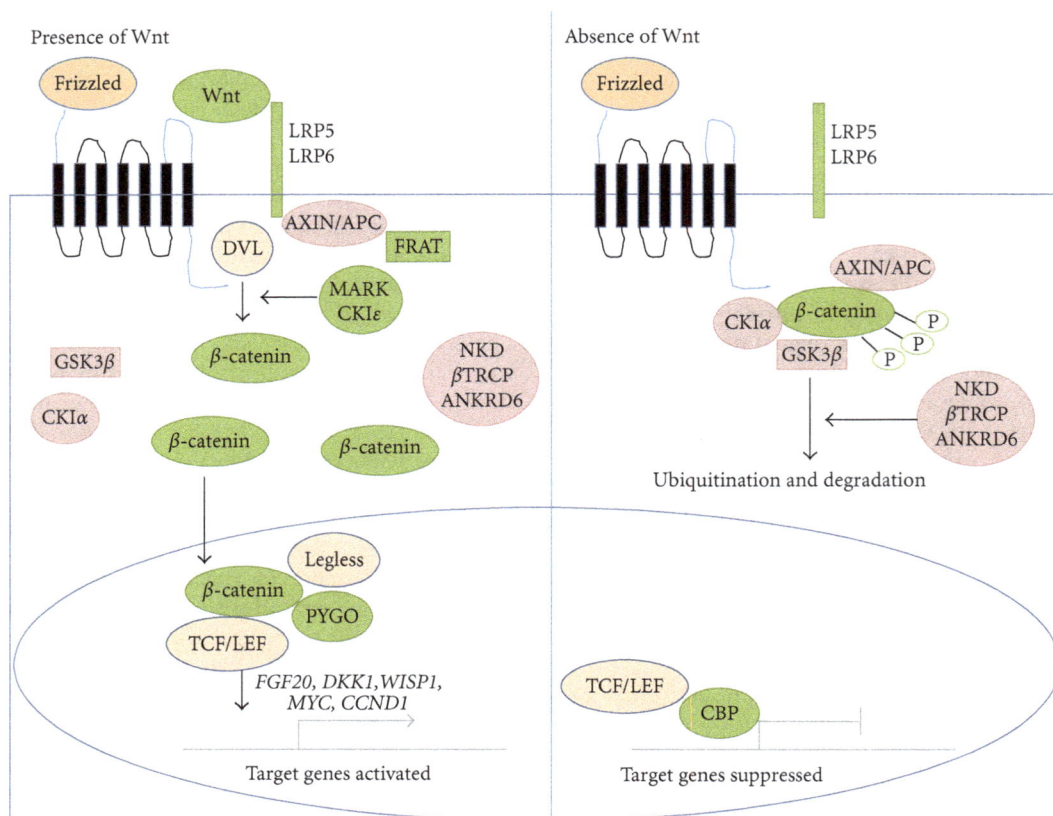

FIGURE 6: A canonical Wnt signaling pathway. In the presence of Wnt, the signals are transduced through Frizzled family receptors and LRP5/LRP6 coreceptor to the β-catenin signaling cascade which then stabilize hypophosphorylated β-catenin and interact with TCF/LEF, Legless and PYGO for target gene activations. MARK and CKIε are the positive regulators of canonical Wnt pathway, while APC, AXIN1, AXIN2, CKIα, NKD1, NKD2, βTRCP1, βTRCP2, and ANKRD6 are negative regulators. In the absence of Wnt, β-catenin-forming complex with AXIN and APC is phosphorylates, leading to be a target for ubiquitination and degradation by proteasome (adapted from [16]).

of molecular mechanisms downstream the signaling cascade of self-renewing and proliferation of HSCs will also provide the knowledge through the new discovery in the treatment of diseases including the development in the performing a large scale preparation of HSCs for clinical transplantation. In addition, the signaling pathways will also provide understanding insight into the cancer stem cells which are now challenging scientists to explore their possible strategy for the treatments.

References

[1] Y. Sera, A. C. LaRue, O. Moussa et al., "Hematopoietic stem cell origin of adipocytes," *Experimental Hematology*, vol. 37, no. 9, pp. 1108.e4–1120.e4, 2009.

[2] M. Pozzobon, S. Bollini, L. Iop et al., "Human bone marrow-derived CD133$^+$ cells delivered to a collagen patch on cryoinjured rat heart promote angiogenesis and arteriogenesis," *Cell Transplantation*, vol. 19, no. 10, pp. 1247–1260, 2010.

[3] N. Elkhafif, H. El Baz, O. Hammam et al., "CD133$^+$ human umbilical cord blood stem cells enhance angiogenesis in experimental chronic hepatic fibrosis," *Acta Pathologica, Microbiologica et Immunologica*, vol. 119, no. 1, pp. 66–75, 2011.

[4] Y. Ebihara, M. Masuya, A. C. LaRue et al., "Hematopoietic origins of fibroblasts: II. In vitro studies of fibroblasts, CFU-F, and fibrocytes," *Experimental Hematology*, vol. 34, no. 2, pp. 219–229, 2006.

[5] S. Khurana and A. Mukhopadhyay, "In vitro transdifferentiation of adult hematopoietic stem cells: an alternative source of engraftable hepatocytes," *Journal of Hepatology*, vol. 49, no. 6, pp. 998–1007, 2008.

[6] S. Sellamuthu, R. Manikandan, R. Thiagarajan et al., "In vitro trans-differentiation of human umbilical cord derived hematopoietic stem cells into hepatocyte like cells using combination of growth factors for cell based therapy," *Cytotechnology*, vol. 63, no. 3, pp. 259–268, 2011.

[7] M. Dominici, C. Pritchard, J. E. Garlits, T. J. Hofmann, D. A. Persons, and E. M. Horwitz, "Hematopoietic cells and osteoblasts are derived from a common marrow progenitor after bone marrow transplantation," *Proceedings of the National Academy of Sciences of the United States of America*, vol. 101, no. 32, pp. 11761–11766, 2004.

[8] M. Mehrotra, M. Rosol, M. Ogawa, and A. C. LaRue, "Amelioration of a mouse model of osteogenesis imperfecta with hematopoietic stem cell transplantation: microcomputed tomography studies," *Experimental Hematology*, vol. 38, no. 7, pp. 593–602, 2010.

[9] H. Minamiguchi, F. Ishikawa, P. A. Fleming et al., "Transplanted human cord blood cells generate amylase-producing

pancreatic acinar cells in engrafted mice," *Pancreas*, vol. 36, no. 2, pp. e30–e35, 2008.

[10] S. Coskun and K. K. Hirschi, "Establishment and regulation of the HSC niche: roles of osteoblastic and vascular compartments," *Birth Defects Research C*, vol. 90, no. 4, pp. 229–242, 2010.

[11] C. Gekas, K. E. Rhodes, B. van Handel, A. Chhabra, M. Ueno, and H. K. A. Mikkola, "Hematopoietic stem cell development in the placenta," *International Journal of Developmental Biology*, vol. 54, no. 6-7, pp. 1089–1098, 2010.

[12] T. Nagasawa, Y. Omatsu, and T. Sugiyama, "Control of hematopoietic stem cells by the bone marrow stromal niche: the role of reticular cells," *Trends in Immunology*, vol. 32, no. 7, pp. 315–320, 2011.

[13] J. Seita and I. L. Weissman, "Hematopoietic stem cell: self-renewal versus differentiation," *Wiley Interdisciplinary Reviews*, vol. 2, no. 6, pp. 640–653, 2010.

[14] F. S. Chou and J. C. Mulloy, "The thrombopoietin/MPL pathway in hematopoiesis and leukemogenesis," *Journal of Cellular Biochemistry*, vol. 112, no. 6, pp. 1491–1498, 2011.

[15] A. E. Geddis, "Megakaryopoiesis," *Seminars in Hematology*, vol. 47, no. 3, pp. 212–219, 2010.

[16] M. Katoh and M. Katoh, "WNT signaling pathway and stem cell signaling network," *Clinical Cancer Research*, vol. 13, no. 14, pp. 4042–4045, 2007.

[17] L. O. Jacobson, E. L. Simmons, E. K. Marks, and J. H. Eldredge, "Recovery from radiation injury," *Science*, vol. 113, no. 2940, pp. 510–511, 1951.

[18] E. Lorenz, D. Uphoff, T. R. REID, and E. Shelton, "Modification of irradiation injury in mice and guinea pigs by bone marrow injections," *Journal of the National Cancer Institute*, vol. 12, no. 1, pp. 197–201, 1951.

[19] J. E. Till and E. A. Mc, "A direct measurement of the radiation sensitivity of normal mouse bone marrow cells," *Radiation Research*, vol. 14, pp. 213–222, 1961.

[20] L. Siminovitch, E. A. Mcculloch, and J. E. Till, "The distribution of colony-forming cells among spleen colonies," *Journal of Cellular Physiology*, vol. 62, pp. 327–336, 1963.

[21] R. Schofield, "The relationship between the spleen colony-forming cell and the haemopoietic stem cell. A hypothesis," *Blood Cells*, vol. 4, no. 1-2, pp. 7–25, 1978.

[22] M. A. Moore and D. Metcalf, "Ontogeny of the haemopoietic system: yolk sac origin of in vivo and in vitro colony forming cells in the developing mouse embryo," *British Journal of Haematology*, vol. 18, no. 3, pp. 279–296, 1970.

[23] B. M. Zeigler, D. Sugiyama, M. Chen, Y. Guo, K. M. Downs, and N. A. Speck, "The allantois and chorion, when isolated before circulation or chorio-allantoic fusion, have hematopoietic potential," *Development*, vol. 133, no. 21, pp. 4183–4192, 2006.

[24] A. Medvinsky and E. Dzierzak, "Definitive hematopoiesis is autonomously initiated by the AGM region," *Cell*, vol. 86, no. 6, pp. 897–906, 1996.

[25] A. M. Müller, A. Medvinsky, J. Strouboulis, F. Grosveld, and E. Dzierzak, "Development of hematopoietic stem cell activity in the mouse embryo," *Immunity*, vol. 1, no. 4, pp. 291–301, 1994.

[26] M. F. T. R. de Bruijn, N. A. Speck, M. C. E. Peeters, and E. Dzierzak, "Definitive hematopoietic stem cells first develop within the major arterial regions of the mouse embryo," *The EMBO Journal*, vol. 19, no. 11, pp. 2465–2474, 2000.

[27] A. Huyhn, M. Dommergues, B. Izac et al., "Characterization of hematopoietic progenitors from human yolk sacs and embryos," *Blood*, vol. 86, no. 12, pp. 4474–4485, 1995.

[28] M. C. Labastie, F. Cortés, P. H. Roméo, C. Dulac, and B. Péault, "Molecular identity of hematopoietic precursor cells emerging in the human embryo," *Blood*, vol. 92, no. 10, pp. 3624–3635, 1998.

[29] M. Tavian, L. Coulombel, D. Luton, H. S. Clemente, F. Dieterlen-Lièvre, and B. Péault, "Aorta-associated CD34+ hematopoietic cells in the early human embryo," *Blood*, vol. 87, no. 1, pp. 67–72, 1996.

[30] M. Tavian, C. Robin, L. Coulombel, and B. Péault, "The human embryo, but not its yolk sac, generates lympho-myeloid stem cells: mapping multipotent hematopoietic cell fate in intraembryonic mesoderm," *Immunity*, vol. 15, no. 3, pp. 487–495, 2001.

[31] M. J. Chen, T. Yokomizo, B. M. Zeigler, E. Dzierzak, and N. A. Speck, "Runx1 is required for the endothelial to haematopoietic cell transition but not thereafter," *Nature*, vol. 457, no. 7231, pp. 887–891, 2009.

[32] M. F. T. R. de Bruijn, X. Ma, C. Robin, K. Ottersbach, M. J. Sanchez, and E. Dzierzak, "Hematopoietic stem cells localize to the endothelial cell layer in the midgestation mouse aorta," *Immunity*, vol. 16, no. 5, pp. 673–683, 2002.

[33] E. Taylor, S. Taoudi, and A. Medvinsky, "Hematopoietic stem cell activity in the aorta-gonad-mesonephros region enhances after mid-day 11 of mouse development," *International Journal of Developmental Biology*, vol. 54, no. 6-7, pp. 1055–1060, 2010.

[34] A. Bárcena, M. Kapidzic, M. O. Muench et al., "The human placenta is a hematopoietic organ during the embryonic and fetal periods of development," *Developmental Biology*, vol. 327, no. 1, pp. 24–33, 2009.

[35] C. Robin, K. Bollerot, S. Mendes et al., "Human placenta is a potent hematopoietic niche containing hematopoietic stem and progenitor cells throughout development," *Cell Stem Cell*, vol. 5, no. 4, pp. 385–395, 2009.

[36] J. C. Cross, "How to make a placenta: mechanisms of trophoblast cell differentiation in mice—a review," *Placenta*, vol. 26, supplement 1, pp. S3–S9, 2005.

[37] P. Georgiades, A. C. Fergyson-Smith, and G. J. Burton, "Comparative developmental anatomy of the murine and human definitive placentae," *Placenta*, vol. 23, no. 1, pp. 3–19, 2002.

[38] B. Cox, M. Kotlyar, A. I. Evangelou et al., "Comparative systems biology of human and mouse as a tool to guide the modeling of human placental pathology," *Molecular Systems Biology*, vol. 5, article 279, 2009.

[39] J. Rossant and J. C. Cross, "Placental development: lessons from mouse mutants," *Nature Reviews Genetics*, vol. 2, no. 7, pp. 538–548, 2001.

[40] C. Corbel, J. Salaün, P. Belo-Diabangouaya, and F. Dieterlen-Lièvre, "Hematopoietic potential of the pre-fusion allantois," *Developmental Biology*, vol. 301, no. 2, pp. 478–488, 2007.

[41] K. E. Rhodes, C. Gekas, Y. Wang et al., "The emergence of hematopoietic stem cells is Initiated in the placental vasculature in the absence of circulation," *Cell Stem Cell*, vol. 2, no. 3, pp. 252–263, 2008.

[42] P. D. F. Murray, "The development in vitro of the blood of the early chick embryo," *Proceedings of the Royal Society*, vol. 111, no. 773, pp. 497–521, 1932.

[43] T. Jaffredo, R. Gautier, A. Eichmann, and F. Dieterlen-Lièvre, "Intraaortic hemopoietic cells are derived from endothelial cells during ontogeny," *Development*, vol. 125, no. 22, pp. 4575–4583, 1998.

[44] S. I. Nishikawa, S. Nishikawa, H. Kawamoto et al., "In vitro generation of lymphohematopoietic cells from endothelial cells purified from murine embryos," *Immunity*, vol. 8, no. 6, pp. 761–769, 1998.

[45] H. M. Eilken, S. I. Nishikawa, and T. Schroeder, "Continuous single-cell imaging of blood generation from haemogenic endothelium," *Nature*, vol. 457, no. 7231, pp. 896–900, 2009.

[46] J. C. Boisset, W. Van Cappellen, C. Andrieu-Soler, N. Galjart, E. Dzierzak, and C. Robin, "In vivo imaging of haematopoietic cells emerging from the mouse aortic endothelium," *Nature*, vol. 464, no. 7285, pp. 116–120, 2010.

[47] E. Oberlin, B. E. Hafny, L. Petit-Cocault, and M. Souyri, "Definitive human and mouse hematopoiesis originates from the embryonic endothelium: a new class of HSCs based on VE-cadherin expression," *International Journal of Developmental Biology*, vol. 54, no. 6-7, pp. 1165–1173, 2010.

[48] T. Ara, K. Tokoyoda, T. Sugiyama, T. Egawa, K. Kawabata, and T. Nagasawa, "Long-term hematopoietic stem cells require stromal cell-derived factor-1 for colonizing bone marrow during ontogeny," *Immunity*, vol. 19, no. 2, pp. 257–267, 2003.

[49] Y. Guo, G. Hangoc, H. Bian, L. M. Pelus, and H. E. Broxmeyer, "SDF-1/CXCL12 enhances survival and chemotaxis of murine embryonic stem cells and production of primitive and definitive hematopoietic progenitor cells," *Stem Cells*, vol. 23, no. 9, pp. 1324–1332, 2005.

[50] T. Xie and A. C. Spradling, "decapentaplegic is essential for the maintenance and division of germline stem cells in the Drosophila ovary," *Cell*, vol. 94, no. 2, pp. 251–260, 1998.

[51] S. K. Nilsson, P. J. Simmons, and I. Bertoncello, "Hemopoietic stem cell engraftment," *Experimental Hematology*, vol. 34, no. 2, pp. 123–129, 2006.

[52] S. Basu, N. T. Ray, S. J. Atkinson, and H. E. Broxmeyer, "Protein phosphatase 2A plays an important role in stromal cell-derived factor-1/CXC chemokine ligand 12-mediated migration and adhesion of CD34+ cells," *Journal of Immunology*, vol. 179, no. 5, pp. 3075–3085, 2007.

[53] C. Lo Celso, H. E. Fleming, J. W. Wu et al., "Live-animal tracking of individual haematopoietic stem/progenitor cells in their niche," *Nature*, vol. 457, no. 7225, pp. 92–96, 2009.

[54] Y. Xie, T. Yin, W. Wiegraebe et al., "Detection of functional haematopoietic stem cell niche using real-time imaging," *Nature*, vol. 457, no. 7225, pp. 97–101, 2009.

[55] Y. Jung, J. Song, Y. Shiozawa et al., "Hematopoietic stem cells regulate mesenchymal stromal cell induction into osteoblasts thereby participating in the formation of the stem cell niche," *Stem Cells*, vol. 26, no. 8, pp. 2042–2051, 2008.

[56] L. M. Calvi, G. B. Adams, K. W. Weibrecht et al., "Osteoblastic cells regulate the haematopoietic stem cell niche," *Nature*, vol. 425, no. 6960, pp. 841–846, 2003.

[57] J. M. Weber, S. R. Forsythe, C. A. Christianson et al., "Parathyroid hormone stimulates expression of the Notch ligand Jagged1 in osteoblastic cells," *Bone*, vol. 39, no. 3, pp. 485–493, 2006.

[58] B. R. Chitteti, Y. H. Cheng, B. Poteat et al., "Impact of interactions of cellular components of the bone marrow microenvironment on hematopoietic stem and progenitor cell function," *Blood*, vol. 115, no. 16, pp. 3239–3248, 2010.

[59] F. Arai, A. Hirao, M. Ohmura et al., "Tie2/angiopoietin-1 signaling regulates hematopoietic stem cell quiescence in the bone marrow niche," *Cell*, vol. 118, no. 2, pp. 149–161, 2004.

[60] R. S. Taichman, "Blood and bone: two tissues whose fates are intertwined to create the hematopoietic stem-cell niche," *Blood*, vol. 105, no. 7, pp. 2631–2639, 2005.

[61] S. Stier, Y. Ko, R. Forkert et al., "Osteopontin is a hematopoietic stem cell niche component that negatively regulates stem cell pool size," *Journal of Experimental Medicine*, vol. 201, no. 11, pp. 1781–1791, 2005.

[62] N. D. Staudt, W. K. Aicher, H. Kalbacher et al., "Cathepsin X is secreted by human osteoblasts, digests CXCL-12 and impairs adhesion of hematopoietic stem and progenitor cells to osteoblasts," *Haematologica*, vol. 95, no. 9, pp. 1452–1460, 2010.

[63] A. P. D. N. de Barros, C. M. Takiya, L. R. Garzoni et al., "Osteoblasts and bone marrow mesenchymal stromal cells control hematopoietic stem cell migration and proliferation in 3D in vitro model," *PLoS ONE*, vol. 5, no. 2, Article ID e9093, 2010.

[64] Y. Nakamura, F. Arai, H. Iwasaki et al., "Isolation and characterization of endosteal niche cell populations that regulate hematopoietic stem cells," *Blood*, vol. 116, no. 9, pp. 1422–1432, 2010.

[65] J. Zhang, C. Niu, L. Ye et al., "Identification of the haematopoietic stem cell niche and control of the niche size," *Nature*, vol. 425, no. 6960, pp. 836–841, 2003.

[66] J. Zhu, R. Garrett, Y. Jung et al., "Osteoblasts support B-lymphocyte commitment and differentiation from hematopoietic stem cell," *Blood*, vol. 109, no. 9, pp. 3706–3712, 2007.

[67] D. Visnjic, Z. Kalajzic, D. W. Rowe, V. Katavic, J. Lorenzo, and H. L. Aguila, "Hematopoiesis is severely altered in mice with an induced osteoblast deficiency," *Blood*, vol. 103, no. 9, pp. 3258–3264, 2004.

[68] M. J. Kiel, G. L. Radice, and S. J. Morrison, "Lack of evidence that hematopoietic stem cells depend on N-cadherin-mediated adhesion to osteoblasts for their maintenance," *Cell Stem Cell*, vol. 1, no. 2, pp. 204–217, 2007.

[69] Y. D. Ma, C. Park, H. Zhao et al., "Defects in osteoblast function but no changes in long-term repopulating potential of hematopoietic stem cells in a mouse chronic inflammatory arthritis model," *Blood*, vol. 114, no. 20, pp. 4402–4410, 2009.

[70] M. J. Kiel, M. Acar, G. L. Radice, and S. J. Morrison, "Hematopoietic stem cells do not depend on N-cadherin to regulate their maintenance," *Cell Stem Cell*, vol. 4, no. 2, pp. 170–179, 2009.

[71] B. Li, A. S. Bailey, S. Jiang, B. Liu, D. C. Goldman, and W. H. Fleming, "Endothelial cells mediate the regeneration of hematopoietic stem cells," *Stem Cell Research*, vol. 4, no. 1, pp. 17–24, 2010.

[72] A. B. Salter, S. K. Meadows, G. G. Muramoto et al., "Endothelial progenitor cell infusion induces hematopoietic stem cell reconstitution in vivo," *Blood*, vol. 113, no. 9, pp. 2104–2107, 2009.

[73] H. Kobayashi, J. M. Butler, R. O'Donnell et al., "Angiocrine factors from Akt-activated endothelial cells balance self-renewal and differentiation of haematopoietic stem cells," *Nature Cell Biology*, vol. 12, no. 11, pp. 1046–1056, 2010.

[74] M. G. Kharas, R. Okabe, J. J. Ganis et al., "Constitutively active AKT depletes hematopoietic stem cells and induces leukemia in mice," *Blood*, vol. 115, no. 7, pp. 1406–1415, 2010.

[75] A. T. Hooper, J. M. Butler, D. J. Nolan et al., "Engraftment and reconstitution of hematopoiesis is dependent on VEGFR2-mediated regeneration of sinusoidal endothelial cells," *Cell Stem Cell*, vol. 4, no. 3, pp. 263–274, 2009.

[76] J. M. Butler, D. J. Nolan, E. L. Vertes et al., "Endothelial cells are essential for the self-renewal and repopulation of notch-dependent hematopoietic stem cells," *Cell Stem Cell*, vol. 6, no. 3, pp. 251–264, 2010.

[77] T. Sugiyama, H. Kohara, M. Noda, and T. Nagasawa, "Maintenance of the hematopoietic stem cell pool by CXCL12-CXCR4 chemokine signaling in bone marrow stromal cell niches," *Immunity*, vol. 25, no. 6, pp. 977–988, 2006.

[78] Y. Nie, Y. C. Han, and Y. R. Zou, "CXCR4 is required for the quiescence of primitive hematopoietic cells," *Journal of Experimental Medicine*, vol. 205, no. 4, pp. 777–783, 2008.

[79] M. Noda, Y. Omatsu, T. Sugiyama, S. Oishi, N. Fujii, and T. Nagasawa, "CXCL12-CXCR4 chemokine signaling is essential for NK-cell development in adult mice," *Blood*, vol. 117, no. 2, pp. 451–458, 2011.

[80] H. Kohara, Y. Omatsu, T. Sugiyama, M. Noda, N. Fujii, and T. Nagasawa, "Development of plasmacytoid dendritic cells in bone marrow stromal cell niches requires CXCL12-CXCR4 chemokine signaling," *Blood*, vol. 110, no. 13, pp. 4153–4160, 2007.

[81] T. Nagasawa, "Microenvironmental niches in the bone marrow required for B-cell development," *Nature Reviews Immunology*, vol. 6, no. 2, pp. 107–116, 2006.

[82] Y. Omatsu, T. Sugiyama, H. Kohara et al., "The essential functions of adipo-osteogenic progenitors as the hematopoietic stem and progenitor cell niche," *Immunity*, vol. 33, no. 3, pp. 387–399, 2010.

[83] B. Sacchetti, A. Funari, S. Michienzi et al., "Self-renewing osteoprogenitors in bone marrow sinusoids can organize a hematopoietic microenvironment," *Cell*, vol. 131, no. 2, pp. 324–336, 2007.

[84] D. Traver, K. Akashi, M. Manz et al., "Development of CD8α-positive dendritic cells from a common myeloid progenitor," *Science*, vol. 290, no. 5499, pp. 2152–2154, 2000.

[85] M. G. Manz, D. Traver, K. Akashi et al., "Dendritic cell development from common myeloid progenitors," *Annals of the New York Academy of Sciences*, vol. 938, pp. 167–174, 2001.

[86] M. G. Manz, D. Traver, T. Miyamoto, I. L. Weissman, and K. Akashi, "Dendritic cell potentials of early lymphoid and myeloid progenitors," *Blood*, vol. 97, no. 11, pp. 3333–3341, 2001.

[87] R. Doyonnas, D. B. Kershaw, C. Duhme et al., "Anuria, omphalocele, and perinatal lethality in mice lacking the CD34-related protein podocalyxin," *Journal of Experimental Medicine*, vol. 194, no. 1, pp. 13–27, 2001.

[88] C. Sassetti, A. Van Zante, and S. D. Rosen, "Identification of endoglycan, a member of the CD34/podocalyxin family of sialomucins," *Journal of Biological Chemistry*, vol. 275, no. 12, pp. 9001–9010, 2000.

[89] C. Sassetti, K. Tangemann, M. S. Singer, D. B. Kershaw, and S. D. Rosen, "Identification of Podocalyxin-like protein as a high endothelial venule ligand for L-selectin: parallels to CD34," *Journal of Experimental Medicine*, vol. 187, no. 12, pp. 1965–1975, 1998.

[90] P. Pranke, J. Hendrikx, G. Debnath et al., "Immunophenotype of hematopoietic stem cells from placental/umbilical cord blood after culture," *Brazilian Journal of Medical and Biological Research*, vol. 38, no. 12, pp. 1775–1789, 2005.

[91] J. P. Hossle, R. A. Seger, and D. Steinhoff, "Gene therapy of hematopoietic stem cells: strategies for improvement," *News in Physiological Sciences*, vol. 17, no. 3, pp. 87–92, 2002.

[92] D. S. Krause, M. J. Fackler, C. I. Civin, and W. S. May, "CD34: structure, biology, and clinical utility," *Blood*, vol. 87, no. 1, pp. 1–13, 1996.

[93] C. M. Baum, I. L. Weissman, A. S. Tsukamoto, A. M. Buckle, and B. Peault, "Isolation of a candidate human hematopoietic stem-cell population," *Proceedings of the National Academy of Sciences of the United States of America*, vol. 89, no. 7, pp. 2804–2808, 1992.

[94] M. Bhatia, J. C. Y. Wang, U. Kapp, D. Bonnet, and J. E. Dick, "Purification of primitive human hematopoietic cells capable of repopulating immune-deficient mice," *Proceedings of the National Academy of Sciences of the United States of America*, vol. 94, no. 10, pp. 5320–5325, 1997.

[95] Q. L. Hao, A. J. Shah, F. T. Thiemann, E. M. Smogorzewska, and G. M. Crooks, "A functional comparison of CD34$^+$ CD38$^-$ cells in cord blood and bone marrow," *Blood*, vol. 86, no. 10, pp. 3745–3753, 1995.

[96] H. Mayani, W. Dragowska, and P. M. Lansdorp, "Characterization of functionally distinct subpopulations of CD34$^+$ cord blood cells in serum-free long-term cultures supplemented with hematopoietic cytokines," *Blood*, vol. 82, no. 9, pp. 2664–2672, 1993.

[97] R. Majeti, C. Y. Park, and I. L. Weissman, "Identification of a hierarchy of multipotent hematopoietic progenitors in human cord blood," *Cell Stem Cell*, vol. 1, no. 6, pp. 635–645, 2007.

[98] F. Notta, S. Doulatov, E. Laurenti, A. Poeppl, I. Jurisica, and J. E. Dick, "Isolation of single human hematopoietic stem cells capable of long-term multilineage engraftment," *Science*, vol. 333, no. 6039, pp. 218–221, 2011.

[99] W. H. Fleming, E. J. Alpern, N. Uchida, K. Ikuta, G. J. Spangrude, and I. L. Weissman, "Functional heterogeneity is associated with the cell cycle status of murine hematopoietic stem cells," *Journal of Cell Biology*, vol. 122, no. 4, pp. 897–902, 1993.

[100] M. Z. Ratajczak, E. Zuba-Surma, M. Kucia, R. Reca, W. Wojakowski, and J. Ratajczak, "The pleiotropic effects of the SDF-1-CXCR4 axis in organogenesis, regeneration and tumorigenesis," *Leukemia*, vol. 20, no. 11, pp. 1915–1924, 2006.

[101] M. Shirozu, T. Nakano, J. Inazawa et al., "Structure and chromosomal localization of the human stromal cell-derived factor 1 (SDF1) gene," *Genomics*, vol. 28, no. 3, pp. 495–500, 1995.

[102] M. Gleichmann, C. Gillen, M. Czardybon et al., "Cloning and characterization of SDF-1γ, a novel SDF-1 chemokine transcript with developmentally regulated expression in the nervous system," *European Journal of Neuroscience*, vol. 12, no. 6, pp. 1857–1866, 2000.

[103] L. Yu, J. Cecil, S. B. Peng et al., "Identification and expression of novel isoforms of human stromal cell-derived factor 1," *Gene*, vol. 374, no. 1-2, pp. 174–179, 2006.

[104] K. Balabanian, B. Lagane, S. Infantino et al., "The chemokine SDF-1/CXCL12 binds to and signals through the orphan receptor RDC1 in T lymphocytes," *Journal of Biological Chemistry*, vol. 280, no. 42, pp. 35760–35766, 2005.

[105] B. Moepps, M. Braun, K. Knopfle et al., "Characterization of a Xenopus laevis CXC chemokine receptor 4: implications for hematopoietic cell development in the vertebrate embryo,"

European Journal of Immunology, vol. 30, no. 10, pp. 2924–2934, 2000.

[106] M. Braun, M. Wunderlin, K. Spieth, W. Knöchel, P. Gierschik, and B. Moepps, "Xenopus laevis stromal cell-derived factor 1: conservation of structure and function during vertebrate development," *Journal of Immunology*, vol. 168, no. 5, pp. 2340–2347, 2002.

[107] H. Zheng, G. Fu, T. Dai, and H. Huang, "Migration of endothelial progenitor cells mediated by stromal cell-derived factor-1α/CXCR4 via PI3K/Akt/eNOS signal transduction pathway," *Journal of Cardiovascular Pharmacology*, vol. 50, no. 3, pp. 274–280, 2007.

[108] D. J. Ceradini, A. R. Kulkarni, M. J. Callaghan et al., "Progenitor cell trafficking is regulated by hypoxic gradients through HIF-1 induction of SDF-1," *Nature Medicine*, vol. 10, no. 8, pp. 858–864, 2004.

[109] Y. Yang, G. Tang, J. Yan et al., "Cellular and molecular mechanism regulating blood flow recovery in acute versus gradual femoral artery occlusion are distinct in the mouse," *Journal of Vascular Surgery*, vol. 48, no. 6, pp. 1546–1558, 2008.

[110] J. I. Yamaguchi, K. F. Kusano, O. Masuo et al., "Stromal cell-derived factor-1 effects on ex vivo expanded endothelial progenitor cell recruitment for ischemic neovascularization," *Circulation*, vol. 107, no. 9, pp. 1322–1328, 2003.

[111] H. Liu, S. Liu, Y. Li et al., "The role of SDF-1-CXCR4/CXCR7 axis in the therapeutic effects of hypoxia-preconditioned mesenchymal stem cells for renal ischemia/reperfusion injury," *PLoS One*, vol. 7, no. 4, Article ID e34608, 2012.

[112] B. Heissig, K. Hattori, S. Dias et al., "Recruitment of stem and progenitor cells from the bone marrow niche requires MMP-9 mediated release of Kit-ligand," *Cell*, vol. 109, no. 5, pp. 625–637, 2002.

[113] Y. S. Tzeng, H. Li, Y. L. Kang, W. G. Chen, W. Cheng, and D. M. Lai, "Loss of Cxcl12/Sdf-1 in adult mice decreases the quiescent state of hematopoietic stem/progenitor cells and alters the pattern of hematopoietic regeneration after myelosuppression," *Blood*, vol. 117, no. 2, pp. 429–439, 2011.

[114] A. H. Reddi and A. Reddi, "Bone morphogenetic proteins (BMPs): from morphogens to metabologens," *Cytokine and Growth Factor Reviews*, vol. 20, no. 5-6, pp. 341–342, 2009.

[115] R. Garimella, S. E. Tague, J. Zhang et al., "Expression and synthesis of bone morphogenetic proteins by osteoclasts: a possible path to anabolic bone remodeling," *Journal of Histochemistry and Cytochemistry*, vol. 56, no. 6, pp. 569–577, 2008.

[116] D. C. Goldman, A. S. Bailey, D. L. Pfaffle, A. Al Masri, J. L. Christian, and W. H. Fleming, "BMP4 regulates the hematopoietic stem cell niche," *Blood*, vol. 114, no. 20, pp. 4393–4401, 2009.

[117] C. Durand, C. Robin, K. Bollerot, M. H. Baron, K. Ottersbach, and E. Dzierzak, "Embryonic stromal clones reveal developmental regulators of definitive hematopoietic stem cells," *Proceedings of the National Academy of Sciences of the United States of America*, vol. 104, no. 52, pp. 20838–20843, 2007.

[118] M. Bhatia, D. Bonnet, D. Wu et al., "Bone morphogenetic proteins regulate the developmental program of human hematopoietic stem cells," *Journal of Experimental Medicine*, vol. 189, no. 7, pp. 1139–1148, 1999.

[119] V. C. Broudy and K. Kaushansky, "Thrombopoietin, the c-mpl ligand, is a major regulator of platelet production," *Journal of Leukocyte Biology*, vol. 57, no. 5, pp. 719–725, 1995.

[120] N. Debili, F. Wendling, D. Cosman et al., "The MpI receptor is expressed in the megakaryocytic lineage from late progenitors to platelets," *Blood*, vol. 85, no. 2, pp. 391–401, 1995.

[121] O. Livnah, E. A. Stura, S. A. Middleton, D. L. Johnson, L. K. Jolliffe, and I. A. Wilson, "Crystallographic evidence for preformed dimers of erythropoietin receptor before ligand activation," *Science*, vol. 283, no. 5404, pp. 987–990, 1999.

[122] J. G. Drachman and K. Kaushansky, "Dissecting the thrombopoietin receptor: functional elements of the Mpl cytoplasmic domain," *Proceedings of the National Academy of Sciences of the United States of America*, vol. 94, no. 6, pp. 2350–2355, 1997.

[123] B. A. Witthuhn, F. W. Quelle, O. Silvennoinen et al., "JAK2 associates with the erythropoietin receptor and is tyrosine phosphorylated and activated following stimulation with erythropoietin," *Cell*, vol. 74, no. 2, pp. 227–236, 1993.

[124] P. J. Tortolani, J. A. Johnston, C. M. Bacon et al., "Thrombopoietin induces tyrosine phosphorylation and activation of the Janus kinase, JAK2," *Blood*, vol. 85, no. 12, pp. 3444–3451, 1995.

[125] H. Yoshihara, F. Arai, K. Hosokawa et al., "Thrombopoietin/MPL signaling regulates hematopoietic stem cell quiescence and interaction with the osteoblastic niche," *Cell Stem Cell*, vol. 1, no. 6, pp. 685–697, 2007.

[126] H. Qian, N. Buza-Vidas, C. D. Hyland et al., "Critical role of thrombopoietin in maintaining adult quiescent hematopoietic stem cells," *Cell Stem Cell*, vol. 1, no. 6, pp. 671–684, 2007.

[127] A. Bersenev, C. Wu, J. Balcerek, and W. Tong, "Lnk controls mouse hematopoietic stem cell self-renewal and quiescence through direct interactions with JAK2," *Journal of Clinical Investigation*, vol. 118, no. 8, pp. 2832–2844, 2008.

[128] A. Rongvaux, T. Willinger, H. Takizawa et al., "Human thrombopoietin knockin mice efficiently support human hematopoiesis in vivo," *Proceedings of the National Academy of Sciences of the United States of America*, vol. 108, no. 6, pp. 2378–2383, 2011.

[129] Y. Gomei, Y. Nakamura, H. Yoshihara et al., "Functional differences between two Tie2 ligands, angiopoietin-1 and -2, in regulation of adult bone marrow hematopoietic stem cells," *Experimental Hematology*, vol. 38, no. 2, pp. 82.e1–89.e1, 2010.

[130] J. J. Trowbridge, M. P. Scott, and M. Bhatia, "Hedgehog modulates cell cycle regulators in stem cells to control hematopoietic regeneration," *Proceedings of the National Academy of Sciences of the United States of America*, vol. 103, no. 38, pp. 14134–14139, 2006.

[131] C. Zhao, A. Chen, C. H. Jamieson et al., "Hedgehog signalling is essential for maintenance of cancer stem cells in myeloid leukaemia," *Nature*, vol. 458, no. 7239, pp. 776–779, 2009.

[132] A. Merchant, G. Joseph, Q. Wang, S. Brennan, and W. Matsui, "Gli1 regulates the proliferation and differentiation of HSCs and myeloid progenitors," *Blood*, vol. 115, no. 12, pp. 2391–2396, 2010.

[133] I. Hofmann, E. H. Stover, D. E. Cullen et al., "Hedgehog signaling is dispensable for adult murine hematopoietic stem cell function and hematopoiesis," *Cell Stem Cell*, vol. 4, no. 6, pp. 559–567, 2009.

[134] J. Gao, S. Graves, U. Koch et al., "Hedgehog signaling is dispensable for adult hematopoietic stem cell function," *Cell Stem Cell*, vol. 4, no. 6, pp. 548–558, 2009.

[135] S. Artavanis-Tsakonas, M. D. Rand, and R. J. Lake, "Notch signaling: cell fate control and signal integration in development," *Science*, vol. 284, no. 5415, pp. 770–776, 1999.

[136] G. L. Lin and K. D. Hankenson, "Integration of BMP, Wnt, and Notch signaling pathways in osteoblast differentiation," *Journal of Cellular Biochemistry*, vol. 112, no. 12, pp. 3491–3501, 2011.

[137] P. Ranganathan, K. L. Weaver, and A. J. Capobianco, "Notch signalling in solid tumours: a little bit of everything but not all the time," *Nature Reviews Cancer*, vol. 11, no. 5, pp. 338–351, 2011.

[138] K. Ohishi, B. Varnum-Finney, and I. D. Bernstein, "Delta-1 enhances marrow and thymus repopulating ability of human CD34+CD38− cord blood cells," *Journal of Clinical Investigation*, vol. 110, no. 8, pp. 1165–1174, 2002.

[139] B. Varnum-Finney, L. M. Halasz, M. Sun, T. Gridley, F. Radtke, and I. D. Bernstein, "Notch2 governs the rate of generation of mouse long- and short-term repopulating stem cells," *Journal of Clinical Investigation*, vol. 121, no. 3, pp. 1207–1216, 2011.

[140] B. Varnum-Finney, C. Brashem-Stein, and I. D. Bernstein, "Combined effects of Notch signaling and cytokines induce a multiple log increase in precursors with lymphoid and myeloid reconstituting ability," *Blood*, vol. 101, no. 5, pp. 1784–1789, 2003.

[141] S. Stier, T. Cheng, D. Dombkowski, N. Carlesso, and D. T. Scadden, "Notch1 activation increases hematopoietic stem cell self-renewal in vivo and favors lymphoid over myeloid lineage outcome," *Blood*, vol. 99, no. 7, pp. 2369–2378, 2002.

[142] J. M. Rowlinson and M. Gering, "Hey2 acts upstream of Notch in hematopoietic stem cell specification in zebrafish embryos," *Blood*, vol. 116, no. 12, pp. 2046–2056, 2010.

[143] I. Maillard, U. Koch, A. Dumortier et al., "Canonical notch signaling is dispensable for the Maintenance of adult hematopoietic stem cells," *Cell Stem Cell*, vol. 2, no. 4, pp. 356–366, 2008.

[144] S. J. C. Mancini, N. Mantei, A. Dumortier, U. Suter, H. R. MacDonald, and F. Radtke, "Jagged1-dependent Notch signaling is dispensable for hematopoietic stem cell self-renewal and differentiation," *Blood*, vol. 105, no. 6, pp. 2340–2342, 2005.

[145] Y. W. Kim, B. K. Koo, H. W. Jeong et al., "Defective Notch activation in microenvironment leads to myeloproliferative disease," *Blood*, vol. 112, no. 12, pp. 4628–4638, 2008.

[146] M. Santaguida, K. Schepers, B. King et al., "JunB protects against myeloid malignancies by limiting hematopoietic stem cell proliferation and differentiation without affecting self-renewal," *Cancer Cell*, vol. 15, no. 4, pp. 341–352, 2009.

[147] W. K. Clements, A. D. Kim, K. G. Ong, J. C. Moore, N. D. Lawson, and D. Traver, "A somitic Wnt16/Notch pathway specifies haematopoietic stem cells," *Nature*, vol. 474, no. 7350, pp. 220–224, 2011.

[148] R. B. Chalamalasetty, W. C. Dunty Jr., K. K. Biris et al., "The Wnt3a/β-catenin target gene Mesogenin1 controls the segmentation clock by activating a Notch signalling program," *Nature Communications*, vol. 2, no. 1, article 390, 2011.

[149] S. Han, N. Dziedzic, P. Gadue, G. M. Keller, and V. Gouon-Evans, "An endothelial cell niche induces hepatic specification through dual repression of Wnt and notch signaling," *Stem Cells*, vol. 29, no. 2, pp. 217–228, 2011.

[150] I. S. Peter and E. H. Davidson, "A gene regulatory network controlling the embryonic specification of endoderm," *Nature*, vol. 474, no. 7353, pp. 635–639, 2011.

[151] D. W. Kim, J. S. Lee, E. S. Yoon, B. I. Lee, S. H. Park, and E. S. Dhong, "Influence of human adipose-derived stromal cells on Wnt signaling in organotypic skin culture," *Journal of Craniofacial Surgery*, vol. 22, no. 2, pp. 694–698, 2011.

[152] N. Sato, L. Meijer, L. Skaltsounis, P. Greengard, and A. H. Brivanlou, "Maintenance of pluripotency in human and mouse embryonic stem cells through activation of Wnt signaling by a pharmacological GSK-3-specific inhibitor," *Nature Medicine*, vol. 10, no. 1, pp. 55–63, 2004.

[153] P. S. Woll, J. K. Morris, M. S. Painschab et al., "Wnt signaling promotes hematoendothelial cell development from human embryonic stem cells," *Blood*, vol. 111, no. 1, pp. 122–131, 2008.

[154] C. H. Wu and R. Nusse, "Ligand receptor interactions in the Wnt signaling pathway in Drosophila," *Journal of Biological Chemistry*, vol. 277, no. 44, pp. 41762–41769, 2002.

[155] H. C. Wong, A. Bourdelas, A. Krauss et al., "Direct binding of the PDZ domain of Dishevelled to a conserved internal sequence in the C-terminal region of Frizzled," *Molecular Cell*, vol. 12, no. 5, pp. 1251–1260, 2003.

[156] N. S. Tolwinski, M. Wehrli, A. Rives, N. Erdeniz, S. DiNardo, and E. Wieschaus, "Wg/Wnt signal can be transmitted through arrow/LRP5,6 and axin independently of Zw3/Gsk3β activity," *Developmental Cell*, vol. 4, no. 3, pp. 407–418, 2003.

[157] T. Kramps, O. Peter, E. Brunner et al., "Wnt/Wingless signaling requires BCL9/legless-mediated recruitment of pygopus to the nuclear β-catenin-TCF complex," *Cell*, vol. 109, no. 1, pp. 47–60, 2002.

[158] M. Katoh and M. Katoh, "Identification and characterization of human BCL9L gene and mouse Bcl9l gene in silico," *International Journal of Molecular Medicine*, vol. 12, no. 4, pp. 643–649, 2003.

[159] J. R. Miller, A. M. Hocking, J. D. Brown, and R. T. Moon, "Mechanism and function of signal transduction by the Wnt/B-catenin and Wnt/Ca2+ pathways," *Oncogene*, vol. 18, no. 55, pp. 7860–7872, 1999.

[160] M. N. Chamorro, D. R. Schwartz, A. Vonica, A. H. Brivanlou, K. R. Cho, and H. E. Varmus, "FGF-20 and DKK1 are transcriptional targets of β-catenin and FGF-20 is implicated in cancer and development," *The EMBO Journal*, vol. 24, no. 1, pp. 73–84, 2005.

[161] D. Pennica, T. A. Swanson, J. W. Welsh et al., "WISP genes are members of the connective tissue growth factor family that are up-regulated in Wnt-1-transformed cells and aberrantly expressed in human colon tumors," *Proceedings of the National Academy of Sciences of the United States of America*, vol. 95, no. 25, pp. 14717–14722, 1998.

[162] T. C. He, A. B. Sparks, C. Rago et al., "Identification of c-MYC as a target of the APC pathway," *Science*, vol. 281, no. 5382, pp. 1509–1512, 1998.

[163] O. Tetsu and F. McCormick, "β-catenin regulates expression of cyclin D1 in colon carcinoma cells," *Nature*, vol. 398, no. 6726, pp. 422–426, 1999.

[164] J. A. Kim, Y. J. Kang, G. Park et al., "Identification of a stroma-mediated Wnt/β-catenin signal promoting self-renewal of hematopoietic stem cells in the stem cell niche," *Stem Cells*, vol. 27, no. 6, pp. 1318–1329, 2009.

[165] T. C. Luis, F. Weerkamp, B. A. E. Naber et al., "Wnt3a deficiency irreversibly impairs hematopoietic stem cell self-renewal and leads to defects in progenitor cell differentiation," *Blood*, vol. 113, no. 3, pp. 546–554, 2009.

[166] M. Scheller, J. Huelsken, F. Rosenbauer et al., "Hematopoietic stem cell and multilineage defects generated by constitutive β-catenin activation," *Nature Immunology*, vol. 7, no. 10, pp. 1037–1047, 2006.

[167] P. Kirstetter, K. Anderson, B. T. Porse, S. E. W. Jacobsen, and C. Nerlov, "Activation of the canonical Wnt pathway leads to loss of hematopoietic stem cell repopulation and multilineage differentiation block," *Nature Immunology*, vol. 7, no. 10, pp. 1048–1056, 2006.

[168] J. J. Trowbridge, A. Xenocostas, R. T. Moon, and M. Bhatia, "Glycogen synthase kinase-3 is an in vivo regulator of hematopoietic stem cell repopulation," *Nature Medicine*, vol. 12, no. 1, pp. 89–98, 2006.

[169] H. E. Fleming, V. Janzen, C. Lo Celso et al., "Wnt signaling in the niche enforces hematopoietic stem cell quiescence and is necessary to preserve self-renewal in vivo," *Cell Stem Cell*, vol. 2, no. 3, pp. 274–283, 2008.

[170] K.-H. Ko, T. Holmes, P. Palladinetti et al., "GSK-3β inhibition promotes engraftment of ex vivo-expanded hematopoietic stem cells and modulates gene expression," *Stem Cells*, vol. 29, no. 1, pp. 108–118, 2011.

[171] M. Kinder, C. Wei, S. G. Shelat et al., "Hematopoietic stem cell function requires 12/15-lipoxygenase-dependent fatty acid metabolism," *Blood*, vol. 115, no. 24, pp. 5012–5022, 2010.

14

NOD2 Polymorphisms and Their Impact on Haematopoietic Stem Cell Transplant Outcome

Neema P. Mayor,[1] **Bronwen E. Shaw,**[1,2] **J. Alejandro Madrigal,**[1,3] **and Steven G. E. Marsh**[1,3]

[1] *Anthony Nolan Research Institute, Royal Free Hospital, Pond Street, London NW3 2QG, UK*
[2] *Section of Haemato-Oncology, Royal Marsden Hospital, Surrey SM2 5PT, UK*
[3] *Department of Haematology, UCL Cancer Institute, Royal Free Campus, London WC1E 6BT, UK*

Correspondence should be addressed to Neema P. Mayor, neema.mayor@anthonynolan.org

Academic Editor: Andrzej Lange

Haematopoietic stem cell transplantation (HSCT) is a valuable tool in the treatment of many haematological disorders. Advances in understanding HLA matching have improved prognoses. However, many recipients of well-matched HSCT develop posttransplant complications, and survival is far from absolute. The pursuit of novel genetic factors that may impact on HSCT outcome has resulted in the publication of many articles on a multitude of genes. Three *NOD2* polymorphisms, identified as disease-associated variants in Crohn's disease, have recently been suggested as important candidate gene markers in the outcome of HSCT. It was originally postulated that as the clinical manifestation of inflammatory responses characteristic of several post-transplant complications was of notable similarity to those seen in Crohn's disease, it was possible that they shared a common cause. Since the publication of this first paper, numerous studies have attempted to replicate the results in different transplant settings. The data has varied considerably between studies, and as yet no consensus on the impact of *NOD2* SNPs on HSCT outcome has been achieved. Here, we will review the existing literature, summarise current theories as to why the data differs, and suggest possible mechanisms by which the SNPs affect HSCT outcome.

1. Introduction

Allogeneic haematopoietic stem cell transplantation (HSCT) is an important treatment option in the management of many diseases including malignant and non-malignant haematological disorders, immune deficiencies and inborn errors [1]. The increased knowledge of transplant biology and the effects of clinical factors and HLA matching have improved outcome. The primary choice of donor is usually an HLA-matched sibling, but the probability of a sibling being HLA identical is only 25%, a problem that is exacerbated due to small family sizes that are usually found today. Alternative allogeneic donor sources are thus often required and have now become an important and viable option. There are currently over 19.8 million volunteer unrelated donors (UDs) that have been recruited to registries around the world, with an additional 543,000 umbilical cord blood units also being available (as of September 2012)

(http://www.bmdw.org/). The improvement in transplant techniques and practice has resulted in similar survival prospects for recipients of a well-matched UD as that using a sibling [2, 3]. However, the risk of posttransplant complications such as graft-versus-host disease (GvHD) and delayed immune reconstitution leading to infection is increased [4].

The vital role of HLA matching in transplant outcome is accepted, but there is still controversy as to which of the six major HLA genes are most important. The current perspective on what constitutes a well-matched donor is a 10/10 HLA allele match that is matched at an allele level for HLA-A, -B, -C, -DRB1, and -DQB1 [3, 5–7]. Comprehensive analyses of UD-HSCT pairs have shown that allelic mismatches are as detrimental to transplant outcome as antigenic mismatches, with a single allelic mismatch at HLA-A, -B, -C, or -DRB1 being associated with an increase in GvHD and a reduction in overall survival. This data has been confirmed in increasingly larger cohorts [8–11]. Mismatches at HLA-DQB1 appear to be better tolerated in the context of an 8/8 HLA-matched background (that is matched for HLA-A, -B, -C, and -DRB1) although there is some suggestion that they have a cumulative effect with any other HLA mismatch [6, 9, 10].

While the current donor selection criteria for matching donors and recipients usually refer to five of the classical HLA genes (HLA-A, -B, -C, -DRB1, and -DQB1), the impact of a sixth gene, HLA-DPB1, on the outcome of UD-HSCT is emerging. Current data suggests that nonpermissive HLA-DPB1 mismatches increase the risk of GvHD and transplant-related mortality [12–15].

Despite the benefit resulting from having a 10/10-matched donor, the survival of such a group of individuals is far from being absolute. Recipients receiving a graft from a well-matched sibling donor can be susceptible to getting GvHD. Conversely, some recipients of ≤9/10 HLA-matched grafts do survive and can achieve full remission of their disease [16]. While clinical factors such as the type of disease, disease stage, and recipient/donor characteristics are most certainly involved, theories have evolved that postulate a role for genes other than HLA in predicting transplant outcome. In recent years, much interest has been shown in the role of SNPs within innate immune response genes on the outcome of HSCT [17, 18]. One of the most prolifically studied genes to date has been the nucleotide-binding oligomerisation domain containing 2 (NOD2) gene (previously known as the caspase recruitment domain, family member 15 (CARD15) gene). The data from these studies is conflicting. Here, we will review the current data, on the impact of NOD2 polymorphisms on the outcome of HSCT, potential causes of differences in the data and possible mechanisms by which the variants affect outcome.

2. NOD2 Gene Structure and Function

The NOD2 gene is located in humans on chromosome 16 (16q21) [19]. It is approximately 36 kb in length (35,938 bp) and encodes a protein of 1040 amino acids. NOD2 encodes the NOD2 protein, a member of the NLR (NOD, leucine-rich repeat (LRR) containing) protein family [20–22]. Other members of this family include apoptosis protease-activating factor-1 (Apaf-1) and the MHC class II transactivator (CIITA) [23]. These proteins are classified by their common tripartite domain structure, namely, a central nucleotide binding domain (NBD, the NOD molecule), an amino terminal effector-binding domain (EBD), and a carboxy-terminal ligand-recognition domain (LRD). While all members of this family contain the central NBD region, the EBD and LRD differ between the different proteins. In NOD2, the central NBD domain is an NOD molecule which is surrounded by two CARD molecules (the EBDs) which enable recruitment of downstream signalling molecules and a series of 11 leucine rich repeats (LRR) which function as the LRD [24–26].

Early functional studies identified NOD2 expression in antigen-presenting cells, specifically intestinal epithelial cells

[27], Paneth cells [28, 29], macrophages, and dendritic cells [21]. An increasing number of studies have demonstrated that NOD2 is expressed in a multitude of tissues including keratinocytes [30], T cells [31], NK cells, and CD34+ bone marrow stem cells [32, 33]. NOD2 is expressed within the cytosol and can be recruited to the cell membrane of intestinal epithelial cells [34, 35], a mechanism that appears to be important in the function of the molecule. Proinflammatory cytokines have been shown to regulate NOD2 expression [36].

The NOD2 protein functions as a regulator of infection by the recognition of pathogenic ligands and the induction inflammatory responses via a number of pathways. The most studied interaction is the response to the bacterial ligand muramyl dipeptide (MDP), a derivative of peptidoglycan, which is a component of both Gram-positive and -negative bacterial cell walls [37, 38]. Recognition of MDP by the LRD of NOD2 initiates a complex change in the structure of the molecule, enabling it to undergo self-oligomerisation via the NBD [25, 26, 39], and subsequently the recruitment of the effector molecule receptor-interacting, CARD-containing serine/threonine kinase (RICK) via homophilic interaction of their CARD domains. This recruitment of RICK by NOD2 causes the effector molecule to be activated, and initiates the downstream signalling events that lead to the induction of the nuclear factor (NF)-κB and mitogen-activated protein kinase pathways [39–41]. In addition to this cytokine response initiated by bacterial infection, it has also been shown that upon exposure to MDP, NOD2 plays a key role in the initiation of the autophagy pathway [42, 43]. NOD2 has also been shown to respond in vitro to viral infection by the recognition of a single-stranded (ss) RNA ligand [44]. Here, ssRNA binds to the LRD of NOD2, but rather than recruiting the RICK as an effector molecule, NOD2 is translocated to the mitochondria where it is able to interact with the mitochondria antivirus signalling protein and initiates downstream signalling of the NF-κB pathway.

3. Genetic Polymorphism of the NOD2 Gene

The NOD2 gene is proving to be highly polymorphic with over 660 single nucleotide polymorphisms (SNPs) reported to date both in the literature [45–47] and in various online databases (http://www.genecards.org/, http://www.ensembl.org/ and http://fmf.igh.cnrs.fr/ISSAID/infevers/) [48–50]. The minor allele frequencies vary from less than 1% to over 30%, although significant differences between different ethnic and geographic populations have been demonstrated.

Early studies to identify possible genetic factors that were affecting the incidence of Crohn's disease, a chronic inflammatory disorder of the gastrointestinal tract that can be complicated by anaemia, stenosis, and fistulae, mapped NOD2 as a susceptibility locus [19]. Further studies identified three polymorphisms (designated nomenclature: SNP 8 (reference SNP (rs) rs2066844), SNP 12 (rs2066845) and SNP 13 (rs41450053)) as disease-associated polymorphisms (Figure 1) [45, 51]. It has been shown that individuals heterozygous for any of the three SNPs have a two- to

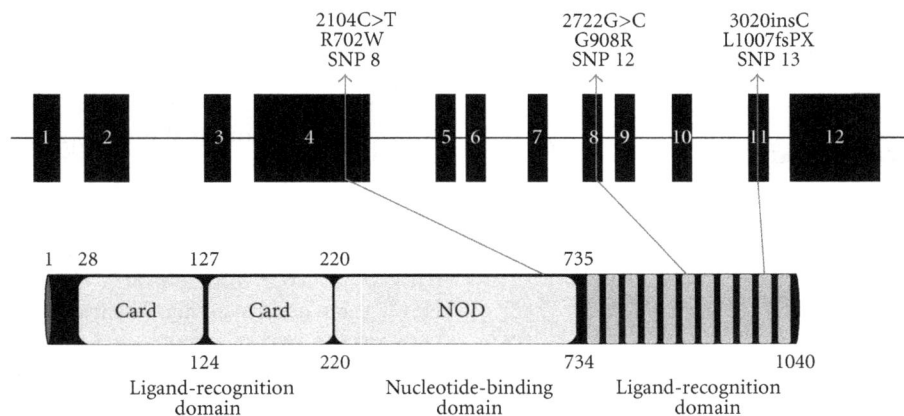

FIGURE 1: The structure of the *NOD2* gene and NOD2 protein. The numbering in the black boxes indicates the exon numbers. The numbering alongside the protein diagram indicates the amino acid positioning. SNPs 8, 12, and 13 are located within exons 4, 8 and 11 respectively, and encode either amino acid substitutions (SNPs 8 and 12) or a frame-shift causing early truncation of the protein (SNP 13).

fourfold increase in the risk of developing Crohn's disease, which increases to approximately twentyfold in individuals who are homozygotes or compound heterozygotes [52]. Other disease-associated studies have also tried to identify the impact of these three polymorphisms with varying results [53]. Subsequently, SNPs 8, 12, and 13 have become some of the most studied and well-characterised SNPs of the *NOD2* gene.

SNPs 8, 12, and 13 are located within *NOD2* exons 4, 8 and 11 respectively. SNPs 8 and 12 are nonsynonymous nucleotide substitutions that result in amino acid changes, SNP 8 (coding (c.) 2104C>T, protein (p.) R702W) and SNP 12 (c. 2722G>C, p. G908R). SNP 13 differs in that it involves the insertion of a nucleotide that results in a frameshift within the coding sequence causing the introduction of an early termination codon and thus a truncated protein (c. 3020CinsC, p. L1007fsPX). SNP 8 is located within the central NBD region of the molecule, while SNPs 12 and 13 are found within LRRs 7 and 10, respectively, of the NOD2 LRD [25, 46].

4. *NOD2* Gene Polymorphisms and Disease

Following the early studies in Crohn's disease, polymorphisms throughout the *NOD2* gene have been implicated in numerous diseases. SNPs 8, 12, and 13 have been correlated with increased risk of ankylosing spondylitis [54], psoriatic arthritis [55], and more recently with early-onset sarcoidosis [56]. Three additional polymorphisms, p. R334W, p. R334Q, and p. L469F, have been associated with Blau syndrome [57]. In addition to these inflammatory disorders, *NOD2* SNPs 8, 12, and 13 have also been correlated with an increased risk of malignant diseases such as colorectal [58], gastric [59], breast, and lung cancer [60] as well with the incidence of non-hodgkin's lymphoma [61], although in most of these studies, the detrimental effects of *NOD2* genotype were limited to the presence of SNP 13. More recently, *NOD2* SNPs have been shown to affect graft survival and mortality

post renal transplantation [62] and coronary artery disease [63].

5. The Functional Consequences of *NOD2* SNPs 8, 12, and 13

SNPs 8, 12, and 13 are thought to reduce the ability of MDP to activate NOD2 and consequently the activation of NF-κB, resulting in reduction in the production of cytokines and antimicrobial peptides [64–66]. These loss-of-function effects caused by the SNPs initially proved controversial, as an enhanced cytokine response is characteristic of Crohn's disease. The publication of data that showed mice with an *NOD2* variant similar to SNP 13 had increased sensitivity to MDP and elevated levels of NF-κB activation when compared to WT mice suggested a gain-of-function effect of *NOD2* SNPs [67, 68]. While this evidence showed a plausible mechanism by which *NOD2* variants contributed to the onset of Crohn's disease, these findings have not been replicated in human studies, and further data has been published that confirm the loss-of-function mechanism [69–72]. Thus, the *NOD2* variants appear to reduce the ability of NOD2 to recognise MDP and consequently to stimulate NF-κB responses. It has been suggested that the inflammatory response seen in Crohn's disease results from the inability of toll-like receptor-2 (TLR-2) to become tolerant to its ligand in the absence of appropriately functioning NOD2, resulting in upregulation of proinflammatory cytokines [73, 74]. In addition to these effects, SNPs 8, 12, and 13 have been associated with increased permeability of the gastrointestinal mucosa and consequently increased levels of bacterial peptides in systemic circulation [75].

The impact of *NOD2* variants other than the three aforementioned SNPs has not been investigated to the same extent. *NOD2* polymorphisms outside of the LRD do not appear to alter the ability of MDP to stimulate NOD2. In the case of the variants associated with Blau syndrome, all of which are located within the central NOD region of the protein, an increase in NF-κB activity has been reported [25, 65]. This gain-of-function mechanism appears to be consistently demonstrated.

6. *NOD2* Polymorphism and the Outcome of HSCT

It was originally postulated that the *NOD2* variants that are purported to increase the risk and severity of Crohn's disease might also contribute to the risk of GvHD, particularly gastrointestinal GvHD, due to their notable similarity in clinical symptoms [76]. In the years following, many groups have published data on their attempts to test this hypothesis in a number of different transplant settings. Table 1 summarises the differences in the cohort characteristics and the clinical observations reported by each group.

In the first published study by Holler et al. [76] 169 HSCT pairs underwent *NOD2* genotyping for SNPs 8, 12 and 13. The cohort consisted of a mix of HLA-matched related donor, unrelated donor and a small number of one HLA antigen-mismatched related donor, transplants. Transplants were performed as a therapy for acute leukaemia, myeloproliferative disorder, lymphoma, or myeloma. Approximately 44% of the cohort underwent T-cell depletion, predominantly with antithymocyte globulin (ATG), while a small number of individuals were treated with alemtuzumab or CD34+ cell selection. The results of this study showed that 29.5% of HSCT pairs in this cohort had at least one of the *NOD2* variants. The authors correlated the presence of any of the three SNPs in the genotype of the pair (recipient, donor or both SNP positive) with increased severe aGvHD, (grades III-IV), severe gastrointestinal aGvHD and nonrelapse mortality [76]. When this was broken down further, severe aGvHD was increased in pairs with SNP-positive donors only, while an increase in severe and gastrointestinal aGvHD was described in pairs where both the recipient and donor were found to have any of the variants. This consequently increased the risk of nonrelapse mortality.

In their subsequent analysis, the authors extended the cohort to 303 HLA-matched sibling HSCT pairs, transplanted at one of five European centres [77]. The underlying disease of the recipients was acute leukaemia, chronic leukaemia, bone marrow failure syndromes, or lymphatic malignancies. The authors did not report the use of T-cell depletion. *NOD2* genotyping of recipients and donors showed similar frequencies of SNPs 8, 12, and 13 to their earlier study and, importantly, between the different cohorts that were included in the study. The data showed that the effect of *NOD2* variants on clinically significant aGvHD (grades III-IV) and gastrointestinal GvHD persisted in this new cohort, while a trend for increased cGvHD was also noted. A dosage effect of the SNPs was seen in this study where individuals with increasing numbers of SNPs correspondingly had an increasing risk of aGvHD. The SNP dosage effect was also seen on the incidence of nonrelapse mortality. Survival was affected, but only when variants were present in the recipient genotype or in both the recipient and donor genotypes. The authors also described how the

use of particular gastrointestinal decontamination agents could reduce the risk of aGvHD and nonrelapse mortality seen with *NOD2* SNPs. Specifically, the effects of *NOD2* variants were only seen in individuals who received either no decontamination or those whose protocol included the antibiotic Ciprofloxacin.

In their third and most recent study, Holler and colleagues have extended their cohorts further to include 358 HLA matched related donor and 342 unrelated donor HSCT pairs [78]. Approximately 55% of the cohort underwent HSCT for acute leukaemia. The use of T-cell depletion varied between the two subgroups that made up the cohort, with 78% of cohort one (HSCT pairs from earlier studies) having some form of T-cell depletion included as compared to only 22% of cohort two (additional HSCT pairs). The impact of *NOD2* variant genotype was analysed separately in the related and unrelated donor cohorts. The presence of any *NOD2* variant in the genotype of the pair was correlated with significantly increased severe aGvHD (grades III-IV), nonrelapse mortality and reduced overall survival in recipients of a related donor HSCT. In the UD-HSCT cohort, aGvHD was the only outcome affected by the presence of any of the three SNPs, while detrimental effects on nonrelapse mortality and survival were associated with the presence of SNP 13 within the donor's genotype. The association of specific gastrointestinal decontamination protocols (either none or Ciprofloxacin-based therapies) with increased effects of *NOD2* variants was confirmed in these cohorts.

Other groups have confirmed the effects of *NOD2* variant genotype on HSCT outcome described by Holler et al. A recent study by a group in The Netherlands described the effects of *NOD2* SNPs 8, 12, and 13 on the outcome of 85 HLA-identical sibling transplants [79]. The cohort included recipients with acute leukaemia, chronic myeloid leukaemia, myeloproliferative disorder, myelodysplastic syndrome, and lymphoma. The entire cohort had a partial T-cell depletion protocol included in their transplant protocols with the most common method being CD34+ cell selection. *NOD2* variant frequencies were similar to those reported in the earlier studies and in the general Dutch population. The authors confirm the detrimental effect of any *NOD2* variant on the risk of clinically significant aGvHD and nonrelapse mortality. As described in the earlier studies, the effect was most profound when both the recipient and donor were positive for any one of the SNPs.

Not all studies have been able to demonstrate an association of *NOD2* polymorphisms with GvHD. Elmaagacli and colleagues published data on the effect of the variants in a cohort of 403 related and unrelated donor transplants [80]. The recipients were transplanted for numerous diseases, predominantly acute leukaemia, chronic myeloid leukaemia, and myelodysplastic syndrome. Approximately 30% of the cohort had T-cell depletion included in the conditioning regimens either with alemtuzumab or with ATG. The frequency of *NOD2* variants in this cohort was similar to those described in other studies. Although an increased risk of aGvHD (grade III-IV) was seen when recipients and donors were both positive for one of the *NOD2* variants, a protective effect was associated with an SNP in the donor

TABLE 1: A comparison of the results published on *NOD2* genotype and haematopoietic stem cell transplant outcome.

Study	Donor source[a]	Recipient diagnosis[b]	T-cell depletion	Effect of *NOD2* SNPs
Holler et al. 2004 [76]	Mixed	Mixed	Yes—*in vivo* 43% WT pairs 48% SNP pairs	Increased severe aGvHD (gr. III-IV) in SNP-positive donors and pairs Increased severe GI aGvHD with SNP-positive pairs; Increased transplant-related mortality in SNP-positive pairs
Holler et al. 2006 [77]	RD	Mixed	—	Reduced overall survival with SNP-positive recipients and when both recipient and donor are SNP positive Increased transplant-related mortality with increasing numbers of SNPs Increased severe (gr. III-IV) and severe GI aGvHD with increasing numbers of SNPs
Elmaagacli et al. 2006 [78]	Mixed	Mixed	Yes ~30%	Lower overall and severe aGvHD (gr. III-IV) with SNP-positive donors Increased severe aGvHD (gr. III-IV) when both recipient and donor are SNP positive Reduced disease relapse when both recipient and donor are SNP-positive
Granell et al. 2006 [81]	RD	Mixed	Yes, 100%	Reduced disease-free survival in SNP positive recipients.
Mayor et al. 2007 [82]	UD	Acute leukaemia	Yes—*in vivo* Alemtuzumab 82% WT pairs 85% SNP pairs	Reduced overall survival in SNP-positive recipients and pairs Increased disease relapse in SNP-positive recipients and pairs Reduced disease-free survival in SNP-positive recipients and pairs
			Yes,	Reduced overall survival in SNP-positive pairs (sibling HSCT) and SNP 13 positive donors (UD)
Holler et al. 2008 [78, 83]	Mixed	Mixed	78% cohort 1, 22% cohort 2	Increased severe aGvHD (gr III-IV) with SNP-positive pairs (sibling and UD) and SNP 13 positive donors (UD) Increased transplant-related mortality with SNP-positive pairs (sibling HSCT) and SNP 13 positive donors (UD)
van der Velden et al. 2009 [79]	RD	Mixed	Yes, 100%	Increased severe aGvHD (gr. III-IV) in SNP-positive pairs Increased transplant-related mortality in SNP-positive pairs
Wermke et al. 2010 [84]	Mixed	Mixed	Yes, *in vivo* ATG for UD, 31.6%	Increased disease relapse in SNP-positive recipients (trend at MV) Trend for less GI aGvHD in SNP-positive recipients (UV only)
Elmaagacli et al. 2011 [85]	RD	AML	None	Increase in overall (gr. I-IV) and severe (gr. III-IV) aGvHD in SNP-positive recipients
Kreyenberg et al. 2011 [86]	Unknown allogeneic	Mixed	—	Reduced overall survival in SNP 13 positive recipients Increased transplant-related mortality in SNP 13 positive recipients
Ditschkowski et al. 2007 [87]	Mixed	Mixed	Yes, 30% *in vivo*	No significant effects on BO or BOOP
Hildebrandt et al. 2008 [88]	Mixed	Mixed	Yes, 37%	BO increased in SNP-positive recipients
Sairafi et al. 2008 [89]	Mixed	Mixed	Yes, 61%	No significant effects
Gruhn et al. 2009 [90]	Mixed	Mixed	None	No significant effects
Nguyen et al. 2010 [91]	UD	Mixed	None	No significant effects
van der Straaten et al. 2011 [92]	Mixed	Mixed	Yes, *in vivo* ATG for UD and HLA-mismatched RD	No significant effects

[a] Mixed as a donor source denotes both related (RD) and unrelated donors (UD) were used.
[b] Mixed as a recipient diagnosis indicates that the included recipients underwent HSCT for any one of a number of diseases.

genotype. The protective effect was also seen on disease relapse in pairs where both the recipient and donor had at least one NOD2 SNP. Unlike previous studies, no effects of NOD2 genotype on nonrelapse mortality or survival were seen. The authors suggested that the possible reason for the lack of association here was due to their routine use of gastrointestinal decontamination with agents to target both Gram-positive and negative bacteria.

In a recent update by this group, the authors have investigated the affects of NOD2 variants in a more homogeneous cohort [85]. NOD2 genotyping was performed on a cohort of 142 AML recipients and their HLA-matched sibling donors. As in previous studies, the reported frequency of SNP-positive recipients and donors was similar to those found elsewhere. The cohort only included recipients who received myeloablative conditioning regimens and T-cell replete grafts. Unlike in their previous study, no protective effects of NOD2 SNPs were associated with GvHD. A significant association was seen between SNP-positive recipients and an increased risk of any aGvHD (grade I–IV) and severe aGvHD (grades III-IV). Interestingly, after multivariate analysis, only a correlation with grade II–IV remained significant (relative risk (RR) 3.7652, $P < 0.002$). No impact on overall survival or nonrelapse mortality was reported.

Granell et al. also failed to correlate NOD2 genotype with increased aGvHD [81]. Here, NOD2 genotyping was performed on 85 HLA-matched sibling HSCT pairs. The underlying diseases of the recipients were acute leukaemia, myeloproliferative disorder, lymphoma, myeloma, myelodysplasia, aplasia, and chronic lymphocytic leukaemia. All recipients had T cell depletion included in their conditioning regimens, although the method was not reported. The authors report an association of recipient NOD2 variant genotype with significantly reduced event-free survival. No other variable was significantly affected [81].

Our group has also reported the effects of NOD2 genotype on HSCT outcome [82]. Here, the impact of NOD2 genotype was investigated in a cohort of 196 recipients of an unrelated donor HSCT for an acute leukaemia. T-cell depletion was included in the conditioning regimens of 83% of recipients, with in vivo alemtuzumab being the preferred method. We reported a significant correlation between SNP-positive pairs (the recipient, the donor, or both had any NOD2 SNP) and increased risks of disease relapse and death. In accordance with the data published by Granell et al. [81], we were also able to show a significant association with event-free survival. Interestingly, although the overall incidence of aGvHD was low in this British cohort due to the near universal use of T-cell depletion, a protective effect of NOD2 SNPs on aGvHD was noted although it remained nonsignificant. Despite failing to achieve statistical significance, this data was in accordance to that reported by Elmaagacli and colleagues [80].

A study published in 2010 from a group in Dresden, Germany also reported a correlation between NOD2 genotype and disease relapse [84]. This single-centre study included 304 HSCT pairs where the predominant diagnoses were AML/MDS (52%) and lymphoma (25.3%). Grafts were from either a ≥8/10 HLA matched unrelated donor (67.1%)

or an HLA-matched related donor. Recipients receiving a graft from an UD had in vivo ATG included in their conditioning regimens. The authors performed extensive analyses to determine if an association between NOD2 genotype and aGvHD could be identified. A trend towards reduced gastrointestinal aGvHD was reported in recipients positive for any NOD2 variant, but this affect was limited to univariate analyses. There were no significant differences in GvHD in any of the other models tested. Recipients positive for any of the three SNPs did have a significantly increased risk of disease relapse, although this was only a trend after multivariate analysis ($P = 0.056$).

A brief communication published last year highlighted the impact of NOD2 SNPs in a large, multicentre, paediatric cohort [86]. A total of 567 HSCT pairs were tested. Donors were both HLA matched (78.7%) and mismatched (21.3%); the type of allogeneic donor was not stated. Transplants were performed for haematological malignancies, nonhaematological malignancies, and nonmalignant disease. The authors describe a significantly increased risk of nonrelapse mortality in recipients positive for SNP 13, an effect that persisted after multivariate analysis (RR 2.01, $P = 0.049$). This study also confirmed the effects of NOD2 genotype on overall survival. A trend for lower survival was reported in pairs where the recipient had at least one of the three variants. Additionally, survival was also lower in recipients only positive for NOD2 SNP 13.

Two studies have specifically reported data on the impact of NOD2 variants on bronchiolitis obliterans (BO) and bronchiolitis obliterans organising Pneumonia (BOOP), two serious late-onset, non-infectious pulmonary complications that can occur after HSCT. Hildebrandt et al. [88] analysed the incidence of BO/BOOP in a heterogeneous cohort of 427 HSCT pairs. Donors were either HLA-matched siblings or UDs. T cell depletion was included in the conditioning protocols of approximately 25% of the cohort although the method varied (ATG, alemtuzumab, or CD34+ selection). The incidence of BO was significantly higher when recipients, donors, or both were positive for NOD2 SNPs, effects that persisted after multivariate analysis. It is important to point out, however, that the overall number of recipients who developed BO was very low in this cohort (11/427, 2.6%). In contrast to this data, Ditschkowski et al. did not find an association between NOD2 genotype and the incidence of BO/BOOP in their cohort of 281 sibling donor HSCT pairs [87]. Transplants were for acute and chronic leukaemia, myelodysplastic syndrome, non-Hodgkin's lymphoma, idiopathic mnyelofibrosis, and multiple myeloma, and approximately 30% protocols included in vivo T cell depletion. As in the previously described study, the overall incidence of BO/BOOP was low (2.1% BO, 3.6% BOOP).

Despite the plethora of data available showing an effect of NOD2 variants, several studies have suggested that there are no significant effects on HSCT outcome. Groups from Sweden [89], Germany [90], the United States [91] and The Netherlands [92] have performed extensive analyses in attempt to replicate the findings of the above-mentioned studies but have shown a lack of association with any of the outcomes measured.

7. Discussion

There does not yet appear to be a consensus on the impact of *NOD2* variants on the outcome of HSCT. It would be reasonable to assume that the potential mechanisms of how the SNPs cause functional irregularities may be common but that the manifestation of the effects differs between groups. Here, we will discuss possible mechanisms by which *NOD2* genotype may affect HSCT outcome.

NOD2 is known to function as a regulator of cytokine production and a mediator of proinflammatory responses upon recognition of the bacterial ligand muramyl dipeptide [40, 93]. Functional changes within the NOD2 protein are seen with SNPs 8, 12, and 13, all resulting in down regulation of cytokine production via the NF-κB pathway [33, 94]. This dysregulation of cytokine production may provide the first mechanism by which *NOD2* variants can affect the outcome of HSCT.

An early event posttransplant is the onset of the "cytokine storm" [95], an extreme increase in cytokine production as a response to both tissue damage in the recipient resulting from conditioning regimens and the activation of donor derived T cells to recipient alloantigens [96]. The result of the cytokine storm is the onset of both GvHD and graft-versus-leukaemia (GvL) responses [97, 98]. These tumour-specific cells are thought to be of T cell origin but data is emerging that suggest other cell types such as NK [99] and NKT cells [100] are also involved. One possible explanation of how *NOD2* genotype causes an effect after HSCT is that the inability of the NOD2 variant proteins to initiate cytokine production could, in theory, lead to a massive disruption of the cytokine storm, resulting in a lack of GvL or GvHD responses.

While the effect of *NOD2* genotype-related dysregulation of cytokine production may not be the only contributing pathway to the cytokine storm, the role of NOD2 and other sensors of bacterial infection has long been proposed as major factors in GvHD responses. Studies that have shown that gastrointestinal mucosa damaged by aggressive treatments such as the conditioning regimens used in HSCT allow bacterial ligands, specifically the MDP homologue Lipopolysaccharide (LPS), to seep into systemic circulation. Once there, T cells specific for these ligands are capable of stimulating cytokine production and eliciting GvHD responses [101–103]. It has been suggested that *NOD2* SNPs can increase the permeability of the gastrointestinal mucosa and potentially increase the ability of bacterial ligands to enter systemic circulation [75]. It is possible that these events in combination with the inability of the variant NOD2 protein to respond efficiently to bacterial infection in recipients with *NOD2* variant genotype result in an increased level of circulating LPS, which are able to prime T cells and thus initiate strong GvHD responses. These effects are in concordance with the data published by numerous groups correlating *NOD2* variant genotype and increased aGvHD.

NOD2 is also known to have a synergistic relationship with TLRs and is thought to provide some regulatory control over their ability to stimulate cytokine production [93, 104–106]. It is possible that the inability of variant NOD2 to regulate or be regulated by TLRs resulted in dysregulation of the cytokine produced, which in turn affected both GvHD and GvL responses. One of the most studied relationships is with TLR2 [107]. NOD2 is known to act as a regulator of IL-12 production via the simultaneous stimulation of NOD2 and TLR2 by their bacterial ligands with both positive and negative regulation occurring dependant on the dose of available ligand [104, 107]. Polymorphisms of *NOD2* are known to cause a reduction in IL-12 production [69]. Interestingly, in the context of HSCT, low IL-12 levels have been correlated with an increase in the incidence of disease relapse [108] without increasing the incidence of aGvHD [108, 109].

NOD2 is expressed both intracellularly and on the cell surface of epithelial cells. It has been suggested that this membrane recruitment of the protein is necessary to initiate a functional response [34, 35]. The repertoire of known cell types showing NOD2 expression is increasing, with both NK cells and CD34+ bone marrow stem cells recently being identified [32, 33]. It is thus feasible to assume that NOD2 is expressed on the cell surface of these other cell types. The presence of SNP 13 has been associated with the failure of the molecule to be expressed on the cell surface, although this has not been reported for the other polymorphisms [34, 35]. It is possible that the failure of leukaemic cells to express NOD2 extracellularly in recipients with *NOD2* variant genotypes results in their evasion of immunesurveillance activity. This escape mechanism would lead to the proliferation of leukaemic cells and thus disease relapse after transplant. This theory is consistent with the observations that *NOD2* polymorphisms cause disruption of GvL responses.

Although no effect of *NOD2* SNPs 8 and 12 on the membrane recruitment of NOD2 has been reported to date, it is possible that they have an alternative mechanism by which they cause cells to evade immune responses. SNP 8 is located within exon 4 of the *NOD2* gene and is found between the NBD and the LRD of the protein [25, 110]. Self-oligomerisation of the protein occurs at the NBD, a process that is fundamental to the ability of the NOD2 protein to function [25, 111]. It is possible that SNP 8 causes a conformational change in the molecule rendering it either incapable of self-binding or causing it to function at a reduced capacity. Alternatively it may render the LRD either unable to or inefficient at binding its ligand. If this is the case, then it is feasible that even if NOD2 is recruited to the cell surface, it is unlikely to initiate a functional response that is adequate to initiate GvL effects. SNP 12 is located within the sixth LRR, which makes up the LRD [110]. The change in protein at this position may alter the ability of the *NOD2* molecule to recognise MDP, leading to the failure of NOD2 to initiate NF-κB signalling and its related downstream events.

A logical explanation for the divergent results could be the heterogeneity in the characteristics and treatment of the recipients, not only between studies but also within each of the cohorts themselves. An obvious difference between the studies is donor source. The advances in transplant techniques and practice have resulted in similar survival prospects for recipients of a well-matched UD and related donor HSCT [2], suggesting that while donor source may contribute to the discrepancies in outcome associations reported, it is more likely that other characteristics of the cohort are correlated with outcome.

A second and strikingly different factor between the cohorts is the use of T-cell depletion within the conditioning regimens. T-cell depletion is used as a mechanism of reducing the risk of GvHD, although a consequence of this may be an increase in disease relapse [98, 112]. While most of the NOD2 SNP association studies reported the use of T-cell depletion in their treatment protocols, several methods (alemtuzumab, ATG and/or CD34+ stem cell selection) were included, and thus it is important to consider the effectiveness of these different methods. For example, the anti-CD52 antibody alemtuzumab targets all human cells of lymphoid lineage, although NK cells appear to be relatively spared [113–115]. CD34+ stem cells are not targeted. Conversely, ATG functions by only targeting cell surface markers including those found specifically on T cells. B and NK cells are also targeted but only in excessive doses of ATG and are thus spared in most transplant protocols [116]. The effects of ATG are also long lasting which results in the specific depletion of T cells from the graft and any reconstituting cells. It is possible that the residual haematopoietic cells or indeed the lack of certain cell types present after different types of T-cell depletion could significantly affect the type and risk of post-transplant complication.

In addition to the method of T-cell depletion used, notable differences in the number of recipients treated varied between the studies (approximately 30–100%). It is interesting to note that a high number of studies that reported a correlation between NOD2 genotype and GvHD were either T-cell replete regimens or included ATG or partial CD34+ cell-selected grafts [76, 78, 79, 85]. Conversely, those studies that correlated NOD2 variants with impaired Graft-versus-leukaemia (GvL) effects included consistently higher numbers of recipients treated with T-cell-depleted protocols (85–100%) and in some cases included alemtuzumab [81, 82, 84].

Gastrointestinal decontamination, a method of using drugs to control levels of bacteria within the gastrointestinal tracts, may also be used all around transplantation as a method of controlling GvHD [103, 117]. Holler and colleagues have suggested that the impact of NOD2 SNPs may be more evident in recipients who received either no decontamination or those who were treated with Ciprofloxacin-based therapy [77, 78]. Elmaagacli et al. (2006) suggested that the lack of correlation between their data and that previously published could be attributed to their universal use of a decontamination protocol that includes a second antibiotic, Metronidazole, in combination with Ciprofloxacin [80]. In addition, the study by van der Velden et al. also highlighted the important role of bacteraemia in the outcome of HSCT in their study [79]. Unfortunately, most of the studies published to date have not included data on the use and/or type of gastrointestinal decontamination in their cohorts, and a few have analysed the effects of NOD2 variants in cohorts stratified by protocol. It would be prudent for future studies

to include this data in their analyses where possible in order for the exact relevance of this information to be obtained.

Several studies, including ours, have demonstrated the effects of NOD2 genotype in recipients diagnosed with an acute leukaemia [82, 83, 85]. We have also reported on the lack of effect in recipients with chronic myeloid leukaemia in our cohort from the UK [118]. Other studies have not fully investigated the suggestion of a disease-specific effect. However, it is interesting that two of the four studies that did not correlate NOD2 genotype with any posttransplant complication had a notably low number of recipients with acute leukaemia in their analyses [91, 92]. A possible explanation for this apparent disease specific effect is that NOD2 SNPs alter the responsiveness of recipients with an acute leukaemia to their treatment. This may occur by modulation of the pathways of disease progression, rendering recipients resistant to treatment. While no direct evidence of the involvement of NOD2 variants in leukaemia progression exists, there is much data to show how it can affect the other diseases that are associated with the polymorphisms. In Crohn's disease, NOD2 SNPs 8, 12, and 13 have been correlated with distinct disease phenotypes, in particular with the site of Crohn's disease within the gastrointestinal tract and with the age of onset [119–122]. NOD2 genotype may also alter the recipient's response to drugs or conditioning therapies. Studies have shown that NOD2 polymorphisms can affect the response to antibiotic treatment of perianal fistulas in Crohn's disease patients. The data showed that patients with an NOD2 WT genotype had a 33% rate of complete response to treatment as compared to none of the patients with NOD2 variant genotypes [77].

While the majority of studies have shown an effect of NOD2 genotype on transplant outcome, data has been published that contradicts these findings [89–92]. As discussed, the lack of effect could be attributed to several characteristics of the cohort, namely the graft source, type of disease, use and method of T-cell depletion, and gastrointestinal decontamination. However, a notable difference between several of these studies and others published is the low incidence of NOD2 SNPs reported. The overall SNP frequencies were between 10–15% lower than reported elsewhere. The difference in the frequency of NOD2 SNPs between different ethnic and geographic populations has been widely discussed [123–127]. Thus, the low prevalence of SNPs in these cohorts may mask any affects that the genotype is having on transplant outcome.

A common feature of many of the studies is the correlation between recipient NOD2 genotype and detrimental posttransplant outcomes. This may imply that cells which express NOD2 and remain in the recipient after their conditioning regimens, such as tissue macrophages, dendritic cells, and Paneth cells, may facilitate GvHD or GvL responses, and that these responses are limited in recipients with NOD2 variant genotypes. The ability of recipient cells, specifically dendritic cells, to initiate GvHD effects has been reported [128]. Additionally, recently published data has demonstrated the importance of recipient NOD2 genotype in murine models of GvHD [129]. Here, murine recipients of bone marrow and/or T cells from either wild-type (WT) or *NOD2* knock-out mice showed no significant differences in the ability of the repopulating cells to proliferate, to be activated, or on their expression of gut-homing molecules. The risk of developing GvHD was similar in the two groups. Conversely, *NOD2* knock-out recipient mice showed significantly higher levels of GvHD than their WT counterparts, and importantly, the organs targeted were the liver and the small and large bowels. Further tests showed that recipient *NOD2* genotype was also able to effect donor T-cell functional capabilities. While the translation of murine studies into human models does not always result in the same findings, these data in combination provide some evidence to substantiate the observation that recipient genotype appears to significantly correlate with HSCT outcome in humans.

The studies that have suggested the *NOD2* genotype results in impaired GvL responses do not fit this model. A possible explanation for this is that recipient cells that are more resistant to the effects of pretransplant conditioning regimens (in these studies, T-cell depletion in particular) are responsible for the lack of GvL effects. NK cells have been shown to be more resistant to the T-cell depletion agent alemtuzumab than other targeted subgroups [115]. The importance of NK cells in this model has been previously suggested [83], and their ability to function as tumour surveillance cells and mediators of antileukaemic responses is widely accepted [100, 130]. Importantly, it has been suggested that autologous NK cells can maintain remission in acute leukaemia patients, although this was described in the context of autologous transplants or chemotherapy induced remission [131]. NK cells have recently been shown to express NOD2 and also to be activated by the recognition of MDP by NOD2 in the presence of costimulatory molecules [32]. It is possible that this mechanism for NK cell activation is of critical importance in mediating early GvL responses after HSCT, but in recipients with *NOD2* variant genotypes, this NK cell activation is limited, resulting in a reduced ability to initiate GvL responses. Interestingly, in our study, where predominant T-cell depletion with alemtuzumab was used, an increase in disease relapse was seen in recipients with *NOD2* polymorphisms.

Finally, it is important to consider what impact *NOD2* polymorphisms other than SNPs 8, 12, and 13 may have on HSCT outcome. It is possible that these SNPs are only markers for detrimental outcomes and that the true association is with one or more untested polymorphisms that may be in linkage disequilibrium with these known variants. As stated previously, *NOD2* is highly polymorphic with some minor allele frequencies reaching 40% in certain populations. It would be prudent for future studies to consider the effects of the previously unstudied variants in any future analyses. It is possible that reanalysis of the published data including novel variants may result in concordance between different groups and potentially elicit an effect of *NOD2* genotype in cohorts where no association has been demonstrated previously.

Despite the many questions that remain even after eight years of investigation into the importance of *NOD2* genotype on HSCT outcome, it must be concluded that the gene and its variants currently indicate an important role in transplant biology. The published data also reaffirms the belief that personalised medicine based on a combination of recipient and donor characteristics, HLA matching, and non-HLA genetics could provide the key to superior outcomes after HSCT.

References

[1] E. A. Copelan, "Hematopoietic stem-cell transplantation," *New England Journal of Medicine*, vol. 354, no. 17, pp. 1813–1826, 2006.

[2] H. D. Ottinger, S. Ferencik, D. W. Beelen et al., "Hematopoietic stem cell transplantation: contrasting the outcome of transplantations from HLA-identical siblings, partially HLA-mismatched related donors, and HLA-matched unrelated donors," *Blood*, vol. 102, no. 3, pp. 1131–1137, 2003.

[3] E. W. Petersdorf, "Risk assessment in haematopoietic stem cell transplantation: histocompatibility," *Best Practice and Research*, vol. 20, no. 2, pp. 155–170, 2007.

[4] B. E. Shaw, J. A. Madrigal, and M. Potter, "Improving the outcome of unrelated donor stem cell transplantation by molecular matching," *Blood Reviews*, vol. 15, no. 4, pp. 167–174, 2001.

[5] P. Loiseau, M. Busson, M. L. Balere et al., "HLA Association with hematopoietic stem cell transplantation outcome: the number of mismatches at HLA-A, -B, -C, -DRB1, or -DQB1 is strongly associated with overall survival," *Biology of Blood and Marrow Transplantation*, vol. 13, no. 8, pp. 965–974, 2007.

[6] Y. Chalandon, J. M. Tiercy, U. Schanz et al., "Impact of high-resolution matching in allogeneic unrelated donor stem cell transplantation in Switzerland," *Bone Marrow Transplantation*, vol. 37, no. 10, pp. 909–916, 2006.

[7] B. E. Shaw, N. P. Mayor, N. H. Russell et al., "Diverging effects of HLA-DPB1 matching status on outcome following unrelated donor transplantation depending on disease stage and the degree of matching for other HLA alleles," *Leukemia*, vol. 24, no. 1, pp. 58–65, 2010.

[8] N. Flomenberg, L. A. Baxter-Lowe, D. Confer et al., "Impact of HLA class I and class II high-resolution matching on outcomes of unrelated donor bone marrow transplantation: HLA-C mismatching is associated with a strong adverse effect on transplantation outcome," *Blood*, vol. 104, no. 7, pp. 1923–1930, 2004.

[9] S. J. Lee, J. Klein, M. Haagenson et al., "High-resolution donor-recipient HLA matching contributes to the success of unrelated donor marrow transplantation," *Blood*, vol. 110, no. 13, pp. 4576–4583, 2007.

[10] E. W. Petersdorf, C. Anasetti, P. J. Martin et al., "Limits of HLA mismatching in unrelated hematopoietic cell transplantation," *Blood*, vol. 104, no. 9, pp. 2976–2980, 2004.

[11] T. Kawase, Y. Morishima, K. Matsuo et al., "High-risk HLA allele mismatch combinations responsible for severe acute graft-versus-host disease and implication for its molecular mechanism," *Blood*, vol. 110, no. 7, pp. 2235–2241, 2007.

[12] B. E. Shaw, T. Gooley, J. A. Madrigal, M. Malkki, S. G. E. Marsh, and E. W. Petersdorf, "Clinical importance of HLA-DPB1 in haematopoietic cell transplantation," *Tissue Antigens*, vol. 69, no. 1, pp. 36–41, 2007.

[13] B. E. Shaw, T. A. Gooley, M. Malkki et al., "The importance of HLA-DPB1 in unrelated donor hematopoietic cell transplantation," *Blood*, vol. 110, no. 13, pp. 4560–4566, 2007.

[14] B. E. Shaw, S. G. E. Marsh, N. P. Mayor, N. H. Russell, and J. A. Madrigal, "HLA-DPB1 matching status has significant

implications for recipients of unrelated donor stem cell transplants," *Blood*, vol. 107, no. 3, pp. 1220–1226, 2006.

[15] K. Fleischhauer, B. E. Shaw, T. Gooley et al., "Effect of T-cell-epitope matching at HLA-DPB1 in recipients of unrelated-donor haemopoietic-cell transplantation: a retrospective study," *The Lancet Oncology*, vol. 13, no. 4, pp. 366–374, 2012.

[16] L. A. Baxter-Lowe, M. Maiers, S. R. Spellman et al., "HLA-A Disparities Illustrate Challenges for Ranking the Impact of HLA Mismatches on Bone Marrow Transplant Outcomes in the United States," *Biology of Blood and Marrow Transplantation*, vol. 15, no. 8, pp. 971–981, 2009.

[17] A. M. Dickinson and E. Holler, "Polymorphisms of cytokine and innate immunity genes and GVHD," *Best Practice and Research*, vol. 21, no. 2, pp. 149–164, 2008.

[18] O. Penack, E. Holler, and M. R. M. Van Den Brink, "Graft-versus-host disease: regulation by microbe-associated molecules and innate immune receptors," *Blood*, vol. 115, no. 10, pp. 1865–1872, 2010.

[19] J. P. Hugot, P. Laurent-Puig, C. Gower-Rousseau et al., "Mapping of a susceptibility locus for Crohn's disease on chromosome 16," *Nature*, vol. 379, no. 6568, pp. 821–823, 1996.

[20] N. Inohara and G. Nuñez, "The NOD: a signaling module that regulates apoptosis and host defense against pathogens," *Oncogene*, vol. 20, no. 44, pp. 6473–6481, 2001.

[21] Y. Ogura, N. Inohara, A. Benito, F. F. Chen, S. Yamaoka, and G. Núñez, "Nod2, a Nod1/Apaf-1 family member that is restricted to monocytes and activates NF-kappaB," *Journal of Biological Chemistry*, vol. 276, no. 7, pp. 4812–4818, 2001.

[22] W. Strober and T. Watanabe, "NOD2, an intracellular innate immune sensor involved in host defense and Crohn's disease," *Mucosal Immunology*, vol. 4, no. 5, pp. 484–495, 2011.

[23] N. Inohara, Y. Ogura, and G. Nuñez, "Nods: a family of cytosolic proteins that regulate the host response to pathogens," *Current Opinion in Microbiology*, vol. 5, no. 1, pp. 76–80, 2002.

[24] P. Enkhbayar, M. Kamiya, M. Osaki, T. Matsumoto, and N. Matsushima, "Structural principles of leucine-rich repeat (LRR) proteins," *Proteins*, vol. 54, no. 3, pp. 394–403, 2004.

[25] T. Tanabe, M. Chamaillard, Y. Ogura et al., "Regulatory regions and critical residues of NOD2 involved in muramyl dipeptide recognition," *EMBO Journal*, vol. 23, no. 7, pp. 1587–1597, 2004.

[26] J. M. Wilmanski, T. Petnicki-Ocwieja, and K. S. Kobayashi, "NLR proteins: integral members of innate immunity and mediators of inflammatory diseases," *Journal of Leukocyte Biology*, vol. 83, no. 1, pp. 13–30, 2008.

[27] O. Gutierrez, C. Pipaon, N. Inohara et al., "Induction of Nod2 in myelomonocytic and intestinal epithelial cells via nuclear factor-κB activation," *Journal of Biological Chemistry*, vol. 277, no. 44, pp. 41701–41705, 2002.

[28] S. Lala, Y. Ogura, C. Osborne et al., "Crohn's disease and the NOD2 gene: a role for paneth cells," *Gastroenterology*, vol. 125, no. 1, pp. 47–57, 2003.

[29] Y. Ogura, S. Lala, W. Xin et al., "Expression of NOD2 in Paneth cells: a possible link to Crohn's ileitis," *Gut*, vol. 52, no. 11, pp. 1591–1597, 2003.

[30] M. Kobayashi, R. Yoshiki, J. Sakabe, K. Kabashima, M. Nakamura, and Y. Tokura, "Expression of toll-like receptor 2, NOD2 and dectin-1 and stimulatory effects of their ligands and histamine in normal human keratinocytes," *British Journal of Dermatology*, vol. 160, no. 2, pp. 297–304, 2009.

[31] M. H. Shaw, T. Reimer, C. Sánchez-Valdepeñas et al., "T cell-intrinsic role of Nod2 in promoting type 1 immunity to Toxoplasma gondii," *Nature Immunology*, vol. 10, no. 12, pp. 1267–1274, 2009.

[32] V. Athié-Morales, G. M. O'Connor, and C. M. Gardiner, "Activation of human NK cells by the bacterial pathogen-associated molecular pattern muramyl dipeptide," *Journal of Immunology*, vol. 180, no. 6, pp. 4082–4089, 2008.

[33] M. Sioud and Y. Fløisand, "NOD2/CARD15 on bone marrow CD34+ hematopoietic cells mediates induction of cytokines and cell differentiation," *Journal of Leukocyte Biology*, vol. 85, no. 6, pp. 939–946, 2009.

[34] N. Barnich, J. E. Aguirre, H. C. Reinecker, R. Xavier, and D. K. Podolsky, "Membrane recruitment of NOD2 in intestinal epithelial cells is essential for nuclear factor-κB activation in muramyl dipeptide recognition," *Journal of Cell Biology*, vol. 170, no. 1, pp. 21–26, 2005.

[35] P. Lécine, S. Esmiol, J. Y. Métais et al., "The NOD2-RICK complex signals from the plasma membrane," *Journal of Biological Chemistry*, vol. 282, no. 20, pp. 15197–15207, 2007.

[36] P. Rosenstiel, M. Fantini, K. Bräutigam et al., "TNF-α and IFN-γ regulate the expression of the NOD2 (CARD15) gene in human intestinal epithelial cells," *Gastroenterology*, vol. 124, no. 4, pp. 1001–1009, 2003.

[37] S. E. Girardin, I. G. Boneca, J. Viala et al., "Nod2 is a general sensor of peptidoglycan through muramyl dipeptide (MDP) detection," *Journal of Biological Chemistry*, vol. 278, no. 11, pp. 8869–8872, 2003.

[38] N. Inohara, Y. Ogura, A. Fontalba et al., "Host recognition of bacterial muramyl dipeptide mediated through NOD2: implications for Crohn's disease," *Journal of Biological Chemistry*, vol. 278, no. 8, pp. 5509–5512, 2003.

[39] L. Franchi, N. Warner, K. Viani, and G. Nuñez, "Function of Nod-like receptors in microbial recognition and host defense," *Immunological Reviews*, vol. 227, no. 1, pp. 106–128, 2009.

[40] W. Strober, P. J. Murray, A. Kitani, and T. Watanabe, "Signalling pathways and molecular interactions of NOD1 and NOD2," *Nature Reviews Immunology*, vol. 6, no. 1, pp. 9–20, 2006.

[41] M. Hedl and C. Abraham, "Distinct roles for Nod2 protein and autocrine interleukin-1β in muramyl dipeptide-induced mitogen-activated protein kinase activation and cytokine secretion in human macrophages," *Journal of Biological Chemistry*, vol. 286, no. 30, pp. 26440–26449, 2011.

[42] R. Cooney, J. Baker, O. Brain et al., "NOD2 stimulation induces autophagy in dendritic cells influencing bacterial handling and antigen presentation," *Nature Medicine*, vol. 16, no. 1, pp. 90–97, 2010.

[43] L. H. Travassos, L. A. M. Carneiro, M. Ramjeet et al., "Nod1 and Nod2 direct autophagy by recruiting ATG16L1 to the plasma membrane at the site of bacterial entry," *Nature Immunology*, vol. 11, no. 1, pp. 55–62, 2010.

[44] A. Sabbah, T. H. Chang, R. Harnack et al., "Activation of innate immune antiviral responses by Nod2," *Nature Immunology*, vol. 10, no. 10, pp. 1073–1080, 2009.

[45] J. P. Hugot, M. Chamaillard, H. Zouali et al., "Association of NOD2 leucine-rich repeat variants with susceptibility to Crohn's disease," *Nature*, vol. 411, no. 6837, pp. 599–603, 2001.

[46] K. King, M. F. Sheikh, A. P. Cuthbert et al., "Mutation, selection, and evolution of the Crohn disease susceptibility gene CARD15," *Human Mutation*, vol. 27, no. 1, pp. 44–54, 2006.

[47] F. Schnitzler, S. Brand, T. Staudinger et al., "Eight novel CARD15 variants detected by DNA sequence analysis of the CARD15 gene in 111 patients with inflammatory bowel disease," *Immunogenetics*, vol. 58, no. 2-3, pp. 99–106, 2006.

[48] M. Rebhan, V. Chalifa-Caspi, J. Prilusky, and D. Lancet, "GeneCards: a novel functional genomics compendium with automated data mining and query reformulation support," *Bioinformatics*, vol. 14, no. 8, pp. 656–664, 1998.

[49] T. Hubbard, D. Barker, E. Birney et al., "The Ensembl genome database project," *Nucleic Acids Research*, vol. 30, no. 1, pp. 38–41, 2002.

[50] I. Touitou, S. Lesage, M. McDermott et al., "Infevers: an evolving mutation database for auto-inflammatory syndromes," *Human Mutation*, vol. 24, no. 3, pp. 194–198, 2004.

[51] Y. Ogura, D. K. Bonen, N. Inohara et al., "A frameshift mutation in NOD2 associated with susceptibility to Crohn's disease," *Nature*, vol. 411, no. 6837, pp. 603–606, 2001.

[52] M. Economou, T. A. Trikalinos, K. T. Loizou, E. V. Tsianos, and J. P. A. Ioannidis, "Differential effects of NOD2 variants on Crohn's disease risk and phenotype in diverse populations: a metaanalysis," *American Journal of Gastroenterology*, vol. 99, no. 12, pp. 2393–2404, 2004.

[53] L. Henckaerts and S. Vermeire, "NOD2/CARD15 disease associations other than Crohn's disease," *Inflammatory Bowel Diseases*, vol. 13, no. 2, pp. 235–241, 2007.

[54] A. M. Crane, L. Bradbury, D. A. Van Heel et al., "Role of NOD2 variants in spondylarthritis," *Arthritis and Rheumatism*, vol. 46, no. 6, pp. 1629–1633, 2002.

[55] P. Rahman, S. Bartlett, F. Siannis et al., "CARD15: a pleiotropic autoimmune gene that confers susceptibility to psoriatic arthritis," *American Journal of Human Genetics*, vol. 73, no. 3, pp. 677–681, 2003.

[56] N. Kanazawa, I. Okafuji, N. Kambe et al., "Early-onset sarcoidosis and CARD15 mutations with constitutive nuclear factor-κB activation: common genetic etiology with Blau syndrome," *Blood*, vol. 105, no. 3, pp. 1195–1197, 2005.

[57] C. Miceli-Richard, S. Lesage, M. Rybojad et al., "CARD15 mutations in Blau syndrome," *Nature Genetics*, vol. 29, no. 1, pp. 19–20, 2001.

[58] G. Kurzawski, J. Suchy, J. Kładny et al., "The NOD2 3020insC mutation and the risk of colorectal cancer," *Cancer Research*, vol. 64, no. 5, pp. 1604–1606, 2004.

[59] S. Angeletti, S. Galluzzo, D. Santini et al., "NOD2/CARD15 polymorphisms impair innate immunity and increase susceptibility to gastric cancer in an Italian population," *Human Immunology*, vol. 70, no. 9, pp. 729–732, 2009.

[60] M. R. Lener, D. Oszutowska, J. Castaneda et al., "Prevalence of the NOD2 3020insC mutation in aggregations of breast and lung cancer," *Breast Cancer Research and Treatment*, vol. 95, no. 2, pp. 141–145, 2006.

[61] M. S. Forrest, C. F. Skibola, T. J. Lightfoot et al., "Polymorphisms in innate immunity genes and risk of non-Hodgkin lymphoma," *British Journal of Haematology*, vol. 134, no. 2, pp. 180–183, 2006.

[62] B. Krüger, C. A. Böger, B. Schröppel et al., "Impact of NOD2/CARD15 haplotypes on the outcome after kidney transplantation," *Transplant International*, vol. 20, no. 7, pp. 600–607, 2007.

[63] S. Galluzzo, G. Patti, G. Dicuonzo et al., "Association between NOD2/CARD15 polymorphisms and coronary artery disease: a case-control study," *Human Immunology*, vol. 72, no. 8, pp. 636–640, 2011.

[64] D. K. Bonen, Y. Ogura, D. L. Nicolae et al., "Crohn's disease-associated NOD2 variants share a signaling defect in response to lipopolysaccharide and peptidoglycan," *Gastroenterology*, vol. 124, no. 1, pp. 140–146, 2003.

[65] M. Chamaillard, D. Philpott, S. E. Girardin et al., "Gene-environment interaction modulated by allelic heterogeneity in inflammatory diseases," *Proceedings of the National Academy of Sciences of the United States of America*, vol. 100, no. 6, pp. 3455–3460, 2003.

[66] J. Wehkamp, J. Harder, M. Weichenthal et al., "NOD2 (CARD15) mutations in Crohn's disease are associated with diminished mucosal α-defensin expression," *Gut*, vol. 53, no. 11, pp. 1658–1664, 2004.

[67] D. A. Van Heel, S. Ghosh, M. Butler et al., "Muramyl dipeptide and toll-like receptor sensitivity in NOD2-associated Crohn's disease," *The Lancet*, vol. 365, no. 9473, pp. 1794–1796, 2005.

[68] S. Maeda, L. C. Hsu, H. Liu et al., "Nod2 mutation in Crohn's disease potentiates NF-κB activity and IL-1β processing," *Science*, vol. 307, no. 5710, pp. 734–738, 2005.

[69] M. Kramer, M. G. Netea, D. J. De Jong, B. J. Kullberg, and G. J. Adema, "Impaired dendritic cell function in Crohn's disease patients with NOD2 3020insC mutation," *Journal of Leukocyte Biology*, vol. 79, no. 4, pp. 860–866, 2006.

[70] M. G. Netea, G. Ferwerda, D. J. De Jong et al., "The frameshift mutation in Nod2 results in unresponsiveness not only to Nod2- but also Nod1-activating peptidoglycan agonists," *Journal of Biological Chemistry*, vol. 280, no. 43, pp. 35859–35867, 2005.

[71] E. Noguchi, Y. Homma, X. Kang, M. G. Netea, and X. Ma, "A Crohn's disease-associated NOD2 mutation suppresses transcription of human IL10 by inhibiting activity of the nuclear ribonucleoprotein hnRNP-A1," *Nature Immunology*, vol. 10, no. 5, pp. 471–479, 2009.

[72] V. Beynon, S. Cotofana, S. Brand et al., "NOD2/CARD15 genotype influences MDP-induced cytokine release and basal IL-12p40 levels in primary isolated peripheral blood monocytes," *Inflammatory Bowel Diseases*, vol. 14, no. 8, pp. 1033–1040, 2008.

[73] M. Hedl, J. Li, J. H. Cho, and C. Abraham, "Chronic stimulation of Nod2 mediates tolerance to bacterial products," *Proceedings of the National Academy of Sciences of the United States of America*, vol. 104, no. 49, pp. 19440–19445, 2007.

[74] T. Watanabe, N. Asano, P. J. Murray et al., "Muramyl dipeptide activation of nucleotide-binding oligomerization domain 2 protects mice from experimental colitis," *Journal of Clinical Investigation*, vol. 118, no. 2, pp. 545–559, 2008.

[75] S. Buhner, C. Buning, J. Genschel et al., "Genetic basis for increased intestinal permeability in families with Crohn's disease: role of CARD15 3020insC mutation?" *Gut*, vol. 55, no. 3, pp. 342–347, 2006.

[76] E. Holler, G. Rogler, H. Herfarth et al., "Both donor and recipient NOD2/CARD15 mutations associate with transplant-related mortality and GvHD following allogeneic stem cell transplantation," *Blood*, vol. 104, no. 3, pp. 889–894, 2004.

[77] E. Holler, G. Rogler, J. Brenmoehl et al., "Prognostic significance of NOD2/CARD15 variants in HLA-identical sibling hematopoietic stem cell transplantation: effect on long-term outcome is confirmed in 2 independent cohorts and may be modulated by the type of gastrointestinal decontamination," *Blood*, vol. 107, no. 10, pp. 4189–4193, 2006.

[78] E. Holler, G. Rogler, J. Brenmoehl et al., "The role of genetic variants of NOD2/CARD15, a receptor of the innate immune system, in GvHD and complications following related and unrelated donor haematopoietic stem cell transplantation,"

International Journal of Immunogenetics, vol. 35, no. 4-5, pp. 381–384, 2008.

[79] W. J. F. M. van der Velden, N. M. A. Blijlevens, F. M. H. M. Maas et al., "NOD2 polymorphisms predict severe acute graft-versus-host and treatment-related mortality in T-cell-depleted haematopoietic stem cell transplantation," *Bone Marrow Transplantation*, vol. 44, no. 4, pp. 243–248, 2009.

[80] A. H. Elmaagacli, M. Koldehoff, H. Hindahl et al., "Mutations in innate immune system NOD2/CARD 15 and TLR-4 (Thr399Ile) genes influence the risk for severe acute graft-versus-host disease in patients who underwent an allogeneic transplantation," *Transplantation*, vol. 81, no. 2, pp. 247–254, 2006.

[81] M. Granell, A. Urbano-Ispizua, J. I. Aróstegui et al., "Effect of NOD2/CARD15 variants in T-cell depleted allogeneic stem cell transplantation," *Haematologica*, vol. 91, no. 10, pp. 1372–1376, 2006.

[82] N. P. Mayor, B. E. Shaw, D. A. Hughes et al., "Single nucleotide polymorphisms in the NOD2/CARD15 gene are associated with an increased risk of relapse and death for patients with acute leukemia after hematopoietic stem-cell transplantation with unrelated donors," *Journal of Clinical Oncology*, vol. 25, no. 27, pp. 4262–4269, 2007.

[83] E. Holler, J. Hahn, R. Andreesen et al., "NOD2/CARD15 polymorphisms in allogeneic stem-cell transplantation from unrelated donors: T depletion matters," *Journal of Clinical Oncology*, vol. 26, no. 2, pp. 338–339, 2008.

[84] M. Wermke, S. Maiwald, R. Schmelz et al., "Genetic variations of interleukin-23R (1143A>G) and BPI (A645G), but not of NOD2, are associated with acute graft-versus-host disease after allogeneic transplantation," *Biology of Blood and Marrow Transplantation*, vol. 16, no. 12, pp. 1718–1727, 2010.

[85] A. H. Elmaagacli, N. Steckel, M. Ditschkowski et al., "Toll-like receptor 9, NOD2 and IL23R gene polymorphisms influenced outcome in AML patients transplanted from HLA-identical sibling donors," *Bone Marrow Transplantation*, vol. 46, no. 5, pp. 702–708, 2011.

[86] H. Kreyenberg, A. Jarisch, C. Bayer et al., "NOD2/CARD15 gene polymorphisms affect outcome in pediatric allogeneic stem cell transplantation," *Blood*, vol. 118, no. 4, pp. 1181–1184, 2011.

[87] M. Ditschkowski, A. H. Eimaagacli, R. Trenschel et al., "T-cell depletion prevents from bronchiolitis obliterans and bronchiolitis obliterans with organizing pneumonia after allogeneic hematopoietic stem cell transplantation with related donors," *Haematologica*, vol. 92, no. 4, pp. 558–561, 2007.

[88] G. C. Hildebrandt, M. Granell, A. Urbano-Ispizua et al., "Recipient NOD2/CARD15 variants: a novel independent risk factor for the development of bronchiolitis obliterans after allogeneic stem cell transplantation," *Biology of Blood and Marrow Transplantation*, vol. 14, no. 1, pp. 67–74, 2008.

[89] D. Sairafi, M. Uzunel, M. Remberger, O. Ringdén, and J. Mattsson, "No impact of NOD2/CARD15 on outcome after SCT," *Bone Marrow Transplantation*, vol. 41, no. 11, pp. 961–964, 2008.

[90] B. Gruhn, J. Intek, N. Pfaffendorf et al., "Polymorphism of interleukin-23 receptor gene but not of NOD2/CARD15 is associated with graft-versus-host disease after hematopoietic stem cell transplantation in children," *Biology of Blood and Marrow Transplantation*, vol. 15, no. 12, pp. 1571–1577, 2009.

[91] Y. Nguyen, A. Al-Lehibi, E. Gorbe et al., "Insufficient evidence for association of NOD2/CARD15 or other inflammatory bowel disease-associated markers on GVHD incidence or other adverse outcomes in T-replete, unrelated donor transplantation," *Blood*, vol. 115, no. 17, pp. 3625–3631, 2010.

[92] H. M. Van der Straaten, M. M. Paquay, M. G. J. Tilanus, N. van Geloven, L. F. Verdonck, and C. Huisman, "NOD2/CARD15 variants are not a risk factor for clinical outcome after nonmyeloablative allogeneic stem cell transplantation," *Biology of Blood and Marrow Transplantation*, vol. 17, no. 8, pp. 1231–1236, 2011.

[93] M. G. Netea, G. Ferwerda, D. J. De Jong et al., "Nucleotide-binding oligomerization domain-2 modulates specific TLR pathways for the induction of cytokine release," *Journal of Immunology*, vol. 174, no. 10, pp. 6518–6523, 2005.

[94] D. J. Philpott and S. E. Girardin, "Crohn's disease-associated Nod2 mutants reduce IL10 transcription," *Nature Immunology*, vol. 10, no. 5, pp. 455–457, 2009.

[95] J. L. M. Ferrara, "Cytokine dysregulation as a mechanism of graft versus host disease," *Current Opinion in Immunology*, vol. 5, no. 5, pp. 794–799, 1993.

[96] G. R. Hill, W. Krenger, and J. L. M. Ferrara, "The role of cytokines in acute graft-versus-host disease," *Cytokines, Cellular and Molecular Therapy*, vol. 3, no. 4, pp. 257–265, 1997.

[97] O. Ringdén, M. Labopin, N. C. Gorin et al., "Is there a graft-versus-leukaemia effect in the absence of graft-versus-host disease in patients undergoing bone marrow transplantation for acute leukaemia?" *British Journal of Haematology*, vol. 111, no. 4, pp. 1130–1137, 2000.

[98] M. M. Horowitz, R. P. Gale, P. M. Sondel et al., "Graft-versus-leukemia reactions after bone marrow transplantation," *Blood*, vol. 75, no. 3, pp. 555–562, 1990.

[99] J. Schetelig, A. Kiani, M. Schmitz, G. Ehninger, and M. Bornhäuser, "T cell-mediated graft-versus-leukemia reactions after allogeneic stem cell transplantation," *Cancer Immunology, Immunotherapy*, vol. 54, no. 11, pp. 1043–1058, 2005.

[100] M. J. Smyth, K. Y. T. Thia, S. E. A. Street et al., "Differential tumor surveillance by natural killer (NK) and NKT cells," *Journal of Experimental Medicine*, vol. 191, no. 4, pp. 661–668, 2000.

[101] G. R. Hill and J. L. M. Ferrara, "The primacy of the gastrointestinal tract as a target organ of acute graft-versus-host disease: rationale for the use of cytokine shields in allogeneic bone marrow transplantation," *Blood*, vol. 95, no. 9, pp. 2754–2759, 2000.

[102] K. R. Cooke, A. Gerbitz, J. M. Crawford et al., "LPS antagonism reduces graft-versus-host disease and preserves graft-versus-leukemia activity after experimental bone marrow transplantation," *Journal of Clinical Investigation*, vol. 107, no. 12, pp. 1581–1589, 2001.

[103] D. W. Beelen, A. Elmaagacli, K. D. Müller, H. Hirche, and U. W. Schaefer, "Influence of intestinal bacterial decontamination using metronidazole and ciprofloxacin or ciprofloxacin alone on the development of acute graft- versus-host disease after marrow transplantation in patients with hematologic malignancies: final results and long-term follow-up of an open-label prospective randomized trial," *Blood*, vol. 93, no. 10, pp. 3267–3275, 1999.

[104] T. Watanabe, A. Kitani, P. J. Murray, and W. Strober, "NOD2 is a negative regulator of Toll-like receptor 2-mediated T helper type 1 responses," *Nature Immunology*, vol. 5, no. 8, pp. 800–808, 2004.

[105] H. Tada, S. Aiba, K. I. Shibata, T. Ohteki, and H. Takada, "Synergistic effect of Nod1 and Nod2 agonists with toll-like

receptor agonists on human dendritic cells to generate interleukin-12 and T helper type 1 cells," *Infection and Immunity*, vol. 73, no. 12, pp. 7967–7976, 2005.

[106] J. H. Fritz, S. E. Girardin, C. Fitting et al., "Synergistic stimulation of human monocytes and dendritic cells by Toll-like receptor 4 and NOD1- and NOD2- activating agonists," *European Journal of Immunology*, vol. 35, no. 8, pp. 2459–2470, 2005.

[107] M. E. A. Borm, A. A. van Bodegraven, C. J. J. Mulder, G. Kraal, and G. Bouma, "The effect of NOD2 activation on TLR2-mediated cytokine responses is dependent on activation dose and NOD2 genotype," *Genes and Immunity*, vol. 9, no. 3, pp. 274–278, 2008.

[108] V. Reddy, A. G. Winer, E. Eksioglu, H. U. Meier-Kriesche, J. D. Schold, and J. R. Wingard, "Interleukin 12 is associated with reduced relapse without increased incidence of graft-versus-host disease after allogeneic hematopoietic stem cell transplantation," *Biology of Blood and Marrow Transplantation*, vol. 11, no. 12, pp. 1014–1021, 2005.

[109] M. Yabe, H. Yabe, K. Hattori et al., "Role of interleukin-12 in the development of acute graft-versus-host disease in bone marrow transplant patients," *Bone Marrow Transplantation*, vol. 24, no. 1, pp. 29–34, 1999.

[110] S. Lesage, H. Zouali, J. P. Cézard et al., "CARD15/NOD2 mutational analysis and genotype-phenotype correlation in 612 patients with inflammatory bowel disease," *American Journal of Human Genetics*, vol. 70, no. 4, pp. 845–857, 2002.

[111] N. Inohara and G. Nuñez, "NODS: intracellular proteins involved in inflammation and apoptosis," *Nature Reviews Immunology*, vol. 3, no. 5, pp. 371–382, 2003.

[112] E. Holler, "Risk assessment in haematopoietic stem cell transplantation: GvHD prevention and treatment," *Best Practice and Research*, vol. 20, no. 2, pp. 281–294, 2007.

[113] G. Hale, S. Bright, and G. Chumbley, "Removal of T cells from bone marrow for transplantation: a monoclonal antilymphocyte antibody that fixes human complement," *Blood*, vol. 62, no. 4, pp. 873–882, 1983.

[114] H. Waldmann, A. Polliak, and G. Hale, "Elimination of graft-versus-host disease by in-vitro depletion of alloreactive lymphocytes with a monoclonal rat anti-human lymphocyte antibody (CAMPATH-1)," *The Lancet*, vol. 2, no. 8401, pp. 483–486, 1984.

[115] R. J. Williams, E. Clarke, A. Blair et al., "Impact on T-cell depletion and CD34+ cell recovery using humanised CD52 monoclonal antibody (CAMPATH-1H) in BM and PSBC collections; Comparison with CAMPATH-1M and CAMPATH-1G," *Cytotherapy*, vol. 2, no. 1, pp. 5–14, 2000.

[116] M. Mohty, "Mechanisms of action of antithymocyte globulin: T-cell depletion and beyond," *Leukemia*, vol. 21, no. 7, pp. 1387–1394, 2007.

[117] J. M. Vossen, P. J. Heidt, H. Van Den Berg, E. J. A. Gerritsen, J. Hermans, and L. J. Dooren, "Prevention of infection and graft-versus-host disease by suppression of intestinal microflora in children treated with allogeneic bone marrow transplantation," *European Journal of Clinical Microbiology and Infectious Diseases*, vol. 9, no. 1, pp. 14–23, 1990.

[118] N. P. Mayor, B. E. Shaw, J. A. Madrigal, and S. G. E. Marsh, "No impact of NOD2/CARD15 on outcome after SCT: a reply," *Bone Marrow Transplantation*, vol. 42, no. 12, pp. 837–838, 2008.

[119] A. P. Cuthbert, S. A. Fisher, M. M. Mirza et al., "The contribution of NOD2 gene mutations to the risk and site of disease in inflammatory bowel disease," *Gastroenterology*, vol. 122, no. 4, pp. 867–874, 2002.

[120] B. Newman, M. S. Silverberg, X. Gu et al., "CARD15 and HLA DRB1 Alleles Influence Susceptibility and Disease Localization in Crohn's Disease," *American Journal of Gastroenterology*, vol. 99, no. 2, pp. 306–315, 2004.

[121] D. Heresbach, V. Gicquel-Douabin, B. Birebent et al., "NOD2/CARD15 gene polymorphisms in Crohn's disease: a genotype-phenotype analysis," *European Journal of Gastroenterology and Hepatology*, vol. 16, no. 1, pp. 55–62, 2004.

[122] S. Brand, T. Staudinger, F. Schnitzler et al., "The role of Toll-like receptor 4 Asp299Gly and Thr399Ile polymorphisms and CARD15/NOD2 mutations in the susceptibility and phenotype of Crohn's disease," *Inflammatory Bowel Diseases*, vol. 11, no. 7, pp. 645–652, 2005.

[123] S. Pugazhendhi, A. Amte, R. Balamurugan, V. Subramanian, and B. S. Ramakrishna, "Common NOD2 mutations are absent in patients with Crohn's disease in India," *Indian Journal of Gastroenterology*, vol. 27, no. 5, pp. 201–203, 2008.

[124] J. P. Hugot, I. Zaccaria, J. Cavanaugh et al., "Prevalence of CARD15/NOD2 mutations in Caucasian healthy people," *American Journal of Gastroenterology*, vol. 102, no. 6, pp. 1259–1267, 2007.

[125] L. Riis, I. Vind, S. Vermeire et al., "The prevalence of genetic and serologic markers in an unselected European population-based cohort of IBD patients," *Inflammatory Bowel Diseases*, vol. 13, no. 1, pp. 24–32, 2007.

[126] M. Ideström, C. Rubio, F. Granath, Y. Finkel, and J. P. Hugot, "CARD 15 mutations are rare in Swedish pediatric Crohn disease," *Journal of Pediatric Gastroenterology and Nutrition*, vol. 40, no. 4, pp. 456–460, 2005.

[127] S. Kugathasan, A. Loizides, U. Babusukumar et al., "Comparative phenotypic and CARD15 mutational analysis among African American, Hispanic, and white children with Crohn's disease," *Inflammatory Bowel Diseases*, vol. 11, no. 7, pp. 631–638, 2005.

[128] U. A. Duffner, Y. Maeda, K. R. Cooke et al., "Host dendritic cells alone are sufficient to initiate acute graft-versus-host disease," *Journal of Immunology*, vol. 172, no. 12, pp. 7393–7398, 2004.

[129] O. Penack, O. M. Smith, A. Cunningham-Bussel et al., "NOD2 regulates hematopoietic cell function during graft-versus-host disease," *Journal of Experimental Medicine*, vol. 206, no. 10, pp. 2101–2110, 2009.

[130] B. Grzywacz, J. S. Miller, and M. R. Verneris, "Use of natural killer cells as immunotherapy for leukaemia," *Best Practice and Research*, vol. 21, no. 3, pp. 467–483, 2008.

[131] M. W. Lowdell, R. Craston, D. Samuel et al., "Evidence that continued remission in patients treated for acute leukaemia is dependent upon autologous natural killer cells," *British Journal of Haematology*, vol. 117, no. 4, pp. 821–827, 2002.

15

Lineage Switching in Acute Leukemias: A Consequence of Stem Cell Plasticity?

Elisa Dorantes-Acosta[1, 2, 3] and Rosana Pelayo[2]

[1] Leukemia Clinic, Mexican Children's Hospital Federico Gómez, 06720 Mexico City, DF, Mexico
[2] Oncology Research Unit, Oncology Hospital, Mexican Institute of Social Security, 06720 Mexico City, DF, Mexico
[3] Medical Sciences Program, National Autonomous University of Mexico, 04510 Mexico City, DF, Mexico

Correspondence should be addressed to Rosana Pelayo, rosana.pelayo@imss.gob.mx

Academic Editor: Amanda C. LaRue

Acute leukemias are the most common cancer in childhood and characterized by the uncontrolled production of hematopoietic precursor cells of the lymphoid or myeloid series within the bone marrow. Even when a relatively high efficiency of therapeutic agents has increased the overall survival rates in the last years, factors such as cell lineage switching and the rise of mixed lineages at relapses often change the prognosis of the illness. During lineage switching, conversions from lymphoblastic leukemia to myeloid leukemia, or vice versa, are recorded. The central mechanisms involved in these phenomena remain undefined, but recent studies suggest that lineage commitment of plastic hematopoietic progenitors may be multidirectional and reversible upon specific signals provided by both intrinsic and environmental cues. In this paper, we focus on the current knowledge about cell heterogeneity and the lineage switch resulting from leukemic cells plasticity. A number of hypothetical mechanisms that may inspire changes in cell fate decisions are highlighted. Understanding the plasticity of leukemia initiating cells might be fundamental to unravel the pathogenesis of lineage switch in acute leukemias and will illuminate the importance of a flexible hematopoietic development.

1. Early Cell Fate Decisions in the Hematopoietic System: Unidirectional and Irreversible?

Mature cells within the hierarchical hematopoietic system, are conventionally classified into two major lineages: lymphoid and myeloid. The lymphoid lineage consists of B, T, and natural killer (NK) cells, whereas the myeloid lineage includes erythrocytes, megakaryocytes, mast cells, granulocytes, monocytes, and macrophages. A number of subtypes of dendritic cells (DC) are generated via the pathways of lymphoid or myeloid differentiation [1–3]. Starting in the very primitive multipotential hematopoietic stem cells (HSC), lineage commitment proceeds after a gradual process of cell differentiation and concomitant series of ordered lineage exclusions. As progenitor cells progress through the pathway, their differentiation capabilities narrow, and at the point where potential limits the fate, the precursors become now-committed [4]. It is believed that once a cell is committed

to a given lineage, its fate must be set due to precise combinations of lineage transcription factors and epigenetic modifications to the chromatin [5]. However, considering that hematopoiesis implies a continuing dialogue between developing cells and the surrounding microenvironmental cues [4], the unidirectional and irreversible nature of the process has been questioned by a number of findings showing redirection of cell fates through various manipulations, highlighting the plasticity of early progenitor cells [5].

HSC give rise to multipotent progenitors (MPP) that no longer retain self-renewal and long-term reconstitution properties (Figure 1). In mice, the lymphoid differentiation program begins in the lymphoid-primed multipotent progenitors (LMPP), a population containing RAG1$^+$ early lymphoid progenitors (ELP) capable of producing all lymphoid-lineage cells as well as components of the innate immune system, including plasmacytoid dendritic cells (pDC) and interferon-producing killer dendritic cells (IKDC) [3, 6, 7]. A further step on the differentiation process results in the production of common lymphoid progenitors (CLP) that are recognized as the major B and NK cell producer (Figure 1). On the other hand, MPP in turn give rise to common myeloid progenitors (CMP) that are responsible of generating granulocyte-monocyte progenitors (GMP) and megakaryocyte-erythroid progenitors (MEP) [8]. Both CLP and CMP lineage precursors have substantially lost the possibility of differentiating into the rest of the lineages and finish their developmental process producing fully committed mature cells that eventually will be exported to peripheral circulation (Figure 1). Human hematopoiesis seems to be generally consistent with the process in mice, except for the cell phenotypes. Development of myeloid and lymphoid cells from HSC also involves a stepwise progression of stem and progenitor cells in the bone marrow [9, 10]. CMP are differentiated from the fraction of multipotent progenitor cells, whereas the earliest lymphoid progenitors may be directly derived from HSC and has been recently designated as multilymphoid progenitor (MLP). A description that fully matches the definition of mouse ELP is still missing, but a counterpart of CLP efficiently differentiates into B and NK cells [10, 11].

Throughout the pathways, a network of transcription factors (TF) is highly important in defining cellular fates. RUNX1, SCL, Ikaros, and GFI-1, among other TF, play a role in early development and during the specification of common myeloid progenitor from HSCs [12]. Downstream, diversification within the CMP fraction correlates with the instructive signals from GATA-1 for the megakaryocyte-erythroid lineage, while myelomonocyte cells are controlled by elevated levels of PU.1, GFI-1, c/EBPα, and/or c/EBPβ [5, 8, 10]. Along the lymphoid pathway, specific NK cell regulation is conducted by Id2 and Zfp105 TF [4]. In B-versus T-lymphoid fate choice, B-cell development is determined by PU.1, E2A, EBF, and Pax5 [13], whereas access to the T-cell fate seems to depend on silencing of Pax5 and expression of GATA-3 and Notch1. Loss of E2A and EBF1 (early B-cell factor) blocks entry into the B cell program, while loss of Pax5 (paired box 5) redirects B-cells into other lineages [14]. Moreover, the enforced expression of EBF1 and Pax5 overcome the developmental block in E2A or IL-7 deficient mice, further illustrating the transcriptional hierarchy of the B-lymphoid program. Acting together with Pax5, EBF drives the expression of B-cell genes, including BLNK, CD79A, RAG, and CD19, among others. The recent report from Singh and colleagues has strikingly established the capability of EBF of repressing lineage-inappropriate genes, upstream and independently of Pax5 [15]. Loss- and gain-of-function experiments with committed lymphoid progenitors demonstrated that EBF regulates B-lymphoid versus myeloid fates by enforcing B-related genes expression while reducing the expression of myeloid-related genes, including PU.1 and EBP.

The genetic manipulation of some of these factors has verified their participation in the lineage decisions, documenting the possibility of cell reprogramming within the hematopoietic system (Figure 1). Conditional deletion of Pax5 in mature B cells can induce conversion to different fates, including macrophages and T cells, potentially through the dedifferentiation of noncommitted progenitors [16, 17]. The absence of EBF allows early progenitors to differentiate into myeloid-lineage cells independently of Pax5, whereas sustained expression of EBF in Pax5-deficient progenitors inhibits their myeloid and T-lineage options [15]. Interestingly, the forced expression of c/EBPs in precursors of B cells results in the activation of specific myeloid genes and a rapid reprogramming to macrophages [5], while PU.1 in fully committed pre-T cells induce formation of myeloid DC, and c/EBPα plus PU.1 convert them to functional macrophages [18]. Iwasaki and colleagues have confirmed the importance of the TF expression timing for a proper early lineage commitment [19]. In their model, CLP could be converted to GMP, as well as basophil and mast cell progenitors by the enforced expression of c/EBPα and GATA-2, respectively. The order of c/EBPα and GATA-2 expression was shown to be critical for CLP to differentiate into eosinophils or into basophils [19].

In addition to transcriptional regulators, inductive environmental signals, including the ones from cytokines and growth factors, are critical for the early cell fate decisions. Of note, when transduced with the GM-CSF receptor, common lymphoid progenitors are able to generate macrophages and granulocytes in response to GM-CSF [20], although this GM-CSF-induced behavior can be redirected by the constant presence of IL-7.

There are other examples of plasticity where progenitor cells can be redirected by extracellular factors, like during infections. Interesting findings indicate that inflammatory cues and infectious stress stimulate stem cells to leave quiescence. Moreover, these seminal cells and developing progenitors express high levels of Toll-like receptors (the receptors concerned with recognizing viral and bacterial components in mammals) and can use them to sense pathogen products, assuming alternative fates and facilitating quick differentiation of innate precursor and effector cells [3, 21–25]. Interaction of TLR2 and TLR4 with their ligands promotes the production of myeloid cells from HSC [26]. Our observations indicate similar elevated levels of TLR9 transcripts in purified fractions of lymphoid progenitors. Furthermore, the generation of DC is strongly favored at expense of B-cell production when TLR9 is ligated on CLP by DNA-CpG motifs or during herpes simplex virus 1 (HSV-1) infection [21]. Together, these data have suggested that the vigorous plasticity of progenitor's genome allow them to be reprogrammed by external signaling cues [27]. Thus, the implications of this phenomenon during lineage adjustments in hematological diseases are crucial to be determined.

2. The Biology of Acute Leukemias

At present, acute leukemias (AL) are the most common cause of childhood cancer worldwide, characterized by the uncontrolled production of hematopoietic precursor cells of the lymphoid or myeloid series within the bone marrow. Of the two types of AL, acute lymphoblastic leukemia (ALL) has the highest frequency, accounting for the 85% of the cases, while acute myeloid leukemia (AML) constitutes 15%

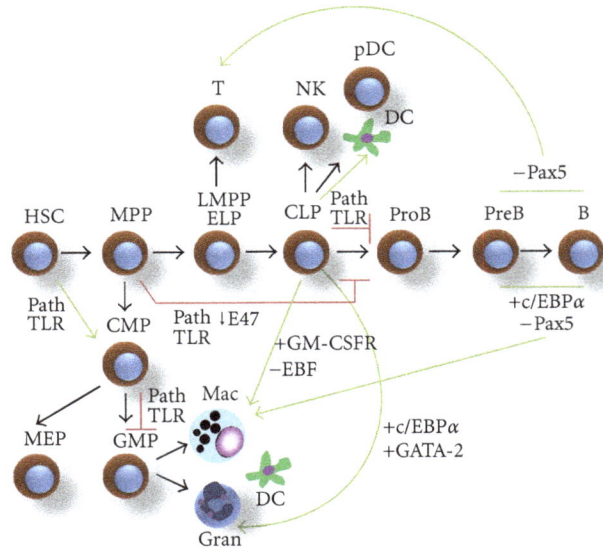

FIGURE 1: Plasticity in the hematopoietic model. Hematopoietic system is organized as a hierarchy of cell types that gradually lose multiple alternate potentials while committing to lineage fates. Ectopic expression or loss of master transcription factors in committed or developing cells, as well as the cell response to microenvironmental cues such as growth factors and pathogen products, can change fate decisions and promote cell conversions. Blue arrows follow the normal hematopoietic model, whereas green arrows follow prospective pathways of plasticity. Red lines indicate differentiation blocking by effect of pathogens or TLR ligation. HSC: hematopoietic stem cells; MPP: multipotent progenitors; LMPP: lymphoid-primed multipotent progenitors; ELP: early lymphoid progenitors; CLP, common lymphoid progenitors; TLR: Toll-like receptors; MEP: megakaryocyte-erythroid progenitors; GMP: granulocyte-monocyte progenitors; Mac: macrophage; Gran: granulocytes; DC: dendritic cells; T, T cells; NK: natural killer cells; pDC: plasmacytoid dendritic cells; GM-CSFR: granulocyte-macrophage colony-stimulating factor receptor.

of them [28]. Nearly 80% of ALL cases have a precursor B-cell immunophenotype and approximately 15% show a T-cell immunophenotype.

There have been several attempts to classify acute leukemias using morphologic, immunophenotypic, and cytogenetic features and the diagnosis criteria have changed according the evolution of diagnosis tools. In 1976, the French-American-British (FAB) Cooperative Group published a morphologic classification of acute leukemias [29, 30]. A revision of this classification was widely used and recognized as the standard for AL classification for over 15 years. For ALL diagnosis, the FAB system defines three categories of lymphoblasts according to cell size, nuclear chromatin, nuclear shape, nucleoli, basophilia of cytoplasm, and cytoplasmic vacuolation (Table 1), whereas for the diagnosis of AML, this system includes eight subtypes (M0 to M7), each characterized by specific morphologic and histochemical features (Table 1). The FAB classification does not correlate particularly well with the immunophenotypic and cytogenetic classification. Nevertheless, Wright-Giemsa staining and application of the FAB criteria is the first step toward the diagnosis of most patients and provides guidance for additional laboratory tests.

On the other hand, the new World Health Organization (WHO) classification proposal defines subsets of AL based on morphologic and cytogenetic characteristics [46], incorporating new information from scientific and clinical studies and adding entities that have only recently

been characterized [46] (Table 1). In order to classify them, the *European Group for the Immunological Classification of Leukemia* (EGIL) [47] has created a scoring system based on the number and specificity degree of lymphoid and myeloid markers expressed by leukemic cells. In keeping with it, biphenotypic/bilineal leukemia are defined when point values are greater than 2 for myeloid and 1 for lymphoid lineages (Table 1). The WHO describes the mixed phenotype acute leukemia (MPAL) classification based on the expression of strictly speci_c T-lymphoid (cytoplasmic CD3) and myeloid (myeloperoxidase (MPO)) antigens, the latter shown by either ow cytometry or cytochemistry and/or clear evidence of monocytic differentiation. Because there is no single antigen strictly specific for B cells, B-cell lineage assignment in MPAL relies on the strong expression of CD19 together with another B cell-associated marker or, in cases with weak CD19, on the expression of at least 3 B-lineage markers. In addition, the WHO recognizes 2 distinct categories: MPAL with the t(9;22)(q34;q11)/BCR-ABL1 and MPAL with t(v;11q23)/MLL rearrangement. The remaining cases are designated as MPAL not otherwise specified [48].

Although, in recent years, studies have reported important advances in the investigation of genetic, molecular, karyotypic and phenotypic aberrations that are prevalent in these diseases, the understanding of the mechanisms that damage the early programs of hematopoietic development remains poor, due in part to the fact that the precise origin of the disease and the susceptibility of primitive leukemic

TABLE 1: Criteria defining acute leukemias according to current classifications.

	Acute lymphoblastic leukemia	Acute myeloid leukemia	Acute leukemias of ambiguous lineage and biphenotypic leukemia
WHO 2008	B lymphoblastic leukemia/lymphoma (i) B lymphoblastic leukemia/lymphoma, NOS (ii) B lymphoblastic leukemia/lymphoma with recurrent genetic abnormalities B lymphoblastic leukemia/lymphoma with t(9;22)(q34;q11.2); BCR-ABL 1 B lymphoblastic leukemia/lymphoma with t(v;11q23); MLL rearranged B lymphoblastic leukemia/lymphoma with t(12;21)(p13;q22) TEL-AML1 (ETV6-RUNX1) B lymphoblastic leukemia/lymphoma with hyperdiploidy B lymphoblastic leukemia/lymphoma with hypodiploidy B lymphoblastic leukemia/lymphoma with t(5;14)(q31;q32) IL3-IGH B lymphoblastic leukemia/lymphoma with t(1;19)(q23;p13.3); TCF3-PBX1 T lymphoblastic leukemia/lymphoma	Acute myeloid leukemia and related neoplasms (i) Acute myeloid leukemia with recurrent genetic abnormalities AML with t(8;21)(q22;q22); RUNX1-RUNX1T1 AML with inv(16)(p13.1q22) or t(16;16)(p13.1;q22); CBFB-MYH11 APL with t(15;17)(q22;q12); PML-RARA AML with t(9;11)(p22;q23); MLLT3-MLL AML with t(6;9)(p23;q34); DEK-NUP214 AML with inv(3)(q21q26.2) or t(3;3)(q21;q26.2); RPN1-EVI1 AML (megakaryoblastic) with t(1;22)(p13;q13); RBM15-MKL1 Provisional entity: AML with mutated NPM1 Provisional entity: AML with mutated CEBPA (ii) Acute myeloid leukemia with myelodysplasia-related changes (iii) Therapy-related myeloid neoplasms (iv) Acute myeloid leukemia, not otherwise specified AML with minimal differentiation AML without maturation AML with maturation Acute myelomonocytic leukemia Acute monoblastic/monocytic leukemia Acute erythroid leukemia Pure erythroid leukemia Erythroleukemia, erythroid/myeloid Acute megakaryoblastic leukemia Acute basophilic leukemia Acute panmyelosis with myelofibrosis (v) Myeloid sarcoma (vi) Myeloid proliferations related to Down syndrome Transient abnormal myelopoiesis Myeloid leukemia associated with Down Syndrome (vii) Blastic plasmacytoid dendritic cell Neoplasm	Acute leukemias of ambiguous lineage (i) Acute undifferentiated leukemia (ii) Mixed phenotype acute leukemia with t(9;22)(q34;q11.2); BCR-ABL1 (iii) Mixed phenotype acute leukemia with t(v;11q23); MLL rearranged (iv) Mixed phenotype acute leukemia, B-myeloid, NOS (v) Mixed phenotype acute leukemia, T-myeloid, NOS (vi) Provisional entity: natural killer (NK) cell lymphoblastic leukemia/lymphoma

TABLE 1: Continued.

	Acute lymphoblastic leukemia	Acute myeloid leukemia	Acute leukemias of ambiguous lineage and biphenotypic leukemia
FAB	L1: lymphoblasts are usually smaller, with scanty cytoplasm and inconspicuous nucleoli L2: lymphoblasts are larger, and they demonstrate considerable heterogeneity in size, prominent nucleoli and more abundant cytoplasm L3: lymphoblasts notable for their deep cytoplasmic basophilia, large, frequently display prominent cytoplasmic vacuolation, morphologically identical to Burkitt's lymphoma cells	M0: undifferentiated. Undifferentiated, large, agranular blasts; >90% blasts MPO−; SBB− M1: acute myeloblastic, no maturation. Undifferentiated; >90% blasts; <10% promyelocytes/monocytes. MPO+;SSB+; PAS− M2: acute myeloblastic with maturation. ≥30% and ≤89% blasts; >105 promyelocytes, myelocytes; <20% monocytic cells. MPO+; SSB+; PAS− M3: acute promyelocytic-hypergranular type. >20% abnormal hypergranular promyelocytes; Auer rods common. MPO+; SSB+; PAS− M3v: acute promyelocytic-hypogranular variant. Fine granularity of cytoplasm in promyelocytes; folded nuclei. MPO+; SSB+; PAS− M4: acute myelomonocytic. ≥30% blasts on nonerythroid series; >20% but <80% monocytic cells; blood monocytes > 5 × 10^9/L; lysozyme >3 × normal. MPO+; NASDA+ M4eo: acute myelomonocytic with eosinophilia. >5% abnormal eosinophils with basophilic granules. MPO+; NASDA+ eosinophils; PAS+ M5a: acute monocytic. >80% of monocytic cells = monoblasts; rest are promonocytes/monocytes. MPO+; NASDA+ M5b: acute monocytic with differentiation. <80% of monocytic cells are monoblasts; rest are promonocytes/monocytes. MPO+; NASDA+ M6: acute erythroleukemia. >30% of nonerythroid cells are blasts; >50% of marrow are erythroblasts. PAS+; ringed sideroblasts with iron stain M7: acute megakaryoblastic. >30% of nonerythroid cells are megakaryoblasts; cytoplasmic blebs; myelofibrosis common. MPO−; SBB−; NASDA+ platelet MPO+ by EM	

TABLE 1: Continued.

	Acute lymphoblastic leukemia	Acute myeloid leukemia	Acute leukemias of ambiguous lineage and biphenotypic leukemia
EGIL			Scoring system for the definition of acute biphenotypic leukemias Scoring lineages points 2: B-lymphoid (CD79a, CD22, cyIgM) T-lymphoid (CD3) myeloid, (MPO) 1: B-lymphoid (CD10, CD19), T-lymphoid (CD2, CD5), myeloid (CD13, CD33) 0.5: B-lymphoid (TdT), T-lymphoid (TdT, CD7), myeloid (CD14, CD15, CD11b, CD11c)

NOS: not otherwise specified, MPO: myeloperoxidase, SSB: Sudan Black B, PAS: periodic acid-Schiff, EM: electron microscopy, NASDA: naphthol-ASD chloroacetate, TdT: Terminal deoxynucleotide transferase, and cy: cytoplasmic.

cells to extrinsic factors are yet to be determined [14, 49]. Even when cancer stem cells (CSC) in myeloid leukemias have been strictly depicted as the cells responsible for tumor maintenance, the identification of a rare, primitive, and malignant cell with intrinsic stem cell properties, and the ability to recapitulate the ALL has been more complicated [50] and is still on debate. Identification of leukemic clones with unrelated DJ rearrangements and cytogenetic abnormalities on lineage negative cells in ALL strongly suggest the existence of oligoclonality and oligolineage, thus the participation of primitive cells in the onset of leukemia [51, 52]. Moreover, data showing that only cells with immature phenotypes are capable of engraftment and reconstitution of leukemia in immunodeficient mice support this notion [53]. However, recent work has remarkably shown that precursor blasts at different differentiation stages can also reestablish leukemic phenotypes *in vivo*, conferring them stem cell properties [50, 54, 55] and the ability to create abnormal bone marrow microenvironments [56]. Furthermore, the combination of genomics and xenotransplant approaches has indicated unsuspected genetic diversity within subclones of leukemia initiating cells, supporting multiclonal evolution of leukemogenesis rather than lineal succession, and outlining the importance of taking account of functional plasticity.

3. Lineage Switching in the Clinic

Analysis of the expression of surface and cytoplasmic and nuclear antigens of leukemia cells has permitted their classification in function of lineage and of maturation stage. Although in the majority of the cases, markers are expressed by which specific lineages can be identified, there are situations in which both lymphoid- and myeloid-lineage markers, or T-cell and B-cell markers, coexist [30].

Some 20–30% of patients with leukemia suffer relapses, during which it is common to find genetic alterations in the same original cell lineage (lymphoid or myeloid). In these individuals, the response to therapies for reinduction is usually of poorer quality and shorter duration. Within this high-risk group, a "lineage switch" phenomenon is occasionally observed, which occurs when acute leukemias that meet the standard FAB (French-American-British) criteria for a lineage (lymphoid or myeloid) at the time of the initial diagnosis meet the criteria for the opposite lineage upon relapse [57, 58]. A lineage switch has been considered an uncommon type of mixed leukemia [59] with a frequency between 6–9% of the cases in relapse [58]. In ALL, the most evident prognostic factor is the time to relapse. An early relapse is associated with a higher rate of nonresponse to treatment, a shorter duration of second complete remission, and a lower event-free survival rate. Most relapses in AML occur during treatment within the first year upon diagnosis. Strikingly, neonate patients that develop lineage switching, present very early relapses and poor event-free survival, that make the prognosis for these patients from variable to bad with no optimal standard treatment for them [39].

A lineage switch may represent either a relapse of the original clone with heterogeneity at the morphological level

or high plasticity attributes, or the emergence of a new leukemic clone [36]. In attempting to explain its etiology, various mechanisms have been postulated, among which reprogramming and/or redirection of the precursor cell fate within bone marrow is prominent, as will be further discussed. Whether lineage switching is a feature of acute leukemia that promotes instability of the hematopoietic lineage or AL genome plasticity is a consequence of the leukemic transformation, are unsolved interesting issues.

4. The Experience of Children's Hospitals

Lineage switching has been reported to occur more frequently in children than adults [42]. Eighteen cases of pediatric lineage switch have been recorded in the literature, and the pertained information is compiled in Table 2, which may provide new insights into the mechanisms of lineage switching.

Cases in Table 2 are ordered by age. Even when most reports classify lineage switching cases into pediatric and adult, there is a group of patients (five out of eighteen) with congenital acute leukemia (CAL). CAL is rare and typically manifests itself within the first 4 weeks of life [31]. Interestingly, the reported clinical outcomes for this group were poor: three of them died, one was alive at the time of publication, and one more was uncertain [31–35]. Overall, approximately 40% CAL cases involve a translocation in chromosome region 11q23, including t(4;11), t(9;11), t(11;19), and other 11q23 abnormalities [60, 61]. This information is congruent with the high frequency (80%) reported for CAL lineage switching.

Furthermore, half of the 18 studied patients had chromosomal aberrations involving 11q rearrangements. As known, the mixed lineage leukemia (MLL) gene participate in more than 50 fusions that might be implicated in transformation of BM cells through regulation of HOX genes. Among them, the fusion MLL-AF9 is associated more commonly with acute myeloid leukemia, whereas the translocation t(4;11)(q21;q23), which produces the fusion of the MLL and AF4 genes, has been documented in up to 80% of infant ALL cases and in near to 2% of children older than 1 year of age [62]. Very recently, a retrospective observational analysis has strikingly shown the high heterogeneity in the disease biology and prognosis of the induction failure (persistence of leukemic blasts in blood, BM or extramedullary sites after 4 to 6 wk of remission-induction therapy) in ALL [63, 64]. Within the induction-failure study group, MLL/11q23 rearrangement was shown to be a poor-risk feature that was overrepresented in those patients with a highly adverse clinical outcome, recording only $16 \pm 5\%$ 10-year survival rate [64].

Despite this information, the role of genetic and chromosomal aberrations in the trigger of lineage switching is unknown, and the possibility of the first leukemic transformation occurring *in utero* during fetal hematopoiesis and the second—concomitant with lineage switch—taking place during the natural evolution of the disease are tempting.

As described in Table 2, in some cases the original karyotype had been replaced by an entirely different abnormal

TABLE 2: Pediatric cases of lineage switching in acute leukemias.

Number of case	Age	Sex	Diagnosis 1st diagnosis	2nd diagnosis at relapse	3rd diagnosis at second relapse	Important findings 1st diagnosis	2nd diagnosis at relapse	3rd diagnosis at second relapse	Time from first diagnosis to relapse	Time from second diagnosis to relapse	Criteria for lineage switching	Clinical outcome	References
1	Neonate	F	ALL L1	AML M5	—	46 XX t(1;6), t(4;11) CD19+ CD22+ CD79a+, MPO− CD34− CD117−	46 XX t(1;6), t(4;11) CD19− CD22− CD79a− CD14+ CD33+ CD13+	—	Day 100 after induction of chemotherapy	—	Morphologic and immunophenotypic	Died	[31]
2	At birth	F	AML M5	B-ALL L1	—	t(9;11)	Karyotype NR	—	12 mo	—	Morphologic	Alive	[32]
3	At birth	F	AML M5	B-ALL	—	t(4;11) MPO− CD33+ CD13+ HLA-DR+ CD14+	t(4;11) CD34+ CD19+ CD22+ HLADR+ CD10−	—	18 dy	—	Morphologic and immunophenotypic	Died	[33]
4	12 dy	?	B-ALL	AML M5	—	MLL rearrangement	MLL rearrangement	—	7 dy	—	Morphologic	NR	[34]
5	21 dy	M	Pro-B ALL	AML	—	t(4;11) MPOX− CD10− CD19+ CD22+ CD34+ CD38+	t(4;11) CD20+ CD13+ CD14+ CD15+ CD33+ CD41+ CD61+	—	8 dy	—	Morphologic and immunophenotypic	Died	[35]
6	3 mo	F	Pre-B cell ALL L1	AML M4	—	t(4;11) PAS+ MPO− ANBE− CD19+ CD34+ TdT+ CD33+	FISH with MLL signal MPO+ ANBE+ CD2+ CD13+ CD14+ CD33+ CD41+ CD65+	—	2 mo	—	Morphologic and immunophenotypic	Alive after allo-HSCT	[36]

TABLE 2: Continued.

Number of case	Age	Sex	Diagnosis 1st diagnosis	Diagnosis 2nd diagnosis at relapse	Diagnosis 3rd diagnosis at second relapse	Important findings 1st diagnosis	Important findings 2nd diagnosis at relapse	Important findings 3rd diagnosis at second relapse	Time from first diagnosis to relapse	Time from second diagnosis to relapse	Criteria for lineage switching	Clinical outcome	References
7	9 mo	M	ALL	AML M5b	—	t(11;16)	t(11;16)	—	8 mo	—	Morphologic	Died	[37]
8	15 mo	M	pro-B ALL L1	AML M0	—	46 XY. CD19+ HLA-DR+	46 XY t(9;11) MPO− CD33+ cyCD13+ cyCD33+ CD117+	—	76 mo	—	Morphologic, immunophenotypic and cytogenetic	Alive after allo-HSCT	[36]
9	25 mo	?	AML	ALL L1	—	46 XY (11q23) PAS+ MPO−	Normal karyotype	—	1 yr	—	Morphologic and cytogenetic	Alive	[38]
10	4 yr	M	AML M5	ALL pro-B	—	Normal karyotype PAX 5 negative when patient was under surveillance CD10+ CD19+ CD13− CD14+ CD15+	Normal karyotype CD10+ CD19+ CD13− CD14− CD15−	—	9 mo	—	Morphologic and immunophenotypic	Died	[39]
11	4 yr	F	ALL L1	AML mo	BM: ALL L1 CNS: AML mo	Normal karyotype BM: MPO− BM: CD13+ CD19+ D22+ CD33+ CD38+ CD34+ HLA DR+	BM: MPO+	Karyotype 47XX+ 18 BM: MPO− BM: CD13− CD19+ D22 NR CD33+ CD38 NR CD34 NR HLA DR+	2 yr after complete remission	1 mo	Morphologic and immunophenotypic	Died	[40]
12	6 yr	M	B-lineage common cell ALL L1	AML M4	—	56 XY HLA-DR+ TdT+ CD10+ CD19+ CD22+	46 XY t(8;16) MPO+ ANBE+ HLA-DR+ CD13+ CD14+ CD33+	—	9 mo	—	Morphologic, immunophenotypic, and cytogenetic	Alive	[36]

TABLE 2: Continued.

Number of case	Age	Sex	Diagnosis 1st diagnosis	Diagnosis 2nd diagnosis at relapse	Diagnosis 3rd diagnosis at second relapse	Important findings 1st diagnosis	Important findings 2nd diagnosis at relapse	Important findings 3rd diagnosis at second relapse	Time from first diagnosis to relapse	Time from second diagnosis to relapse	Criteria for lineage switching	Clinical outcome	References
13	7 yr	F	B-lineage ALL L2	T cell ALL	AML M1	46, XX MPO− HLA-DR+, cyIgM+ CD33.+ PAS+ NSE−	Trisomy 13 CD2+ CD5+ CD7+ CD34+ HLA-DR+ CD33+	ANBE−. MPO+. CD13+, CD33+, CD34+ HLA-DR+ CD7+	14 mo	45 dy	Morphologic, immunophenotypic and cytogenetic	Died	[36]
14	8 yr	M	AML	ALL	—	Karyotype NR	Normal karyotype	—	13 mo	—	Morphologic	Alive	[41]
15	9 yr	M	ALL L1	AML M4	—	56 XY	46 XY t(8;16)	—	9 mo	—	Morphologic and cytogenetic	Alive	[42]
16	13 yr	F	Common B-cell ALL	AML M4/M5	—	t(12;21) amplification of RUNX1	Amplification of RUNX1	—	5 yr	—	Morphologic	Alive	[43]
17	16 yr	F	T-cell ALL	AML M0	—	46 XX MPO− CD7+ CD4+ CD8+ CD1− TdT+	46 ~ 62, XX, + X, MPO− CD19+ CD117+ CD33+ CD34+ CD56+	—	13 mo	—	Morphologic, immunophenotypic, and cytogenetic	Died	[44]
18	20 yr	M	T-ALL	AML	—	52 XY MPO− cytCD3+, CD5+ CD2+ TdT+ CD7+ CD3− CD1a− CD10− CD33− CD117− CD19− CD13±	MPO− CD117+ CD33+ CD13+ CD56+ TdT− CD7− cyCD3− CD2− CD5− CD19+	—	21 mo	—	Morphologic and immunophenotypic	Died	[45]

M: male, F: female, BM: bone marrow, CNS: central nervous system, FISH: fluorescence *in situ* hybridization, ANBE: α-naphthyl-butyrate esterase, PAS: periodic acid-Schiff, NSE: nonspecific esterase, MPO: myeloperoxidase, TdT: terminal deoxynucleotide transferase, yr: year, mo: months, dy: days, cy: cytoplasmic, and NR: not reported.

karyotype, while in other patients, the lineage switch may represent a relapse of the same leukemic clone.

Interestingly, the case of a mixed leukemia may correspond to two types of leukemia, and the phenotype switched from one lineage to another between the time of diagnosis and relapse [40]. This phenomenon could have occurred due to a clonal selection because chemotherapy eradicates the dominant clone present at diagnosis, thus permitting the expansion of a secondary clone with a different phenotype.

Of note, most cases involve the conversion of ALL to AML, and cases of conversion from AML to ALL are extremely rare, with only five cases being reported in the English literature (Table 2). Among them, two correspond to CAL, and three correspond to pediatric AML. The time from diagnosis to conversion was approximately 1 year, and almost all patients within this group achieved remission after conversion. For our reported case of AML to ALL conversion [39], the immunocytochemistry for PAX5 suggested no expression of a transcription factor of lymphoid origin, at least at the time of remission. Moreover, between the first and second leukemias there was no evidence of lymphoid malignancy for a period of time until the patient relapsed. The absence of a lymphoid transcription factor at the beginning of surveillance suggested that the lineage switch occurred upon relapse, opening an intriguing possibility of development of de novo lymphoid leukemia after myeloid leukemia.

In the switch case presented by Podgornik and colleagues, the first course of chemotherapy successfully eradicated the t(12;21). However, a second cell line with AML1 amplification may have remained latent during the time of complete remission, and then reappeared showing a different immunophenotype [43].

On the other hand, lineage switching may be part of the biological spectrum of mixed-lineage leukemias. Pui and colleagues have previously suggested that loss of CD10 might be related to the malignant transformation of multipotent stem cells occurring after eradication of the original stem cell line with chemotherapy. The precise significance of this finding remains unknown [65].

5. Potential Mechanisms of Lineage Conversion

Several hypotheses have been suggested to explain lineage conversion in acute leukemia, but its precise mechanism remains unclear. An examination of some known physiological plasticity mechanisms may help to understand the cell and molecular biology behind this phenomenon.

Physiological plasticity has been defined as the capacity of changing cell fate without altering genotype [66]. Thus, epigenetic modifications might be of great importance in regulating phenotype cell conversions in response to changes in the microenvironment.

Accordingly, the fate of cells having the plasticity attribute as a part of their normal developmental program, is then potentially able to be redirected [66]. Under pathological circumstances, including acute leukemias, different routes might exist, other than transformation, to allow "plastic"

differentiating cells to give rise to other cells different from themselves. According to Rothenberg's view, changes in cell potentials can be explained by mechanisms operating at different levels: at the cell-intrinsic level, clearly defined by transcription factors and possible epigenetic cues; and at the cell/environment interface where modification of TF activities take place in response to inductive environmental signals [4].

5.1. Bi- and Oligopotential Progenitors. According to the classical model of hierarchical hematopoiesis, blood cells arising from HSC can be subdivided into two major lineages, a myeloerythroid and a lymphoid lineage. However, a number of recent studies indicate that the divergence lymphoid-myeloid is less abrupt than previously believed. An alternative "myeloid-based model" has been proposed by Kawamoto and Katsura in which myeloid potential is retained in erythroid, T-, and B-cell branches even after these lineages have segregated from each other [67, 68].

The presence of early bipotential B-macrophage progenitors in the bone marrow and the fact that MLL-positive B-ALL show gene expression profiles consistent with early hematopoietic progenitors have raised the possibility that early bipotential or oligopotential progenitor cells are target for leukemogenic translocations, and constitute the origin of lineage switching events [65] (Figure 2, upper panel). Alternatively, in a subset of cases, the MLL translocation might lead to a stem/progenitor cell phenotype, irrespective of the cell lineage targeted by the translocation, and the cellular environment might allow for lineage interconversions [58].

For Palomero and colleagues, leukemic transformation may occur in early progenitors and be influenced by external and internal cues [69]. Although apparently Notch signaling is essential to open the T-cell differentiation pathway but does not initiate the T-cell program itself [70], mutations occurring in the Notch1 TF in leukemic stem cells that precede both myeloid and T-lineage commitment seems to be responsible for T-cell/myeloid lineage switching, highlighting the participation of a putative common progenitor [69].

Interestingly, leukemic blasts from a group of ALL and AML patients often express cell markers of more than one lineage while retaining characteristics that demonstrate a strong commitment to a single lineage, a phenomenon denominated lineage infidelity. According to St Jude Children's Hospital, AL with aberrant antigen expression can be classified into ALL that express myeloid-associated antigens (My+ALL) and AML that express lymphoid-associated antigens (Ly+AML). Large studies of patients with My+ALL and Ly+AML suggest that lineage infidelity does not have an apparent prognostic significance [71]. By contrast, mixed-lineage acute leukemias (or acute leukemias of ambiguous lineage) represent a heterogeneous category of rare, poorly differentiated acute leukemias possessing characteristics of both lymphoid and myeloid precursor cells [72]. These divergent morphologic and immunophenotypic features may be uniformly present in one blast population (biphenotypic leukemia) or may be seen on distinct blast populations in a single patient (bilineal leukemia). Leukemias that switch their lineage of origin during therapy or show poorly differentiated or undifferentiated features are also included in this category. As mentioned before, the *European Group for the Immunological Classification of Leukemia* (EGIL) [47] has created a scoring system based on the number and specificity degree of lymphoid and myeloid markers expressed by the leukemic cells. In keeping with it, a biphenotypic/bilineal leukemia is considered when point values are greater than 2 for the myeloid and then 1 for the lymphoid lineages.

Because the leukemic cells can aberrantly express other lineage markers, an accurate subclassification of the disease, along with a clear cut diagnosis are critical to define lineage switch. Moreover, investigation of a precursor-product relationship between bipotential progenitors and the "faithless" cells, or between bipotential progenitors and bilineal leukemias, is required and will be valuable to further understand lineage switch origins.

5.2. Cell Reprogramming and Dedifferentiation. Genetic and epigenetic activities are suggested to be directly implicated in lineage redirection, as modifications affecting chromatin structure are important for the expression of genes involved in cell fate decisions and in the maintenance of cell-differentiated states [73]. Apparently, any reprogramming implying a change towards a new cellular identity may involve epigenetic regulation [66].

Using a very interesting model for instability in leukemic cells, Messina and colleagues have found an aberrant expression of activation-induced cytidine deaminase (AICDA) in BCR/ABL1+ B-ALL [74] that upregulate DNA repair/replication and cell cycle genes, and suggested its participation in the genetic instability of BCR/ABL1+ B-ALL. Lineage conversion in ALL can be promoted by significant copy number alterations of "stemness" modulators, such as deletions in peak regions from MYC, TCF3, RB1, CDKN1A, and deletions in CDKN1B [75].

As discussed in earlier sections of this paper, lineage commitment in blood cells is controlled by transcription factors such as PU.1 and C/EBPα for the commitment of myeloid cells, and Notch1, GATA3, and Pax5, which mediate T- and B-cell development, respectively [5]. The ectopic expression or deletion of these master regulators mostly result in lineage reprogramming, with or without reversion of cells back to a multipotent stage [66] (Figure 2). The now-functional TF in the reprogrammed cells may be able to establish a new epigenetic program and to remove the original one.

The introduction of c/EBPα into B- or T-cells converts them into functional macrophages [5, 18, 76]. While the expression of GATA-1 can reprogram common B- and T-progenitor cells to differentiate into megakaryocytic/erythroid cells [19]. Furthermore, loss of Pax5 in fully committed B cells allows them to revert to a multipotential cell and to take alternate differentiation routes upon specific stimuli [66]. An integral activity of Pax5 is pivotal for normal and neoplastic B lymphopoiesis [77, 78]. It will be crucial to investigate a correlation between genetic/epigenetic abnormalities in Pax5 and lineage switching in acute leukemias.

In addition to genetic changes, dynamic epigenetic remodeling may take place over the course of the reprogramming processes. We have learned from *in vitro* reprogramming of somatic cells into embryonic stem cells (ESC) [79] that the ectopic expression of the four pluripotency-associated transcription factors (c-Myc, Oct-4, Klf4 and Sox2) is made possible by a variety of epigenetic changes that take place during the process, that permit the reactivation of key pluripotency-related genes, establish the appropriate bivalent chromatin domains and hypomethylate genomic heterochromatic regions. Thus, an epigenetic reorganization is central to get a cell reprogrammed [72, 80, 81].

Of note, dedifferentiation may co-function as a mechanism for lineage conversion, where cells lacking a master TF revert to a primitive stage before committing to a second lineage fate [17]. It remains to be addressed if the cases like the *in vivo* conversion of T-ALL reported by Mantadakis et al. [44], with an early thymocyte to AML result from dedifferentiation programs.

5.3. Clonal Selection. This mechanism, which would involve heterogeneous populations of developing cells, is believed to occur at relapse in patients with a persistent TEL/AML1+ preleukemic/leukemic clone [82]. Interestingly, karyotype analyses do not often show cytogenetic alterations, and lineage switch may represent the emergence of a new leukemic clone. Chemotherapy might suppress or eradicate the leukemic clone that is apparent at the time of diagnosis, thereby permitting the expansion of a subclone with a different phenotype (Figure 2).

5.4. Seeding of Donor Cells. Although no biological cell conversion could be explained by this mechanism, its impact on the clinical lineage switch is a fact. There have been reported around 40 cases making a lineage change at relapse after hematopoietic stem cell transplantation (HSCT), as a consequence of leukemia relapse occurring in donor cells. This so-called donor cell leukemia (DCL) seems to be an uncommon and possibly underreported complication after allogeneic HSCT [83]. A major problem in the analysis of DCL is the demonstration of the donor cell origin of leukemic relapse after allogeneic transplantation, which includes cytogenetic detection of marker chromosomes, fluorescent *in situ* hybridization for the identification of sex-related chromosomes (XY-FISH), detection of Y chromosome-specific sequences (YCS-PCR) and detection of polymorphic markers like minisatellites or variable number tandem repeats (VNTRs: repeats of 10–100 bp) [84, 85].

Possible causes of DCL include oncogenic alteration or premature aging of transplanted donor cells in immunosuppressed individuals, aberrant homeostasis promoting transformation, impaired immune surveillance, chemotherapy-induced mutagenesis/transformation, replicative stress and a first "hit" in donor followed by second "hit" in recipient [86]. Both intrinsic cell factors and external signals from the recipient, as a proinflammatory or immunocompromised microenvironment may contribute to the leukemic clone expansion (Figure 2).

5.5. The Role of the Hematopoietic Environment. Hematopoietic stem and progenitor cells do not grow as self-supporting units; rather they are completely surrounded by the microenvironment of the BM and have a continuing dialogue with signals provided by it [4]. A network of mesenchymal cells, osteoblasts, fibroblasts, adipocytes, macrophages, endothelial cells, and reticular cells building the endosteal, vascular and reticular niches, forms a highly organized three-dimensional scaffold and supports hematopoietic differentiation [62]. Clearly, the very early fate decisions in hematopoiesis are influenced by environmental cues in physiological conditions. While it has long been recognized that intrinsic abnormalities may cause leukemia, it has also become clear that changes in microenvironment composition might lead to disease. A number of seminal studies have highlighted the microenvironment-hematopoietic relationship in leukemia, and led to propose at least three mechanisms to explain possible niche contributions to oncogenesis: competition of tumor cells for the niche, manipulation of the environment, and disruption of the HSC-niche communication [62]. How any of these alterations would allow or promote lineage switching in leukemia is currently a topical question.

Heuser and colleagues have shown that although genetic disruption of Flt3 and c-Kit does not affect the MN1-induced leukemogenesis in the MN1 model of acute myeloid leukemia, it is important to preserve a switch from the myeloid to erythroid phenotype [87], highlighting the relevance of microenvironmental signals controlling myeloid-erythroid lineage choices.

Interesting studies on acute leukemias harboring MLL (mixed lineage leukemia) rearrangements have suggested that the fusion partner may instruct lineage decisions. For example, MLL-AF9 and MLL-AF6 are related more commonly with acute myeloid leukemia (AML), while the fusion MLL-AF4 and MLL-ENL has been mostly documented in ALL [88]. The capability of MLL-GAS7 cells to generate distinct leukemias in mice models, including an acute biphenotypic leukemia, supports the existence of a multipotent leukemia-initiating cell that may give rise to both AML and ALL [89]. Moreover, using a human-based MLL leukemia mouse model, the role of microenvironment has been shown to be critical to the lineage outcome, with manipulation of the *in vivo* cytokine milieu influencing the commitment of both lineage-restricted and multipotent LIC [90]. Again, these findings underline the plasticity of leukemic MLL-target cells and their critical vulnerability to environmental cues.

Finally, our prior observations suggest that in normal conditions, human and mouse HSC and lymphoid progenitors in bone marrow respond to stimulation by microbial components through Toll-like receptors (TLR), thereby redirecting their differentiation potentials [3, 21] (Vadillo et al., unpublished data). Thus, there is a strong possibility that their TLR-expressing counterparts in leukemia represent the beginning of instability of the lineage. The *in vitro* TLR ligation on CD34+ cells from ALL pediatric patients induce cell proliferation and redirection of cell fates (Dorantes-Acosta et al., unpublished data). Along with recurrent infections, increasing evidence suggests the prevalence of inflammatory environments in hematological abnormalities such as acute leukemias [56, 91], remaining to be addressed if overproduction of inflammatory cytokines impacts the HSC niches and can stimulate aberrant cell fate decisions.

5.6. Prospective Signaling Pathways in Lineage Conversion. A comprehensive model for the molecular and signaling pathways involved in both nonleukemic and leukemic cell fate conversions is not yet available. Canonical routes participating in the regulation of lineage decisions may function as platforms for abnormal activities of transcription factors, oncoproteins or rearranged genes. MLL trithorax domain participate in the methylation of H3K4, activating the transcription of leukemogenesis- and cell fate-associated genes like HOX [13]. HOX deregulation is the most relevant factor for MLL fusion-induced leukemogenesis. HOX proteins, in particular HOXA9 and its partner MEIS1, are oncoproteins substantially overexpressed in leukemias, can function through activation of the protooncogene c-Myb [92]. On the other hand, an elegant model of MLL-AF9-induced AML showing the significance of the microenvironment in providing instructive signals for leukemic lineage fates, has suggested that the signaling through the small GTPase Rac1 pathway is critical to leukemia development within this particular lineage promiscuity scenario [86].

Proliferation and apoptosis are defining features of the hematopoietic development, and the NF-κB signaling pathway participates in their regulation [93]. The effects of NEMO inactivation in both mice and human strengthen the role of NF-κB in lymphopoiesis—in the absence of NEMO-dependent NFκB signaling, B and T cells fail to develop. However, whether NF-κB contributes to early lineage cell decisions or just play a survival role is yet to be determined [93].

EBF1 is critical to B-lineage commitment, driving the expression of genes relevant to B-cell differentiation and function at both genetic and epigenetic levels. EBF alterations are common in patients with poor outcomes and are particularly frequent (25%) in relapsed children [14]. A recent report from Sigvardsson has shown an increase lineage plasticity and low expression of Ebf-1 on committed lymphoid progenitors in the absence of IL-7, supporting the notion that Ebf is crucial for lineage restriction [94]. Despite their findings position this transcription factor downstream of IL-7 in the developmental hierarchy, the role of STAT5 in fate conversions is uncertain. A regulatory circuit with EBF as determinant of B-lymphoid versus myeloid fates has been proposed from the Ebf$^{-/-}$ reporter mouse model, where EBF regulates expression of myeloid-related transcription factors and can reprogram early progenitor cells [15]. EBF induction is controlled by PU.1, E2A, and IL-7R, and its promoter is responsive to STAT5, which is conventionally phosphorilated as result of JAK activation. Interestingly, genetic alterations of members of the JAK family are particularly prominent in acute leukemias [95]. Of note, STAT5 is also a critical node in the signaling pathway of BCR/ABL, and we have recently learned from the model of BCR/ABL-tumour initiation that

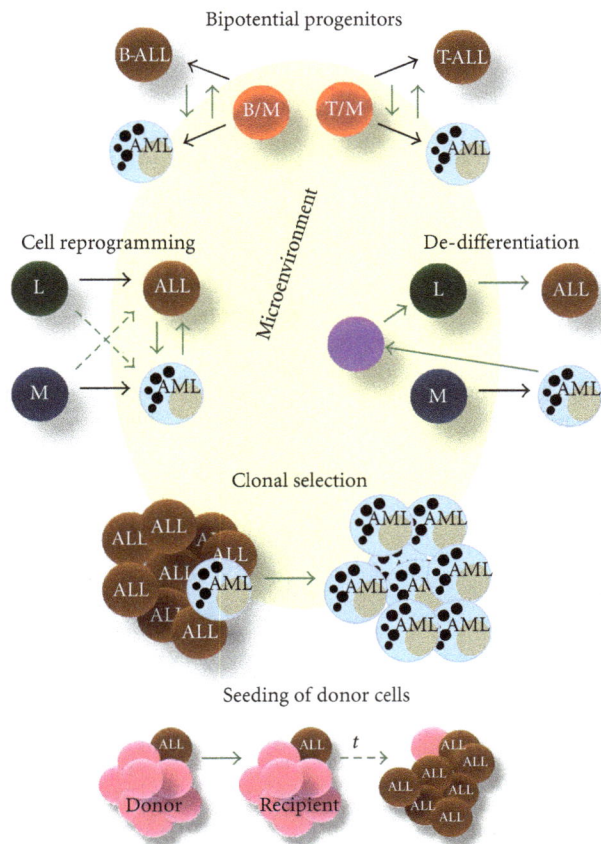

FIGURE 2: Potential mechanisms of lineage switching in acute leukemias. The existence of bipotential progenitors, cell reprogramming, dedifferentiation, clonal selection, and seeding of donor cells are proposed to participate in leukemic cell fates conversion. Microenvironment may influence all proposed mechanisms by modulating the genome plasticity of the cells and change the leukemia outcome at relapse. Black arrows follow normal differentiation, whereas green arrows indicate potential mechanisms of lineage switching. Bipotential progenitors might be responsible for fate interconversions from mixed lymphoid-myeloid leukemias. Genetic and epigenetic changes in transcription factors of fully committed or developing cells are the basis of cellular reprogramming. During dedifferentiation, a cellular change occurs in a differentiated state which in turn get back to a more primitive and less committed stage. Clonal selection is based on the existence of an oligoclonal disease, and the selection of a distinct and chemoresistant clone. In seeding of donor cell leukemia after allografts from bone marrow, a first "hit" may take place in donor followed by a second "hit" in the recipient, along with a clonal selection upon time. B/M: bipotent B and myeloid progenitor; T/M: bipotent T and myeloid progenitor; AML: acute myeloid leukemia; B-ALL: acute lymphoblastic leukemia from B precursors; T-ALL: acute lymphoblastic leukemia from T precursors; L: lymphoid progenitors; M: myeloid progenitors; *t*: time.

its activity may influence the ultimate leukaemia phenotype [96].

6. Concluding Remarks

Lineage switching is an example of the lineage heterogeneity that exists in acute leukemias, representing a relapse of the original clone with high attributes of plasticity, or the emergence of new leukemic clones. As this phenomenon clearly correlates with very bad prognosis and resistance to therapy, further sequential phenotypic and cytogenetic studies may yield valuable insights into the mechanisms of leukemic recurrence and possible implications for treatment selection. Despite tremendous progress in the knowledge of the pathogenesis of acute leukemias, much remains to be addressed about the mechanisms driving lineage switching at

relapse. Aberrant function of specific fusion genes and surrounding microenvironmental cues might guide leukemia phenotype conversion through modulation of plasticity within leukemia initiating cells. Moreover, clinical features could play important roles in establishing environmental scenarios proper for cell conversion events. Although we have much to learn about what controls and coordinate the mechanisms of action in lineage exclusions and switching, clearly leukemia-initiating cells are considerably more plastic in their developmental potential than previously envisioned, challenging the notion of limited lineage fates in these diseases.

Abbreviations

AICDA: Activation-induced cytidine deaminase
AL: Acute leukemias

ALL:	Acute lymphoblastic leukemia
AML:	Acute myeloid leukemia
ANBE:	α-naphthyl-butyrate esterase
B-ALL:	B-cell acute lymphoblastic leukemia
BM:	Bone marrow
B/M:	Bipotent B and myeloid progenitor
CAL:	Congenital acute leukemia
CLP:	Common lymphoid progenitors
CMP:	Common myeloid progenitors
CNS:	Central nervous system
CSC:	Cancer stem cells
DC:	Dendritic cells
DCL:	Donor cell leukemia
EGIL:	European Group for the Immunological Classification of Leukemia
ELP:	Early lymphoid progenitors
ESC:	Embryonic stem cells
FAB:	French-American-British
FISH:	Fluorescence in situ hybridization
GM-CSF:	Granulocyte-macrophage colony-stimulating factor
GM-CSFR:	Granulocyte-macrophage colony-stimulating factor receptor
GMP:	Granulocyte-monocyte progenitors
Gran:	Granulocytes
HSC:	Hematopoietic stem cells
HSCT:	Hematopoietic stem cell transplantation
HSV-1:	Herpes simplex virus 1
IKDC:	Interferon-producing killer dendritic cells
LMPP:	Lymphoid-primed multipotent progenitors
Ly+AML:	AML with lymphoid-associated antigens
MEP:	Megakaryocyte-erythroid progenitors
MLL:	Mixed lineage leukemia
MLP:	Multilymphoid progenitor
MPAL:	Mixed phenotype acute leukemia
MPO:	Myeloperoxidase
MPP:	Multipotent progenitors
My+ALL:	ALL with myeloid-associated antigens
NASDA:	Naphthol-ASD chloroacetate
NK:	Natural killer cells
NSE:	Nonspecific esterase
PAS:	Periodic Acid Schiff
pDC:	Plasmacytoid dendritic cells
SSB:	Sudan Black B
T-ALL:	T-cell acute lymphoblastic leukemia
TdT:	Terminal deoxynucleotide transferase
TF:	Transcription factors
TLR:	Toll-like receptors
T/M:	Bipotent T and myeloid progenitor
VNTRs:	Variable number tandem repeats
WHO:	World Health Organization
XY-FISH:	Fluorescent in situ hybridization for sex-related chromosomes
YCS-PCR:	Y chromosome-specific sequences.

Acknowledgments

The authors apologize to investigators whose work could not be discussed due to space limitation. The authors thank the members of the Lymphopoiesis Lab from UIMEO, Dr. Aurora Medina, and Dr. Onofre Muñoz for critical input and academic support. R. Pelayo is recipient of funding from the National Council of Science and Technology, CONACYT (Grant CB-2010-01-152695) and the Mexican Institute for Social Security, IMSS (Grants 2008-785-044 and FIS/IMSS/852). E. Dorantes-Acosta is a scholarship holder from CONACYT.

References

[1] R. Pelayo, R. Welner, S. S. Perry et al., "Lymphoid progenitors and primary routes to becoming cells of the immune system," *Current Opinion in Immunology*, vol. 17, no. 2, pp. 100–107, 2005.

[2] R. Pelayo, K. Miyazaki, J. Huang, K. P. Garrett, D. G. Osmond, and P. W. Kincade, "Cell cycle quiescence of early lymphoid progenitors in adult bone marrow," *Stem Cells*, vol. 24, no. 12, pp. 2703–2713, 2006.

[3] R. S. Welner, R. Pelayo, and P. W. Kincade, "Evolving views on the genealogy of B cells," *Nature Reviews Immunology*, vol. 8, no. 2, pp. 95–106, 2008.

[4] E. V. Rothenberg, "T cell lineage commitment: identity and renunciation," *Journal of Immunology*, vol. 186, no. 12, pp. 6649–6655, 2011.

[5] H. Xie and S. H. Orkin, "Immunology: changed destiny," *Nature*, vol. 449, no. 7161, pp. 410–411, 2007.

[6] R. Pelayo, J. Hirose, J. Huang et al., "Derivation of 2 categories of plasmacytoid dendritic cells in murine bone marrow," *Blood*, vol. 105, no. 11, pp. 4407–4415, 2005.

[7] R. S. Welner, R. Pelayo, K. P. Garrett et al., "Interferon-producing killer dendritic cells (IKDCs) arise via a unique differentiation pathway from primitive c-kitHiCD62L+ lymphoid progenitors," *Blood*, vol. 109, no. 11, pp. 4825–4931, 2007.

[8] H. Iwasaki and K. Akashi, "Hematopoietic developmental pathways: on cellular basis," *Oncogene*, vol. 26, no. 47, pp. 6687–6696, 2007.

[9] B. Blom and H. Spits, "Development of human lymphoid cells," *Annual Review of Immunology*, vol. 24, pp. 287–320, 2006.

[10] S. Doulatov, F. Notta, E. Laurenti, and J. E. Dick, "Hematopoiesis: a human perspective," *Cell Stem Cell*, vol. 10, no. 2, pp. 120–136, 2012.

[11] S. Doulatov, F. Notta, K. Eppert, L. T. Nguyen, P. S. Ohashi, and J. E. Dick, "Revised map of the human progenitor hierarchy shows the origin of macrophages and dendritic cells in early lymphoid development," *Nature Immunology*, vol. 11, no. 7, pp. 585–593, 2010.

[12] Y. Baba, R. Pelayo, and P. W. Kincade, "Relationships between hematopoietic stem cells and lymphocyte progenitors," *Trends in Immunology*, vol. 25, no. 12, pp. 645–649, 2004.

[13] P. Perez-Vera, A. Reyes-Leon, and E. M. Fuentes-Panana, "Signaling proteins and transcription factors in normal and malignant early B cell development," *Bone Marrow Research*, vol. 2011, Article ID 502751, 2011.

[14] R. Pelayo, E. Dorantes-Acosta, E. Vadillo, and E. Fuentes-Panana, "From HSC to B-lymphoid cells in normal and malignant hematopoiesis," in *Advances in Hematopoietic Stem Cell Research*, R. Pelayo, Ed., InTech, 2012.

[15] J. M. Pongubala, D. L. Northrup, D. W. Lancki et al., "Transcription factor EBF restricts alternative lineage options

and promotes B cell fate commitment independently of Pax5," *Nature Immunology*, vol. 9, no. 2, pp. 203–215, 2008.

[16] S. L. Nutt, B. Heavey, A. G. Rolink, and M. Busslinger, "Commitment to the B-lymphoid lineage depends on the transcription factor Pax5," *Nature*, vol. 401, no. 6753, pp. 556–562, 1999.

[17] C. Cobaleda, W. Jochum, and M. Busslinger, "Conversion of mature B cells into T cells by dedifferentiation to uncommitted progenitors," *Nature*, vol. 449, no. 7161, pp. 473–477, 2007.

[18] C. V. Laiosa, M. Stadtfeld, H. Xie, L. de Andres-Aguayo, and T. Graf, "Reprogramming of committed T cell progenitors to macrophages and dendritic cells by C/EBP alpha and PU.1 transcription factors," *Immunity*, vol. 25, no. 5, pp. 731–744, 2006.

[19] H. Iwasaki, S. I. Mizuno, Y. Arinobu et al., "The order of expression of transcription factors directs hierarchical specification of hematopoietic lineages," *Genes and Development*, vol. 20, no. 21, pp. 3010–3021, 2006.

[20] M. Kondo, D. C. Scherer, T. Miyamoto et al., "Cell-fate conversion of lymphoid-committed progenitors by instructive actions of cytokines," *Nature*, vol. 407, no. 6802, pp. 383–386, 2000.

[21] R. S. Welner, R. Pelayo, Y. Nagai et al., "Lymphoid precursors are directed to produce dendritic cells as a result of TLR9 ligation during herpes infection," *Blood*, vol. 112, no. 9, pp. 3753–3761, 2008.

[22] M. T. Baldridge, K. Y. King, N. C. Boles, D. C. Weksberg, and M. A. Goodell, "Quiescent haematopoietic stem cells are activated by IFN-γ in response to chronic infection," *Nature*, vol. 465, no. 7299, pp. 793–797, 2010.

[23] J. R. Boiko and L. Borghesi, "Hematopoiesis sculpted by pathogens: toll-like receptors and inflammatory mediators directly activate stem cells," *Cytokine*, vol. 57, no. 1, pp. 1–8, 2012.

[24] K. De Luca, V. Frances-Duvert, M. J. Asensio et al., "The TLR1/2 agonist PAM3CSK4 instructs commitment of human hematopoietic stem cells to a myeloid cell fate," *Leukemia*, vol. 23, no. 11, pp. 2063–2074, 2009.

[25] M. Sioud and Y. Floisand, "TLR agonists induce the differentiation of human bone marrow CD34+ progenitors into CD11c+ CD80/86+ DC capable of inducing a Th1-type response," *European Journal of Immunology*, vol. 37, no. 10, pp. 2834–2846, 2007.

[26] Y. Nagai, K. P. Garrett, S. Ohta et al., "Toll-like receptors on hematopoietic progenitor cells stimulate innate immune system replenishment," *Immunity*, vol. 24, no. 6, pp. 801–812, 2006.

[27] P. G. Heyworth, D. Noack, and A. R. Cross, "Identification of a novel NCF-1 (p47-phox) pseudogene not containing the signature GT deletion: significance for A47 degrees chronic granulomatous disease carrier detection," *Blood*, vol. 100, no. 5, pp. 1845–1851, 2002.

[28] M. L. Perez-Saldivar, A. Fajardo-Gutiérrez, R. Bernáldez-Ríos et al., "Childhood acute leukemias are frequent in Mexico City: descriptive epidemiology," *British Medical Journal*, vol. 11, article 355, 2011.

[29] J. M. Bennett, D. Catovsky, M.-T. Daniel et al., "Proposals for the classification of the acute leukaemias. French-American-British (FAB) co-operative group," *British Journal of Haematology*, vol. 33, no. 4, pp. 451–458, 1976.

[30] J. M. Bennett, D. Catovsky, M. T. Daniel et al., "Proposed revised criteria for the classification of acute myeloid leukemia.

A report of the French-American-British Cooperative Group," *Annals of Internal Medicine*, vol. 103, no. 4, pp. 620–625, 1985.

[31] J. G. Jiang, E. Roman, S. V. Nandula, V. V. S. Murty, G. Bhagat, and B. Alobeid, "Congenital MLL-positive B-cell acute lymphoblastic leukemia (B-ALL) switched lineage at relapse to acute myelocytic leukemia (AML) with persistent t(4;11) and t(1;6) translocations and JH gene rearrangement," *Leukemia and Lymphoma*, vol. 46, no. 8, pp. 1223–1227, 2005.

[32] H. Shimizu, S. J. Culbert, A. Cork, and J. J. Iacuone, "A lineage switch in acute monocytic leukemia. A case report," *American Journal of Pediatric Hematology/Oncology*, vol. 11, no. 2, pp. 162–166, 1989.

[33] M. Krawczuk-Rybak, J. Zak, and B. Jaworowska, "A lineage switch from AML to ALL with persistent translocation t(4;11) in congenital leukemia," *Medical and Pediatric Oncology*, vol. 41, no. 1, pp. 95–96, 2003.

[34] S. A. Ridge, M. E. Cabrera, A. M. Ford et al., "Rapid intraclonal switch of lineage dominance in congenital leukaemia with a MLL gene rearrangement," *Leukemia*, vol. 9, no. 12, pp. 2023–2026, 1995.

[35] H. Sakaki, H. Kanegane, K. Nomura et al., "Early lineage switch in an infant acute lymphoblastic leukemia," *International Journal of Hematology*, vol. 90, no. 5, pp. 653–655, 2009.

[36] M. Park, K. N. Koh, B. E. Kim et al., "Lineage switch at relapse of childhood acute leukemia: a report of four cases," *Journal of Korean Medical Science*, vol. 26, no. 6, pp. 829–831, 2011.

[37] C. Stasik, S. Ganguly, M. T. Cunningham, S. Hagemeister, and D. L. Persons, "Infant acute lymphoblastic leukemia with t(11;16)(q23;p13.3) and lineage switch into acute monoblastic leukemia," *Cancer Genetics and Cytogenetics*, vol. 168, no. 2, pp. 146–149, 2006.

[38] M. L. Bernstein, D. W. Esseltine, J. Emond, and M. Vekemans, "Acute lymphoblastic leukemia at relapse in a child with acute myeloblastic leukemia," *American Journal of Pediatric Hematology/Oncology*, vol. 8, no. 2, pp. 153–157, 1986.

[39] E. Dorantes-Acosta, F. Arreguin-Gonzalez, C. A. Rodriguez-Osorio, S. Sadowinski, R. Pelayo, and A. Medina-Sanson, "Acute myelogenous leukemia switch lineage upon relapse to acute lymphoblastic leukemia: a case report," *Cases Journal*, vol. 2, article 154, 2009.

[40] Y. Ikarashi, T. Kakihara, C. Imai, A. Tanaka, A. Watanabe, and M. Uchiyama, "Double leukemias simultaneously showing lymphoblastic leukemia of the bone marrow and monocytic leukemia of the central nervous system," *American Journal of Hematology*, vol. 75, no. 3, pp. 164–167, 2004.

[41] A. Emami, Y. Ravindranath, and S. Inoue, "Phenotypic change of acute monocytic leukemia to acute lymphoblastic leukemia on therapy," *American Journal of Pediatric Hematology/Oncology*, vol. 5, no. 4, pp. 341–343, 1983.

[42] H. J. Chung, C. J. Park, S. Jang, H. S. Chi, E. J. Seo, and J. J. Seo, "A case of lineage switch from acute lymphoblastic leukemia to acute myeloid leukemia," *The Korean Journal of Laboratory Medicine*, vol. 27, no. 2, pp. 102–105, 2007.

[43] H. Podgornik, M. Debeljak, D. Žontar, P. Černelč, V. V. Prestor, and J. Jazbec, "RUNX1 amplification in lineage conversion of childhood B-cell acute lymphoblastic leukemia to acute myelogenous leukemia," *Cancer Genetics and Cytogenetics*, vol. 178, no. 1, pp. 77–81, 2007.

[44] E. Mantadakis, V. Danilatou, E. Stiakaki, G. Paterakis, S. Papadhimitriou, and M. Kalmanti, "T-cell acute lymphoblastic leukemia relapsing as acute myelogenous leukemia," *Pediatric Blood and Cancer*, vol. 48, no. 3, pp. 354–357, 2007.

[45] W. van den Ancker, M. Terwijn, J. Regelink et al., "Uncommon lineage switch warrants immunophenotyping even in relapsing leukemia," *Leukemia Research*, vol. 33, no. 7, pp. e77–e80, 2009.

[46] J. W. Vardiman, J. Thiele, D. A. Arber et al., "The 2008 revision of the World Health Organization (WHO) classification of myeloid neoplasms and acute leukemia: rationale and important changes," *Blood*, vol. 114, no. 5, pp. 937–951, 2009.

[47] M. C. Bene, G. Castoldi, W. Knapp et al., "Proposals for the immunological classification of acute leukemias," *Leukemia*, vol. 9, no. 10, pp. 1783–1786, 1995.

[48] E. Matutes, W. F. Pickl, M. V. Veer et al., "Mixed-phenotype acute leukemia: clinical and laboratory features and outcome in 100 patients defined according to the WHO 2008 classification," *Blood*, vol. 117, no. 11, pp. 3163–3171, 2011.

[49] K. Akashi, "Lymphoid lineage fate decision of hematopoietic stem cells," *Annals of the New York Academy of Sciences*, vol. 1176, pp. 18–25, 2009.

[50] S. Bomken, K. Fišer, O. Heidenreich, and J. Vormoor, "Understanding the cancer stem cell," *British Journal of Cancer*, vol. 103, no. 4, pp. 439–445, 2010.

[51] F. Davi, C. Gocke, S. Smith, and J. Sklar, "Lymphocytic progenitor cell origin and clonal evolution of human B-lineage acute lymphoblastic leukemia," *Blood*, vol. 88, no. 2, pp. 609–621, 1996.

[52] T. Stankovic, V. Weston, C. M. McConville et al., "Clonal diversity of Ig and T-cell receptor gene rearrangements in childhood B-precursor acute lymphoblastic leukaemia," *Leukemia and Lymphoma*, vol. 36, no. 3-4, pp. 213–224, 2000.

[53] C. V. Cox, P. Diamanti, R. S. Evely, P. R. Kearns, and A. Blair, "Expression of CD133 on leukemia-initiating cells in childhood ALL," *Blood*, vol. 113, no. 14, pp. 3287–3296, 2009.

[54] O. Heidenreich and J. Vormoor, "Malignant stem cells in childhood ALL: the debate continues," *Blood*, vol. 113, no. 18, pp. 4476–4477, 2009.

[55] C. le Viseur, M. Hotfilder, S. Bomken et al., "In childhood acute lymphoblastic leukemia, blasts at different stages of immunophenotypic maturation have stem cell properties," *Cancer Cell*, vol. 14, no. 1, pp. 47–58, 2008.

[56] A. Colmone, M. Amorim, A. L. Pontier, S. Wang, E. Jablonski, and D. A. Sipkins, "Leukemic cells create bone marrow niches that disrupt the behavior of normal hematopoietic progenitor cells," *Science*, vol. 322, no. 5909, pp. 1861–1865, 2008.

[57] G. A. Gagnon, C. C. Childs, A. LeMaistre et al., "Molecular heterogeneity in acute leukemia lineage switch," *Blood*, vol. 74, no. 6, pp. 2088–2095, 1989.

[58] S. Stass, J. Mirro, and S. Melvin, "Lineage switch in acute leukemia," *Blood*, vol. 64, no. 3, pp. 701–706, 1984.

[59] O. Imataki, H. Ohnishi, G. Yamaoka et al., "Lineage switch from precursor B cell acute lymphoblastic leukemia to acute monocytic leukemia at relapse," *International Journal of Clinical Oncology*, vol. 15, no. 1, pp. 112–115, 2010.

[60] D. Bresters, A. C. W. Reus, A. J. P. Veerman, E. R. Van Wering, A. Van Der Does-Van Den Berg, and G. J. L. Kaspers, "Congenital leukaemia: the Dutch experience and review of the literature," *British Journal of Haematology*, vol. 117, no. 3, pp. 513–524, 2002.

[61] M. C. Fernandez, B. Weiss, S. Atwater, K. Shannon, and K. K. Matthay, "Congenital leukemia: successful treatment of a newborn with t(5;11)(q31;q23)," *Journal of Pediatric Hematology/Oncology*, vol. 21, no. 2, pp. 152–157, 1999.

[62] J. Purizaca, I. Meza, and R. Pelayo, "Early lymphoid development and microenvironmental cues in B-cell acute lymphoblastic leukemia," *Archives of Medical Research*, vol. 43, no. 2, pp. 89–101, 2012.

[63] K. R. Rabin, "Attacking remaining challenges in childhood leukemia," *The New England Journal of Medicine*, vol. 366, no. 15, pp. 1445–1446, 2012.

[64] M. Schrappe, S. P. Hunger, C.-H. Pui et al., "Outcomes after induction failure in childhood acute lymphoblastic leukemia," *The New England Journal of Medicine*, vol. 366, no. 15, pp. 1371–1381, 2012.

[65] C. H. Pui, S. C. Raimondi, and F. G. Behm, "Shifts in blast cell phenotype and karyotype at relapse of childhood lymphoblastic leukemia," *Blood*, vol. 68, no. 6, pp. 1306–1310, 1986.

[66] C. Cobaleda, "Reprogramming of B cells," *Methods in Molecular Biology*, vol. 636, pp. 233–250, 2010.

[67] H. Kawamoto and Y. Katsura, "A new paradigm for hematopoietic cell lineages: revision of the classical concept of the myeloid-lymphoid dichotomy," *Trends in Immunology*, vol. 30, no. 5, pp. 193–200, 2009.

[68] J. J. Bell and A. Bhandoola, "The earliest thymic progenitors for T cells possess myeloid lineage potential," *Nature*, vol. 452, no. 7188, pp. 764–767, 2008.

[69] T. Palomero, K. McKenna, J. O-Neil et al., "Activating mutations in NOTCH1 in acute myeloid leukemia and lineage switch leukemias," *Leukemia*, vol. 20, no. 11, pp. 1963–1966, 2006.

[70] F. Weerkamp, T. C. Luis, B. A. E. Naber et al., "Identification of Notch target genes in uncommitted T-cell progenitors: no direct induction of a T-cell specific gene program," *Leukemia*, vol. 20, no. 11, pp. 1967–1977, 2006.

[71] J. E. Rubnitz, M. Onciu, S. Pounds et al., "Acute mixed lineage leukemia in children: the experience of St Jude Children's Research Hospital," *Blood*, vol. 113, no. 21, pp. 5083–5089, 2009.

[72] E. G. Weir, M. A. Ansari-Lari, D. A. S. Batista et al., "Acute bilineal leukemia: a rare disease with poor outcome," *Leukemia*, vol. 21, no. 11, pp. 2264–2270, 2007.

[73] G. Zardo, G. Cimino, and C. Nervi, "Epigenetic plasticity of chromatin in embryonic and hematopoietic stem/ progenitor cells: therapeutic potential of cell reprogramming," *Leukemia*, vol. 22, no. 8, pp. 1503–1518, 2008.

[74] M. Messina, S. Chiaretti, I. Iacobucci et al., "AICDA expression in BCR/ABL1-positive acute lymphoblastic leukaemia is associated with a peculiar gene expression profile," *British Journal of Haematology*, vol. 152, no. 6, pp. 727–732, 2011.

[75] R. Strauss, P. Hamerlik, A. Lieber, and J. Bartek, "Regulation of stem cell plasticity: mechanisms and relevance to tissue biology and cancer," *Molecular Therapy*, vol. 20, no. 5, pp. 887–897, 2012.

[76] T. Graf, "Differentiation plasticity of hematopoietic cells," *Blood*, vol. 99, no. 9, pp. 3089–3101, 2002.

[77] B. Falini and D. Y. Mason, "Proteins encoded by genes involved in chromosomal alterations in lymphoma and leukemia: clinical value of their detection by immunocytochemistry," *Blood*, vol. 99, no. 2, pp. 409–426, 2002.

[78] E. Smith and M. Sigvardsson, "The roles of transcription factors in B lymphocyte commitment, development, and transformation," *Journal of Leukocyte Biology*, vol. 75, no. 6, pp. 973–981, 2004.

[79] M. Wernig, A. Meissner, R. Foreman et al., "In vitro reprogramming of fibroblasts into a pluripotent ES-cell-like state," *Nature*, vol. 448, no. 7151, pp. 318–324, 2007.

[80] K. Takahashi and S. Yamanaka, "Induction of pluripotent stem cells from mouse embryonic and adult fibroblast cultures by defined factors," *Cell*, vol. 126, no. 4, pp. 663–676, 2006.

[81] R. Jaenisch and R. Young, "Stem cells, the molecular circuitry of pluripotency and nuclear reprogramming," *Cell*, vol. 132, no. 4, pp. 567–582, 2008.

[82] E. R. Panzer-Grümayer, G. Cazzaniga, V. H. J. Van Der Velden et al., "Immunogenotype changes prevail in relapses of young children with TEL-AML1-positive acute lymphoblastic leukemia and derive mainly from clonal selection," *Clinical Cancer Research*, vol. 11, no. 21, pp. 7720–7727, 2005.

[83] G. J. Ruiz-Argüelles, A. Ruiz-Argüelles, and J. Garcés-Eisele, "Donor cell leukemia: a critical review," *Leukemia and Lymphoma*, vol. 48, no. 1, pp. 25–38, 2007.

[84] S. A. Schichman, P. Suess, A. M. Vertino, and P. S. Gray, "Comparison of short tandem repeat and variable number tandemrepeat genetic markers for quantitative determination of allogeneic bone marrow transplant engraftment," *Bone Marrow Transplantation*, vol. 29, no. 3, pp. 243–248, 2002.

[85] I. Buño, P. Nava, A. Simón et al., "A comparison of fluorescent in situ hybridization and multiplex short tandem repeat polymerase chain reaction for quantifying chimerism after stem cell transplantation," *Haematologica*, vol. 90, no. 10, pp. 1373–1379, 2005.

[86] C. M. Flynn and D. S. Kaufman, "Donor cell leukemia: insight into cancer stem cells and the stem cell niche," *Blood*, vol. 109, no. 7, pp. 2688–2692, 2007.

[87] M. Heuser, G. Park, Y. Moon et al., "Extrinsic signals determine myeloid-erythroid lineage switch in MN1 leukemia," *Experimental Hematology*, vol. 38, no. 3, pp. 174–179, 2010.

[88] A. G. Muntean and J. L. Hess, "MLL-AF9 leukemia stem cells: hardwired or taking cues from the microenvironment?" *Cancer Cell*, vol. 13, no. 6, pp. 465–467, 2008.

[89] C. W. So, H. Karsunky, E. Passegué, A. Cozzio, I. L. Weissman, and M. L. Cleary, "MLL-GAS7 transforms multipotent hematopoietic progenitors and induces mixed lineage leukemias in mice," *Cancer Cell*, vol. 3, no. 2, pp. 161–171, 2003.

[90] J. Wei, M. Wunderlich, C. Fox et al., "Microenvironment determines lineage fate in a human model of MLL-AF9 leukemia," *Cancer Cell*, vol. 13, no. 6, pp. 483–495, 2008.

[91] L. Espinoza-Hernández, J. Cruz-Rico, H. Benítez-Aranda et al., "In vitro characterization of the hematopoietic system in pediatric patients with acute lymphoblastic leukemia," *Leukemia Research*, vol. 25, no. 4, pp. 295–303, 2001.

[92] D. Mueller, M. P. García-Cuéllar, C. Bach, S. Buhl, E. Maethner, and R. K. Slany, "Misguided transcriptional elongation causes mixed lineage leukemia," *PLoS Biology*, vol. 7, no. 11, Article ID e1000249, 2009.

[93] M. S. Hayden and S. Ghosh, "NF-κB in immunobiology," *Cell Research*, vol. 21, no. 2, pp. 223–244, 2011.

[94] P. Tsapogas, S. Zandi, J. Åhsberg et al., "IL-7 mediates Ebf-1-dependent lineage restriction in early lymphoid progenitors," *Blood*, vol. 118, no. 5, pp. 1283–1290, 2011.

[95] E. Chen, L. M. Staudt, and A. R. Green, "Janus kinase deregulation in leukemia and lymphoma," *Immunity*, vol. 36, no. 4, pp. 529–541, 2012.

[96] B. Kovacic, A. Hoelbl, G. Litos et al., "Diverging fates of cells of origin in acute and chronic leukaemia," *EMBO Molecular Medicine*, vol. 4, no. 4, pp. 283–297, 2012.

16

Autologous Stem Cell Transplant for AL Amyloidosis

Vivek Roy

Division of Hematology/Oncology, Mayo Clinic, 4500 San Pablo Road, Jacksonville, FL 32224, USA

Correspondence should be addressed to Vivek Roy, roy.vivek@mayo.edu

Academic Editor: Gordon Cook

AL amyloidosis is caused by clonal plasma cells that produce immunoglobulin light chains which misfold and get deposited as amyloid fibrils. Therapy directed against the plasma cell clone leads to clinical benefit. Melphalan and corticosteroids have been the mainstay of treatment for a number of years and the recent availability of other effective agents (IMiDs and proteasome inhibitors) has increased treatment options. Autologous stem cell transplant (ASCT) has been used in the treatment of AL amyloidosis for many years. It is associated with high rates of hematologic response and improvement in organ function. However, transplant carries considerable risks. Careful patient selection is important to minimize transplant related morbidity and mortality and ensure optimal patient outcomes. As newer more affective therapies become available the role and timing of ASCT in the overall treatment strategy of AL amyloidosis will need to be continually reassessed.

1. Introduction

Amyloidosis is a disease of protein misfolding in which the involved protein acquires an abnormal beta-pleated sheet configuration rather than the native alpha helical state [1]. The amyloid protein is insoluble, and its deposition in various tissues causes tissue damage and organ dysfunction. Amyloidosis can be of various types based on the precursor protein involved in amyloid formation. More than 20 different human fibrillar amyloid proteins have been described [2], and accurate identification of the type is crucial to treatment planning. It is also important to distinguish localized from systemic amyloidosis since patients presenting with localized amyloidosis generally do not need systemic treatment. The most common type of systemic amyloidosis (primary amyloidosis or AL amyloidosis) is caused by production of immunoglobulin light chain or light chain fragment secondary to an underlying plasma cell dyscrasia. Other systemic amyloidoses (secondary amyloidoses) include AA amyloid (caused as a result of chronic inflammatory disease), ATTR caused by alteration in transthyretin (TTR) protein because of one of several mutations (familial amyloid) or misfolding of wild-type transthyretin protein (senile amyloidosis), and dialysis-related amyloidosis (deposition of beta 2 microglobulin).

Primary amyloidosis is the only type of systemic amyloidosis that responds to cytotoxic chemotherapy directed against the abnormal plasma cell clone, the source of amyloidogenic light chains. Other treatment strategies to prevent amyloid formation by altering the equilibrium between soluble precursor and insoluble fibrils, destabilizing the amyloid fibril protein, or antibodies directed against amyloid fibrils are being investigated and show promise but are not available for clinical use [3–5].

This paper will focus on the role of autologous hematopoietic stem cell transplantation for primary systemic amyloidosis.

2. Treatment of Amyloidosis

The ultimate goal of treatment of amyloidosis is to improve organ function, prolong survival, and enhance quality of life. The mainstay of treatment is cytotoxic chemotherapy directed against the plasma cells to decrease the level of circulating amyloid causing light chains. This, in turn, can be expected to slow down further amyloid deposition and improve the prospects for mobilization or dissolution of already deposited amyloid and reversal of organ damage. Treatment of AL amyloid has evolved over the years and has closely paralleled the developments in multiple myeloma therapy since the fundamental underlying problem in both these conditions is the same. Early studies established melphalan as an effective agent. In randomized controlled trials comparing melphalan plus prednisone to colchicine in patients with AL amyloidosis, the melphalan and prednisone combination was associated with objective responses and prolonged survival compared to colchicine [6, 7]. Melphalan has continued to be a key agent in the treatment of amyloidosis. Melphalan combined with dexamethasone is considered a "standard" first line therapy. Palladini et al. showed that this combination results in high response rates, 67% hematologic response including 33% complete response, and 48% of patients had objective organ function response. Responses were durable, and CR was maintained in 9 of 15 patients after a median of 4.8 years. Six-year progression-free survival was 40%, and median overall survival was 5.1 years [8, 9]. Other studies with oral or intravenous melphalan combined with dexamethasone have shown less robust responses with complete response rates of 11 and 13%, likely because of different patient characteristics especially cardiac involvement [10, 11]. The development of free immunoglobulin light chain (FLC) assay allowed quantitation of circulating amyloidogenic light chains. Reduction in FLC with treatment was subsequently shown to be associated with decrease in amyloid load, clinical improvement, and survival benefit [12]. The introduction of new agents (IMiDs and bortezomib) in the last 10 years has revolutionized the treatment of multiple myeloma and improved survival [13]. Since the underlying problem in amyloidosis is also plasma cell dyscrasia, it is logical to expect that these agents will also be effective in the treatment of primary amyloidosis. Studies with thalidomide, lenalidomide, and bortezomib indeed demonstrate activity of these agents. Bortezomib appears to be highly effective with hematologic response rates of 50%– 94% and CR rates of 20–44% in different studies [14–16].

3. Autologous Stem Cell Transplant (ASCT)

High-dose chemotherapy followed by ASCT reliably produces hematologic complete remissions in a sizable proportion of patients with multiple myeloma. Because plasma cell dyscrasia is the underlying cause of AL amyloidosis, ASCT has also been adopted for the treatment of AL amyloidosis. Early studies of ASCT reported significant toxicity including mortality rate of over 40% in one small study [17]. Subsequent studies showed better results and showed that with careful patient selection transplant can be performed with acceptable toxicity [18, 19]. Autologous stem cell transplant has remained an important treatment option for systemic AL amyloidosis.

3.1. Selection of Patients. Although mortality from autologous stem cell transplant has continued to decrease over time, [20, 21] the procedure remains high risk, and careful selection of patients is critical for good outcomes. Best results were obtained in patients with nephrotic syndrome as the predominant manifestation of amyloidosis. Patients with multiple organ involvement, particularly those with cardiac dysfunction, fare poorly with high risk of morbidity and mortality [22]. Many patients with primary amyloidosis are too sick to undergo autologous stem cell transplant.

Predictors of poor prognosis in patients with amyloidosis include the number of organs involved, cardiac involvement evidenced by clinical cardiac dysfunction or elevation of cardiac biomarkers (troponin-T and N-terminal brain natriuretic peptide (NT-pro-BNP)), pretransplant free light chain ratio, and elevated serum uric acid [23–26]. The number of organs involved and the extent of cardiac dysfunction are by far the dominant predictors of prognosis with or without transplant [22, 26]. Excessive fluid retention during stem cell mobilization and harvest may be a reflection of limited cardiac and/or renal reserve and is associated with poor outcomes during transplant [27]. Although older individuals are more likely to have comorbidities, age per se is not a contraindication, and older individuals can successfully undergo autologous HSCT [28]. A risk-adapted approach to transplant has been suggested wherein the melphalan dose in the conditioning regimen is lowered for individuals considered at high risk for transplant toxicity. However, the risk-adjusted lowering of conditioning chemotherapy is associated with reduced response rates [29]. The risks and benefits of transplant have to be carefully evaluated for each individual patient to ensure optimal balance between efficacy and toxicity.

3.2. Outcomes. Autologous stem cell transplant is associated with substantial likelihood of hematologic response including organ function improvement. Long-term posttransplant follow-up studies show the durability of responses and better survival of responders. Cibeira et al. reported longterm outcomes of 421 AL patients transplanted between 1994 and 2008. Hematologic CR rate was 43%, and 78% of complete responders had improvement in organ function. For patients achieving a CR the median event free survival (EFS) and overall survival (OS) were 8.3 and 13.2 years compared to organ response rate of 52%, EFS of 2 years, and OS of 5.9 years in those who did not achieve hematologic CR [20]. Investigators from Mayo Clinic reported their experience with 434 transplants since 1996. Hematologic response rate of 76% (CR rate 38.7%) and organ response rate of 46.8% were described. Median OS was not reached for patients achieving hematologic CR and was 107 months and 32 months, respectively, for those with partial response and no response [30]. Outcomes of 107 recipients of ASCT performed at 48 centers between 1995 and 2001 were reported by Center for International Blood & Marrow Transplant Research (CIBMTR) investigators. A relatively high transplant-related mortality of 18% at 30 days was noted. One-year and 3-year survival rates were 66% and 56%, respectively. The outcomes were better in patients transplanted in later years possibly related to better patient selection, improved supportive care and/or physician experience [31]. These and other studies show that hematologic response, particularly CR is associated with better survival and improvement in organ function, including renal and cardiac functions in substantial proportion of patients [32–34]. Histologic regression of amyloid has been shown but seems to occur only in patients who achieve normalization of free light chains [35].

4. Hematopoietic Stem Cell Transplant versus Other Therapies

The exact role of autologous stem cell transplant in the treatment of primary AL amyloidosis and the benefit relative to other available therapies continues to be debated. It has been argued that apparent superior outcomes of patients undergoing transplant are a function of selection bias since only healthier patients, who are destined to do better, are selected to undergo transplant. A retrospective study looked at outcomes of patients who were transplant eligible but did not undergo transplant. Transplant eligibility itself identified a good risk group who did better than transplant ineligible patients even with nontransplant therapy [36]. A case control study compared the overall survival of 63 ASCT recipients with matched controls not undergoing transplant. The groups were matched for age, gender, time to presentation, left ventricular function, serum creatinine, interventricular septal thickness, nerve involvement, and 24-hour proteinuria). One-, 2-, and 4-year overall survival rates for the transplant versus non-transplant groups were 89% versus 71%, 81% versus 55%, and 77% versus 41%, respectively [37]. These data showing better overall survival as well as studies demonstrating improved quality of life [38] provide strong arguments in support of the role of autologous HSCT for AL amyloidosis. However, randomized trials have not substantiated the benefit of autologous transplant. In a randomized control trial 100 patients with AL amyloidosis aged 18–70 years were randomized between HSCT and conventional therapy. The overall survival was similar in the two arms [39]. High transplant-related mortality of 24% in this study is a notable concern. The publication generated many letters to the journal highlighting concerns about patient selection, inclusion of high-risk patients which necessitated reduction in melphalan dose in 10 of 37 patients, lack of information about cardiac biomarkers, and whether transplants performed at low volume centers in this multicenter study may have biased the results against ASCT [40–42]. A systematic review and meta-analysis of 1 randomized control trial, 2 other control studies, and 9 single arm studies also did not provide a conclusive answer. The study did not find a survival benefit with transplant but the authors commented that the quality of evidence was low, indicating a need for well-designed and adequately powered trials to better address the role of AHCT in AL amyloidosis [43].

Therapeutic options for AL amyloidosis are constantly changing. As newer, more effective therapies become available, and the role of transplant will need to be reevaluated. Modern, bortezomib-based therapies are associated with response rates approaching those obtained by transplant. Bortezomib as monotherapy or with other agents is active in AL amyloidosis, and produces rapid responses and high rates of hematologic and organ response [44–46]. The durability of these responses is unclear at present since only relatively short followup is available. A phase III, multicenter study evaluating melphalan and dexamethasone with or without bortezomib in patients with previously untreated systemic AL amyloidosis is currently ongoing (NCT01078454). Bortezomib has also been used for amyloidosis relapsing after transplant. It is effective in that setting and can lead to normalization of free light chains and potentially render patients previously not candidates for transplant safe to undergo high-dose therapy [47].

The availability of multiple very active treatment options for patients is clearly welcome news for patients with this devastating disorder. Conventional therapy with bortezomib or other agents and ASCT should not be seen as competitive but rather additive or complementary in nature. Achieving a CR is a key predictor of overall survival. ASCT after a bortezomib-based induction regimen may improve the proportion of patients achieving complete remission. However, that remains to be shown in clinical trials. Amyloidosis is a heterogeneous disease with a large variation in the range and severity of clinical presentations, tempo of disease progression, and comorbidities. The challenge for the physicians is to individualize treatment by selecting the optimal combination or sequence of the various therapies to achieve best possible results for the patient. Clearly, optimal approach will be different for each patient depending on their disease status (number of organs involved, organ function), overall health status and co-morbidities, and their personal choice and goals.

5. Conclusions

ASCT is an effective therapy for primary amyloidosis. It is associated with consistently high hematologic response rates, which lead to improvement in organ function, quality of life, and survival. Best results are obtained in patients with 1-2 organ involvement and no cardiac dysfunction. Patients with multiple (more than 2) organ involvement, particularly advanced cardiac involvement and renal insufficiency, are not suitable candidates for this therapy. The question whether ASCT should be the preferred therapy for patients who are healthy enough to tolerate it has not been answered definitely. In the consensus opinion of physicians at the Mayo Clinic experienced in the treatment of amyloidosis the answer to this question is yes [48]. The importance of patient selection to ensure safety and optimal outcomes cannot be overemphasized. The role of HSCT in the overall treatment of AL amyloidosis is likely to evolve as new, more effective therapies become available and will need to be continually assessed in future prospective trials.

References

[1] R. H. Falk, R. L. Comenzo, and M. Skinner, "The systemic amyloidoses," *New England Journal of Medicine*, vol. 337, no. 13, pp. 898–909, 1997.

[2] J. D. Sipe, M. D. Benson, J. N. Buxbaum et al., "Amyloid fibril protein nomenclature: 2010 recommendations from

the nomenclature committee of the International Society of Amyloidosis," *Amyloid*, vol. 17, no. 3-4, pp. 101–104, 2010.

[3] K. Bodin, S. Ellmerich, M. C. Kahan et al., "Antibodies to human serum amyloid P component eliminate visceral amyloid deposits," *Nature*, vol. 468, no. 7320, pp. 93–97, 2010.

[4] J. S. Wall, S. J. Kennel, A. C. Stuckey et al., "Radioimmunodetection of amyloid deposits in patients with AL amyloidosis," *Blood*, vol. 116, no. 13, pp. 2241–2244, 2010.

[5] L. M. Dember, P. N. Hawkins, B. P. C. Hazenberg et al., "Eprodisate for the treatment of renal disease in AA amyloidosis," *New England Journal of Medicine*, vol. 356, no. 23, pp. 2349–2360, 2007.

[6] M. Skinner, J. J. Anderson, R. Simms et al., "Treatment of 100 patients with primary amyloidosis: a randomized trial of melphalan, prednisone, and colchicine versus colchicine only," *American Journal of Medicine*, vol. 100, no. 3, pp. 290–298, 1996.

[7] R. A. Kyle, M. A. Gertz, P. R. Greipp et al., "A trial of three regimens for primary amyloidosis: colchicine alone, melphalan and prednisone, melphalan, prednisone, and colchicine," *New England Journal of Medicine*, vol. 336, no. 17, pp. 1202–1207, 1997.

[8] G. Palladini, V. Perfetti, L. Obici et al., "Association of melphalan and high-dose dexamethasone is effective and well tolerated in patients with AL (primary) amyloidosis who are ineligible for stem cell transplantation," *Blood*, vol. 103, no. 8, pp. 2936–2938, 2004.

[9] G. Palladini, P. Russo, M. Nuvolone et al., "Treatment with oral melphalan plus dexamethasone produces long-term remissions in AL amyloidosis," *Blood*, vol. 110, no. 2, pp. 787–788, 2007.

[10] S. Dietrich, S. O. Schönland, A. Benner et al., "Treatment with intravenous melphalan and dexamethasone is not able to overcome the poor prognosis of patients with newly diagnosed systemic light chain amyloidosis and severe cardiac involvement," *Blood*, vol. 116, no. 4, pp. 522–528, 2010.

[11] D. Lebovic, J. Hoffman, B. M. Levine et al., "Predictors of survival in patients with systemic light-chain amyloidosis and cardiac involvement initially ineligible for stem cell transplantation and treated with oral melphalan and dexamethasone," *British Journal of Haematology*, vol. 143, no. 3, pp. 369–373, 2008.

[12] H. J. Lachmann, R. Gallimore, J. D. Gillmore et al., "Outcome in systemic AL amyloidosis in relation to changes in concentration of circulating free immunoglobulin light chains following chemotherapy," *British Journal of Haematology*, vol. 122, no. 1, pp. 78–84, 2003.

[13] S. K. Kumar, S. V. Rajkumar, A. Dispenzieri et al., "Improved survival in multiple myeloma and the impact of novel therapies," *Blood*, vol. 111, no. 5, pp. 2516–2520, 2008.

[14] E. Kastritis, A. Anagnostopoulos, M. Roussou et al., "Treatment of light chain (AL) amyloidosis with the combination of bortezomib and dexamethasone," *Haematologica*, vol. 92, no. 10, pp. 1351–1358, 2007.

[15] D. E. Reece, V. Sanchorawala, U. Hegenbart et al., "Weekly and twice-weekly bortezomib in patients with systemic AL amyloidosis: results of a phase 1 dose-escalation study," *Blood*, vol. 114, no. 8, pp. 1489–1497, 2009.

[16] A. D. Wechalekar, H. J. Lachmann, M. Offer, P. N. Hawkins, and J. D. Gillmore, "Efficacy of bortezomib in systemic AL amyloidosis with relapsed/refractory clonal disease," *Haematologica*, vol. 93, no. 2, pp. 295–298, 2008.

[17] P. Moreau, V. Leblond, P. Bourquelot et al., "Prognostic factors for survival and response after high-dose therapy and autologous stem cell transplantation in systemic AL amyloidosis: a report on 21 patients," *British Journal of Haematology*, vol. 101, no. 4, pp. 766–769, 1998.

[18] R. L. Comenzo, E. Vosburgh, R. H. Falk et al., "Dose-intensive melphalan with blood stem-cell support for the treatment of AL (amyloid light-chain) amyloidosis: survival and responses in 25 patients," *Blood*, vol. 91, no. 10, pp. 3662–3670, 1998.

[19] M. A. Gertz, M. Q. Lacy, D. A. Gastineau et al., "Blood stem cell transplantation as therapy for primary systemic amyloidosis (AL)," *Bone Marrow Transplantation*, vol. 26, no. 9, pp. 963–969, 2000.

[20] M. T. Cibeira, V. Sanchorawala, D. C. Seldin et al., "Outcome of AL amyloidosis after high-dose melphalan and autologous stem cell transplantation: long-term results in a series of 421 patients," *Blood*, vol. 118, pp. 4346–4352, 2011.

[21] M. A. Gertz, M. Q. Lacy, A. Dispenzieri et al., "Trends in day 100 and 2-year survival after auto-SCT for AL amyloidosis: outcomes before and after 2006," *Bone Marrow Transplantation*, vol. 46, no. 7, pp. 970–975, 2011.

[22] M. A. Gertz, M. Q. Lacy, A. Dispenzieri et al., "Stem cell transplantation for the management of primary systemic amyloidosis," *American Journal of Medicine*, vol. 113, no. 7, pp. 549–555, 2002.

[23] A. Dispenzieri, M. A. Gertz, R. A. Kyle et al., "Prognostication of survival using cardiac troponins and N-terminal pro-brain natriuretic peptide in patients with primary systemic amyloidosis undergoing peripheral blood stem cell transplantation," *Blood*, vol. 104, no. 6, pp. 1881–1887, 2004.

[24] S. Kumar, A. Dispenzieri, J. A. Katzmann et al., "Serum immunoglobulin free light-chain measurement in primary amyloidosis: prognostic value and correlations with clinical features," *Blood*, vol. 116, no. 24, pp. 5126–5129, 2010.

[25] S. Kumar, A. Dispenzieri, M. Q. Lacy et al., "Serum uric acid: novel prognostic factor in primary systemic amyloidosis," *Mayo Clinic Proceedings*, vol. 83, no. 3, pp. 297–303, 2008.

[26] G. Palladini, C. Campana, C. Klersy et al., "Serum N-terminal pro-brain natriuretic peptide is a sensitive marker of myocardial dysfunction in AL amyloidosis," *Circulation*, vol. 107, no. 19, pp. 2440–2445, 2003.

[27] N. Leung, T. R. Leung, S. S. Cha, A. Dispenzieri, M. Q. Lacy, and M. A. Gertz, "Excessive fluid accumulation during stem cell mobilization: a novel prognostic factor of first-year survival after stem cell transplantation in AL amyloidosis patients," *Blood*, vol. 106, no. 10, pp. 3353–3357, 2005.

[28] D. C. Seldin, J. J. Anderson, M. Skinner et al., "Successful treatment of AL amyloidosis with high-dose melphalan and autologous stem cell transplantation in patients over age 65," *Blood*, vol. 108, no. 12, pp. 3945–3947, 2006.

[29] M. A. Gertz, M. Q. Lacy, A. Dispenzieri et al., "Risk-adjusted manipulation of melphalan dose before stem cell transplantation in patients with amyloidosis is associated with a lower response rate," *Bone Marrow Transplantation*, vol. 34, no. 12, pp. 1025–1031, 2004.

[30] M. A. Gertz, M. Q. Lacy, A. Dispenzieri et al., "Autologous stem cell transplant for immunoglobulin light chain amyloidosis: a status report," *Leukemia and Lymphoma*, vol. 51, no. 12, pp. 2181–2187, 2010.

[31] D. H. Vesole, W. S. Pérez, M. Akasheh, C. Boudreau, D. E. Reece, and C. N. Bredeson, "High-dose therapy and autologous hematopoietic stem cell transplantation for patients with primary systemic amyloidosis: a Center for International Blood and Marrow Transplant Research study," *Mayo Clinic Proceedings*, vol. 81, no. 7, pp. 880–888, 2006.

[32] N. Leung, A. Dispenzieri, F. C. Fervenza et al., "Renal response after high-dose melphalan and stem cell transplantation is a favorable marker in patients with primary systemic amyloidosis," *American Journal of Kidney Diseases*, vol. 46, no. 2, pp. 270–277, 2005.

[33] M. Skinner, V. Sanchorawala, D. C. Seldin et al., "High-dose melphalan and autologous stem-cell transplantation in patients with AL amyloidosis: an 8-year study," *Annals of Internal Medicine*, vol. 140, no. 2, pp. 85–93, 2004.

[34] S. Madan, S. K. Kumar, A. Dispenzieri et al., "High-dose melphalan and peripheral blood stem cell transplantation for light-chain amyloidosis with cardiac involvement," *Blood*, vol. 46, no. 5, pp. 1117–1122.

[35] I. I. Van Gameren, M. H. Van Rijswijk, J. Bijzet, E. Vellenga, and B. P. Hazenberg, "Histological regression of amyloid in AL amyloidosis is exclusively seen after normalization of serum free light chain," *Haematologica*, vol. 94, no. 8, pp. 1094–1100, 2009.

[36] A. Dispenzieri, M. Q. Lacy, R. A. Kyle et al., "Eligibility for hematopoietic stem-cell transplantation for primary systemic amyloidosis is a favorable prognostic factor for survival," *Journal of Clinical Oncology*, vol. 19, no. 14, pp. 3350–3356, 2001.

[37] A. Dispenzieri, R. A. Kyle, M. Q. Lacy et al., "Superior survival in primary systemic amyloidosis patients undergoing peripheral blood stem cell transplantation: a case-control study," *Blood*, vol. 103, no. 10, pp. 3960–3963, 2004.

[38] D. C. Seldin, J. J. Anderson, V. Sanchorawala et al., "Improvement in quality of life of patients with AL amyloidosis treated with high-dose melphalan and autologous stem cell transplantation," *Blood*, vol. 104, no. 6, pp. 1888–1893, 2004.

[39] A. Jaccard, P. Moreau, V. Leblond et al., "High-dose melphalan versus melphalan plus dexamethasone for AL amyloidosis," *New England Journal of Medicine*, vol. 357, no. 11, pp. 1083–1093, 2007.

[40] S. Kumar, A. Dispenzieri, and M. A. Gertz, "High-dose melphalan versus melphalan plus dexamethasone for AL amyloidosis," *New England Journal of Medicine*, vol. 358, no. 1, p. 91, 2008.

[41] J. Mehta, "High-dose melphalan versus melphalan plus dexamethasone for AL amyloidosis," *New England Journal of Medicine*, vol. 358, no. 1, p. 91, 2008.

[42] R. L. Comenzo, R. M. Steingart, and A. D. Cohen, "High-dose melphalan versus melphalan plus dexamethasone for AL amyloidosis," *New England Journal of Medicine*, vol. 358, no. 1, p. 92, 2008.

[43] R. Mhaskar, A. Kumar, M. Behera, M. A. Kharfan-Dabaja, and B. Djulbegovic, "Role of high-dose chemotherapy and autologous hematopoietic cell transplantation in primary systemic amyloidosis: a systematic review," *Biology of Blood and Marrow Transplantation*, vol. 15, no. 8, pp. 893–902, 2009.

[44] E. Kastritis, A. D. Wechalekar, M. A. Dimopoulos et al., "Bortezomib with or without dexamethasone in primary systemic (light chain) amyloidosis," *Journal of Clinical Oncology*, vol. 28, no. 6, pp. 1031–1037, 2010.

[45] C. Gasparetto, V. Sanchorawala, R. M. Snyder et al., "Use of melphalan (M)/dexamethasone (D)/bortezomib in AL amyloidosis," *Journal of Clinical Oncology*, vol. 28, abstract 8024, 2010.

[46] V. Jimenez-Zepeda, C. B. Reeder, J. R. Mikhael et al., "Cyclophosphamide, bortezomib and dexamethasone (CyBORD) induces rapid and complete responses in patients with amyloidosis not eligible for peripheral blood stem cell transplant," *Blood*, vol. 114, abstract 1857, 2010.

[47] M. W. Brunvand and M. Bitter, "Amyloidosis relapsing after autologous stem cell transplantation treated with bortezomib: normalization of detectable serum-free light chains and reversal of tissue damage with improved suitability for transplant," *Haematologica*, vol. 95, no. 3, pp. 519–521, 2010.

[48] Mayo Consensus on AL Amyloidosis: Diagnosis and Treatment, 2011, http://www.msmart.org/msmart_mar09_002 .htm.

17

Role of HLA in Hematopoietic Stem Cell Transplantation

Meerim Park[1] and Jong Jin Seo[2]

[1] *Department of Pediatrics, College of Medicine, Chungbuk National University, Cheongju, Republic of Korea*
[2] *Department of Pediatrics, Asan Medical Center Children's Hospital, University of Ulsan College of Medicine, Seoul, Republic of Korea*

Correspondence should be addressed to Jong Jin Seo, jjseo@amc.seoul.kr

Academic Editor: Andrzej Lange

The selection of hematopoietic stem cell transplantation (HSCT) donors includes a rigorous assessment of the availability and human leukocyte antigen (HLA) match status of donors. HLA plays a critical role in HSCT, but its involvement in HSCT is constantly in flux because of changing technologies and variations in clinical transplantation results. The increased availability of HSCT through the use of HLA-mismatched related and unrelated donors is feasible with a more complete understanding of permissible HLA mismatches and the role of killer-cell immunoglobulin-like receptor (KIR) genes in HSCT. The influence of nongenetic factors on the tolerability of HLA mismatching has recently become evident, demonstrating a need for the integration of both genetic and nongenetic variables in donor selection.

1. Introduction

Allogeneic hematopoietic stem cell transplantation (HSCT) has been established as a mode of curative therapy for hematologic malignancies and other hematologic or immune disorders. Hematopoietic stem cell donor selection has been almost exclusively based on selecting an human leukocyte antigen (HLA) identical donor or near-identical donor; however, not all patients are able to find a suitable donor. Advances in HLA testing and matching and understanding donor selection factors are therefore important to improve outcomes of unrelated donor (UD) HSCT. HLAs can elicit an immune response either by presentation of variable peptides or by recognition of polymorphic fragments of foreign HLA molecules. HLA disparity has been associated with graft failure, delayed immune reconstitution, graft-versus-host disease (GVHD), and mortality. Since many patients lack HLA-matched donors, current research is focused on the identifying permissible HLA mismatches. Recently, extensive research has accumulated evidence on the role of each HLA locus mismatch on clinical outcome for UD HSCT, making it easy to search for and select a partially matched donor [1, 2].

In this paper, we will focus on the current understanding of HLA typing and its clinical implications on UD HSCT.

2. HLA Typing

HLA class I and II loci are the most polymorphic genes in the human genome, with a highly clustered and patchwork pattern of sequence motifs [3]. Each individual carries 10 to 12 genes that encode the HLA-A, -B, -C, -DR, -DQ, and -DP. Most of these genes are highly polymorphic, ranging from 13 (HLA-DRB4) to 699 (HLA-B) alleles per locus [4]. Extensive allelic diversity has made, and continues to make, high-resolution HLA-DNA typing very challenging. Over the past three decades, the remarkable extent of allelic diversity at these loci has been shown by molecular genetic analyses, made possible by the development of recombinant DNA technology, chain-termination Sanger sequencing, and PCR amplification [3].

Initially, HLA-DNA typing involved restriction fragment length polymorphism (RFLP) analysis, but this approach had many limitations in terms of workflow and resolution and represented at best a complement to, rather than a replacement for, serological typing [5]. The development of PCR in 1985 allowed for the amplification of the polymorphic exons of the HLA class I and II genes and for the analysis of polymorphic sequence motifs with sequence-specific oligonucleotide (SSO) hybridization probes. Currently available methods to identify specific polymorphisms or nucleotide motifs include SSO probe hybridization, sequence-specific primer (SSP) amplification, sequencing-based typing (SBT), and reference-strand-based conformation analysis [3, 6]. Both PCR-SSP and PCR-SSO rely on the use of oligonucleotide primers or probes to react and/or detect specific and previously known polymorphic sequence motifs present within the amplified HLA-allele fragment. A major disadvantage is that such methods rely on the screening of a limited number of previously known polymorphisms. Therefore, when a novel allele is present a sample, mistyping can occur, depending on whether the allele possesses a different polymorphism or different arrangement of known polymorphisms. However, SBT uses generic oligonucleotide primers directed towards conserved regions of a locus to amplify the polymorphic exons of all alleles. Although SBT is able to detect previously unknown HLA alleles, it is not entirely capable of resolving novel arrangements of known polymorphisms, a limitation known as ambiguity. This problem can be overcome by separating the alleles by groups or allele-specific PCR, cloning, or by the use of conformational techniques. Conformational methods, such as the Reference-Strand-mediated Conformational Analysis (RSCA), have shown to achieve high-resolution results without the ambiguities seen in the previously mentioned methods [7].

HLA-typing methods convey certain advantages and present various limitations. Matching by high-resolution HLA typing, a more recent and sophisticated method, certainly reduces the risk of immune complications, namely, graft rejection and GVHD along with increased chance of finding a suitable donor [2]. As such, the choice of method is dependent on the intended application and on establishing an appropriate balance of what level of resolution is needed with regards to speed of typing, cost, and human intervention [8].

3. Effect of HLA on Clinical Outcomes after HSCT

3.1. Number of HLA Mismatches. Advances in HLA-typing techniques allowing better matching of donor-to-recipient have improved the prognosis of HSCT. A recent prospective study investigating outcomes after transplant with 10/10 allelic-matched unrelated donors (MUDs) and HLA-identical sibling grafts for patients with standard-risk hematological malignancies showed that overall survival, disease-free survival, transplantation-related mortality (TRM), relapse, and acute GVHD were not dependent on donor type [9]. The similar outcome values for different donor types suggest that well-selected UDs can perform as well as HLA-identical sibling donors. Immune genetic disparity in the donor-recipient pair is associated with a worse patient outcome, mainly due to the high incidence of transplantation-related complications. A direct assessment of the number of HLA mismatches between the donor and the recipient has highlighted its great importance in UD HSCT. As the number of class I and II HLA mismatches increases, the risks of graft failure, GVHD, and mortality increase [10–12]. Indeed,

a recent analysis by the Center for International Blood and Marrow Transplant Research (CIBMTR) on patients with hematological malignancies, mainly transplanted with bone marrow cells, has shown that, as compared to patients transplanted from a donor matched at the allelic level for HLA-A, -B, -C, and -DRB1, patients given an allograft from a donor with a single antigenic or allelic disparity had an increased risk of both acute GVHD and TRM [2]. Disparities at two or more loci compounded this risk.

3.2. Permissible Mismatches. The need to broaden the availability of UD HSCT for patients who lack a matched donor has provided a rationale to define permissible HLA mismatches. The most important HLA loci influencing posttransplant outcome of patients given HSCT from UDs are HLA-A, -B, -C and -DRB1 [13, 14]. There have been several large-scale analyses on the role of each HLA locus in non-T-cell-depleted UD HSCT (Table 1). The Japan Marrow Donor Program (JMDP) showed the effect of matching HLA class I alleles on the development of severe acute GVHD and the importance of HLA-A and -B allele matching for better survival [10, 15]. The Fred Hutchinson Cancer Research Center (FHCRC) and the US National Marrow Donor Program (NMDP) reported the importance of HLA class II matching to prevent GVHD and to increase survival [13, 16]. An analysis of NMDP in 2004 indicated that HLA-A allele level mismatching, HLA-B serological mismatching, and DRB1 mismatching are significant risk factors for severe acute GVHD and that disparity in HLA class I and/or HLA-DRB1 increases the incidence of mortality [14]. An analysis of NMDP published in 2007 showed that the impact of HLA-A or -DRB1 mismatch on overall survival was more marked than a mismatch at HLA-B or -C [2]. And recent analysis of Korean data showed the importance of HLA-B and -C locus matching for better survival [11]. However, the above-mentioned reports, as well as others, have produced considerable conflicting results on the causal role of HLA mismatch locus on clinical outcomes.

The significance of HLA mismatching may be related to population-based locus- and allele-specific differences that distinguish ethnically diverse transplant donors and recipients. The International Histocompatibility Working Group (IHWG) studied the impact of individual locus mismatches in different populations [17]. The authors found that a single HLA-A mismatch was poorly tolerated in JMDP transplant recipients, but less detrimental in the non-JMDP population. Conversely, mismatches at HLA-C were well tolerated among the JMDP patients, but poorly tolerated among non-JMDP patients. One explanation for this may be differences in the actual allele mismatches in these separate populations. Morishima et al. [18] reported that the most frequent mismatch found in Japanese patients was HLA-A*0201 and HLA-A*0206 and that this mismatch was deleterious. By contrast, the most common HLA-A*02 mismatch in Caucasians was found to be HLA-A*0201 and HLA-A*0205, and an adverse relationship between this mismatch and transplantation outcomes was not found. The identification of a nonpermissive HLA-allele mismatch combination

TABLE 1: Effect of HLA mismatching on survival.

Study	Mismatched HLA locus			
	A	B	C	DRB1
Petersdorf et al. [13]	Merged A, B, and C Decreased			Decreased
Morishima et al. [10]	Decreased	Decreased	None	None
Flomenberg et al. [14]	Decreased	Decreased	Decreased	Decreased
Lee et al. [2]	Decreased	None	Decreased	Decreased
Park et al. [11]	None	Decreased	Decreased	None

indicates that the ethnic diversity of the recipient and donor can translate into molecular differences based on HLA alleles, indicating that it is essential to reconcile differences in HLA risk observed among ethnically diverse transplant groups. Analysis of HLA-DPB1 mismatches in this way has lead to interesting findings [19, 20]. Crocchiolo et al. [21] reported a significantly higher 2-year survival in transplants with permissive as compared to nonpermissive HLA-DPB1 mismatches (54.8% versus 39.1%, $P = 0.005$). Similarly, Zino et al. [20] found a significantly higher risk of mortality in patients with nonpermissive DPB1 mismatches compared to those without such mismatches.

3.3. HLA-DQ and HLA-DP. The importance of HLA-A, -B, -C, and -DR in HSCT has been well described, whereas there have been conflicting results as to the clinical significance of HLA-DP and -DQ. Less than 20% of transplants matched for HLA-A, -B, -C, -DRB1, and -DQB1 are also compatible for HLA-DPB1, due to the very weak linkage disequilibrium existing between the DR/DQ loci and the DP locus. Therefore, over 80% of unrelated transplants are performed across the HLA-DPB1 barrier [2, 22]. Furthermore, the low frequency of fortuitous HLA-DP matching hinders a precise analysis of the true independent effects of HLA-DP mismatching except in cases of very large numbers of transplants. Early investigations were conflicting as to the significance of HLA-DP as a classical transplantation determinant. In a recent analysis of 627 HLA-identical sibling transplants, of which 30 were HLA-DP-mismatched due to recombination, HLA-DP mismatch was an independent risk factor for GVHD [23]. Furthermore, Schaffer et al. [24] reported that mismatching for HLA-DP was a risk factor for increased mortality compared to DP matching. Most studies now agree that HLA-DQB1 does not need to be considered in a well-matched donor [10], but evidence supports that there may be an additive effect of a DQB1 mismatch if a mismatch at another locus is present [25]. Taken together, roles of the HLA-DQ and DP loci remain not fully elucidated. However, previous results suggest that when patients have a choice of equivalently matched donors, selection of an HLA-DQB1-matched donor over a mismatched donor may decrease posttransplant complications.

3.4. Level of HLA Disparity. The level of HLA disparity (antigenic or allele level) affects HSCT outcome differently [26–28]. Sequence analyses show that antigenic disparity is frequently associated with more than ten amino acid substitutions in HLA molecules, which can be easily recognized by immunocompetent cells, thereby stimulating an immune response [26]. Allele level disparity most frequently concerns only one or a few amino acid substitutions, which should produce weaker immune stimulations. A linear increase in the number of amino acid substitutions in the disparate HLA molecule may cause significant deleterious effects or be irrelevant in HSCT [26, 29]. However, there are conflicting data concerning the value of selecting an allelic mismatch over an antigenic mismatch. According to Lee et al. [2], there were no significant differences in survival depending on whether the mismatch was allelic or antigenic, except at HLA-C, in which an antigenic mismatch increased transplant risks while an allelic mismatch did not. Similarly, a single-center study from Seattle could not find any apparent difference between allele and antigen mismatches with respect to the number of deaths from transplants, suggesting that donors with a single HLA allele of antigen mismatch may be used for HSCT when a fully MUD is not available for patients with severe diseases not permitting time for a lengthy search [25]. However, the NMDP study found that antigenic mismatch was associated with higher mortality compared to allelic mismatch [14]. They indicated that selection of donors with high-resolution mismatches over those with low-resolution mismatches may lower the rate of posttransplant complications. The analysis of large transplant populations with a diversity of mismatches is needed to further define potential differences between allele and antigen mismatches in post-HSCT complications.

3.5. Tolerable Mismatches. Although HLA-identical donors are now known to be the gold standard, using a donor with a single-allele mismatch has been associated with an equally favorable outcome in certain situations. According to the report of Teshima et al. [30], reduced intensity conditioning (RIC) transplantation from a two- to three-loci-mismatched donor resulted in poor outcome, as shown in conventional HSCT. However, the 2-year overall survival after one-locus-mismatched RIC transplantation was comparable with that of HLA-matched RIC transplantation in high-risk malignancies. In a study of T-cell-depleted RIC transplants, there was no significant difference in overall survival between matched or one-antigen-mismatched grafts [31]. A recent report from the United Kingdom, in recipients of T-cell-depleted RIC transplantation protocols using Alemtuzumab, showed that transplant outcomes were similar between HLA-matched and, mismatched pairs [32]. As listed above, in settings of T-cell depletion and/or RIC transplantation, the impact of HLA matching may differ and these conditions require further investigation.

3.6. Importance of Disease Stage. It is important to note that the effect of a single-allele mismatch may vary with the underlying diagnosis. In a recent publication on 948 donor-recipient pairs at the FHCRC, it was found that a single-allele mismatch conferred a higher risk of death, but only for low-risk patients, defined as those with chronic myeloid leukemia (CML) within 2 years of diagnosis [25]. By contrast, a single-allele mismatch had no effect on survival among higher-risk patients, such as those with more advanced CML, acute leukemia, or myelodysplastic syndrome. Similar outcomes are reported in a recent report from an Italian group [33]. When only a single HLA mismatch (9/10 matched pairs) was present, the mortality risk was higher than among 10/10 matched pairs in patients transplanted with acute leukemia in the first CR (early stage disease), but not in patients with advanced diseases. These results suggest that the potential benefit of HLA matching was offset by the negative impact of advanced disease. Therefore, if a donor search is highly unlikely to yield matched donors in the early phases of disease, the increased mortality associated with a longer time interval from diagnosis to transplantation must be weighed carefully against the increased mortality associated with earlier HSCT with a mismatched donor, as well as against the chance of disease progression during the prolonged donor search.

4. The Role of Anti-HLA Antibodies

Donor-specific anti-HLA antibodies (DSHAs) have been implicated in graft rejection in solid-organ transplantation, but their role in allogeneic HSCT remains under investigation [34–36]. Controversy exists as to whether DSHAs actually mediate graft rejection or if they are surrogate markers for cellular immunity that cause graft failure [37]. DSHAs cause graft failures in animal models of allogenic HSCT, mainly because the cognate HLA antigens are expressed on hematopoietic stem cells and hematopoietic precursors [38].

The complement-dependent microlymphocytotoxicity assay (CDC) has been the standard method for the detection of anti-HLA antibodies for the last 30 years [39]. The recent introduction of solid-phase assays enabled a reassessment of the role of both HLA class I and II antibodies in organ rejection. Spellman et al. [40] tested archived pretransplantation sera from graft failure patients and a matched-control cohort to evaluate the role of DSHAs in UD HSCT. The presence of DSHAs was significantly associated with graft failure (odds ratio = 22.84; 95% CI, 3.57–infinity), indicating that the presence of pretransplantation DSHAs in recipients of UD HSCT should be considered in donor selection. Similarly, Ciurea et al. [41] found that DSHAs were associated with a high rate of graft rejection in patients undergoing haploidentical HSCT. On the basis of the

previously mentioned findings, DSHA identification should be performed in HSCT settings where HLA matching is not complete [42]. Immunoadsorption and plasmapheresis could be considered to desensitize the recipient when no alternative donor is available.

5. Killer Immunoglobulin-Like Receptor (KIR) Ligand Incompatibility

Natural killer (NK) cells and subpopulations of T cells express NK cell receptors. The activity of NK cells is controlled by the recognition of HLA class I molecules on the target cells by NK cell inhibitory and activating receptors [43, 44]. Depending on the type of KIR, ligation by HLA can stimulate or inhibit the ability of NK cells to kill foreign cells, including tumor cells [45]. The coexistence of the incompatibility of both types on the same HLA molecules makes it difficult to show the advantages of KIR-ligand mismatches clearly. The strong immune reactions provoked by T-cell recognition elements on incompatible HLA molecule can probably override the favorable effect of the simultaneous KIR-ligand mismatch [46]. In fact, Farag et al. [47] investigated the effect of KIR-ligand mismatching on the outcome of UD HSCT in the T-replete setting. In that study, patients who received grafts from donors mismatched at the KIR ligand and at HLA-B and/or C but matched at the KIR ligand had similar rates of TRM, treatment failure, and overall mortality. By contrast, Giebel et al. [48] investigated UD HSCT in 130 patients with acute myeloid leukemia (AML), acute lymphoblastic leukemia (ALL), or CML, who received unmanipulated grafts. The results of that study showed that transplant from KIR-incompatible donors resulted in enhanced overall survival, decreased disease relapse, and increased probability of disease-free survival. When myeloid leukemia patients were selected for analysis, these effects became more prominent, suggesting that patients with myeloid malignancies were more responsive to treatment. More recently, Cooley et al. [49, 50] analyzed the outcomes of 1,409 patients, taking into account the role of KIR-gene variability. Donor KIR genotype influenced transplantation outcomes for patients with AML but not for those with ALL. Compared to donors without KIR mismatches, donors having KIR mismatches showed reduced incidences of relapse and improved disease-free survival. Furthermore, KIR-ligand incompatibility in the graft-versus-host direction in haplotype-mismatched transplants suggests a possible clinical benefit as it may allow early recovery of donor alloreactive NK cells with enhanced antileukemia activity in AML [51].

If KIR mismatch results in graft versus tumor (GVT) effects, one may assume that several mismatches would result in further enhances in the GVT effect. Previous transplant studies commented upon the impact of numerous mismatches compared to one mismatch. Clausen et al. [52] demonstrated that relapse risk was decreased in patients who underwent HLA-identical sibling HSCT who both received high NK cell dose and lacked at least one HLA-B or HLA-C ligand to a present donor's inhibitory KIR. In that study, transplants with more than two different activating donor KIRs were associated with an increased risk for nonrelapse morality. Similarly, Willemze et al. [53] reported that a higher number of HLA disparities resulted in a decreased incidence of relapse in patients who received umbilical cord blood transplantation.

Collectively, it is clear that the exploitation of NK cell alloreactivity as a therapeutic advantage in HSCT is promising, and certain patients with myeloid malignancies have benefited from allogeneic HSCT. KIR genotyping of several best HLA-matched potential UDs may change clinical practice in the future [54].

6. Conclusion

A donor's HLA match status should be considered to help the physician and patient in transplantation-related risk assessment and in planning treatment options based on those risks. The benefits of high-resolution HLA class I and II typing have been well demonstrated, particularly for posttransplant survival. The current gold standard is a donor matched for 8/8 alleles; however, it is clear that mismatches may be tolerated with regards to survival in some transplant settings and that evidence for permissive mismatches exists. Permissiveness depends not only on the potential adverse effects of HLA mismatches, but also on the urgency of the HSCT, the desirable GVT effect, and the potential efficacy of the alternative therapy available for the patient. Further knowledge on DSHAs, NK cell alloreactivity, and KIR receptors will aid HSCT in becoming safer and more efficacious.

Conflict of Interests

The authors declare they have no conflict of interests.

Acknowledgment

This study was supported by a Grant from the National R&D Program for Cancer Control, Ministry for Health and Welfare, Republic of Korea (0520290-3).

References

[1] T. Kawase, Y. Morishima, K. Matsuo et al., "High-risk HLA allele mismatch combinations responsible for severe acute graft-versus-host disease and implication for its molecular mechanism," *Blood*, vol. 110, no. 7, pp. 2235–2241, 2007.

[2] S. J. Lee, J. Klein, M. Haagenson et al., "High-resolution donor-recipient HLA matching contributes to the success of unrelated donor marrow transplantation," *Blood*, vol. 110, no. 13, pp. 4576–4583, 2007.

[3] H. Erlich, "HLA DNA typing: past, present, and future," *Tissue Antigens*, vol. 80, no. 1, pp. 1–11, 2012.

[4] S. G. E. Marsh, E. D. Albert, W. F. Bodmer et al., "Nomenclature for factors of the HLA system, 2004," *Tissue Antigens*, vol. 65, no. 4, pp. 301–369, 2005.

[5] P. Parham, "Histocompatibility typing—Mac is back in town," *Immunology Today*, vol. 9, no. 5, pp. 127–130, 1988.

[6] J. R. Argüello and J. A. Madrigal, "HLA typing by Reference Strand Mediated Conformation Analysis (RSCA)," *Reviews in immunogenetics*, vol. 1, no. 2, pp. 209–219, 1999.

[7] J. R. Argüellol, A. M. Little, A. L. Pay et al., "Mutation detection and typing of polymorphic loci through double-strand conformation analysis," *Nature Genetics*, vol. 18, no. 2, pp. 192–194, 1998.

[8] B. E. Shaw, R. Arguello, C. A. Garcia-Sepulveda, and J. A. Madrigal, "The impact of HLA genotyping on survival following unrelated donor haematopoietic stem cell transplantation," *British Journal of Haematology*, vol. 150, no. 3, pp. 251–258, 2010.

[9] I. Yakoub-Agha, F. Mesnil, M. Kuentz et al., "Allogeneic marrow stem-cell transplantation from human leukocyte antigen-identical siblings versus human leukocyte antigen-allelic-matched unrelated donors (10/10) in patients with standard-risk hematologic malignancy: a prospective study from the French society of bone marrow transplantation and cell therapy," *Journal of Clinical Oncology*, vol. 24, no. 36, pp. 5695–5702, 2006.

[10] Y. Morishima, T. Sasazuki, H. Inoko et al., "The clinical significance of human leukocyte antigen (HLA) allele compatibility in patients receiving a marrow transplant from serologically HLA-A, HLA-B, and HLA-DR matched unrelated donors," *Blood*, vol. 99, no. 11, pp. 4200–4206, 2002.

[11] M. Park, K. N. Koh, B. E. Kim et al., "The impact of HLA matching on unrelated donor hematopoietic stem cell transplantation in Korean children," *Korean Journal of Hematology*, vol. 46, no. 1, pp. 11–17, 2011.

[12] E. W. Petersdorf, J. A. Hansen, P. J. Martin et al., "Major-histocompatibility-complex class I alleles and antigens in hematopoietic-cell transplantation," *New England Journal of Medicine*, vol. 345, no. 25, pp. 1794–1800, 2001.

[13] E. W. Petersdorf, T. A. Gooley, C. Anasetti et al., "Optimizing outcome after unrelated marrow transplantation by comprehensive matching of HLA class I and II alleles in the donor and recipient," *Blood*, vol. 92, no. 10, pp. 3515–3520, 1998.

[14] N. Flomenberg, L. A. Baxter-Lowe, D. Confer et al., "Impact of HLA class I and class II high-resolution matching on outcomes of unrelated donor bone marrow transplantation: HLA-C mismatching is associated with a strong adverse effect on transplantation outcome," *Blood*, vol. 104, no. 7, pp. 1923–1930, 2004.

[15] T. Sasazuki, T. Juji, Y. Morishima et al., "Effect of matching of class I HLA alleles on clinical outcome after transplantation of hematopoietic stem cells from an unrelated donor," *New England Journal of Medicine*, vol. 339, no. 17, pp. 1177–1185, 1998.

[16] E. W. Petersdorf, C. Kollman, C. K. Hurley et al., "Effect of HLA class II gene disparity on clinical outcome in unrelated donor hematopoietic cell transplantation for chronic myeloid leukemia: the US National Marrow Donor Program experience," *Blood*, vol. 98, no. 10, pp. 2922–2929, 2001.

[17] E. W. Petersdorf, T. Gooley, M. Malkki, and M. Horowitz, "Clinical significance of donor-recipient HLA matching on survival after myeloablative hematopoietic cell transplantation from unrelated donors," *Tissue Antigens*, vol. 69, supplement 1, pp. 25–30, 2007.

[18] Y. Morishima, T. Kawase, M. Malkki, and E. W. Petersdorf, "Effect of HLA-A2 allele disparity on clinical outcome in hematopoietic cell transplantation from unrelated donors," *Tissue Antigens*, vol. 69, supplement 1, pp. 31–35, 2007.

[19] K. Fleischhauer, E. Zino, B. Mazzi et al., "Peripheral blood stem cell allograft rejection mediated by CD4$^+$ T lymphocytes

recognizing a single mismatch at HLA-DPβ1*0901," *Blood*, vol. 98, no. 4, pp. 1122–1126, 2001.

[20] E. Zino, G. Frumento, S. Marktel et al., "A T-cell epitope encoded by a subset of HLA-DPB1 alleles determines non-permissive mismatches for hematologic stem cell transplantation," *Blood*, vol. 103, no. 4, pp. 1417–1424, 2004.

[21] R. Crocchiolo, E. Zino, L. Vago et al., "Nonpermissive HLA-DPB1 disparity is a significant independent risk factor for mortality after unrelated hematopoietic stem cell transplantation," *Blood*, vol. 114, no. 7, pp. 1437–1444, 2009.

[22] E. W. Petersdorf, T. Gooley, M. Malkki et al., "The biological significance of HLA-DP gene variation in haematopoietic cell transplantation," *British Journal of Haematology*, vol. 112, no. 4, pp. 988–994, 2001.

[23] D. Gallardo, S. Brunet, A. Torres et al., "HLA-DPB1 mismatch in HLA-A-B-DRB1 identical sibling donor stem cell transplantation and acute graft-versus-host disease," *Transplantation*, vol. 77, no. 7, pp. 1107–1110, 2004.

[24] M. Schaffer, A. Aldener-Cannavá, M. Remberger, O. Ringdén, and O. Olerup, "Roles of HLA-B, HLA-C and HLA-DPA1 incompatibilities in the outcome of unrelated stem-cell transplantation," *Tissue Antigens*, vol. 62, no. 3, pp. 243–250, 2003.

[25] E. W. Petersdorf, C. Anasetti, P. J. Martin et al., "Limits of HLA mismatching in unrelated hematopoietic cell transplantation," *Blood*, vol. 104, no. 9, pp. 2976–2980, 2004.

[26] H. T. Greinix, I. Faé, B. Schneider et al., "Impact of HLA class I high-resolution mismatches on chronic graft-versus-host disease and survival of patients given hematopoietic stem cell grafts from unrelated donors," *Bone Marrow Transplantation*, vol. 35, no. 1, pp. 57–62, 2005.

[27] C. Liao, J. Y. Wu, Z. P. Xu et al., "Indiscernible benefit of high-resolution HLA typing in improving long-term clinical outcome of unrelated umbilical cord blood transplant," *Bone Marrow Transplantation*, vol. 40, no. 3, pp. 201–208, 2007.

[28] M. B. A. Heemskerk, J. J. Cornelissen, D. L. Roelen et al., "Highly diverged MHC class I mismatches are acceptable for haematopoietic stem cell transplantation," *Bone Marrow Transplantation*, vol. 40, no. 3, pp. 193–200, 2007.

[29] G. B. Ferrara, A. Bacigalupo, T. Lamparelli et al., "Bone marrow transplantation from unrelated donors: the impact of mismatches with substitutions at position 116 of the human leukocyte antigen class I heavy chain," *Blood*, vol. 98, no. 10, pp. 3150–3155, 2001.

[30] T. Teshima, K. Matsuo, K. Matsue et al., "Impact of human leucocyte antigen mismatch on graft-versus-host disease and graft failure after reduced intensity conditioning allogeneic haematopoietic stem cell transplantation from related donors," *British Journal of Haematology*, vol. 130, no. 4, pp. 575–587, 2005.

[31] B. E. Shaw, N. H. Russell, S. Devereux et al., "The impact of donor factors on primary non-engraftment in recipients of reduced intensity conditioned transplants from unrelated donors," *Haematologica*, vol. 90, no. 11, pp. 1562–1569, 2005.

[32] A. J. Mead, K. J. Thomson, E. C. Morris et al., "HLA-mismatched unrelated donors are a viable alternate graft source for allogeneic transplantation following alemtuzumab-based reduced-intensity conditioning," *Blood*, vol. 115, no. 25, pp. 5147–5153, 2010.

[33] R. Crocchiolo, F. Ciceri, K. Fleischhauer et al., "HLA matching affects clinical outcome of adult patients undergoing haematopoietic SCT from unrelated donors: a study from the Gruppo Italiano Trapianto di Midollo Osseo and Italian Bone Marrow Donor Registry," *Bone Marrow Transplantation*, vol. 44, no. 9, pp. 571–577, 2009.

[34] F. H. Claas, "Clinical relevance of circulating donor-specific HLA antibodies," *Current Opinion in Organ Transplantation*, vol. 15, no. 4, pp. 462–466, 2010.

[35] C. Lefaucheur, C. Suberbielle-Boissel, G. S. Hill et al., "Clinical relevance of preformed HLA donor-specific antibodies in kidney transplantation," *Contributions to Nephrology*, vol. 162, pp. 1–12, 2009.

[36] E. M. Van Den Berg-Loonen, E. V. A. Billen, C. E. M. Voorter et al., "Clinical relevance of pretransplant donor-directed antibodies detected by single antigen beads in highly sensitized renal transplant patients," *Transplantation*, vol. 85, no. 8, pp. 1086–1090, 2008.

[37] R. Storb, "B cells versus T cells as primary barrier to hematopoietic engraftment in allosensitized recipients," *Blood*, vol. 113, no. 5, p. 1205, 2009.

[38] M. Gabbianelli, G. Boccoli, S. Petti et al., "Expression and in-vitro modulation of HLA antigens in ontogenic development of human hemopoietic system," *Annals of the New York Academy of Sciences*, vol. 511, pp. 138–147, 1987.

[39] P. I. Terasaki, M. R. Mickey, D. P. Singal, K. K. Mittal, and R. Patel, "Serotyping for homotransplantation. XX. Selection of recipients for cadaver donor transplants," *New England Journal of Medicine*, vol. 279, no. 20, pp. 1101–1103, 1968.

[40] S. Spellman, R. Bray, S. Rosen-Bronson et al., "The detection of donor-directed, HLA-specific alloantibodies in recipients of unrelated hematopoietic cell transplantation is predictive of graft failure," *Blood*, vol. 115, no. 13, pp. 2704–2708, 2010.

[41] S. O. Ciurea, M. De Lima, P. Cano et al., "High risk of graft failure in patients with anti-hla antibodies undergoing haploidentical stem-cell transplantation," *Transplantation*, vol. 88, no. 8, pp. 1019–1024, 2009.

[42] D. Focosi, A. Zucca, and F. Scatena, "The role of anti-HLA antibodies in hematopoietic stem cell transplantation," *Biology of Blood and Marrow Transplantation*, vol. 17, no. 11, pp. 1585–1588, 2011.

[43] L. Moretta and A. Moretta, "Killer immunoglobulin-like receptors," *Current Opinion in Immunology*, vol. 16, no. 5, pp. 626–633, 2004.

[44] P. Parham, "MHC class I molecules and KIRS in human history, health and survival," *Nature Reviews Immunology*, vol. 5, no. 3, pp. 201–214, 2005.

[45] M. A. Cook, D. W. Milligan, C. D. Fegan et al., "The impact of donor KIR and patient HLA-C genotypes on outcome following HLA-identical sibling hematopoietic stem cell transplantation for myeloid leukemia," *Blood*, vol. 103, no. 4, pp. 1521–1526, 2004.

[46] E. J. Lowe, V. Turner, R. Handgretinger et al., "T-cell alloreactivity dominates natural killer cell alloreactivity in minimally T-cell-depleted HLA-non-identical paediatric bone marrow transplantation," *British Journal of Haematology*, vol. 123, no. 2, pp. 323–326, 2003.

[47] S. S. Farag, A. Bacigalupo, M. Eapen et al., "The effect of KIR ligand incompatibility on the outcome of unrelated donor transplantation: a report from the center for international blood and marrow transplant research, the European blood and marrow transplant registry, and the Dutch registry," *Biology of Blood and Marrow Transplantation*, vol. 12, no. 8, pp. 876–884, 2006.

[48] S. Giebel, F. Locatelli, T. Lamparelli et al., "Survival advantage with KIR ligand incompatibility in hematopoietic stem cell transplantation from unrelated donors," *Blood*, vol. 102, no. 3, pp. 814–819, 2003.

[49] S. Cooley, E. Trachtenberg, T. L. Bergemann et al., "Donors with group B KIR haplotypes improve relapse-free survival

after unrelated hematopoietic cell transplantation for acute myelogenous leukemia," *Blood*, vol. 113, no. 3, pp. 726–732, 2009.

[50] S. Cooley, D. J. Weisdorf, L. A. Guethlein et al., "Donor selection for natural killer cell receptor genes leads to superior survival after unrelated transplantation for acute myelogenous leukemia," *Blood*, vol. 116, no. 14, pp. 2411–2419, 2010.

[51] L. Ruggeri, M. Capanni, E. Urbani et al., "Effectiveness of donor natural killer cell aloreactivity in mismatched hematopoietic transplants," *Science*, vol. 295, no. 5562, pp. 2097–2100, 2002.

[52] J. Clausen, D. Wolf, A. L. Petzer et al., "Impact of natural killer cell dose and donor killer-cell immunoglobulin-like receptor (KIR) genotype on outcome following human leucocyte antigen-identical haematopoietic stem cell transplantation," *Clinical and Experimental Immunology*, vol. 148, no. 3, pp. 520–528, 2007.

[53] R. Willemze, C. A. Rodrigues, M. Labopin et al., "KIR-ligand incompatibility in the graft-versus-host direction improves outcomes after umbilical cord blood transplantation for acute leukemia," *Leukemia*, vol. 23, no. 3, pp. 492–500, 2009.

[54] H. J. Pegram, D. S. Ritchie, M. J. Smyth et al., "Alloreactive natural killer cells in hematopoietic stem cell transplantation," *Leukemia Research*, vol. 35, no. 1, pp. 14–21, 2011.

18

Curability of Multiple Myeloma

Raymond Alexanian, Kay Delasalle, Michael Wang, Sheeba Thomas, and Donna Weber

University of Texas MD Anderson Cancer Center, Houston, TX 77030-4009, USA

Correspondence should be addressed to Raymond Alexanian, ralexani@mdanderson.org

Academic Editor: Luciano J. Costa

Among 792 patients with multiple myeloma treated from 1987 to 2010 and assessed after 18 months, there were 167 patients with complete remission. For those 60 patients treated between 1987–1998 and with long followup, the latest relapse occurred after 11.8 years, so that 13 patients have remained in sustained complete remission for longer than 12 years (range 12–22 years). These results suggest that 3% of all patients treated during that period may be cured of multiple myeloma. In addition to immunofixation, more sensitive techniques for the detection of residual disease should be applied more consistently in patients with apparent complete remission in order to identify those with potential cure.

1. Introduction

In recent years, there have been major advances in the treatment of multiple myeloma, due to new agents, superior drug combinations, and widespread use of intensive therapy supported by autologous stem cells [1–5]. Thus, remission of disease has been achieved in 85–90% of currently treated patients, including 30–40% with complete remission (CR) [5–8]. This paper assessed the potential for curability among 792 patients with newly diagnosed myeloma treated at a single center over a long time span.

2. Patients and Methods

Between 1987–2010, we identified 792 newly diagnosed patients treated with primary, intermittent, high-dose dexamethasone-based regimens in sequential protocols (e.g., VAD, combinations with thalidomide, bortezomib, etc.) [1–3, 7, 8]. Patients older than 65 were excluded in order to assess results among those more likely to receive intensive therapy. Patients with nonsecretory or "hyposecretory" disease (e.g., only Bence Jones protein <50 mg/day) were excluded in order to define remission status clearly (Table 1). In order to assess the impact of improved treatments and the impact of prolonged complete remission (CR), we assessed

outcomes separately for those treated initially between 1987–1998 or 1999–2010. None of the patients treated between 1987–1998 had received thalidomide, lenalidomide, or bortezomib at diagnosis, but approximately 25% had received at least one of these drugs upon relapse; in contrast, all of the 330 patients treated between 1999–2010 had received at least one of those drugs as part of primary or salvage therapy. Cytogenetics was not evaluated since few patients were studied during the early treatment period.

Among all patients, intensive therapy (HDT) supported by autologous stem cells had been given within 1 year to 35% of those treated between 1987–1998 and to 82% of those treated later ($P < .01$). Details of these treatments have been described [9, 10]. All patients who received the different primary therapies were combined in the analysis, as were all patients who received the different HDT. (Most patients who had not received HDT had been denied insurance coverage, especially prior to 2000). Written permission for this retrospective review was provided by our Institutional Review Board, in accordance with an assurance approved by the Department of Health and Human Services.

3. Clinical Response and Statistical Methods

Partial response (PR) was defined as reduction of serum myeloma protein by >50% and of Bence Jones protein by

TABLE 1: Patient population (1987–2010).

No. patients	1070		
Age > 65	−246		
Non secretory or hyposecretory	−32		
No. studied	792		
	1987–1998 (%)	1999–2010 (%)	P
No. patients	462	330	
Deaths < 18 mo	96 (21)	35 (11)	<.01
No. HDT < 12 mo	162 (35)	272 (82)	<.01
Response status at 18 mo (%)			
No. patients	366	295	
NR	57 (16)	13 (5)	
PR	249 (68)	175 (59)	<.01
CR	60 (16)	107 (36)	
Duration of CR	No. (% of CR)		
>3 years	43 (72)	60 (56)	
>12 years	13 (22)	n.a.	

>90%. CR required disappearance of myeloma protein by immunofixation for at least 2 months [11]. Duration of CR was calculated from onset of CR to earliest sign of relapse, such as myeloma protein recurrence by immunofixation, new bone lesions, or marrow plasmacytosis.

Survival was calculated using the Kaplan and Meier method and differences between groups compared using the log-rank test [12, 13]. Since we desired to compare survival for patients with different degrees of response, landmark analysis was conducted after 18 months to avoid the potential bias of guaranteed survival. For 12 patients with onsets of PR or CR to later rescue treatments, survival and remission were censored at such change in status [14]; survival and remission were also censored at the last electrophoresis or immunofixation for 6 patients with CR or PR who died of unrelated diseases. Thus, 131 patients who died within 18 months were excluded from the survival analysis, including 80 patients with NR, 48 patients with PR, and 3 patients with CR; 42 of the 131 patients had received HDT with treatment-related deaths in 13 patients.

4. Results

4.1. Remission and Survival. The best remission status at 18 months following primary treatment was defined for all 661 patients alive at that time and subsequent survival by landmark analysis was assessed for each group based on response status. Among recently treated patients, there were significantly higher frequencies of CR (36 versus 16%) and lower frequencies of NR (5 versus 16%), in comparison with earlier patients (Table 1). Figure 1 not only depicts the longer survival for all patients treated since 1999 in comparison with the earlier group, but also the similar survival for each response status among those treated in the different time frames.

4.2. Complete Remission. We focused on long-term outcomes for the 167 patients with CR at 18 months among whom 86% had received HDT, in comparison with 51% of those with NR or PR (P < .01). Figure 2 shows the duration of CR for 60 patients treated between 1987–1998 and for 107 patients treated between 1999–2010, with longer duration among those treated during the earlier period (a); after landmark of 3 years following primary treatment, the differences were not significant (b). For the early treatment period, relapse of myeloma has not been seen in any patient after 12 years of CR, identifying 13 patients with sustained CR > 12 years (3% of all patients and 22% of those with CR). Clear plateaus in survival (Figure 1(a)) and in duration of CR (Figure 2(a)) were evident in patients with CR > 12 years. Yet, the higher frequency of CR with recent therapies was associated with a shorter remission time. All 13 patients with prolonged CR showed levels of uninvolved IgM that were either normal at diagnosis (>40 mg/dL) (9 patients) or had recovered to this level within 1 year of CR (4 patients).

We assessed various clinical features that might distinguish the 13 patients with CR > 12 years from the remaining 47 patients with shorter CR. There were no apparent differences in age, stage of disease, the frequency of HDT, or the pathway to reach CR with or without HDT. In addition, there was no correlation of prolonged CR with pretreatment levels of serum B_2M, LDH, and uninvolved IgA.

5. Discussion

In the past, criteria for improved treatments for multiple myeloma had focused on the achievement of higher response rates and longer survival. With the wider application of new drugs and intensive therapies, progressively higher frequencies of CR have been observed in recent years [6–8, 15–17]. Among all patients treated, frequencies of CR have increased from approximately 5% prior to 1987, to approximately 15% for those treated between 1987–1998, and to approximately 30% for those treated in recent year [4–8, 15–18]. Our paper focused on long-term outcomes and the potential for cure among patients with prolonged CR.

Criteria for complete remission, based on negative immunofixation sustained for at least 2 months [11], have been accepted for several years [11]. Greater sensitivities for the definition of CR have also been proposed using criteria that include the disappearance of clonal plasma cells by negative phenotype, normal molecular studies, and normal PET-scanning studies [19–21]. Further studies in large numbers of patients followed for long periods are required to clarify the added value of these procedures.

There has been recent controversy concerning the prospect of cure for patients with multiple myeloma [22–24]. The differences expressed have focused on the definition of CR and the uncertainty concerning the duration of CR. In regard to the definition of CR, many centers have considered patients with "near" CR as equivalent to CR, while others have included some patients with PR after reasoning that the residual monoclonal component may represent an MGUS

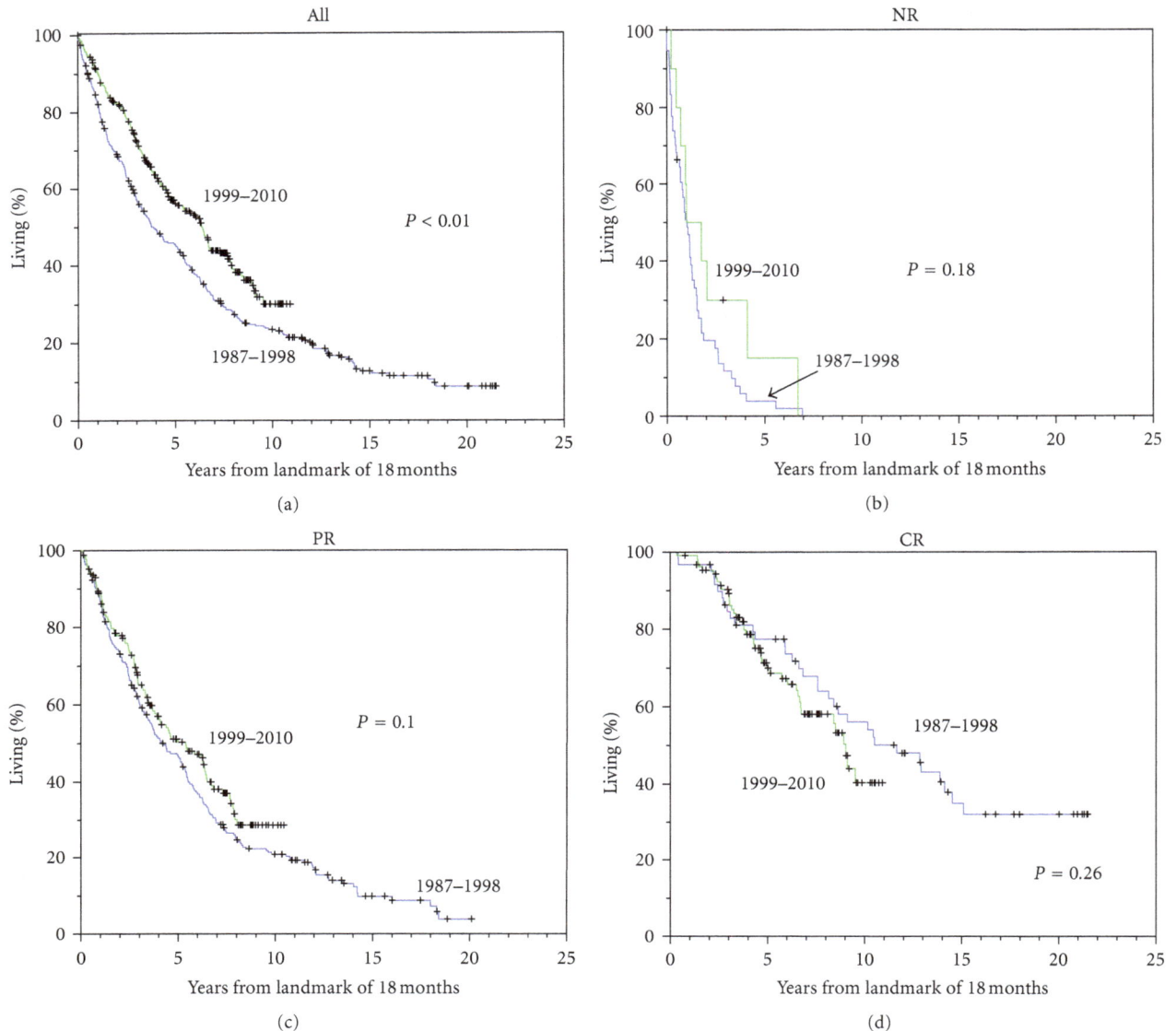

FigURE 1: Survival after landmark of 18 months for all patients (a) and for those with NR, PR, or CR as best response at 18 months, with patients separated by early versus later treatment period. Note: longer survival among all patients treated recently but similar survival for patients with the same response status.

status that preceded multiple myeloma [6, 22–24]. Even though many patients with "near" CR or PR have long survival, there is no evidence of a plateau in survival times for such patients, such as we describe here and others have described previously for patients with CR defined by negative immunofixation [25]. Definitions of CR that are not rigorous inflate the true frequency of CR and handicap the identification of those with meaningful potential for cure. Furthermore, Lahuerta et al. and Martinez-Lopez et al. have described significant differences in survival among patients with CR, near CR, or very good PR [5, 25]. Barlogie et al. have also shown that the implications of CR may be overrated since the duration of CR may be short (i.e., <3 years) due to early relapse of a more proliferative clone [18].

Following the sequence of conventional primary therapy followed by HDT supported by autologous stem cells, we observed a clear plateau in duration of CR and in survival for patients with CR sustained for at least 12 years. These findings affirm those described recently by Martinez-Lopez et al. who observed that patients treated from 1989–1998 and with sustained CR for longer than 11 years may be cured [25]. In our study, the higher frequency of CR with recent therapies was associated with shorter remission time, but this difference was not evident after requiring a landmark survival of 3 years. The validity of these findings are uncertain since the 2 groups of patients with CR were not comparable in terms of their primary therapies, the frequencies of HDT, and the unknown cytogenetic profiles.

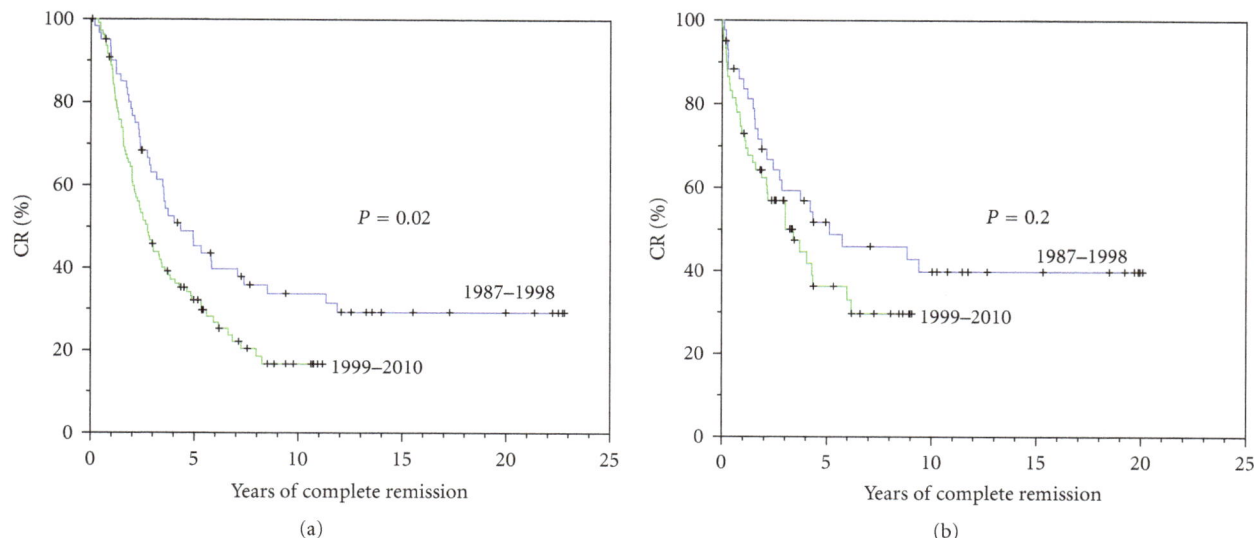

FIGURE 2: Durations of complete remission for 60 patients treated from 1987 to 1998 and for 107 patients treated from 1999 to 2010 (a). Durations of complete remission for the same group of patients after landmark of 3 years following primary therapy (b).

Also, Barlogie et al. have associated high frequencies of CR after intensive therapy with short durations in many patients, such as observed among many of our patients treated recently [18]. However, despite the more frequent use of HDT and new agents in the more recent cohort, the durations of CR appeared to be shorter so that CR as now defined may not be as predictive of cure as had appeared previously.

In view of the long CR in many patients and the potential for cure in some, maintenance therapy for CR remains controversial unless prognostic factors identify those who are more likely to have short CR. Until such guidelines become available, prolonged maintenance therapy may increase the likelihood of side effects, increase the cost, and promote resistance to later drug combinations upon relapse.

6. Conclusion

In this retrospective review of a large number of patients with multiple myeloma, we have not observed disease relapse in any patient with CR sustained for at least 12 years. For 13 such patients, who represented 3% of those treated from 1987 to 1998, there were clear plateaus in the duration of CR and in survival that were consistent with apparent cure of multiple myeloma.

Acknowledgment

The authors are indebted to Lisa Foucheaux-Heider for typing this paper.

References

[1] R. Alexanian, B. Barlogie, and S. Tucker, "VAD-based regimens as primary treatment for multiple myeloma," *American Journal of Hematology*, vol. 33, no. 2, pp. 86–89, 1990.

[2] R. Alexanian, M. A. Dimopoulos, K. Delasalle, and B. Barlogie, "Primary dexamethasone treatment of multiple myeloma," *Blood*, vol. 80, no. 4, pp. 887–890, 1992.

[3] D. Weber, K. Rankin, M. Gavino, K. Delasalle, and R. Alexanian, "Thalidomide alone or with dexamethasone for previously untreated multiple myeloma," *Journal of Clinical Oncology*, vol. 21, no. 1, pp. 16–19, 2003.

[4] M. Attal, J. L. Harousseau, T. Facon et al., "Single versus double autologous stem-cell transplantation for multiple myeloma," *New England Journal of Medicine*, vol. 349, no. 26, pp. 2495–2502, 2003.

[5] J. J. Lahuerta, M. V. Mateos, J. Martínez-Lopez et al., "Influence of pre- and post-transplantation responses on outcome of patients with multiple myeloma: sequential improvement of response and achievement of complete response are associated with longer survival," *Journal of Clinical Oncology*, vol. 26, no. 35, pp. 5775–5782, 2008.

[6] J. L. Harousseau, H. Avet-Loiseau, M. Attal et al., "Achievement of at least very good partial response is a simple and robust prognostic factor in patients with multiple myeloma treated with high-dose therapy: long-term analysis of the IFM 99-02 and 99-04 trials," *Journal of Clinical Oncology*, vol. 27, no. 34, pp. 5720–5726, 2009.

[7] M. Wang, S. Giralt, K. Delasalle, B. Handy, and R. Alexanian, "Bortezomib in combination with thalidomide-dexamethasone for previously untreated multiple myeloma," *Hematology*, vol. 12, no. 3, pp. 235–239, 2007.

[8] M. Wang, K. Delasalle, S. Giralt, and R. Alexanian, "Rapid control of previously untreated multiple myeloma with bortezomib-lenalidomide-dexamethasone (BLD)," *Hematology*, vol. 15, no. 2, pp. 70–73, 2010.

[9] R. Alexanian, D. Weber, S. Giralt et al., "Impact of complete remission with intensive therapy in patients with responsive multiple myeloma," *Bone Marrow Transplantation*, vol. 27, no. 10, pp. 1037–1043, 2001.

[10] R. Alexanian, D. Weber, K. Delasalle, B. Handy, R. Champlin, and S. Giralt, "Clinical outcomes with intensive therapy for patients with primary resistant multiple myeloma," *Bone Marrow Transplantation*, vol. 34, no. 3, pp. 229–234, 2004.

[11] J. Blade, D. Samson, D. Reece et al., "Criteria for evaluating disease response and progression in patients with multiple myeloma treated by high-dose therapy and haemopoietic stem cell transplantation," *British Journal of Haematology*, vol. 102, no. 5, pp. 1115–1123, 1998.

[12] E. Kaplan and P. Meier, "Nonparametric estimation from incomplete observations," *Journal of the American Statistical Association*, vol. 53, no. 282, pp. 457–481, 1958.

[13] N. Mantel, "Evaluation of survival data and two new rank order statistics arising in its consideration," *Cancer Chemotherapy Reports*, vol. 50, no. 3, pp. 163–170, 1966.

[14] J. R. Anderson, K. C. Cain, and R. D. Gelber, "Analysis of survival by tumor response," *Journal of Clinical Oncology*, vol. 1, no. 11, pp. 710–719, 1983.

[15] M. Wang, K. Delasalle, L. Feng et al., "CR represents an early index of potential long survival in multiple myeloma," *Bone Marrow Transplantation*, vol. 45, no. 3, pp. 498–504, 2010.

[16] R. Desikan, B. Barlogie, J. Sawyer et al., "Results of high-dose therapy for 1000 patients with multiple myeloma: durable complete remissions and superior survival in the absence of chromosome 13 abnormalities," *Blood*, vol. 95, no. 12, pp. 4008–4010, 2000.

[17] B. Barlogie, G. J. Tricot, F. Van Rhee et al., "Long-term outcome results of the first tandem autotransplant trial for multiple myeloma," *British Journal of Haematology*, vol. 135, no. 2, pp. 158–164, 2006.

[18] B. Barlogie, E. Anaissie, J. Haessler et al., "Complete remission sustained 3 years from treatment initiation is a powerful surrogate for extended survival in multiple myeloma," *Cancer*, vol. 113, no. 2, pp. 355–359, 2008.

[19] J. F. S. San Miguel, J. Almeida, G. Mateo et al., "Immunophenotypic evaluation of the plasma cell compartment in multiple myeloma: a tool for comparing the efficacy of different treatment strategies and predicting outcome," *Blood*, vol. 99, no. 5, pp. 1853–1856, 2002.

[20] M. Ladetto, G. Pagliano, S. Ferrero et al., "Major tumor shrinking and persistent molecular remissions after consolidation with bortezomib, thalidomide, and dexamethasone in patients with autografted myeloma," *Journal of Clinical Oncology*, vol. 28, no. 12, pp. 2077–2084, 2010.

[21] D. van Lammeren-Venema, J. Regelink, I. Riphagen, S. Zweegman, H. Otto, and J. Zijlstra, "F-fluoro-deoxyglucose position emission tomography in assessment of myeloma-related bone disease," *Cancer*, vol. 11, pp. 1–11, 2011.

[22] S. V. Rajkumar, "Treatment of myeloma: cure vs control," *Mayo Clinic Proceedings*, vol. 83, no. 10, pp. 1142–1145, 2008.

[23] A. Fassas, J. Shaughnessy, and B. Barlogie, "Cure of myeloma: hype or reality?" *Bone Marrow Transplantation*, vol. 35, no. 3, p. 215–224, 2005.

[24] P. Hari, M. C. Pasquini, and D. H. Vesole, "Cure of multiple myeloma—more hype, less reality," *Bone Marrow Transplantation*, vol. 37, no. 1, pp. 1–18, 2006.

[25] J. Martinez-Lopez, J. Blade, M.-V. Mateos et al., "Long-term prognostic significance of response in multiple myeloma after stem cell transplantation," *Blood*, vol. 118, no. 3, pp. 529–534, 2011.

19

Index of CD34+ Cells and Mononuclear Cells in the Bone Marrow of Spinal Cord Injury Patients of Different Age Groups: A Comparative Analysis

Vidyasagar Devaprasad Dedeepiya,[1,2] **Yegneswara Yellury Rao,**[3]
Gosalakkal A. Jayakrishnan,[4] **Jutty K. B. C. Parthiban,**[1] **Subramani Baskar,**[1,2]
Sadananda Rao Manjunath,[1,2] **Rajappa Senthilkumar,**[1,2] **and Samuel J. K. Abraham**[1,5]

[1] Division of Translational Medicine, Nichi-In Centre for Regenerative Medicine (NCRM), C 16 & 17,
  Vijaya Health Centre Premises, 175 NSK Salai, Vadapalani, Chennai-600026, Tamil Nadu, India
[2] Department of Biotechnology, Acharya Nagarjuna University, Nagarjuna Nagar, Guntur 522 510, India
[3] Department of Medicine, KG Hospital, Arts College Road, Coimbatore 641018, India
[4] Department of Cardiothoracic Surgery, Omega Hospital, Mangalore, Mahaveera Circle, Kankanady, Mangalore 575002, India
[5] Department of Surgery, Faculty of Medicine, University of Yamanashi, 1110 Shimokato, Yamanashi, Chuo 409-3898, Japan

Correspondence should be addressed to Samuel J. K. Abraham, drabrahamsj@ybb.ne.jp

Academic Editor: Mark R. Litzow

Introduction. Recent evidence of safety and efficacy of Bone Marrow Mononuclear Cells (BMMNC) in spinal cord injury makes the Bone Marrow (BM) CD34+ percentage and the BMMNC count gain significance. The indices of BM that change with body mass index and aging in general population have been reported but seldom in Spinal Cord Injury (SCI) victims, whose parameters of relevance differ from general population. Herein, we report the indices of BMMNC in SCI victims. *Materials and Methods.* BMMNCs of 332 SCI patients were isolated under GMP protocols. Cell count by Trypan blue method and CD34+ cells by flow cytometry were documented and analysed across ages and gender. *Results.* The average BMMNC per ml in the age groups 0–20, 21–40, 41–60, and 61–80 years were 4.71, 4.03, 3.67, and 3.02 million and the CD34+ were 1.05%, 1.04%, 0.94%, and 0.93% respectively. The decline in CD34+ was sharp between 20–40 and 40–60 age groups. Females of reproductive age group had lesser CD34+. *Conclusion.* The BMMNC and CD34+ percentages decline with aging in SCI victims. Their lower values in females during reproductive age should be analysed for relevance to hormonal influence. This study offers reference values of BMMNC and CD34+ of SCI victims for successful clinical application.

1. Introduction

With a reported global prevalence ranging from 236 to 1009 per million [1], Spinal Cord Injury (SCI) continues to be a devastating problem with no definite solutions. Spinal Cord Injury may be due to both traumatic (e.g., road traffic accidents) or nontraumatic causes (e.g., infections, congenital causes, tumours, etc.). In traumatic spinal cord injury, primary injury caused by compression or traction causes direct injury to neural elements due to the displaced bone fragments, ligaments, and disc material which leads to damage

of the axons, neural cell bodies, and blood vessels. The spinal cord swells occupying the entire diameter of the spinal canal and ischemia results. The ischemia by releasing toxins gives rise to a cascade of secondary events ultimately leading to damage of the neighbouring healthy neurons [2]. The current mainline approaches of treatment involve removal of the bone fragments or other components to decompress the swollen spinal cord with the primary approach being limiting the secondary damage, followed by rehabilitation to assist in spontaneous recovery [2]. However the recovery is only limited in most of the cases. Hence, newer therapeutic options are being explored which might aid in complete recovery of the injured spinal cord. In this context, in addition to pharmacological treatment for improving the regeneration of the neurons using antiapoptotic agents, growth factors, and so forth [2], cell-based therapies are being sought for, as a promising approach to the condition. Several works of literature have reported the application of Bone Marrow Mononuclear Cell transplantation in Spinal Cord Injury with varying success rates [3–12]. It should be noted that CD34+ Hematopoietic Stem Cell (HSC) quantity is important because it has been reported that CD34 + cell quantity is an important dosage indicator for the success of BMMNC cell therapy [13]. Since clinical success of therapy might be attributed to the cell composition, an analysis of the same is needed to predict the success of such cell-based therapies. There are several works of literature on the composition of progenitor cell components in blood and bone marrow of healthy donors [14–16], but seldom in patients. In particular, the composition and other characteristics of bone marrow stem cells in spinal cord injury patients might be different from healthy individuals and even in patients with other kinds of organ dysfunctions, because spinal cord injury patients differ from the rest, in characteristics such as sedentary life style, body mass index, changes in neuronal control over hematopoiesis after the injury, and so forth [17–20]. This revelation can be drawn from works of literature like the study by Chernykh et al., which has compared the phenotypical and functional characteristics of bone marrow stem cells from spinal cord injury patients and healthy donors. In that study, it is stated that the percentage of CD34+CD38− hematopoietic stem cells is elevated in these patients compared to donors [21]. Also, Wright et al. published a study in which they examined the growth in cell culture of MSCs isolated from individuals with SCI, compared with non-SCI donors and they reported that age, level of spinal injury, and cell-seeding density were all related to the growth kinetics of MSC cultures *in vitro* [22].

In this study, we present a retrospective analysis of the data on BMMNC and HSC quantity obtained from 332 spinal cord injury patients admitted for autologous BMSC application over five years and we arrived at various indices such as BMMNC present in per mL of BM and percentage of CD34+ HSC in these patients.

2. Materials and Methods

2.1. Patients. All the procedures were carried in accordance with the local and national regulatory guidelines. The procedures followed were in accordance with the ethical standards described by the Helsinki Declaration.

Three hundred and thirty-two bone marrow samples were included in the study. The bone marrow samples were obtained from spinal cord injury patients who were admitted to various hospitals for autologous application of BMMNC, after ethics committee approvals from the respective hospitals and after proper informed consent. Males were predominant, with a total of 267 against 65 females. The age of the patients ranged from 1 to 76 years. The level of injury varied, ranging from C1 to S1 level. The samples were grouped

into four based on the age: 0 to 20 years—Group I, 21–40 years—Group II, 41–60 years—Group III and 61–80 years—Group IV. The time from injury to stem cell application ranged from one month to twenty years. The samples were included only if the patients' vital parameters were in the normal physiological range and they did not have any other abnormalities in their blood forming system such as an associated autoimmune disease or malignancy.

2.2. Bone Marrow Aspiration and Cell Isolation. The cell processing was done in a single institute for all the five years. Ninety to hundred mL (average 95 mL) of bone marrow aspirated from the ileac crest in all the patients was transported in an anticoagulant solution under cold chain and on reaching the lab the samples were subjected to processing immediately. The samples were processed under cGMP SOP's class 10000 clean room and class 100 Biosafety cabinets. The samples were subjected to Ficoll gradient centrifugation procedure and the BMMNCs were collected by removing the buffy coat. The viability of the cells was checked using Trypan blue and cell count was done by using Neubaur's Haemocytometer. The quantity of BMMNC per mL was calculated. A portion of the isolated BMMNCs from each sample was sent for Immunophenotyping (IP Typing) analysis to analyze the quantity of CD34+ cells by flow cytometry (BD FACS Calibur, USA).

3. Results

The results are presented in Table 1. The average BMMNC per mL in patients of age group 0–20 years was 4.71 million; in 21–40 years it was 4.03 million; in 41–60 years it was 3.67 million; in 61–80 it was 3.02 million. The average BMMNC per mL in all the 332 patients ranged from a minimum of 1.47 million to a maximum of 15.36 million. The percentage of CD34+ cells in those patients belonging to the age group of 0–20 years was 1.05; in 21–40 year group 1.04; in 41–60 year group 0.94; in 61–80 year group 0.93. The average BMMNC per mL in males was 3.86 million, while in females it was 3.66 million. The average CD34% in males was 1.01, while in females it was 0.925. A slight decrease in the BMMNC per mL and CD34+ quantity was observed with increase in the age but they were not stastically significant (Figures 1 and 2). The decline in CD34+ was sharp between the groups 20–40 and 40–60, and particularly, females in the reproductive age group had a lesser CD34+ HSC and BMMNC quantity compared to males of similar age. Clinical observations of the patients till date showed that there are no adverse reactions in any of the patients and further followup is underway.

4. Discussion

Bone marrow mononuclear cell transplantation for spinal cord injury is a promising approach with several studies reporting varying efficacies in animal models and in humans. [3–12]. The mechanisms by which these cells contribute to spinal cord injury repair are still not understood to the fullest. The proposed mechanisms by which the injected cells may act are by transdifferentiation into neuronal lineage,

TABLE 1: Age and genderwise quantity of Bone Marrow Mononuclear Cells (BMMNC) and percentage of CD34+ cells in Spinal Cord Injury (SCI) victims.

Groups	Age (years)	No. of patients	No. of males	No. of females	Average quantity of BM-aspirated (mL)	Average quantity of BMMNC isolated ($\times 10^6$)	Average CD34+ HSC%	Average BMMNC per mL index	Average CD34+ HSC% in males	Average CD34+ HSC% in females	Average BMMNC per mL index in males	Average BMMNC per mL index in females
Group I	0–20	35	24	11	92	434	1.05	4.71	1.02	1.12	4.5	5.39
Group II	21–40	203	165	38	100	403	1.04	4.03	1.08	0.91	4.1	3.6
Group III	41–60	83	70	13	100	367	0.94	3.67	0.95	0.9	3.87	2.59
Group IV	61–80	11	8	3	100	302	0.93	3.02	0.99	0.77	3	3.09

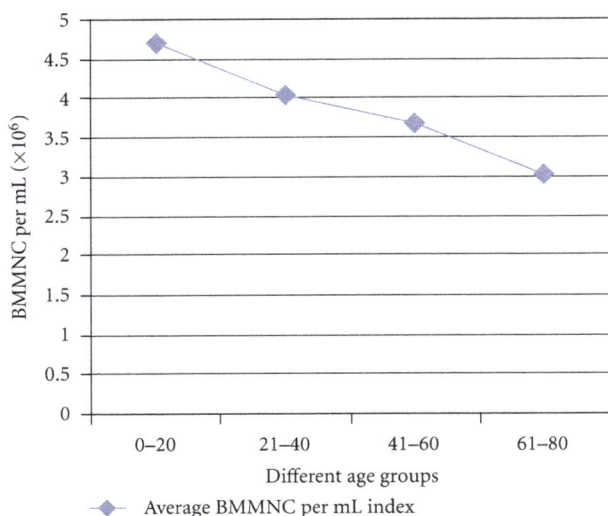

FIGURE 1: Average quantity of Bone Marrow Mononuclear Cells (BMMNC) per mL across various age groups of bone marrow samples from Spinal Cord Injury (SCI) victims.

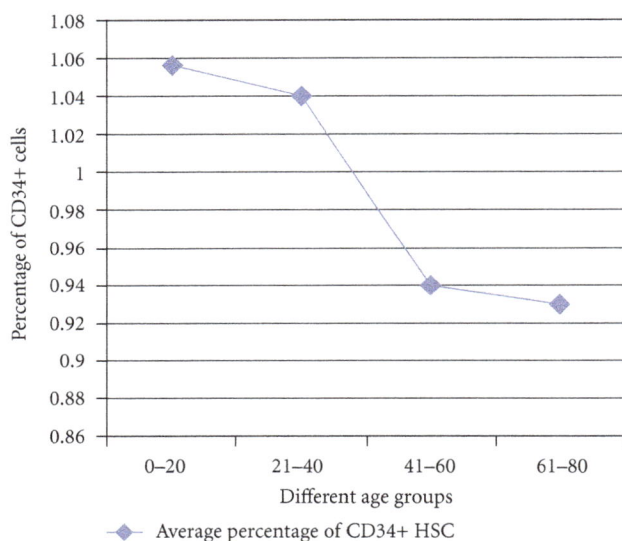

FIGURE 2: Average quantity of CD34+ Hematopoietic Stem Cell (HSC) percentage across various age groups of bone marrow samples from Spinal Cord Injury (SCI) victims.

inducing cells in the region neighbouring the spinal cord injury to regenerate or replace the injured neurons, secretion of neurotrophic factors, and altering the *in vivo* milieu in favour of regeneration [23]. Though BMMNC is a comprehensive cell population, particular importance has been attached to the CD34+ HSC quantity as several studies have reported that it is an important dosage indicator for success of bone marrow cell therapy [7–9].

There are several works of literature on the quantity of Mononuclear Cells (MNCs) and CD34+ HSCs in per mL or the whole bone marrow. Table 2 gives the details of some of the literature on such parameters based on our search. It has

been found that works of literature reporting such data are very limited, which can serve as a valuable reference on the quantity of BMMNC or CD34+ HSC across different age groups of individuals, especially in spinal cord injury patients. Chernykh et al. have reported a similar study in spinal cord injury patients but the sample size is limited [21]. Our study on samples obtained from 332 spinal cord injury victims can thus serve as a very valuable literature for future studies on evaluation of quantity of bone marrow for optimal cell isolation and dosing studies on stem cells in spinal cord injury.

Body mass index has a significant role to play in progenitor cell population and their mobilization with majority of the reports indicating that higher BMI and obesity are associated with increased CD34+ cell counts [16, 24, 25]. It is noticed that spinal cord injury victims generally have higher BMI due to their sedentary lifestyle and higher food intake [17–19]. Hence, it is logical to expect the CD34+ cell percentage to be higher in them. Another reason stated for higher CD34+ HSC count in spinal cord injury patients is the increase in the proliferative potential of CD34+ HSCs rising from the impaired innervation resulting in attenuation of negative control over HSC proliferation from the nervous system [21]. Spinal cord injury leads to secondary complications like alterations in lipid and glucose metabolism, which may lead to increased body fat. Chronic spinal cord injury also has been shown to increase the level of cytokines and interleukins thereby leading to increased inflammatory activity, which may also be a possible mechanism behind the increased CD34+ HSC proliferation in spinal cord injury. The increased progenitor levels in spinal cord injury may have a positive effect in improving tissue repair and regeneration in spinal cord injury following stem cell application [20]. A study in a chick embryo concluded that HSCs produce neurons more efficiently in a regenerating spinal cord due to favourable microenvironment [26]. All these studies imply that autologous HSCs from the spinal cord injury patients can be of a therapeutic advantage in these patients. However, increased inflammation combined with decreased immunity observed in spinal cord injury patients may also lead to increased risk of cancer incidence in these patients as reported [20]. The average BMMNC per mL and CD34+ HSC % obtained in the present study was 3.85 million, which is relatively less compared to that reported by Chernykh et al. [21], but the number of study subjects is substantially high in the present study. Also, the large difference in age, level of injury, and time of bone marrow harvest since time of injury between the patients may influence the average values obtained. The present study provides information of the index of quantity of BMMNC present per mL of bone marrow in different age groups of patients with spinal cord injury which is a worthy reference for future studies.

The influence of donor characteristics on the yield of BMMNC and the percentage of hematopoietic stem cells in the BMMNC population have been the objective of various studies described in works of literature [15, 16]. Variables such as gender, genetics, sleep, and circadian rhythm have been found to influence the quantity and other

TABLE 2: Data of the quantity of Bone Marrow Mononuclear Cells (BMMNC) and CD34+ Hematopoietic Stem Cells (HSC) from the literatures based on our search.

S. No.	Author	Year of Publication	No. of Samples	Patients or Donors	Parameters assessed	Mean Quantity of MNC/ml	Mean CD34%	Mean CD34+ cell count
1	Ema et al. [32]	1990	12	Donors	CD34%	NA	$1.05\% \pm 0.44\%^*$	
2	Chernykh et al. [21]	2006	10	Donors	MNC, count and CD34%	$7.5 \pm 2.2 \times 10^6$	5.40 ± 1.35	
3	Chernykh et al. [21]	2006	16	Spinal Cord injury Patients	MNC count and CD34 percentage	$11.0 \pm 1.1 \times 10^6$	5.4 ± 0.6	
4	Mohamadnejad et al. [33]	2007	4	Liver Cirrhosis patients	MNC and CD34 percentage	3.13×10^8		5.25×10^6
5	Hernández et al. [34]	2007	12	Critical limb Ischemia patients	MNC and CD34+ cell counts	$1.74 \pm 1.23 \times 10^9$ in group A (Separation done using blood cell separator) and $2.47 \pm 1.48 \times 10^9$ in group B (Separation done by density gradient by Ficoll-Hypaque)		$8.14 \pm 6.67 \times 10^7$ in group A and $7.90 \pm 5.46 \times 10^7$ in group B
6	Kaparthi et al. [35]	2008	5	Cardiac Disease patients	MNC and CD34+ cell count and percentage	9.16×10^7	0.348	3.68×10^5
7	Harting et al. [36]	2009	36	10 paediatric and 26 adult Non-cancer patients	MNC counts	Paediatric patients -2.1×10^6/mL and in older patients -3.2×10^6/mL		
8	Zhang et al. [16]	2010	104	Donors	CD34+ cell count and Circulating Immature Cells (CIC) count	$CIC = 9\cdot4\ (4\cdot3–21\cdot1) \times 10^9\ L^{-1}$		Total CD34+ cell count $(\times 10^6)$ is $395\cdot7$ $(102–1282)$
9	Perseghin and Incontri [37]	2010	10	Patients-nine with chronic GvHD and one with bullous pemphigoid	MNC	$5.9 \pm 2.19 \times 10^9$ in the separation done by Spectra cell separator and $5.29 \pm 2.39 \times 10^9$ in the separation done by Amicus cell separator		

*% mentioned is that of gated cells.

characteristics of BMMNC and CD34+ cells [27–31]. We have assessed the quantity of BMMNC and CD34+ HSCs in relation to age and gender in this study.

The slight decrease in CD34+ cell quantity with increasing age in our study, though statistically not significant (Figure 2), needs thorough analysis taking into consideration other parameters of significance, which are beyond the scope of this study. On the influence of age on BMMNC and CD34+ cell count, there are conflicting reports as in few of the works of literature; it has been reported that there is indeed a decrease in CD34+ cell quantity with increasing age [30, 31, 38–40], but few other works have indicated that though the functionality of HSC decreases with increasing age, there is not much difference in the HSC number with increasing age [41, 42] including reports that there is an increase in multipotent CD34(+) CD38(−) population in the bone marrow of elderly individuals above 70 years of

age. Also, in the same study it was reported that CD34(+) CD38(+) CD90(−) CD45RA(+/−) CD10(−) and CD34(+) CD33(+) myeloid progenitors persist at the same level in the bone marrow, while the frequency of early CD34(+) CD38(+) CD90(−) CD45RA(+) CD10(+) and committed CD34(+) CD19(+) B-lymphoid progenitors decreases with age [43]. Cho et al. suggests that there are several subsets in HSCs, which are very different from each other, each possessing distinct self-renewal capacities, differentiation abilities, life span, and repopulation kinetics and with aging, lymphoid-biased HSCs are decreased, while the myeloid-biased HSCs accumulate, indicating that aging instead of affecting the HSC in general changes the clonal composition of the HSC compartment [44]. In another study, it was reported that in hematopoietic stem cell transplantation (HSCT), 0–20 year-old donors were yielding relatively higher Mesenchymal Stem Cells (MSCs) in shorter duration and their biological characteristics were superior to that of older age groups [40]. It should be understood that in our study the CD34+ cells as a whole have been studied and not the clonal proliferative capability. It has been reported that there is a strong genetic component that contributes to the changes in stem cell numbers during aging [30]. Thus, it will be ideal to analyse not only the CD34+ cell quantity as a whole, but also the clonal populations in the different age groups of such patients as it will serve as an accurate indicator of the variations in bone marrow functionality with increasing age. This analysis will help in predicting the success of cell transplantation in different age groups of patients with spinal cord injury.

On the influence of gender on BMMNC and CD34+ HSC, in an article by Newman et al. on the yield of nucleated cells from marrow derived from cadaveric vertebral bodies, it has been reported that female donors yielded lower cell numbers independent of age and male donors less than 30 years of age yielded the highest number of cells [27]. There are also studies to show that male infants have significantly higher median CD34+ cell concentrations than female infants, which are reflected in an increased number of colony-forming cells, erythroblastic colonies, and granulocyte-macrophage colonies in their peripheral blood [45, 46]. It has also been suggested, based on literary evidence, that "17β-estradiol exerts negative influence on the production of B-lineage cells by modifying the differentiation, proliferation, and survival of early B-cell precursors and androgens exert an inhibitory effect on B lymphopoiesis but enhance erythropoietic differentiation and thrombocytopoiesis." [46]. Thus, it can be understood that sex hormones may influence HSC and hematopoiesis but the effects of different sex hormones on individual cell populations of the bone marrow need further analysis. In our study, a steady decrease in the BMMNC per mL can be seen with increasing age but it is not of statistical significance. The decline in CD34+ was sharp between the 20–40 and the 40–60 age groups and particularly females in the reproductive age group had a lesser CD34 and BMMNC quantity compared to males though statistically insignificant. The lesser BMMNC per mL and CD34+ HSC in females compared to males might be due to the influence of sex hormones, which exert their effects on hematopoiesis in the bone marrow and this effect of female sex hormones will possibly be more pronounced in the reproductive age group of females appreciated by the sharp decline of BMMNC per mL and CD34+ HSC in Figures 3 and 4. However, the number of females is several times lesser than the number of males in each age group in this study and hence, further investigation on these lines is warranted in studies with equal number of samples from both the genders.

Clinical observations in the patients showed that there were no adverse reactions in any of the patients. The interim results of six-month followup on 108 patients out of these 332 patients revealed that "14.11% of patients reported at least 2 grades of improvement in motor power and 4.7% of patient were able to walk independently. 16.47% of patients reported subjective sensory improvement; none of the patients had abnormal sensations such as Allodynia

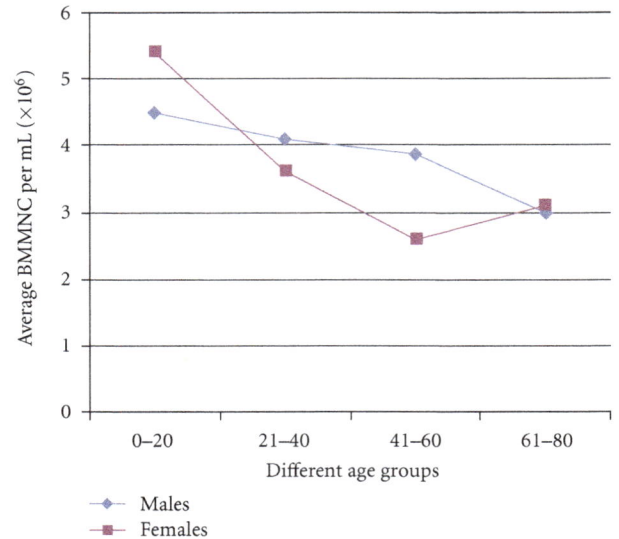

FIGURE 3: Comparison of average quantity of Bone Marrow Mononuclear Cells (BMMNC) per mL between male and female Spinal Cord Injury (SCI) victims.

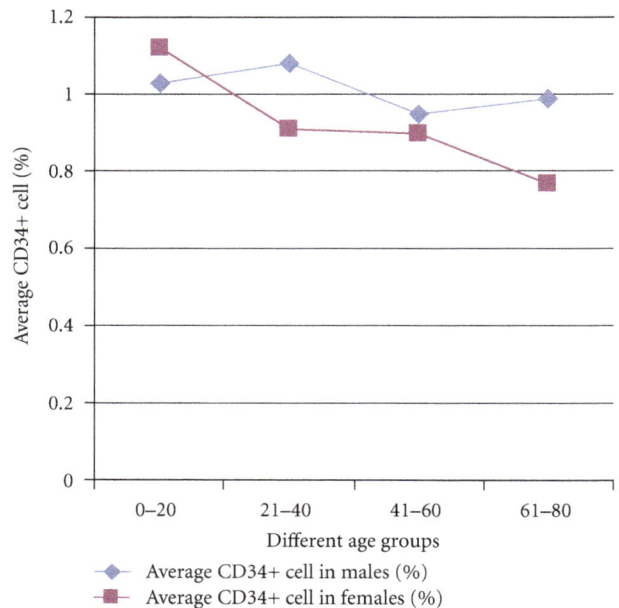

FIGURE 4: Comparison of CD34+ Hematopoietic Stem Cell (HSC) percentage between male and female Spinal Cord Injury (SCI) victims.

and 9.41% of patients had improvement as documented by Urodynamic studies." [47]. Since the main aim of the present study is evaluation of characteristics of the bone marrow in these patients, results of clinical evaluation will be out of scope of the current study.

The two indices described above, namely, the BMMNC index, that is, quantity of BMMNC per mL of bone marrow and the CD34+ cell index, that is, percentage of CD34+ cells in a given bone marrow sample can also be used for quantification studies to assess the approximate quantity of bone marrow to be harvested from spinal cord injury patients for therapeutic application. Though CD34+ cell quantity is widely used as a predictor of engraftment, a recent study done on 435 Cord Blood Transplants has suggested that the CFU dose is a better predictor of engraftment [48]. Further studies should be done on analysing this triad of parameters: the BMMNC per mL, CD34+ cell quantity per mL, and CFU in bone marrow samples in various age groups of patients with spinal cord injury also with healthy donors to arrive at data, based on which this triad can be made as a gold standard testing method in accurately predicting the functionality and quality of the bone marrow for application in spinal cord injuries.

5. Conclusion

We have described two useful indices for assessment of BMMNC and CD34+ HSC quantity in bone marrow based on data obtained from spinal cord injury patients with normal vital physiological parameters. In our evaluation, the average BMMNC per mL and the percentage of CD34+ cells show a decline with aging in spinal cord injury victims of both males and females. The BMMNC and CD34+ HSC are relatively lower in females than males and there is a sharp decline of CD34+ HSC in females in the reproductive age group. The fact that the characteristics of BMMNCs and HSCs will differ in spinal cord injury patients compared to normal patients due to the differences in lifestyle and other parameters makes these findings important, as the values of BMMNC and CD34+ HSC from this study may be used as a reference for future studies. The decreased BMMNC and CD34+ HSC in females will have to be analysed for their relevance to hormonal influence. The Colony Forming Unit (CFU) analysis, which is more relevant as physiological indicator, when assessed may throw further light and add significance.

Acknowledgments

The authors acknowledge Dr. Ryuji Hata for his technical advice, Dr. Preethy Senthilkumar for her assistance in preparation of the paper, M/S Hope Foundation (Trust) Chennai, India for funding the study.

References

[1] R. A. Cripps, B. B. Lee, P. Wing, E. Weerts, J. MacKay, and D. Brown, "A global map for traumatic spinal cord injury epidemiology: towards a living data repository for injury prevention," Spinal Cord, vol. 49, no. 4, pp. 493–501, 2011.

[2] J. W. McDonald and C. Sadowsky, "Spinal-cord injury," The Lancet, vol. 359, no. 9304, pp. 417–425, 2002.

[3] A. Sharma, N. Gokulchandran, G. Chopra et al., "Administration of autologous bone marrow-derived mononuclear cells in children with incurable neurological disorders and injury is safe and improves their quality of life," Cell Transplantation, vol. 21, supplement 1, pp. S79–S90, 2012.

[4] A. F. Samdani, C. Paul, R. R. Betz, I. Fischer, and B. Neuhuber, "Transplantation of human marrow stromal cells and mononuclear bone marrow cells into the injured spinal cord: a comparative study," Spine, vol. 34, no. 24, pp. 2605–2612, 2009.

[5] E. Syková, A. Homola, R. Mazanec et al., "Autologous bone marrow transplantation in patients with subacute and chronic spinal cord injury," Cell Transplantation, vol. 15, no. 8-9, pp. 675–687, 2006.

[6] T. Yoshihara, M. Ohta, Y. Itokazu et al., "Neuroprotective effect of bone marrow-derived mononuclear cells promoting functional recovery from spinal cord injury," Journal of Neurotrauma, vol. 24, no. 6, pp. 1026–1036, 2007.

[7] J. B. William, R. Prabakaran, S. Ayyappan et al., "Functional recovery of spinal cord injury following application of intralesional bone marrow mononuclear cells embedded in polymer scaffold—two year follow-up in a Canine," Journal of Stem Cell Research & Therapy, vol. 1, p. 110, 2011.

[8] H. C. Park, Y. S. Shim, Y. Ha et al., "Treatment of complete spinal cord injury patients by autologous bone marrow cell transplantation and administration of granulocyte-macrophage colony stimulating factor," Tissue Engineering, vol. 11, no. 5-6, pp. 913–922, 2005.

[9] F. Callera and R. X. Do Nascimento, "Delivery of autologous bone marrow precursor cells into the spinal cord via lumbar puncture technique in patients with spinal cord injury: a preliminary safety study," Experimental Hematology, vol. 34, no. 2, pp. 130–131, 2006.

[10] S. H. Yoon, Y. S. Shim, H. P. Yong et al., "Complete spinal cord injury treatment using autologous bone marrow cell transplantation and bone marrow stimulation with granulocyte macrophage-colony stimulating factor: phase I/II clinical trial," Stem Cells, vol. 25, no. 8, pp. 2066–2073, 2007.

[11] H. Deda, M. C. Inci, A. Kurekçi et al., "Treatment of chronic spinal cord injured patients with autologous bone marrow-derived hematopoietic stem cell transplantation: 1-year follow-up," Cytotherapy, vol. 10, no. 6, pp. 565–574, 2008.

[12] L. F. Geffner, P. Santacruz, M. Izurieta et al., "Administration of autologous bone marrow stem cells into spinal cord injury patients via multiple routes is safe and improves their quality of life: comprehensive case studies," Cell Transplantation, vol. 17, no. 12, pp. 1277–1293, 2008.

[13] S. Yasuhara, Y. Yasunaga, T. Hisatome et al., "Efficacy of bone marrow mononuclear cells to promote bone regeneration compared with isolated CD34+ cells from the same volume of aspirate," Artificial Organs, vol. 34, no. 7, pp. 594–599, 2010.

[14] D. F. Stroncek, M. E. Clay, J. Smith et al., "Composition of peripheral blood progenitor cell components collected from healthy donors," Transfusion, vol. 37, no. 4, pp. 411–417, 1997.

[15] W. Bouwmeester, M. M. Fechter, M. W. Heymans, J. W. R. Twisk, L. J. Ebeling, and A. Brand, "Prediction of nucleated cells in bone marrow stem cell products by donor characteristics: a retrospective single centre analysis," Vox Sanguinis A, vol. 98, no. 3, pp. e276–e283, 2010.

[16] C. Zhang, X. H. Chen, X. Zhang et al., "Stem cell collection in unmanipulated HLA-haploidentical/mismatched related transplantation with combined granulocyte-colony stimulating factor-mobilised blood and bone marrow for patients with haematologic malignancies: the impact of donor characteristics and procedural settings," Transfusion Medicine, vol. 20, no. 3, pp. 169–177, 2010.

[17] S. L. Groah, M. S. Nash, I. H. Ljungberg et al., "Nutrient intake and body habitus after spinal cord injury: an analysis by sex and level of injury," Journal of Spinal Cord Medicine, vol. 32, no. 1, pp. 25–33, 2009.

[18] Y. Chen, Y. Cao, V. Allen, and J. S. Richards, "Weight matters: physical and psychosocial well being of persons with spinal cord injury in relation to body mass index," *Archives of Physical Medicine and Rehabilitation*, vol. 92, no. 3, pp. 391–398, 2011.

[19] D. A. Crane, J. W. Little, and S. P. Burns, "Weight gain following spinal cord injury: a pilot study," *Journal of Spinal Cord Medicine*, vol. 34, no. 2, pp. 227–232, 2011.

[20] E. Kostovski, P. O. Iversen, and N. Hjeltnes, "Complications of chronic spinal cord injury," *Tidsskr Nor Laegeforen*, vol. 130, no. 12, pp. 1242–1245, 2010.

[21] E. R. Chernykh, E. Y. Shevela, O. Y. Leplina et al., "Characteristics of bone marrow cells under conditions of impaired innervation in patients with spinal trauma," *Bulletin of Experimental Biology and Medicine*, vol. 141, no. 1, pp. 117–120, 2006.

[22] K. T. Wright, W. E. Masri, A. Osman et al., "The cell culture expansion of bone marrow stromal cells from humans with spinal cord injury: implications for future cell transplantation therapy," *Spinal Cord*, vol. 46, no. 12, pp. 811–817, 2008.

[23] K. T. Wright, W. El Masri, A. Osman, J. Chowdhury, and W. E. B. Johnson, "Concise review: bone marrow for the treatment of spinal cord injury: mechanisms and clinical applications," *Stem Cells*, vol. 29, no. 2, pp. 169–178, 2011.

[24] S. H. Chen, S. H. Yang, S. C. Chu et al., "The role of donor characteristics and post-granulocyte colony-stimulating factor white blood cell counts in predicting the adverse events and yields of stem cell mobilization," *International Journal of Hematology*, pp. 1–8, 2011.

[25] C. F. Bellows, Y. Zhang, P. J. Simmons, A. S. Khalsa, and M. G. Kolonin, "Influence of BMI on level of circulating progenitor cells," *Obesity*, vol. 19, no. 8, pp. 1722–1726, 2011.

[26] O. E. Sigurjonsson, M. C. Perreault, T. Egeland, and J. C. Glover, "Adult human hematopoietic stem cells produce neurons efficiently in the regenerating chicken embryo spinal cord," *Proceedings of the National Academy of Sciences of the United States of America*, vol. 102, no. 14, pp. 5227–5232, 2005.

[27] H. Newman, J. A. Reems, T. H. Rigley, D. Bravo, and D. M. Strong, "Donor age and gender are the strongest predictors of marrow recovery from cadaveric vertebral bodies," *Cell Transplantation*, vol. 12, no. 1, pp. 83–90, 2003.

[28] Y. J. Chang, X. Y. Zhao, M. R. Huo, X. H. Luo, and X. J. Huang, "CD34 cells and T cell subsets in recombinant human granulocyte colony-stimulating factor primed bone marrow grafts from donors with different characteristics," *Zhonghua Xue Ye Xue Za Zhi*, vol. 29, no. 8, pp. 512–516, 2008.

[29] L. D. Guariniello, P. Vicari, K. S. Lee, A. C. de Oliveira, and S. Tufik, "Bone marrow and peripheral white blood cells number is affected by sleep deprivation in a murine experimental model," *Journal of Cellular Physiology*, vol. 227, no. 1, pp. 361–366, 2012.

[30] G. de Haan and G. Van Zant, "Dynamic changes in mouse hematopoietic stem cell numbers during aging," *Blood*, vol. 93, no. 10, pp. 3294–3301, 1999.

[31] O. Tsinkalovsky, R. Smaaland, B. Rosenlund et al., "Circadian variations in clock gene expression of human bone marrow CD34+ cells," *Journal of Biological Rhythms*, vol. 22, no. 2, pp. 140–150, 2007.

[32] H. Ema, T. Suda, Y. Miura, and H. Nakauchi, "Colony formation of clone-sorted human hematopoietic progenitors," *Blood*, vol. 75, no. 10, pp. 1941–1946, 1990.

[33] M. Mohamadnejad, M. Namiri, M. Bagheri et al., "Phase 1 human trial of autologous bone marrow-hematopoietic stem cell transplantation in patients with decompensated cirrhosis," *World Journal of Gastroenterology*, vol. 13, no. 24, pp. 3359–3363, 2007.

[34] P. Hernández, L. Cortina, H. Artaza et al., "Autologous bone-marrow mononuclear cell implantation in patients with severe lower limb ischaemia: a comparison of using blood cell separator and Ficoll density gradient centrifugation," *Atherosclerosis*, vol. 194, no. 2, pp. e52–e56, 2007.

[35] P. L. N. Kaparthi, G. Namita, L. K. Chelluri et al., "Autologous bone marrow mononuclear cell delivery to dilated cardiomyopathy patients: a clinical trial," *African Journal of Biotechnology*, vol. 7, no. 3, pp. 207–210, 2008.

[36] M. T. Harting, C. S. Cox, M. C. Day et al., "Bone marrow-derived mononuclear cell populations in pediatric and adult patients," *Cytotherapy*, vol. 11, no. 4, pp. 480–484, 2009.

[37] P. Perseghin and A. Incontri, "Mononuclear cell collection in patients treated with extracorporeal photochemotherapy by using the off-line method: a comparison between COBE Spectra AutoPbsc version 6.1 and Amicus cell separators," *Journal of Clinical Apheresis*, vol. 25, no. 6, pp. 310–314, 2010.

[38] I. Stelzer, R. Fuchs, E. Schraml et al., "Decline of bone marrow-derived hematopoietic progenitor cell quality during aging in the rat," *Experimental Aging Research*, vol. 36, no. 3, pp. 359–370, 2010.

[39] H. Vaziri, W. Dragowska, R. C. Allsopp, T. E. Thomas, C. B. Harley, and P. M. Lansdorp, "Evidence for a mitotic clock in human hematopoietic stem cells: loss of telomeric DNA with age," *Proceedings of the National Academy of Sciences of the United States of America*, vol. 91, no. 21, pp. 9857–9860, 1994.

[40] K. Huang, D. H. Zhou, S. L. Huang, and S. H. Liang, "Age-related biological characteristics of human bone marrow mesenchymal stem cells from different age donors," *Zhongguo Shi Yan Xue Ye Xue Za Zhi*, vol. 13, no. 6, pp. 1049–1053, 2005.

[41] S. J. Morrison, A. M. Wandycz, K. Akashi, A. Globerson, and I. L. Weissman, "The aging of hematopoietic stem cells," *Nature Medicine*, vol. 2, no. 9, pp. 1011–1016, 1996.

[42] L. Berkahn and A. Keating, "Hematopoiesis in the elderly," *Hematology*, vol. 9, no. 3, pp. 159–163, 2004.

[43] K. Kuranda, J. Vargaftig, P. de la Rochere et al., "Age-related changes in human hematopoietic stem/progenitor cells," *Aging Cell*, vol. 10, no. 3, pp. 542–546, 2011.

[44] R. H. Cho, H. B. Sieburg, and C. E. Muller-Sieburg, "A new mechanism for the aging of hematopoietic stem cells: aging changes the clonal composition of the stem cell compartment but not individual stem cells," *Blood*, vol. 111, no. 12, pp. 5553–5561, 2008.

[45] P. Aroviita, K. Teramo, V. Hiilesmaa, and R. Kekomäki, "Cord blood hematopoietic progenitor cell concentration and infant sex," *Transfusion*, vol. 45, no. 4, pp. 613–621, 2005.

[46] R. Ray, N. M. Novotny, P. R. Crisostomo, T. Lahm, A. Abarbanell, and D. R. Meldrum, "Sex steroids and stem cell function," *Molecular Medicine*, vol. 14, no. 7-8, pp. 493–501, 2008.

[47] S. Abraham, S. Manjunath, S. Baskar et al., "Autologous stem cell injections for spinal cord injury-a multicentric study with 6 month follow up of 108 patients. 7th Annual Meeting of Japanese Society of Regenerative Medicine, Nagoya, Japan, 13-14 March 2008. Saisei-iryo (Regenerative Medicine)," *Journal of Japanese Society of Regenerative Medicine*, vol. 7, supplement 1, 2008, abstract No O-13-7.

[48] K. M. Page, L. Zhang, A. Mendizabal et al., "Total colony-forming units are a strong, independent predictor of neutrophil and platelet engraftment after unrelated umbilical cord blood transplantation: a single-center analysis of 435 cord blood transplants," *Biology of Blood and Marrow Transplantation*, vol. 17, no. 9, pp. 1362–1374, 2011.

20

Both Optimal Matching and Procedure Duration Influence Survival of Patients after Unrelated Donor Hematopoietic Stem Cell Transplantation

Sylwia Mizia,[1] **Dorota Dera-Joachimiak,**[1] **Malgorzata Polak,**[1] **Katarzyna Koscinska,**[1] **Mariola Sedzimirska,**[1] **and Andrzej Lange**[1, 2]

[1] *Division of the National Bone Marrow Donor Registry, Lower Silesian Center for Cellular Transplantation, Grabiszynska 105, 53-439 Wroclaw, Poland*
[2] *Institute of Immunology and Experimental Therapy, Polish Academy of Sciences, 53-114 Wroclaw, Poland*

Correspondence should be addressed to Andrzej Lange, lange@iitd.pan.wroc.pl

Academic Editor: Colette Raffoux

Eighty-six patients suffering from hematological malignancies, immunodeficiencies, and aplastic anemias received alloHSCT from unrelated donors. Donors were selected from the BMDW files and further matching was performed according to the confirmatory typing procedure with the use of PCR SSP and that based on sequencing. The time from the clinical request of the donor search to the final decision of clinicians accepting the donor was from 0.3 to 17.8 months (median 1.6). Matching was analyzed at the allele level, and 50, 27, and 9 donor-recipient pairs were 10/10 matched, mismatched in one or more alleles, respectively. In an univariate analysis we found better survival if patients were transplanted: (i) from donors matched 10/10 ($P = 0.025$), (ii) not from female donor to male recipient ($P = 0.037$), (iii) in female donation from those with ≤ 1 pregnancy than multiparous ($P = 0.075$). Notably, it became apparent that duration of the confirmatory typing process affected the survival (HR = 1.138, $P = 0.013$). In multivariate analysis only the level of matching and the duration of the matching procedure significantly affected the survival. In conclusion, the duration of the matching procedure in addition to the level of matching should be considered as an independent risk factor of survival.

1. Introduction

The number of allogeneic hematopoietic stem cell transplantations (alloHSCTs) from unrelated donors has increased over the years and in Europe reached 7098 in 2010 (EBMT Survey on Transplant Activity 2010). This was possible due to the improvement in international cooperation in donor-recipient matching procedures facilitated by the Bone Marrow Donors Worldwide (BMDW) files [1] and implementation of the European Marrow Donor Information System (EMDIS) in a number of countries. The priority of the search procedure is to identify the optimally matched donor for patients badly needing hematopoietic stem cell transplantation (HSCT). Quite recently the pace of the matching procedure has improved due to the use of computer-assisted communication systems including the EMDIS. However, still some time is needed, especially when the process of searching for a fully matched donor is prolonged. Previously published studies showed that the time needed to identify an acceptable donor is associated with a profile of HLA alleles being prolonged in cases with rare haplotypes [2–4]. Prolonged search may result in postponing transplantation in some cases that become medically unfit in the meantime. This may be due to various medical reasons including relapse and consequently, unless successfully treated, advancing in the stage of the disease. Tiercy et al. [4] showed that patients categorized in the group with a high probability of finding an optimal 10/10 matched donor have better survival than

TABLE 1: Patients' characteristics.

Recipient age (y), median (range)		28.5 (0.6–59)
Diagnosis, no. (%)	Hematological malignancy	73 (80)
	Immunodeficiency	9 (15)
	Aplastic anemia	4 (5)
Donor age (y), median (range)		34 (19–59)
Donor-recipient sex match, no. (%)	Female to male	23 (27)
	Other	63 (73)
Number of pregnancies in female donors, no. (%)	0-1	21 (54)
	>1	18 (46)
Donor-recipient CMV serostatus match, no. (%)	Positive-negative	10 (38)
	Negative-positive	26 (72)
Donor origin, no. (%)	Poland registry	14 (17)
	Europe foreign registry	63 (73)
	Other world registries	9 (10)
Donor-recipient HLA matching, no. (%)	Matched	50 (58)
	Mismatched	36 (42)
Number of CT procedures, no. (%)	≤2	58 (73)
	>2	22 (27)
Duration of the matching procedure (mth), median (range)		1.6 (0.27–17.8)
Hematopoietic stem cell source, no. (%)	Bone marrow	6 (7)
	Peripheral blood	80 (93)

those with intermediate or low probability. Here, we study the impact of the actual length of the search procedure on the outcome of alloHSCT.

2. Materials and Methods

2.1. Patients. In this study we analyze the outcome of 86 patients transplanted in our institution from unrelated donors in years 2004–2010. The patients suffered from hematological malignancies (80%), immunodeficiencies (15%), and aplastic anemias (5%). The group consisted of 39 (45%) females and 47 (55%) males aged from 0.6 to 59 years (median 28.5) and received marrow (6) or PBPC (80) from female (40) and male (46) donors (Table 1).

2.2. Histocompatibility Testing and Search Strategy. The donor-recipient matching procedure commissioned to the National Polish Bone Marrow Donor Registry (NPBMDR), a part of the Lower Silesian Center for Cellular Transplantation, was conducted according to two principles: (i) a donor should be compatible in human leukocyte antigen (HLA) with a patient at a high-resolution level of typing considering five loci (A, B, C, DR, and DQ) and (ii) among donors with similar HLA characteristics, residents of Poland, and if absent those from neighboring countries are chosen with priority [5, 6]. Donors were selected from the BMDW files with an HLA-compatible potential with a priority according to the distance principle policy. Further matching procedures were performed as follow: (1) registries having potential donors

are conducted to confirm the donor availability and if so a blood sample is requested for confirmatory typing (CT), (2) as soon as blood is received high resolution typing of a potential donor is performed with the use of PCR SSP and that based on sequencing, and the same procedure is applied to the recipient, (3) the transplant center is asked for acceptance of a donor which may result in a request for further search, (4) the above procedures are performed in an iterative manner.

The time from the beginning of the search process, the level of matching and the outcome of transplantation were recorded and statistically evaluated.

2.3. Data Collection. The outcome of transplantation was followed and registered in a database according to the EBMT Med-A form requirements. The overall survival of patients receiving alloHSCT from unrelated donor was evaluated using the already known factors including level of HLA matching, female-to-male donation, number of female donor pregnancies, age of donors and CMV serostatus and in addition the duration of the matching procedure.

2.4. Statistical Analysis. Statistical analysis was conducted using STATISTICA v.10. The associations between two variables were tested by Chi-square test, with Yates' correction if appropriate, for categorical variables and Mann-Whitney U test for categorical and continuous variables. The overall survival was analyzed by the Kaplan-Meier method, log-rank

TABLE 2: Univariate analysis (discrete variables).

		No.	Overall survival (2-yr survival, %)	P-value
Donor-recipient HLA matching	Matched	50	58.9	0.025
	Mismatched	36	37.7	
Donor-recipient sex match	F-M	23	31.8	0.037
	Other	63	56.6	
Number of pregnancies in female donors	0-1	21	52.5	0.075
	>1	18	38.9	
Donor-recipient CMV serostatus match	Positive-negative	10	58.3	0.479
	Negative-positive	26	48.8	

test, and parametric survival models [7, 8]. The likelihood of committing a type 1 error was set to 0.05.

3. Results

All patients were typed at the level of a primary workup in a majority of cases. However, in 15% of cases patients were typed when it was clinically apparent that the transplant was badly needed. The time of the donor search varied from 0.3 to 17.8 months (median 1.6). Analysis of the level of matching at the point of clinical acceptance revealed that 50, 27, and 9 donor-recipient pairs were 10/10 matched, mismatched in one or more alleles, respectively.

The overall survival was significantly higher for patients transplanted from donors matched at the level of 10 specificities (2-year survival rates of matched and mismatched donors: 59% versus 38%, respectively; log-rank test $P = 0.025$) and transplanted other than from female donor to male recipient (2-year survival rates: 57% versus 32%, respectively; log-rank test $P = 0.037$). Survival curves of patients transplanted from female donors with no or 1 pregnancy tended to be higher than those reflecting the effect of donation from multiparous women (2-year survival rates: 53% versus 39%; log-rank test $P = 0.075$).

Notably, it became apparent that duration of the searching process (mth) affected the survival (Cox model: hazard ratio HR = 1.138, $P = 0.013$). The results of univariate statistical analysis are shown in Tables 2 and 3.

In multivariate analysis only the level of matching and the duration of the matching procedure significantly affected the survival in an independent fashion (Cox model: HR = 2.422, $P = 0.007$ and HR = 1.109, $P = 0.045$, resp.) (Table 4). Multivariate analysis was used to calculate the coefficients reflecting the impact of different variables on the overall survival. More thorough analysis of the study group revealed that the duration of the searching process was significantly longer in patients having as compared to those lacking the presence of rare haplotypes and/or rare B-C or DR-DQ associations defined according to our published study (median: 3.1 versus 1.5 months, Mann-Whitney U test $P = 0.001$) [5]. Only 10% of patients with common HLA haplotypes waited longer than 3 months for a conclusion of the search process due to the prolonged donor activation time resulted, for example, from a withdrawal of a donor

TABLE 3: Univariate analysis (continuous variables).

	HR	P value
Donor age (y)	1.004	0.775
Duration of the matching procedure (mth)	1.138	0.013

TABLE 4: Multivariate analysis.

	HR	P value
Donor-recipient HLA matching (mismatched)	2.422	0.007
Duration of the matching procedure (mth)	1.109	0.045

from the registry. In addition, we analyzed the presence of the progression in stage of the disease during the search process. It became apparent that proportions of patients who advance in stage of the disease were similar in patients with a short and a longer search process (median cut-point: 11% versus 14%, Chi-square test $P = 0.865$). This shows that in both groups there were patients with diseases at similar levels of relapse/progression potential. Time from the diagnosis to transplantation is influenced by several factors, including biology of underlying diseases and willingness of patients to undergo transplantation as an optional treatment. However, patients with a long time between the diagnosis and transplantation in the more homogeneous group of acute leukemias had more frequently rare alleles and/or B-C or DR-DQ associations than those being transplanted sooner after diagnosis (1-year cut-point: 50% versus 14%, Chi-square test $P = 0.035$). Therefore, length of the search process and the level of matching are major factors affecting post-HSCT survival. It enabled the development of a model predicting survival according to the level of matching and the time of the search process. Figures 1 and 2 show the predicted survival curves.

In addition we investigated whether time of the search procedure was affected by the number of matching attempts. It became apparent that more than two CT procedures resulted in a significant prolongation of the donor search completion (median: 1.5 versus 2.7 months, Mann-Whitney U test $P = 0.0002$; Figure 3).

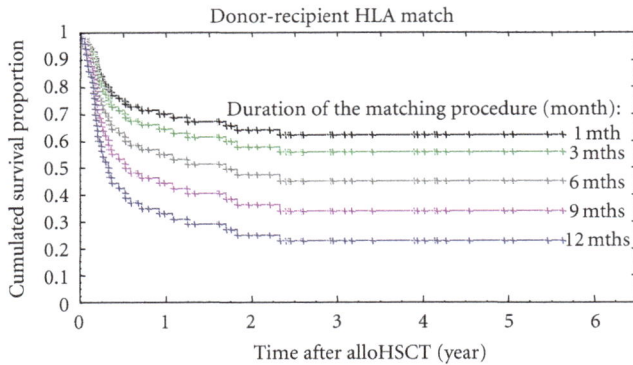

FIGURE 1: Survival curves of patients receiving alloHSCT from matched unrelated donor with respect to the duration of the matching procedure (as predicted according to the model).

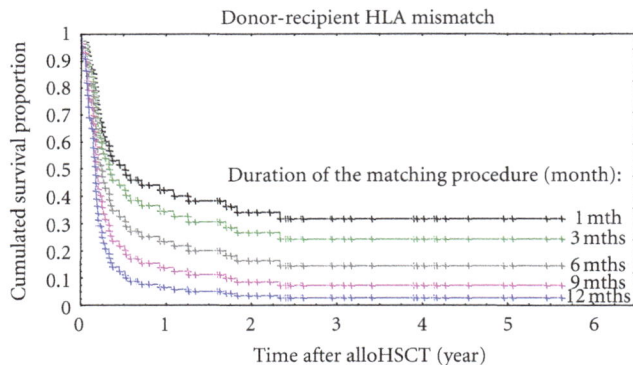

FIGURE 2: Survival curves of patients receiving alloHSCT from mismatched unrelated donor with respect to the duration of the matching procedure (as predicted according to the model).

4. Conclusions

Data recorded in this study enabled us to confirm already known factors, namely, number of pregnancies and female-to-male donation, as those affecting survival after HSCT. This observation, concordant with other studies [9], shows that the donor-recipient pairs presented in this paper share similar characteristics with other reported HSCT groups of donors and recipients. Also it is apparent from the present study that the level of HLA matching plays an important role. This is also a well-known observation [10]. Keeping in mind the latter data, transplant centers frequently focus on the level of matching, neglecting the time needed for a prolonged procedure if the matching process is rather complex. Indeed, the time from the beginning until the completion of the search significantly depends on the number of confirmatory typing procedures performed. The novel aspect of the present paper is the finding that time needed for optimal match adversely affects the survival. Therefore, an optimal match reached after prolonged time results in a similar survival as that not optimal but completed promptly. Several previously published studies suggested ways to predict the length of the process on the basis of the

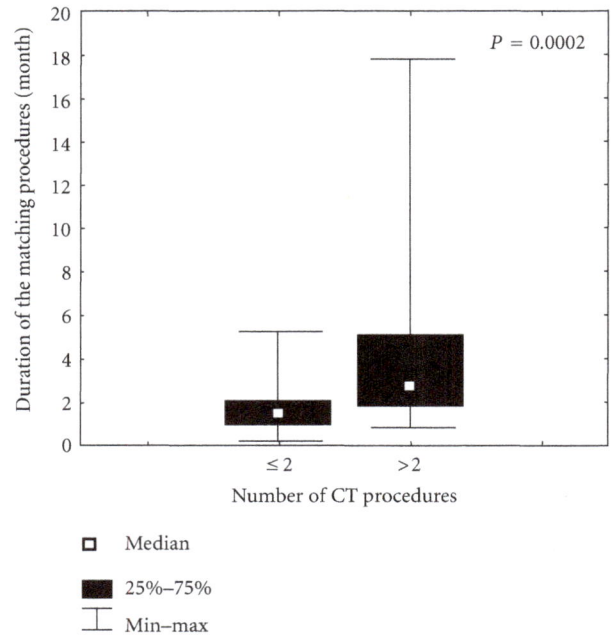

FIGURE 3: The duration of the matching procedure with respect to the number of CT procedures.

HLA specificity profile in patients. This was also shown in the present group as patients with HLA rarities waited longer. Tiercy et al. [4] documented poorer survival in patients with rare alleles and B-C or DR-DQ associations. In the present study survival was analyzed not according to the HLA specificities associated with prediction but independently of any specific factors; just length of the search process was taken as a variable. Indeed, HLA rarities play an important role, but also other factors may be associated. Ten percent of patients with rather common HLA specificities waited for the search conclusion longer than 3 months. The reason of such delay is not entirely clear, but withdrawal of a potential donor from the registry may serve as an example.

The present study offers a rationale for the observation in the paper by Heemskerk et al. [11] that to achieve transplant results in the range of sibling transplantations the search procedure should be similarly time consuming.

Acknowledgments

This work was supported by Grant no. N R13 0082 06 from the Polish Ministry of Science & Higher Education.

References

[1] http://www.bmdw.org/.

[2] K. Hirv, K. Bloch, M. Fischer et al., "Prediction of duration and success rate of unrelated hematopoietic stem cell donor searches based on the patient's HLA-DRB1 allele and DRB1-DQB1 haplotype frequencies," Bone Marrow Transplantation, vol. 44, no. 7, pp. 433–440, 2009.

[3] B. Pédron, V. Guérin-El Khourouj, J. H. Dalle et al., "Contribution of HLA-A/B/C/DRB1/DQB1 common haplotypes to

donor search outcome in unrelated hematopoietic stem cell transplantation," *Biology of Blood and Marrow Transplantation*, vol. 17, no. 11, pp. 1612–1628, 2011.

[4] J. M. Tiercy, G. Nicoloso, J. Passweg et al., "The probability of identifying a 10/10 HLA allele-matched unrelated donor is highly predictable," *Bone Marrow Transplantation*, vol. 40, no. 6, pp. 515–522, 2007.

[5] A. Lange, D. Dera-Joachimiak, S. Madej et al., "Activity of the National Polish Bone Marrow Donor Registry—analysis of the matching process successfully completed with hematopoietic stem cell transplantation," *Transplantation Proceedings*, vol. 42, no. 8, pp. 3316–3318, 2010.

[6] A. Lange, M. Polak, M. Dudkiewicz et al., "Activity of the National Polish Bone Marrow Donor Registry," in *Standardization of Donor-Recipient Matching in Transplantation*, A. Lange, Ed., pp. 93–101, Nova Science Publishers, 2006.

[7] M. Labopin and S. Iacobelli, "Statistical guidelines for EBMT," 2003, http://www.ebmt.org/1WhatisEBMT/Op_Manual/OP-MAN_StatGuidelines_oct2003.pdf.

[8] R. Szydlo, "Statistical evaluation of HSCT data," in *Haematopoietic Stem Cell Transplantation, The EBMT Handbook*, pp. 328–339, 5th edition, 2008.

[9] A. Devergie, "Graft versus host disease," in *Haematopoietic Stem Cell Transplantation, The EBMT Handbook*, pp. 218–235, 5th edition, 2008.

[10] J. M. Tiercy, "The role of HLA in HSCT," in *Haematopoietic Stem Cell Transplantation, The EBMT Handbook*, pp. 46–65, 5th edition, 2008.

[11] M. B. Heemskerk, S. M. van Walraven, J. J. Cornelissen et al., "How to improve the search for an unrelated haematopoietic stem cell donor. Faster is better than more!," *Bone Marrow Transplantation*, vol. 35, no. 7, pp. 645–652, 2005.

21

Controversies and Recent Advances in Hematopoietic Cell Transplantation for Follicular Non-Hodgkin Lymphoma

Abraham S. Kanate,[1] Mohamed A. Kharfan-Dabaja,[2] and Mehdi Hamadani[1, 3]

[1] *Myeloma and Lymphoma Service, Osborn Hematopoietic Malignancy and Transplantation Program, West Virginia University, Morgantown, WV 26506, USA*
[2] *Blood and Marrow Transplantation, Moffitt Cancer Center, Tampa, FL 33612, USA*
[3] *Division of Hematology and Oncology, West Virginia University, P.O. Box 9162, 1 Medical Center Drive, Morgantown, WV 26506, USA*

Correspondence should be addressed to Mehdi Hamadani, mehdi.hamadani@gmail.com

Academic Editor: Joseph H. Antin

Commonly designated as an indolent non-Hodgkin lymphoma, follicular lymphoma (FL) presents with striking pathobiological and clinical heterogeneity. Initial management strategies for FL have evolved to involve combination chemoimmunotherapy and/or radio-immunoconjugates. Unfortunately even with the best available nontransplant treatment, which nowadays results in higher frequency of response, FL remains incurable. Although considered a feasible therapeutic option, the use of hematopoietic cell transplantation (HCT) remains controversial. The appropriate timing, graft source, and intensity of HCT conditioning regimens in FL are often matters of debate. Herein we review the available published data pertaining to the use of autologous or allogeneic HCT in patients with FL across different stages of the disease, discuss major recent advances in the field, and highlight avenues for future research. The current literature does not support a role of HCT for FL in first remission, but in the relapsed setting autologous HCT remains appropriate for patients with early chemosensitive relapses, while allogeneic transplantation remains the sole curative modality for this disease, in relatively younger patients without significant comorbidities.

1. Introduction

Follicular lymphoma (FL) is the second most common type of non-Hodgkin lymphoma (NHL) in the western hemisphere accounting for 22% of all cases [1]. The median age at diagnosis is generally in the 6th decade, with a slight female preponderance. Being an indolent lymphoma, the disease course of FL is one of remissions and relapses with conventional chemoimmunotherapies followed not infrequently by development of resistance and/or transformation into a more aggressive histology. A subset of FL patients has a more aggressive clinical course, with approximately 15% mortality at 2 years resulting from progressive or transformed disease [2]. While clinical prognostic systems such as FL international prognostic index (FLIPI) are good in estimating overall survival (OS) [3, 4], they have limited predictive value in identifying patient groups that may (or may not) benefit from aggressive initial therapy.

Management strategies include surveillance, combination chemoimmunotherapy, radio-immunotherapy, and autologous or allogeneic hematopoietic cell transplantation (HCT). The addition of rituximab to conventional chemotherapy regimens has resulted in improved progression-free survival (PFS) and OS [5–7] in several studies.

Despite improved outcomes achieved with incorporation of monoclonal antibodies, namely, rituximab, or introduction of radio-immunoconjugates, namely, iodine I-131 tositumomab or ibritumomab tiuxetan, FL remains incurable. The role and timing of HCT in the management of FL is a controversial issue. While high-dose therapy (HDT) and autologous HCT (auto-HCT) has low treatment-related mortality (TRM) and morbidity, disease relapse remains a major concern. Myeloablative (MA) allogeneic HCT (allo-HCT) is a potentially curative modality; however, it is often associated with prohibitive TRM, particularly in more frail patients. Factors to be considered while assessing patients' eligibility for HCT include but are not limited to patient- and disease-related characteristics, optimal timing of HCT, type of HCT (autologous versus allogeneic), and selecting intensity of preparative regimens (MA or reduced-intensity conditioning (RIC)) in case an allograft is pursued [8, 9].

Herein we review the available published data pertaining to the role and optimal timing of HCT in patients with FL. To identify relevant publications, PubMed and Medline (the Web sites developed by the National Center of Biotechnology Information at the National Library of Medicine of the NIH), were searched using the search terms "follicular lymphoma" and "transplantation" limited to "English language," and a publication date of 1992 or later. In addition to the online database search, a manual search of the reference lists of reviews and included articles was conducted. Papers that did not include FL patients or the ones that included fewer than 25 FL patients were excluded. Also excluded were editorials, letters to the editor, reviews, consensus conference papers, practice guidelines, and laboratory studies with no clinical correlates. National or international meetings' abstracts (American Society of Hematology, American Society of Blood and Marrow Transplantation, American Society of Clinical Oncology, European Hematology Association, and European Group for Blood and Marrow Transplantation) from January 2010 onwards and http://www.clinicaltrials.gov/ were searched to identify important ongoing trials. The goal of the paper is to critically analyze the current data pertaining to HCT in FL, in order to provide practical recommendation about the preferred graft source, conditioning regimen intensity, optimal timing, and the role of this modality in FL.

2. Role of Transplantation for FL in First Remission

Several studies have explored the use of HCT as consolidation after initial chemotherapy for FL, with the ultimate goal of improving the depth of response, disease control, and possibly OS.

2.1. Autologous HCT for FL in First Remission. Single center data from Dana-Farber Cancer Institute (DFCI), demonstrating prolonged disease-free survival in approximately 40% of FL patients undergoing purged bone marrow autografts, provided preliminary evidence for auto-HCT as consolidation for FL in first remission [10].

Four-randomized-controlled trials (RCT) have evaluated the role auto-HCT as consolidation for FL in first remission (Table 1) [11–14]. One German (German Low Grade Lymphoma Study Group (GLSG)) and two French (Groupe d'Etude des Lymphomes de l'Adulte (GELA) Groupe Ouest-Est des Leucémies et Autres Maladies du Sang (GOELAMS)) cooperative group studies randomized newly diagnosed, younger (≤60 years), advanced stage FL patients to receive consolidation with auto-HCT or interferon maintenance, after first-line chemotherapy with CHOP (cyclophosphamide, doxorubicin, vincristine, and prednisone) or CHOP-like regimens [11–13]. As shown in

Table 1, a significant PFS benefit was demonstrated in favor of auto-HCT in the GLSG and GOELAMS trials, but not in the GELA protocol. To date no OS benefit has been reported in any published study. Despite a relatively low TRM after autografting in the GLSG trial, this modality, however, was associated with a significantly higher incidence of secondary hematological malignancies (3.8% versus 0%, P = 0.02) [11, 15]. Similarly, significantly higher frequency of second malignancies was also seen in the GOELAMS study. A major limitation of these three trials is that they were conducted in the prerituximab era, hence questioning the applicability and relevance of these results in current practice. Interestingly, the PFS of FL patients receiving rituximab-based 1st line chemoimmunotherapy in contemporary cooperative group trials is roughly similar to the PFS reported in auto-HCT arm of GELA and GLSG studies [6, 7, 16].

To address the role of auto-HCT in upfront consolidation of FL in the rituximab era, the Gruppo Italiano Trapianto di Midollo Osseo/Intergruppo Italiano Linfomi (GITMO/IIL) trial compared chemoimmunotherapy with R-CHOP to rituximab supplemented HDT and auto-HCT. While rates of complete remission (CR), molecular remission, and event-free survival (EFS) were significantly better with Auto-HCT, no difference in OS was seen. A trend towards more secondary myelodysplasia/acute myeloid leukemia (sMDS/AML) was observed in the HDT arm, albeit not statistically significant (6.6% versus 1.7%; P = 0.111). Lack of survival benefit, despite better disease control in the auto-HCT arm, is likely due to subsequent salvage of patients relapsing after R-CHOP alone with an autograft in second (or later) remission, among other reasons [17]. Two recently published meta-analyses of aforementioned clinical trials confirmed the PFS benefit with autografting of FL patients in first remission, but no benefit in OS was described [18, 19].

In view of recent advances in the treatment of patients with newly diagnosed FL, including strategies such as consolidation with radio-immunotherapy [20], rituximab maintenance [21], and/or rituximab retreatment [22], routine use of autologous transplantation as consolidation in first remission for patients with FL cannot be recommended, especially as the latter is associated with development of secondary malignancies without a benefit in OS.

2.2. Allogeneic HCT for FL in First Remission. Allo-HCT offers several advantages such as a lymphoma-free graft, and the immunologic graft-versus-lymphoma (GVL) effect mediated by alloreactive donor T cells. It is a potentially curative treatment modality for patients with FL, who would be otherwise incurable with conventional chemoimmunotherapy or auto-HCT. However, there are no randomized controlled data available to support allografting in chemosensitive FL patients in first remission. Limited single-institution data are available for allo-HCT in a small subset of high risk FL patients with primary refractory disease, despite multiple treatment attempts [23, 24]. Such high-risk FL patients with primary refractory disease can be considered for an allo-HCT, ideally within the context of a clinical trial. At our institution, refractory FL patients are offered allo-HCT as part of an ongoing prospective study evaluating

TABLE 1: Randomized prospective trials addressing the role of autologous transplantation in follicular lymphoma patients in first remission.

Study group (year)	Number of patients	TRM in HDT versus C	EFS/PFS in HDT versus C (years)	OS in HDT versus C (years)	Comments
GLSG (2004)	307	<2.5% in both arms	64% versus 33%; $P < 0.0001$ [5]	Not reported	Significantly more sMDS/AML with HDT (3.5% versus 0%; $P = 0.02$)
GELA (2006)	402	Not reported	38% versus 28%; $P = 0.11$ [7]	76% versus 71%; $P = 0.53$ [7]	Secondary malignancy similar in both groups—14 with chemotherapy and 11 with HDT
GOELAMS (2009)	166	Not reported	64% versus 39%; $P = 0.004$ [9]	76% versus 80%; $P = 0.55$ [9]	Significantly more secondary malignancies with HDT ($n = 12$ versus 1; $P = 0.01$)
GITMO (2008)	136	$n = 3$ versus $n = 2$ at 100 days	61% versus 28%; $P < 0.01$ [4]	81% versus 80%; $P = 0.96$ [4]	4-year MDS/AML was higher with HDT (6.6% versus 1.7%)

Abbreviations: GLSG: german low grade lymphoma study group; GELA: groupe d'etude des lymphomes de l'adulte; GOELAMS: groupe ouest-est des leucémies et autres maladies du sang; GITMO: gruppo italiano trapianto di midollo osseo; TRM: treatment-related mortality; HDT: high-dose therapy and autologous HCT arm; C: chemotherapy arm; EFS/PFS: event/progression-free survival; OS: overall survival; sMDS: secondary myelodysplastic syndrome; AML: acute myeloid leukemia.

the role of pharmacokinetically guided reduced-toxicity conditioning allo-HCT for refractory aggressive lymphomas (http://www.clinicaltrials.gov/, NCT01203020).

3. HCT for Relapsed FL

Although the majority of FL patients respond to initial therapy, the vast majority of such patients eventually experience disease progression. HCT, autologous or allogeneic, is often considered in patients with relapsed disease, particularly after multiple lines of therapies. The role, optimal timing, and preferred transplant modality (autologous versus allogeneic) in the relapsed setting remain a matter of controversy.

3.1. Autologous Transplantation for Relapsed FL. Auto-HCT has long been available for patients with relapsed chemosensitive disease. Early single-institution, retrospective studies showed encouraging data for patients with relapsed disease [25, 26]. Large prospective trials comparing auto-HCT with chemotherapy are lacking, adding to the existing controversy about the role of this treatment modality in relapsed FL. The European Blood and Marrow Transplant (EBMT) group reported the only RCT in this setting (CUP trial). The CUP trial compared chemotherapy alone to chemotherapy followed by either unpurged or purged autografts. This trial was closed early because of poor accrual. Notwithstanding the small number of patients that was randomized (n = 89), the trial showed a significant PFS and OS benefit following HDT [27]. There was no reported difference in outcomes of purged compared to unpurged autografts. However, since this trial was conducted in the pre-rituximab era, its significance and clinical relevance to contemporary clinical practice is questioned.

To address the role of auto-HCT versus salvage chemotherapy alone in the rituximab-era, Sebban et al. conducted a *post hoc* analysis of patients enrolled on two GELF (Groupe d'Etude des Lymphomes Folliculaires) protocols that subsequently relapsed and received various salvage therapies including auto-HCT. In patients who received rituximab-containing salvage therapies, no statistically significant EFS or OS benefits were reported after HDT and auto-HCT when compared to patients who did not undergo autografting [28]. In a different study, the combined retrospective data from DFCI and St. Bartholomew's Hospital suggested prolonged remissions in a subset of FL patients after HDT; however, this benefit appeared restricted mostly to patients in second CR [29]. Conceptually, HDT and autologous transplantation at such an early point in relapsed FL could be uniformly offered, if it was curative and devoid of long-term serious complications. Auto-HCT, unfortunately, cannot be considered a curative modality for majority of the patients with FL. Large registry data from EBMT [30] and Center for International Blood and Marrow Transplant Research (CIBMTR) show no plateau in risk of disease relapse after autografting [31]. More importantly the risks of second cancers and sMDS/AML after auto-HCT are not insignificant, ranging from 5 to 15% in several large studies [29, 30]. While acknowledging the limitations of HDT in relapsed FL, it is also prudent

to highlight the fact about a third of carefully selected chemosensitive FL patients that can experience durable responses following auto-HCT (31% PFS at 10 years in the EBMT registry data) [30].

In order to solve the problem of autograft contamination by lymphoma cells, several studies have examined the role of *ex vivo* purging (by monoclonal antibodies, CD34+ cell selection, etc.) [32, 33] and *in vivo* purging (e.g., rituximab with mobilization) [34, 35] of autologous stem cell products with encouraging results. However, the lack of randomized data to prove the superiority or curative potential of purged auto-HCT [27], and a possible increase in infectious complications with *ex vivo* purging [36, 37], has prevented the uniform acceptance to this modality by transplant centers. In the rituximab era, the decision to offer an autologous transplant should take into account several factors including patient's age, associated comorbidities, risk of secondary cancers, and presence of chemosensitive disease. Heavily pretreated patients with refractory disease are unlikely to benefit from HDT and should preferably be considered for participation in clinical trials. Outside the setting of a clinical trial, the decision to offer an auto-HCT for FL should be made on a case-by-case basis. Auto-HCT is best reserved for chemosensitive, relapsed FL patients after 2-3 lines of prior chemoimmunotherapies (ideally at least one doxorubicin-based line, and a bendamustine-based regimen), who are not candidates for curative therapies, namely, allo-HCT, because of donor unavailability, associated comorbidities, or patient preference. Whether postauto-HCT rituximab maintenance will improve patient outcomes is an area of active investigation and at the moment, it cannot be considered a standard option [38, 39].

3.2. Myeloablative Allogeneic Transplantation for Relapsed FL. Adoptive immunotherapy in the form of allo-HCT is potentially curative for patients with FL. The GVL effects mediated by the donor T-lymphocytes are beneficial in patients with lymphoid malignancies [40, 41]. One of the most compelling evidence for a clinically relevant GVL effect in relapsed FL comes from the success of allo-HCT after an autograft failure [42–44]. Unlike auto-HCT where relapse-risk posttransplant does not decrease overtime, registry data from CIBMTR and EBMT [31, 45] clearly show that a plateau in relapse risk is achievable in 2-3 years after allografting, indicating that a substantial proportion of these patients can be cured with MA allo-HCT. However, in both CIBMTR and EBMT studies, despite impressively low relapse rates (20–25% at 5 years) after MA allo-HCT, compared to rates following auto-HCT (50–55% at 5 years), no difference in OS was seen, primarily due to unacceptably high rates of TRM following MA allografts (approximately 35–40% compared to 8–15% after auto-HCT). Moreover, since the median age at diagnosis for FL is the sixth decade of life, a significant number of such patients are not appropriate candidates for MA conditioning. Whether there is a benefit of MA allo-HCT in younger patients with chemorefractory disease, over less ablative, so-called RIC regimens, is not known. It is unlikely that a prospective clinical trial will be performed to compare MA conditioning with RIC allogeneic transplantation in patients with FL, as the latter has been broadly adopted as the preferred regimen to use when considering allografting. In the absence of robust prospective data to prove otherwise, MA allo-HCT should not be considered as the regimen of choice in patients with FL, especially for those with advanced age and/or with associated medical comorbidities and poor performance status.

3.3. RIC Transplantation for Relapsed FL. RIC regimens were developed to improve applicability of allo-HCT to older, heavily pretreated patients, particularly those with associated medical comorbidities. These regimens aim at reducing procedure-related toxicities and rely more heavily on GVL immunologic effects. While no prospective trials have compared MA conditioning against RIC transplantation in FL, registry data from EBMT and CIBMTR, with their inherent limitations [31, 45], have established the feasibility of this approach by demonstrating acceptable rates TRM [46], albeit at the possible expense of higher relapse rates [47] and comparable OS and PFS with RIC allo-HCT compared to MA allografts.

Several phase II studies have prospectively assessed the feasibility of RIC HCT in patients with relapsed FL (Table 2) [42, 48–51]. Khouri et al. have recently reported updated M.D. Anderson Cancer Center (MDACC) experience with 47 chemosensitive FL patients conditioned with fludarabine, cyclophosphamide, and high-dose rituximab. The 11-year PFS and OS were 72% and 78%, respectively. The incidence of grade 2–4 acute GVHD was 11% [48, 52]. This updated report from MDACC also includes 26 patients (38% with chemorefractory disease) who received novel conditioning with ^{90}Y-ibritumomab tiuxetan. The 3-year PFS rates for patients with chemorefractory and chemosensitive disease were 80% and 87%, respectively [52]. The Cancer and Leukemia Group B (CALGB) also reported encouraging outcomes of FL patients with RIC in a smaller, but multicenter prospective study [51]. The Blood and Marrow Transplant Clinical Trials Network (BMT CTN) Protocol 0701 is currently conducting a multicenter study using the RIC reported by Khouri et al. It is important to point out that the CALGB study and 2008 publication by Khouri et al. comprised almost exclusively of patients undergoing matched sibling donor HCT. To mitigate the higher rates GVHD associated with unrelated donor (URD) HCT, Thomson et al. employed *in vivo* T-cell depletion with alemtuzumab. In this large multicenter study, 52% of the patients underwent URD transplantation. Ten percent of cases had refractory disease. The 4-year rates of PFS, OS, and TRM were 76%, 76%, and 15%, respectively, with clinically significant acute GVHD noted in 13% [49]. Nevertheless, relapse rates were slightly high (26%) and donor lymphocyte infusions were frequently needed, likely because of the use of T-cell depletion.

3.4. Autologous versus RIC Allogeneic Transplant for Relapsed FL. A commonly encountered question in the clinic is whether to offer auto- or RIC allo-HCT to patients with FL relapsing after multiple lines of prior therapies. An adequately powered prospective trial comparing these two

options is lacking [1]. Unfortunately, the very important BMT CTN 0202 trial comparing auto-HCT to RIC allo-HCT in FL was closed early due to poor accrual (N for auto-HCT = 22 and N for allo-HCT = 8) [53]. For the 30 patients enrolled in the BMT CTN 0202 study, the 3-year OS was 73% with auto-HCT versus 100% following allo-HCT, and 3 year PFS was 63% in the auto-HCT group versus 86% in the allo-HCT cohort. No patient had grade II–IV acute GVHD. Three auto-HCT recipients died from nonrelapse causes. The Canadian group recently reported 3-year PFS and OS of 96%, with a novel approach of auto-HCT followed by a tandem RIC allo-HCT, with low rate of TRM [54]. Whether a tandem auto/allo-HCT approach is truly superior to the current clinical practice of effective cytoreduction with chemoimmunotherapy followed by allo-HCT is not known, and at the present time a tandem auto/allo-HCT should be considered investigational. While acknowledging the scarcity of good quality clinical trial data, it appears that TRM rate with RIC allo-HCT [48, 49, 51] is relatively low, with much lower risk of disease relapse and no risk of sMDS/AML, when compared against auto-HCT. Considering these facts, it is appropriate to offer RIC allo-HCT for appropriately selected and clinically fit FL patients with an available suitable adult donor, when curative intent is pursued. While the timing remains controversial, we consider this option mainly in patients who have progressed after 2-3 lines of prior therapies (including at least one with anthracyclines and/or fludarabine), provided that the disease remains chemosensitive and patients are not candidates for clinical trials. Auto-HCT can be considered for patients who are medically unfit for RIC allografting or those without an adult or alternative donor, with the understanding that cure may not be achievable.

4. Transplantation for Transformed FL

Histological transformation of FL (HT-FL) to aggressive NHL is not uncommon with up to 30% of FL patients undergoing transformation, at an annual rate of 3% [55]. Studies evaluating the role of HCT in this setting are limited by a small sample size and unavailability of prospective data. Table 3 details selected studies evaluating auto-HCT for HT-FL, that involved at least 20 patients [56–60]. The EBMT reported the largest study, involving 50 patients, all with chemosensitive, disease. The 5-year PFS and OS rates were 30% and 51% respectively [61]. The Norwegian group recently published the only prospective trial of auto-HCT in HT-FL. This study showed 5-year PFS and OS rates of 32% and 47%, respectively, in 30 patients [60]. Short followup and patient selection (with majority of patients with minimal disease at transplantation) is a limitation to consider when interpreting these results. An often overlooked clinical problem in this setting is the possibility of developing late relapses, mostly involving the indolent histologic component after auto-HCT, indicating that while HDT might potentially eradicate the large cell component, the (nontransformed) FL component appears less curable in this setting.

To circumvent this problem, and to salvage patients with chemorefractory disease, limited data is available for

TABLE 2: Results of prospective, phase II trials evaluating allogeneic hematopoietic cell transplantation after reduced intensity conditioning.

Author (Year)	Number of patients	Age (range)	Conditioning regimen	TRM	EFS/PFS	OS	Comments
Khouri et al. [48, 52] (2008 and 2012)	47	53 (33–68)	FCR +/– ATG	15% (5 years)	72% (11 years)	78% (11 years)	Grades 2–4 acute GVHD in 11%. All had chemosensitive disease. High-dose rituximab (1000 mg/m^2) used.
Thomson et al. [49] (2010)	82	45 (26–65)	FMC	15% (4 years)	76% (4 years)	76% (4 years)	Grades 2–4 acute GVHD in 13%. Included 26% with prior auto-HCT and 9% with refractory disease.
Piñana et al. [50] (2010)	37	50 (34–62)	FM	35%*	57% (4 years)	54% (4 years)	Grades 2–4 acute GVHD in 47%. Included 46% with prior auto-HCT.
Shea et al. [51] (2011)	44 (16 had FL)	53 (39–68)	FC	9% (3 years)	75% (3 years)	81% (3 years)	All were sibling donors and none had prior auto-HCT.

Abbreviations: FL: follicular lymphoma; FCR: fludarabine, cyclophosphamide, rituximab; ATG: antithymocyte globulin; F: fludarabine, M: melphalan, C: campath; FC: fludarabine, cyclophosphamide; TRM: treatment-related mortality; EFS/PFS: event/progression-free survival; OS: overall survival; GVHD: graft versus host disease; auto-HCT: autologous hematopoietic cell transplantation. *TRM estimated from numbers in the publication.

TABLE 3: Autologous hematopoietic cell transplantation for follicular lymphoma that has undergone histological transformation to large cell lymphoma.

Author (year)	Number of patients	Age (range)	Conditioning regimen	TRM	PFS	OS	Comments
Friedberg et al. [56] (1999)	21	44 (29–58)	TBI/CY	NA	46% (5 years)	58% (5 years)	All had minimal disease state. Purged autograft used.
Chen et al. [58] (2001)	25[a]	48 (36–64)	Mel/TBI/VP	28%	36% (5 years)	37% (5 years)	All had chemosensitive disease.
Williams et al. [57, 61] (2001)	50	40 (26–52)	Various regimens	8% (100 days)	30% (5 years)	51% (5 years)	100% had chemo-sensitive disease. High LDH led to poor outcomes.
Hamadani et al. [59] (2008)	24	56 (47–68)	BU/CY BCNU based	8% (100 days)	40% (3 years)	52% (3 years)	17% had bulky disease and no purged autografts used.
Eide et al. [60] (2011)	30[b]	55 (31–65)	BEAM	NA	32% (5 years)	47% (5 years)	The only prospective trial. All 30 had chemosensitive disease.

Abbreviations: TBI: total body irradiation; CY: cyclophosphamide; Mel: melphalan; VP: etoposide; BU: busulfan; BCNU: carmustine; TRM: treatment-related mortality; PFS: progression-free survival; OS: overall survival; LDH: lactate dehydrogenase; BEAM: BCNU, etoposide, cytarabine, melphalan.
[a]Of the 35 patients in the sample, only 25 had true histological transformation to diffuse large B-cell lymphoma. [b]Of the 47 patients enrolled, only 30 underwent autologous hematopoietic cell transplantation.

TABLE 4: Recommendations based on current evidence and expert opinion, on the role of hematopoietic cell transplantation in follicular lymphoma.

Status of FL	Type of HCT	Recommendations
First remission as consolidative therapy	HDT-autologous HCT	Not recommended.
	Allogeneic HCT	Not recommended.
Relapsed/refractory FL	HDT-autologous HCT	Consider for patients with chemosensitive disease, and ≤2-3 lines of prior therapies.
	Myeloablative allogeneic HCT	Best reserved for medically fit younger patients with refractory disease.
	RIC allogeneic HCT	Recommended for appropriately selected relapsed/refractory patients.
FL after histological transformation	HDT-autologous HCT	Appropriate for patients with chemosensitive disease. Ideally on a clinical trial.
	Allogeneic HCT	Consider for fit patients with refractory relapse, bone marrow involvement, and history of prior autologous HCT. Ideally on a clinical trial.

Abbreviations: FL: follicular lymphoma; HCT: hematopoietic cell transplantation; HDT: high-dose therapy; RIC: reduced intensity conditioning; RCT: randomized controlled trials; OS: overall survival; PFS: progression-free survival; TBI: total body irradiation; TRM: treatment-related mortality; URD: unrelated donor.

allo-HCT in HT-FL. One study evaluated the role of RIC in 16 patients with HT-FL and reported a dismal 3-year TRM, PFS, and OS rates of 43%, 21%, and 18% respectively [62]. A South African report, which included HT-FL patients ($n = 11$) who received MA conditioning, showed OS of 64% [63]. Hamadani et al. reported a 100-day TRM of 12% and 5-year PFS and OS of 56% and 66%, respectively, in a cohort of 8 HT-FL patients that included bulky disease ($n = 3$) and/or chemorefractory disease ($n = 3$) [59]. At this time, HT-FL is best managed within the context of a clinical trial. At our institution, elderly transformed patients with minimal disease are typically offered auto-HCT, while the younger patients with minimal comorbidities and those with refractory transformed disease are offered participation on an ongoing allo-HCT clinical trial (http://www.clinicaltrials.gov/, NCT01203020).

5. Conclusions

Table 4 documents recommendations on the role of HCT in FL based on aforementioned reviewed data and expert opinion [64]. FL is a heterogeneous disease entity with variable presentation and clinical course. Currently, no predictive clinical or molecular markers to guide role of HCT therapy exist and this issue remains an area of active research. With improvements seen in management of newly diagnosed FL, including immunochemotherapy and rituximab maintenance [21], HCT is unlikely to play a role in the frontline setting. In the relapsed setting, prospective cooperative group effort is certainly needed to elucidate the optimal timing and overall role of HCT. Ongoing clinical trials are assessing the role of rituximab, for *in vivo* purging prior to auto HCT (NCT00856245) and radio-immunotherapy for disease control in the peri-transplant period. Whether the encouraging, but limited, data of tandem autologous and

RIC allo-HCT [54] in FL will play a role in future awaits confirmation with a randomized control study. For allo-HCT to become a more widely accepted curative modality for majority of FL patients it will require development of safer and less toxic conditioning regimens, more effective ways of augmenting the beneficial GVL without increasing the incidence and severity of GVHD, and improving supportive care measures after transplantation. The BMT CTN protocol 0701 (NCT00912223) is a step in the right direction, but the need remains for more robust randomized, clinical trials. While slow accrual has led to premature closure of several key clinical trials [53], continued cooperative efforts are necessary.

Acknowledgments

This work is supported in part by Conquer Cancer Foundation of ASCO Career Development Award (MH) and ASBMT New Investigator Award (MH).

References

[1] E. Ayala and M. Tomblyn, "Hematopoietic cell transplantation for lymphomas," *Cancer Control*, vol. 18, pp. 246–257, 2011.

[2] L. H. Sehn, T. S. Fenske, and G. G. Laport, "Follicular lymphoma: prognostic factors, conventional therapies, and hematopoietic cell transplantation," *Biology of Blood and Marrow Transplantation*, vol. 18, pp. S82–S91, 2012.

[3] P. Solal-Celigny, P. Roy, P. Colombat et al., "Follicular lymphoma international prognostic index," *Blood*, vol. 104, no. 5, pp. 1258–1265, 2004.

[4] C. Buske, E. Hoster, M. Dreyling, J. Hasford, M. Unterhalt, and W. Hiddemann, "The follicular lymphoma international prognostic index (FLIPI) separates high-risk from intermediate- or low-risk patients with advanced-stage follicular lymphoma treated front-line with rituximab and the combination of

cyclophosphamide, doxorubicin, vincristine, and prednisone (R-CHOP) with respect to treatment outcome," *Blood*, vol. 108, no. 5, pp. 1504–1508, 2006.

[5] M. S. Czuczman, R. Weaver, B. Alkuzweny, J. Berlfein, and A. J. Grillo-López, "Prolonged clinical and molecular remission in patients with low-grade or follicular non-Hodgkin's lymphoma treated with rituximab plus CHOP chemotherapy: 9-Year follow-up," *Journal of Clinical Oncology*, vol. 22, no. 23, pp. 4711–4716, 2004.

[6] W. Hiddemann, M. Kneba, M. Dreyling et al., "Frontline therapy with rituximab added to the combination of cyclophosphamide, doxorubicin, vincristine, and prednisone (CHOP) significantly improves the outcome for patients with advanced-stage follicular lymphoma compared with therapy with CHOP alone: results of a prospective randomized study of the German Low-Grade Lymphoma Study Group," *Blood*, vol. 106, no. 12, pp. 3725–3732, 2005.

[7] R. Marcus, K. Imrie, P. Solal-Celigny et al., "Phase III study of R-CVP compared with cyclophosphamide, vincristine, and prednisone alone in patients with previously untreated advanced follicular lymphoma," *Journal of Clinical Oncology*, vol. 26, no. 28, pp. 4579–4586, 2008.

[8] M. L. Sorror, S. Giralt, B. M. Sandmaier et al., "Hematopoietic cell transplantation-specific comorbidity index as an outcome predictor for patients with acute myeloid leukemia in first remission: combined FHCRC and MDACC experiences," *Blood*, vol. 110, no. 13, pp. 4606–4613, 2007.

[9] M. Hamadani, M. Craig, F. T. Awan, and S. M. Devine, "How we approach patient evaluation for hematopoietic stem cell transplantation," *Bone Marrow Transplantation*, vol. 45, no. 8, pp. 1259–1268, 2010.

[10] J. R. Brown, Y. Feng, J. G. Gribben et al., "Long-term survival after autologous bone marrow transplantation for follicular lymphoma in first remission," *Biology of Blood and Marrow Transplantation*, vol. 13, no. 9, pp. 1057–1065, 2007.

[11] G. Lenz, M. Dreyling, E. Schiegnitz et al., "Myeloablative radiochemotherapy followed by autologous stem cell transplantation in first remission prolongs progression-free survival in follicular lymphoma: results of a prospective, randomized trial of the German Low-Grade Lymphoma Study Group," *Blood*, vol. 104, no. 9, pp. 2667–2674, 2004.

[12] C. Sebban, N. Mounier, N. Brousse et al., "Standard chemotherapy with interferon compared with CHOP followed by high-dose therapy with autologous stem cell transplantation in untreated patients with advanced follicular lymphoma: the GELF-94 randomized study from the Groupe d'Etude des Lymphomes de l'Adulte (GELA)," *Blood*, vol. 108, no. 8, pp. 2540–2544, 2006.

[13] E. Gyan, C. Foussard, P. Bertrand et al., "High-dose therapy followed by autologous purged stem cell transplantation and doxorubicin-based chemotherapy in patients with advanced follicular lymphoma: a randomized multicenter study by the GOELAMS with final results after a median follow-up of 9 years," *Blood*, vol. 113, no. 5, pp. 995–1001, 2009.

[14] M. Ladetto, F. De Marco, F. Benedetti et al., "Prospective, multicenter randomized GITMO/IIL trial comparing intensive (R-HDS) versus conventional (CHOP-R) chemoimmunotherapy in high-risk follicular lymphoma at diagnosis: the superior disease control of R-HDS does not translate into an overall survival advantage," *Blood*, vol. 111, no. 8, pp. 4004–4013, 2008.

[15] G. Lenz, M. Dreyling, E. Schiegnitz et al., "Moderate increase of secondary hematologic malignancies after myeloablative radiochemotherapy and autologous stem-cell transplantation

in patients with indolent lymphoma: results of a prospective randomized trial of the German Low Grade Lymphoma Study Group," *Journal of Clinical Oncology*, vol. 22, no. 24, pp. 4926–4933, 2004.

[16] G. Salles, N. Mounier, S. De Guibert et al., "Rituximab combined with chemotherapy and interferon in follicular lymphoma patients: results of the GELA-GOELAMS FL2000 study," *Blood*, vol. 112, no. 13, pp. 4824–4831, 2008.

[17] M. Ladetto, F. De Marco, F. Benedetti et al., "Prospective, multicenter randomized GITMO/IIL trial comparing intensive (R-HDS) versus conventional (CHOP-R) chemoimmunotherapy in high-risk follicular lymphoma at diagnosis: the superior disease control of R-HDS does not translate into an overall survival advantage," *Blood*, vol. 111, no. 8, pp. 4004–4013, 2008.

[18] M. Al Khabori, J. R. de Almeida, G. H. Guyatt et al., "Autologous stem cell transplantation in follicular lymphoma: a systematic review and meta-analysis," *Journal of the National Cancer Institute*, vol. 104, pp. 18–28, 2012.

[19] M. Schaaf, M. Reiser, P. Borchmann, A. Engert, and N. Skoetz, "High-dose therapy with autologous stem cell transplantation versus chemotherapy or immuno-chemotherapy for follicular lymphoma in adults," *Cochrane Database of Systematic Reviews*, vol. 1, Article ID CD007678, 2012.

[20] F. Morschhauser, J. Radford, A. Van Hoof et al., "Phase III trial of consolidation therapy with yttrium-90-ibritumomab tiuxetan compared with no additional therapy after first remission in advanced follicular lymphoma," *Journal of Clinical Oncology*, vol. 26, no. 32, pp. 5156–5164, 2008.

[21] G. Salles, J. F. Seymour, F. Offner et al., "Rituximab maintenance for 2 years in patients with high tumour burden follicular lymphoma responding to rituximab plus chemotherapy (PRIMA): a phase 3, randomised controlled trial," *The Lancet*, vol. 377, no. 9759, pp. 42–51, 2011.

[22] B. Kahl, F. Hong, M. E. Williams et al., "Results of eastern cooperative oncology group protocol E4402 (RESORT): a randomized phase III study comparing two different rituximab dosing strategies for low tumor burden follicular lymphoma," *Blood*, vol. 118, LBA-6, no. 21, 2011.

[23] A. K. Gopal, K. A. Guthrie, J. Rajendran et al., "⁹⁰Y-Ibritumomab tiuxetan, fludarabine, and TBI-based nonmyeloablative allogeneic transplantation conditioning for patients with persistent high-risk B-cell lymphoma," *Blood*, vol. 118, no. 4, pp. 1132–1139, 2011.

[24] M. Hamadani, D. M. Benson Jr., C. C. Hofmeister et al., "Allogeneic stem cell transplantation for patients with relapsed chemorefractory aggressive non-hodgkin lymphomas," *Biology of Blood and Marrow Transplantation*, vol. 15, no. 5, pp. 547–553, 2009.

[25] P. J. Bierman, J. M. Vose, J. R. Anderson, M. R. Bishop, A. Kessinger, and J. O. Armitage, "High-dose therapy with autologous hematopoietic rescue for follicular low-grade non-Hodgkin's lymphoma," *Journal of Clinical Oncology*, vol. 15, no. 2, pp. 445–450, 1997.

[26] T. M. Cao, S. J. Horning, R. S. Negrin et al., "High-dose therapy and autologous hematopoietic-cell transplantation for follicular lymphoma beyond first remission: The Stanford University experience," *Biology of Blood and Marrow Transplantation*, vol. 7, no. 5, pp. 294–301, 2001.

[27] H. C. Schouten, W. Qian, S. Kvaloy et al., "High-dose therapy improves progression-free survival and survival in relapsed follicular non-Hodgkin's lymphoma: results from the randomized European CUP trial," *Journal of Clinical Oncology*, vol. 21, no. 21, pp. 3918–3927, 2003.

[28] C. Sebban, P. Brice, R. Delarue et al., "Impact of rituximab and/or high-dose therapy with autotransplant at time of relapse in patients with follicular lymphoma: a GELA study," *Journal of Clinical Oncology*, vol. 26, no. 21, pp. 3614–3620, 2008.

[29] A. Z. S. Rohatiner, L. Nadler, A. J. Davies et al., "Myeloablative therapy with autologous bone marrow transplantation for follicular lymphoma at the time of second or subsequent remission: long-term follow-up," *Journal of Clinical Oncology*, vol. 25, no. 18, pp. 2554–2559, 2007.

[30] S. Montoto, C. Canals, A. Z. S. Rohatiner et al., "Long-term follow-up of high-dose treatment with autologous haemato-poietic progenitor cell support in 693 patients with follicular lymphoma: an EBMT registry study," *Leukemia*, vol. 21, no. 11, pp. 2324–2331, 2007.

[31] K. Van Besien, F. R. Loberiza, R. Bajorunaite et al., "Comparison of autologous and allogeneic hematopoietic stem cell transplantation for follicular lymphoma," *Blood*, vol. 102, no. 10, pp. 3521–3529, 2003.

[32] A. S. Freedman, D. Neuberg, P. Mauch et al., "Long-term follow-up of autologous bone marrow transplantation in patients with relapsed follicular lymphoma," *Blood*, vol. 94, no. 10, pp. 3325–3333, 1999.

[33] C. Tarella, P. Corradini, M. Astolfi et al., "Negative immun-omagnetic ex vivo purging combined with high-dose chemotherapy with peripheral blood progenitor cell autograft in follicular lymphoma patients: evidence for long-term clinical and molecular remissions," *Leukemia*, vol. 13, no. 9, pp. 1456–1462, 1999.

[34] C. Tarella, M. Zanni, M. Magni et al., "Rituximab improves the efficacy of high-dose chemotherapy with autograft for high-risk follicular and diffuse large B-cell lymphoma: a multicenter gruppo italiano terapie innnovative nei linfomi survey," *Journal of Clinical Oncology*, vol. 26, no. 19, pp. 3166–3175, 2008.

[35] L. Arcaini, F. Montanari, E. P. Alessandrino et al., "Immun-ochemotherapy with *in vivo* purging and autotransplant induces long clinical and molecular remission in advanced relapsed and refractory follicular lymphoma," *Annals of Oncology*, vol. 19, no. 7, pp. 1331–1335, 2008.

[36] F. Crippa, L. Holmberg, R. A. Carter et al., "Infectious complications after autologous CD34-selected peripheral blood stem cell transplantation," *Biology of Blood and Marrow Transplantation*, vol. 8, no. 5, pp. 281–289, 2002.

[37] L. K. Hicks, A. Woods, R. Buckstein et al., "Rituximab purging and maintenance combined with auto-SCT: long-term molecular remissions and prolonged hypogammaglobulinemia in relapsed follicular lymphoma," *Bone Marrow Transplantation*, vol. 43, no. 9, pp. 701–708, 2009.

[38] R. Pettengell, N. Schmitz, C. Gisselbrecht et al., "Randomized study of rituximab in patients with relapsed or resistant follicular lymphoma prior to high-dose therapy as in vivo purging and to maintain remission following high-dose therapy," *Journal of Clinical Oncology*, vol. 28, no. 15, p. 8005, 2010.

[39] M. Magni, M. Di Nicola, C. Carlo-Stella et al., "High-dose sequential chemotherapy and in vivo rituximab-purged stem cell autografting in mantle cell lymphoma: a 10-year update of the R-HDS regimen," *Bone Marrow Transplantation*, vol. 43, no. 6, pp. 509–511, 2009.

[40] C. M. P. W. Mandigers, L. F. Verdonck, J. P. P. Meijerink, A. W. Dekker, A. V. M. B. Schattenberg, and J. M. M. Raemaekers, "Graft-versus-lymphoma effect of donor lymphocyte infusion in indolent lymphomas relapsed after allogeneic stem cell transplantation," *Bone Marrow Transplantation*, vol. 32, no. 12, pp. 1159–1163, 2003.

[41] P. Armand, H. T. Kim, V. T. Ho et al., "Allogeneic transplantation with reduced-intensity conditioning for hodgkin and non-hodgkin lymphoma: importance of histology for outcome," *Biology of Blood and Marrow Transplantation*, vol. 14, no. 4, pp. 418–425, 2008.

[42] I. F. Khouri, "Allogeneic stem cell transplantation in follicular lymphoma," *Best Practice and Research*, vol. 24, no. 2, pp. 271–277, 2011.

[43] M. P. Escalón, R. E. Champlin, R. M. Saliba et al., "Non-myeloablative allogeneic hematopoietic transplantation: a promising salvage therapy for patients with non-Hodgkin's lymphoma whose disease has failed a prior autologous transplantation," *Journal of Clinical Oncology*, vol. 22, no. 12, pp. 2419–2423, 2004.

[44] K. Branson, R. Chopra, P. D. Kottaridis et al., "Role of nonmy-eloablative allogeneic stem-cell transplantation after failure of autologous transplantation in patients with lymphoprolifera-tive malignancies," *Journal of Clinical Oncology*, vol. 20, no. 19, pp. 4022–4031, 2002.

[45] A. J. Peniket, M. C. Ruiz de Elvira, G. Taghipour et al., "An EBMT registry matched study of allogeneic stem cell transplants for lymphoma: allogeneic transplantation is associated with a lower relapse rate but a higher procedure-related mortality rate than autologous transplantation," *Bone Marrow Transplantation*, vol. 31, no. 8, pp. 667–678, 2003.

[46] I. Avivi, S. Montoto, C. Canals et al., "Matched unrelated donor stem cell transplant in 131 patients with follicular lymphoma: an analysis from the Lymphoma Working Party of the European Group for Blood and Marrow Transplantation," *British Journal of Haematology*, vol. 147, no. 5, pp. 719–728, 2009.

[47] P. Hari, J. Carreras, M. J. Zhang et al., "Allogeneic transplants in follicular lymphoma: higher risk of disease progression after reduced-intensity compared to myeloablative conditioning," *Biology of Blood and Marrow Transplantation*, vol. 14, no. 2, pp. 236–245, 2008.

[48] I. F. Khouri, P. McLaughlin, R. M. Saliba et al., "Eight-year experience with allogeneic stem cell transplantation for relapsed follicular lymphoma after nonmyeloablative conditioning with fludarabine, cyclophosphamide, and rituximab," *Blood*, vol. 111, no. 12, pp. 5530–5536, 2008.

[49] K. J. Thomson, E. C. Morris, D. Milligan et al., "T-cell-depleted reduced-intensity transplantation followed by donor leukocyte infusions to promote graft-versus-lymphoma activity results in excellent long-term survival in patients with multiply relapsed follicular lymphoma," *Journal of Clinical Oncology*, vol. 28, no. 23, pp. 3695–3700, 2010.

[50] J. L. Piñana, R. Martino, J. Gayoso et al., "Reduced intensity conditioning HLA identical sibling donor allogeneic stem cell transplantation for patients with follicular lymphoma: long-term follow-up from two prospective multicenter trials," *Haematologica*, vol. 95, no. 7, pp. 1176–1182, 2010.

[51] T. Shea, J. Johnson, P. Westervelt et al., "Reduced-intensity allogeneic transplantation provides high event-free and overall survival in patients with advanced indolent B cell malignancies: CALGB 109901," *Biology of Blood and Marrow Transplantation*, vol. 17, pp. 1395–1403, 2011.

[52] I. F. Khouri, R. M. Saliba, W. D. Erwin et al., "Nonmyeloab-lative allogeneic transplantation with or without 90yttrium ibritumomab tiuxetan is potentially curative for relapsed follicular lymphoma: 12-year results," *Blood*, vol. 119, pp. 6373–6378, 2012.

[53] M. R. Tomblyn, M. Ewell, C. Bredeson et al., "Autologous versus reduced-intensity allogeneic hematopoietic cell transplantation for patients with chemosensitive follicular Non-Hodgkin lymphoma beyond first complete response or first partial response," *Biology of Blood and Marrow Transplantation*, vol. 17, no. 7, pp. 1051–1057, 2011.

[54] S. Cohen, T. Kiss, S. Lachance et al., "Tandem autologous-allogeneic nonmyeloablative sibling transplantation in relapsed follicular lymphoma leads to impressive progression-free survival with minimal toxicity," *Biology of Blood and Marrow Transplantation*, vol. 18, pp. 951–957, 2012.

[55] A. J. Al-Tourah, K. K. Gill, M. Chhanabhai et al., "Population-based analysis of incidence and outcome of transformed non-hodgkin's lymphoma," *Journal of Clinical Oncology*, vol. 26, no. 32, pp. 5165–5169, 2008.

[56] J. W. Friedberg, D. Neuberg, J. G. Gribben et al., "Autologous bone marrow transplantation after histologic transformation of indolent B cell malignancies," *Biology of Blood and Marrow Transplantation*, vol. 5, no. 4, pp. 262–268, 1999.

[57] C. D. Williams, C. N. Harrison, T. A. Lister et al., "High-dose therapy and autologous stem-cell support for chemosensitive transformed low-grade follicular non-Hodgkin's lymphoma: a case-matched study from the European bone marrow transplant registry," *Journal of Clinical Oncology*, vol. 19, no. 3, pp. 727–735, 2001.

[58] C. I. Chen, M. Crump, R. Tsang, A. Keith Stewart, and A. Keating, "Autotransplants for histologically transformed follicular non-Hodgkin's lymphoma," *British Journal of Haematology*, vol. 113, no. 1, pp. 202–208, 2001.

[59] M. Hamadani, D. M. Benson, T. S. Lin, P. Porcu, K. A. Blum, and S. M. Devine, "High-dose therapy and autologous stem cell transplantation for follicular lymphoma undergoing transformation to diffuse large B-cell lymphoma," *European Journal of Haematology*, vol. 81, no. 6, pp. 425–431, 2008.

[60] M. B. Eide, G. F. Lauritzsen, G. Kvalheim et al., "High dose chemotherapy with autologous stem cell support for patients with histologically transformed B-cell non-Hodgkin lymphomas. A Norwegian multi centre phase II study," *British Journal of Haematology*, vol. 152, no. 5, pp. 600–610, 2011.

[61] C. D. Williams, C. N. Harrison, T. A. Lister et al., "High-dose therapy and autologous stem-cell support for chemosensitive transformed low-grade follicular non-Hodgkin's lymphoma: a case-matched study from the European bone marrow transplant registry," *Journal of Clinical Oncology*, vol. 19, no. 3, pp. 727–735, 2001.

[62] A. R. Rezvani, L. Norasetthada, T. Gooley et al., "Non-myeloablative allogeneic haematopoietic cell transplantation for relapsed diffuse large B-cell lymphoma: a multicentre experience," *British Journal of Haematology*, vol. 143, no. 3, pp. 395–403, 2008.

[63] N. Novitzky and V. Thomas, "Allogeneic stem cell transplantation with T cell-depleted grafts for lymphoproliferative malignancies," *Biology of Blood and Marrow Transplantation*, vol. 13, no. 1, pp. 107–115, 2007.

[64] D. M. Oliansky, L. I. Gordon, J. King et al., "The role of cytotoxic therapy with hematopoietic stem cell transplantation in the treatment of follicular lymphoma: an evidence-based review," *Biology of Blood and Marrow Transplantation*, vol. 16, no. 4, pp. 443–468, 2010.

22

Unrelated Hematopoietic Stem Cell Donor Matching Probability and Search Algorithm

J.-M. Tiercy

National Reference Laboratory for Histocompatibility, Transplantation Immunology Unit,
Department of Medical Specialties and Department of Genetics and Laboratory Medicine, Geneva University Hospitals,
University of Geneva, 1211 Geneva, Switzerland

Correspondence should be addressed to J.-M. Tiercy, jean-marie.tiercy@unige.ch

Academic Editor: Andrzej Lange

In transplantation of hematopoietic stem cells (HSCs) from unrelated donors a high HLA compatibility level decreases the risk of acute graft-versus-host disease and mortality. The diversity of the HLA system at the allelic and haplotypic level and the heterogeneity of HLA typing data of the registered donors render the search process a complex task. This paper summarizes our experience with a search algorithm that includes at the start of the search a probability estimate (high/intermediate/low) to identify a HLA-A, B, C, DRB1, DQB1-compatible donor (a 10/10 match). Based on 2002–2011 searches about 30% of patients have a high, 30% an intermediate, and 40% a low probability search. Search success rate and duration are presented and discussed in light of the experience of other centers. Overall a 9-10/10 matched HSC donor can now be identified for 60–80% of patients of European descent. For high probability searches donors can be selected on the basis of DPB1-matching with an estimated success rate of >40%. For low probability searches there is no consensus on which HLA incompatibilities are more permissive, although HLA-DQB1 mismatches are generally considered as acceptable. Models for the discrimination of more detrimental mismatches based on specific amino acid residues rather than specific HLA alleles are presented.

1. Introduction

An increasing number of transplantations are now performed with hematopoietic stem cells (HSC) from unrelated volunteer donors. This trend has been largely facilitated by the impressive growth of volunteer donor registries in the last decade: 8 million donors in 2002 and more than 20 million in 2012. The implementation of recipient and donor HLA high resolution genotyping in the clinical practice has clearly contributed to improve the success of transplantation through a better matching [1, 2]. On the other hand the polymorphism of HLA genes turns out to be much higher than anticipated, resulting in larger difficulties in identifying a perfectly matched donor. Because most donors in the Bone Marrow Donor Worldwide (BMDW) registry are of European descent, searches for patients of other ethnic backgrounds have a lower success rate, particularly for those patients with a mixed origin.

HLA matching is commonly based on exons 2 and 3 polymorphism for class I loci and on exon 2 polymorphism for class II loci. The nature of HLA polymorphism with reshuffling of gene segments coding for just a few amino acids has rendered HLA typing a challenging task. The HLA typing techniques currently used in the clinical laboratories often lead to ambiguities because alleles share sequence motifs and because a number of alleles are not resolved by the methods in use. Most typing techniques rely on a locus-specific generic amplification (of one or several exons) which makes it sometimes difficult ot detect whether two polymorphic segments are in *cis* or in *trans* in heterozygous individuals. Furthermore the extension of sequencing techniques to additional exons has disclosed many new alleles, thereby contributing to increase the difficulty of HLA matching. The deleterious impact of single HLA disparities between patient and donor has been largely documented [1–3]. Matching for HLA-A, B, C, DRB1, and DQB1 alleles, a so-called 10/10 match [1–3], and more recently for HLA-DPB1 [2, 4, 5], has been shown to decrease the risk of acute graft-versus-host disease (aGVHD) and mortality after HSCT.

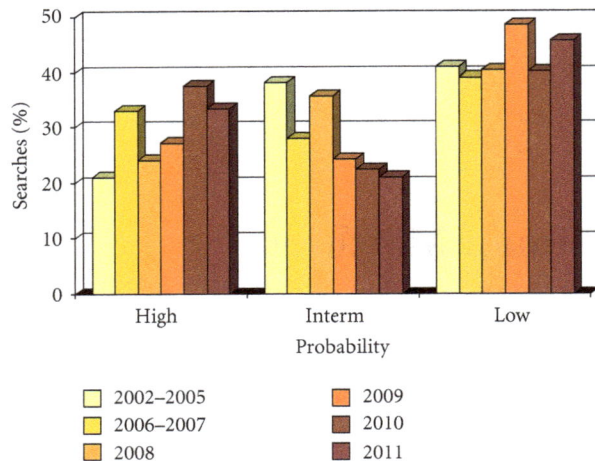

FIGURE 1: Relative distribution of 1244 high, intermediate, and low probability searches run from 2002 to 2011. The 2002–2005 probability estimates have been reported previously [6].

In 2002 we have introduced at the very start of the search an estimation of the probability to identify a perfectly matched donor, that is, compatible for the HLA-A, B, C, DRB1/B3/B5, and DQB1 loci. The probabilities were classified in 3 categories: high (>95% chance), intermediate (about 50%), and low (<5%). As computed from 350 searches (2002–2005) the positive and negative predictive values were 96% and 88%, respectively [6]. This paper reviews our experience in unrelated HSC donor searches as a follow-up of the search algorithm applied in our laboratory since 2002 [6]. A recent evaluation of the success rate and of the time frame for the identification of a suitable donor as well as the impact of the inclusion of DPB1 matching in the algorithm are presented and compared to those reported by other centers. Criteria that negatively impact the matching probability rate, and HLA-linked parameters that could be taken into account for selecting a mismatched donor, are reviewed. Clinical and functional relevance of HLA disparities is reviewed and possible models for the identification of more detrimental mismatches based on specific amino acid positions are discussed.

2. Search Probabilities

According to the search algorithm initiated in 2002 on a national basis, search probabilities are assigned as high, intermediate, or low based on patients HLA-A, B, C, DRB1/B3/B5,DQB1 haplotypes and on interrogation of the BMDW database [6]. Parameters that are taken into account for the probability assignment are presented in the next section. For each consecutive year the relative ratios of high/intermediate/low probabilities have been computed. All donors were requested by the national registry Swiss Blood Stem Cells (SBSC) and tested by the national reference laboratory for histocompatibility (LNRH). Usually 4–6 donors were requested, taking into account a >20% donor unavailability rate.

As compared to the initial observations of 2002–2005, the ratio of high probability searches has increased from 21% to 33–37% in the last 2 years (Figure 1). However the ratio of low probability searches remained stable around 40%. The absolute increase of the registered donors in BMDW, the implementation of HLA typing data (higher resolution level and additional loci tested) of the newly registered donors, and our increased knowledge on HLA haplotypic frequencies [7–12] have also allowed more precise probability estimates. Indeed the ratio of searches qualified as intermediate probability searches (i.e., the most difficult to assign) has decreased from 38% to 21-22% in the last 2 years (Figure 1). Predictive algorithms based on population HLA allele and haplotype frequencies are used by other centers: Haplogic by the National Marrow Donor Program (NMDP), Optimatch by the German Registry or EasyMatch by the French Registry.

3. Impact of Rare Alleles and Haplotypes on the Search

Based on our experience of the last 10 years, still 2–5% of the patients do have a unique phenotype (not necessarily including a rare HLA variant) that is not represented in the 20 million donors-BMDW registry. A German study based on 2008-2009 searches reported a 3.3% rate [13]. The ratio is expected to be higher for patients of non-European ancestry. In our experience, among 55 patients with 0 donor in BMDW some serotypes occurred more frequently, such as A25, A33, A68, B18, B53, B58, or B72. HLA-DRB1*09:01-, *10:01-, *14:01, *15:02- and *04:02/03/05/06/07/08-positive haplotypes also occurred more frequently (data not shown).

Criteria that negatively impact the probability to identify a 10/10 compatible donor are summarized in Table 1 and are obviously linked to patients allele/haplotype frequencies [6, 10, 11, 13]. Searches for patients with a rare allele (e.g., B*07:04 or DRB1*11:58 as encountered in patients analysed in our laboratory) have a low probability of success. Even searches for patients with alleles that represent 5–10% of all alleles within a serotype such as B*35:02 or DRB1*13:03, may have a low probability estimate depending on the extended HLA-A, B, DRB1 haplotype. For example matching for A*02:05 will be much easier if the patient has the A2-B50-DR7 haplotype [11] when compared to the A2-B50-DR3 haplotype. Rare alleles are often associated with a well-defined HLA-A-B-DRB1 haplotype, presumably because of a more recent origin of the allele. A few examples are illustrated in Table 2. A most representative case is the A*02:151 allele, initially described as A*9251 [14], that was subsequently confirmed in 17 individuals (http://www.ebi.ac.uk/imgt/hla/): in 13/17 confirmations this allele was identified on the haplotype A*02:151-B*07:02-C*07:02-DRB1*15:01. Consequently, the presence of a rare allele on a given haplotype might not necessarily mean that search will not be successful. Recently sequenced new alleles that differ outside exons 2 and 3 (for class I) and exon 2 (for class II) may also impact on matching probability. A classic example is the DRB1*14:01 versus *14:54 incompatibility. However the clinical relevance of such

TABLE 1: Parameters that contribute to define a low probability estimate.

HLA, ethnicity, nb donors	Examples and comments
≤3 donors in BMDW	
Non-European ancestry	
Rare[1] allele at any locus	A*02:17, B*44:05, DRB1*11:03
Rare B-C association	B*18:01-C*02:02, B*51:01-C*16:02
Rare DRB1-DQB1 association	DRB1*15:01-DQB1*06:03, DRB1*0701-DQB1*03:02
B*15:01, B*18:01, B*27:05, B*51:01-positive haplotypes	Higher risk of C MM
B*35:02/35:03/35:08-positive haplotypes	Higher risk of B*35 allele MM

[1] <5% of the alleles included a given serotype.

TABLE 2: Examples of conserved haplotypes with rare HLA class I alleles.

Rare allele	First assigned	Extended haplotype
A*02:151	2008	A*02:151-B*07:02-C*07:02-DRB1*15:01
A*03:20	2005	A*03:20-B*51:08-C*16:02-DRB1*11:04
A*03:50	2009	A*03:50-B*35:01-C*04:01-DRB1*01:01
A*03:96	2010	A*03:96-B*07:02-C*07:02-DRB1*15:01
A*03:102	2010	A*03:102-B*18:01-C*02:02-DRB1*13:01
B*07:20	1999	A*24:02-B*07:20-C*07:02-DRB1*16:01
B*27:70	2010	A*02:01-B*27:70-C*02:02-DRB1*04:01/04:04
B*51:43	2006	A*02:01-B*51:43-C*14:02-DRB1*04:01
C*05:14	2006	A*02:01-B*51:01-C*05:14-DRB1*04:04
C*15:13	2004	A*02:01-B*51:01-C*15:13-DRB1*04:02

disparities is unknown. Unusual B-C and DRB1-DQB1 [6, 11, 13, 15] associations involving common alleles also lead to low probability searches. In such cases the transplant physician should rapidly consider a 9/10 matched donor with a C or DQB1 mismatch, respectively.

4. Search Algorithm and DPB1 Matching

An outline of the search algorithm as a function of the probability estimate is represented in Table 3. Requesting >2 donors for the high probability searches has also proven to be useful for the rapid identification of a "back-up donor" since the availability rate of selected donors has slightly decreased in the past years. As a major implementation of our initial algorithm [6], we have recently included HLA-DPB1 typing in the algorithm for a fraction of the high probability searches. Selection according to HLA-DPB1 matching was evaluated on 33 patients for whom >1 potential 10/10 matched donor could be identified (January–July 2012). Based on 33 searches we could identify a DPB1 matched donor for 42.4% of the patients (including one DPB1 mismatched pair in rejection direction only), with an average of 2.7 donors tested/patient (range 1–5, 90 donors tested). Although calculated on a limited number of searches that include essentially patients of European ancestry, this is the first evaluation of the success rate of prospective DPB1 typing aiming at the identification of a 12/12 matched donor. If no DPB1-matched donor can be identified, donors can

be selected according the T-cell epitope (TCE)3 matching algorithm [4].

5. Efficiency of the Searches

Efficiency of the search is detemined by the likelihood to identify a "matched" donor by testing a "reasonable" number of donors (i.e., in a cost-efficient manner) and by the the time required for the process. Data in the literature on "successful" searches and on search duration are scarce and are difficult to compare mainly because HLA matching criteria vary between the centers. Depending on risk factors such as patient's age, disease stage, or urgency of transplant, a 9/10 matched donor would be considered a suitable donor in center A, but not in center B.

A detailed Dutch study of 212 searches run in 1996–2000 showed that a suitable donor (9-10/10, or <9/10 in 13% cases) could be identified for 69% of the patients with a median search time of 2.5 months [16]. A study from the UK based on 60 unrelated donor searches run in 2005 reported that a 9-10/10 donor could be identified for 72% of the patients with a median time to donor availability of 11 weeks if donor was registered in the UK and of 14 weeks if the donor had to be searched in the international registry [17]. A retrospective evaluation of 549 searches run in 2005 for 23 German transplant centers reported the identification of a 10/10 matched donor for 61.6% of the patients [13]. Overall median search duration was 20 days (7–330), 45 days

TABLE 3: Unrelated donor search algorithm for high, intermediate, and low probability categories aiming at the identification of 12/12, 10/10, or 9/10 matched donors. This algorithm is based on requesting blood sample from BMDW registries, and histocompatibility testing in the laboratory serving the transplant center(s). Alternatively HLA typing can be performed by the laboratory linked to each registry at the request of the transplant center. Intermediate resolution typing must resolve the main allele groups, for example, B*44:02 versus B*44:03 groups or C*07:01 versus 07:02 groups.

Probability	Steps	Procedure
High	1	Urgent transplant: (i) select 2–4 donors (incl. "back-up donor") according to age, sex, CMV status, blood group (ii) type for HLA-A, B, C, DRB1/B3/B5, DQB1 at a high resolution level[1]
	2	Nonurgent transplant: consider DPB1 matching (a 12/12 match is possible for >1/3 patients) (i) type for HLA-A, B, C, and DRB1, DQB1 at an intermediate resolution level (ii) type for DRB3 if DRB3 MM risk (i.e. DRB1*13:01 haplotypes)[1] (iii) if DPB1 matched donor found: complete high resolution typing for all HLA loci
Interm	1	Select 4–6 potential donors and type for HLA-A, B, C, DRB1, and DQB1 at an intermediate level >1 potentially matched donor identified: select according non HLA criteria and complete high resolution typing
	2	no matched donor identified and urgent transplant: select according non HLA criteria and complete high resolution typing
	3	no matched donor identified and non-urgent transplant: request another set of 4–6 donors
Low	1	Consider a mismatch early in the search and request 4–6 donors: (i) type for HLA-A, B, C, DRB1/B3/B5, DQB1 at an intermediate resolution level
	2	No matched donor identified and urgent transplant: (i) select a donor among potential donors with single MM and complete high resolution typing
	3	No matched donor identified and nonurgent transplant: (i) request another 4–6 donors and type for HLA-A, B, C, DRB1/B3/B5, and DQB1 at an intermediate resolution level
	4	If no potential donors available in BMDW: (i) select donor(s) with a mismatch located at the locus where the patient's rare allele is found (ii) if B MM: select donors with B MM associated with same HLA-C (e.g., B35:08 versus B*53:01 or B*13:01 versus B*57:01) (iii) if DRB1 MM: select donors with DRB1 mismatches associated with same DQB1 allele (e.g., DRB1*11:03 versus DRB1*12:01)
	5	If no mismatch accepted consider another HSC source (cord blood, haplo-identical donor) or a nontransplant protocol

[1] HLA-A, B, C, DRB1, and DQB1 testing is performed by PCR-SSO on microbeads arrays (luminex technology, OneLambda HD reagents) by PCR-SSP (Genovision), and by mono-allelic PCR-SBT (Protrans). HLA-DRB3, DRB5, and DPB1 typing is performed by PCR-SSP.
MM: mismatches.

TABLE 4: Donor matching grade for 274 consecutive searches run from 1.1.2010 to 31.8.2012.

Category[1]	Nb patients	Nb donors tested	Mean nb don/patient	10/10	9/10[2]	≤8/10 or non evaluable
High	103	331	3.2	102 (99%)	1 (1%)	0
Interm	61	333	5.45	38 (62.2%)	20 (32.8%)	3 (5%)
Low	110	744	6.76	19 (17.3%)	44 (40%)	47 (42.7%)
Total	274	1408	5.14	159 (58%)	65 (23.7%)	50 (18.3%)

[1] For 26 patients classified with a high ($n = 7$), intermediate ($n = 5$), and low ($n = 14$) probability a formal search was not initiated or no donor could be requested or analysed during the same time frame.
[2] DRB3 disparities were counted as a mismatch.

TABLE 5: Time frame of donor searches run from 1.1.2010 to 31.8.2012 for transplanted patients with different search probability estimates.

Category	Nb patients	Time for donor identification (days)	Time to HSCT (days)	Mean nb donor tested/patient
High[1]	66	54 (20–208)	101 (24–428)	4.92
Interm	30	73 (34–217)	76 (11–170)	5.13
Low	36	83 (33–308)	94 (12–298)	5.05

[1] For 98/99 high probability searches a 10/10 matched donor could be identified with a mean duration of 56 days (20–208), a transplant date was not (yet) available for 18 patients, 5 patients declined transplantation, 6 patients died, 1 relapsed, 1 was transplanted abroad, 1 was transplanted with a haplo-identical donor.

(7–1225), and 477 (2–2870) days in patients groups with high, low and very low search success probabilities, respectively [13]. A recent Austrian study reported that a 9-10/10 (exceptionally a 8/10) matched donor could be identified for 78.3% of the patients (87.7% of European origin) in 2008–2010 searches, with a mean search time of 1.84 months in 2010 [18].

Not surprisingly ethnic origin of the patients has a major influence on the likelihood to find a matched donor because of the underrepresentation of "non-Caucasian" donors in the international registry. For example, based on the NMDP data, "Asian" patients have a two-fold higher probability to have a mismatched donor compared to "Caucasian" patients [19]. In a single center the donor (7-8/8 match) identification rate was about 90% for patients classified as "US or European Caucasians", 76% for "Hispanics", 62% for "Black/African American", and 33% for "Asians" [20].

In our experience we could identify a 10/10 or 9/10 matched donor in 71.2% patients in 2002–2005 (350 searches, mean 4.9 donors tested/patient) [6], and in 81.8% patients in 2010-2011 (274 searches, mean 5.1 donors tested/patient) (Table 4). In 2011 the average number of tested donors/patient was similar for all 3 categories (4 donors/patient), but lower than in 2010 (data not shown). The efficiency of searches run at the LNRH in 2010-2011 was evaluated by computing the time frame between the start of the search and the date of the HLA report providing the best matched donor, that is, a 10/10 matched donor for the high probability searches, or 9-10/10 matched donor for the low/intermediate searches, and with date of transplantation. For the high probability searches run in 2010-2011 that led to a transplant the average time to propose a donor to the transplant center was 54 days (Table 5). This is comparable to the 1.4 months median search time reported for Northwestern European patients [16] and the 1.7 months time reported

for Austrian patients [21]. This duration was however longer than the 21-days mean time reported for successful searches run by the German study [13]. Considering the nontransplanted patients with a high probability estimate the time frame for donor identification was identical. For the intermediate probability searches the time frame was 73 (34–217) days, and for the low probability searches the time frame was 83 (33–308) days (data not shown). For these 2 categories the search time was therefore longer than the average time reported in other studies [13, 21], but comparable to the duration reported by the U.K. study of searches run in 2005 [17]. Interestingly the time to transplant was similar for high and low probability searches, but slightly lower for intermediate probability searches (Table 5).

6. Clinical and Functional Relevance of Single HLA Mismatches

Whereas there is a consensus on the negative impact of single mismatches at HLA-A, B, C, DRB1 loci, the most difficult issue in selecting a 9/10 matched donor concerns the nature of the accepted mismatch. HLA-DQB1 incompatibilities are usually more readily accepted [1–3, 22]. In the NMDP study [3] HLA-A and -DRB1 mismatches were reported to have a more detrimental impact on overall survival than HLA-B and -C mismatches. On the other hand a recent analysis of unrelated donor peripheral blood HSC transplants from NMDP reported that only HLA-C antigen and HLA-B allele or antigen mismatches were associated with mortality [23]. In the Japan Marrow Donor Program (JMDP) study, HLA-A/B mismatches, but not HLA-C/DRB1/DQB1, were found to be significantly associated with reduced overall survival [24]. HLA disparities might reveal a stronger negative impact in those patients that have less advanced disease [1–3, 25] or other risk factors. There are no conclusive data showing a difference between allele-level and antigen-level mismatches [3, 26]. Furthermore, one should be careful in interpreting the permissivity of a given locus as identified in retrospective studies, because of possible bias in the accepted mismatches. For example, the role of DRB1 incompatibilities could be underestimated in patients study groups if a significant number of DRB1*11:01 versus *11:04 mismatched pairs are included. It is perhaps not a surprise that the negative impact of HLA-C mismatches is reported with a high statistical significance, as compared to A,B,DRB1 mismatches, since incompatibilities do occur more frequently at HLA-C locus and are often more readily accepted by the transplant centers. A hierarchy in the relevance of HLA incompatibilities must be considered in light of other patient/donor risk factors, as proven by the high predictive value of the EBMT risk score [27, 28]. *A fortiori* the ranking of individual permissive mismatches will be impossible to define unless extremely large patients cohorts can be analysed [29]. Some HLA incompatibilities have been shown to be potential permissive mismatches by *in vitro* cytotoxic T lymphocyte precursor (CTLp) frequency assays, as exemplified by the C*03:03 versus *03:04 disparity [30, 31].

7. Evaluation of HLA Mismatches at the Amino Acid Level

Other strategies for disclosing less detrimental mismatches have focused on the nature of the mismatch at the amino acid (aa) level. The HistoCheck scoring system for HLA class I mismatches, based on functional similarity of aa involved in antigenic peptides and T-cell receptor binding turned out not to be predictive of clinical outcome [32]. An evaluation of the impact of individual HLA mismatches, such as those reported in the JMDP study [33] may not be applicable in other populations which show a much larger heterogeneity in HLA disparities and therefore fewer mismatches of similar nature [29]. Using a novel statistical methodology, Marino et al. [34] have reported 13 aa substitutions associated with increased mortality at day 100 in low/intermediate risk patients transplanted with HSC from a single HLA class I mismatched donor. In a recent study [35], the alloreactive CTLp frequency determined in single HLA-A and -C incompatibilities was associated with the aa differences between the mismatched alleles. The probability of a negative CTLp was higher in pairs with >9 aa differences compared to pairs with 0–5 aa differences in the α-helices and β-sheet. Eight aa (62, 63, 73, 80, 116, 138, 144, 163) were most predictive for a negative CTLp frequency analysis. It is however difficult to compare this model with the random forest analysis mentioned above since 7 of the 12 aa substitutions associated with a negative CTLp outcome are reported to be associated with lower 100 day-survival in the NMDP analysis [34]. At least these models should be tested on independent patients cohorts. CD8+ T-cell alloreactivity, as determined by intracellular staining for IFN-γ, has been reported to be higher for HLA-B than for HLA-A mismatches [36]. This observation is not consistent with the more detrimental impact of HLA-A disparities reported in the NMDP study [3].

8. Conclusion

As evaluated in searches for patients mainly of European ancestry, a 9-10/10 HLA matched donor can be identified for 60–80% patients. Many transplant centers are now using search algorithms based on allele/haplotype frequencies in order to take earlier decisions to transplant with a mismatched donor or to select an alternative donor (e.g., cord blood, haplo-identical donor) or a nontransplant strategy. In our preliminary experience, the inclusion of prospective HLA-DPB1 typing in the search algorithm for those patients with more than one 10/10 allele matched donor has allowed to identify a 12/12 matched donor for about 40% patients. The challenge remains to reliably predict the functional relevance of individual mismatches for low probability searches, but at least some models are testable. Considering the multiple clinical variables in HSCT, as represented partially by the EBMT risk score [27], it is likely that only clinical studies with more homogenous patients cohorts will be informative. Parameters such as urgency of the transplantation, T-cell depletion, and reduced intensity conditioning might well impact on the role of HLA disparities. At the present time the ranking of HLA-A, B, C, or DRB1 mismatches still appears elusive. We consider the possibility that an *in vitro* functional assay may be used in the algorithm provided it is simple enough, requires limited amount of blood, and is quantitatively highly reproducible. MHC-linked non-HLA genetic polymorphisms that do impact clinical outcome [5, 37, 38] could also be included in the algorithm, primarily for the high probability searches, if validated by larger scale studies.

Acknowledgments

The author is grateful to L. Quiquerez, M. Bujan, and the technicians of the LNRH, and to Dr. G. Nicoloso from Swiss Blood Stem Cells for their expert collaboration. He also acknowledges the most efficient collaboration with Professor J. Passweg, Professor Y. Chalandon, Dr. U. Schanz, and Dr. T. Güngör, heads of the four Swiss centers for allogenic HSCT. This work has been supported by Grant 320030_130483 from the Swiss National Science Foundation.

References

[1] E. W. Petersdorf, "Optimal HLA matching in hematopoietic cell transplantation," *Current Opinion in Immunology*, vol. 20, no. 5, pp. 588–593, 2008.

[2] B. E. Shaw, R. Arguello, C. A. Garcia-Sepulveda, and J. A. Madrigal, "The impact of HLA genotyping on survival following unrelated donor haematopoietic stem cell transplantation: review," *British Journal of Haematology*, vol. 150, no. 3, pp. 251–258, 2010.

[3] S. J. Lee, J. Klein, M. Haagenson et al., "High-resolution donor-recipient HLA matching contributes to the success of unrelated donor marrow transplantation," *Blood*, vol. 110, no. 13, pp. 4576–4583, 2007.

[4] K. Fleischhauer, B. E. Shaw, T. Gooley, M. Malkki, P. Bardy, and J. D. Bignon, "Effect of T-cell epitope matching at HLA-DPB1 in recipients of unrelated-donor haematopoietic-cell-transplantation : a retrospective study," *Lancet Oncology*, vol. 13, pp. 366–374, 2012.

[5] F. Bettens, J. Passweg, U. Schanz, Y. Chalandon, D. Heim, and T. Güngör, "Impact of HLA-DPB1 haplotypes on outcome of 10/10 matched unrelated hematopoietic stem cell donor transplantation depends on MHC-linked microsatellite polymorphisms," *Biology of Blood and Marrow Transplantation*, vol. 18, pp. 608–616, 2012.

[6] J. M. Tiercy, G. Nicoloso, J. Passweg et al., "The probability of identifying a 10/10 HLA allele-matched unrelated donor is highly predictable," *Bone Marrow Transplantation*, vol. 40, no. 6, pp. 515–522, 2007.

[7] M. Maiers, L. Gragert, and W. Klitz, "High-resolution HLA alleles and haplotypes in the United States population," *Human Immunology*, vol. 68, no. 9, pp. 779–788, 2007.

[8] H. P. Eberhard, U. Feldmann, W. Bochtler et al., "Estimating unbiased haplotype frequencies from stem cell donor samples typed at heterogeneous resolutions: a practical study based on over 1 million German donors," *Tissue Antigens*, vol. 76, no. 5, pp. 352–361, 2010.

[9] A. H. Schmidt, U. V. Solloch, D. Baier et al., "Regional differences in HLA antigen and haplotype frequency distributions in Germany and their relevance to the optimization of hematopoietic stem cell donor recruitment," *Tissue Antigens*, vol. 76, no. 5, pp. 362–379, 2010.

[10] A. Balas, F. García-Sánchez, and J. L. Vicario, "Allelic and haplotypic HLA frequency distribution in Spanish hematopoietic patients. Implications for unrelated donor searching," *Tissue Antigens*, vol. 77, no. 1, pp. 45–53, 2011.

[11] B. Pédron, V. Guérin-El Khourouj, J. H. Dalle et al., "Contribution of HLA-A/B/C/DRB1/DQB1 common haplotypes to donor search outcome in unrelated hematopoietic stem cell transplantation," *Biology of Blood and Marrow Transplantation*, vol. 17, pp. 1612–1618, 2011.

[12] S. Buhler, J. M. Nunes, G. Nicoloso, J. Tiercy -M, and A. Sanchez-Mazas, "the heterogeneous genetic makeup of the Swiss population," *Plos ONE*, vol. 7, Article ID e41400, 2012.

[13] K. Hirv, K. Bloch, M. Fischer, B. Einsiedler, H. Schrezenmeier, and J. Mytilineos, "Prediction of duration and success rate of unrelated hematopoietic stem cell donor searches based on the patient's HLA-DRB1 allele and DRB1-DQB1 haplotype frequencies," *Bone Marrow Transplantation*, vol. 44, no. 7, pp. 433–440, 2009.

[14] B. Kervaire, A. H. Schmidt, J. Villard, and J. M. Tiercy, "Sequence of a novel HLA-A2 allele in a haematopoietic stem cell donor of the international registry," *Tissue Antigens*, vol. 74, no. 3, pp. 248–249, 2009.

[15] F. Bettens, G. Nicoloso De Faveri, and J. M. Tiercy, "HLA-B51 and haplotypic diversity of B-Cw associations: implications for matching in unrelated hematopoietic stem cell transplantation," *Tissue Antigens*, vol. 73, no. 4, pp. 316–325, 2009.

[16] M. B. A. Heemskerk, S. M. van Walraven, J. J. Cornelissen et al., "How to improve the search for an unrelated haematopoietic stem cell donor. Faster is better than more!," *Bone Marrow Transplantation*, vol. 35, no. 7, pp. 645–652, 2005.

[17] S. Querol, G. J. Mufti, S. G. E. Marsh et al., "Cord blood stem cells for hematopoietic stem cell transplantation in the uk:how big should the bank be?" *Haematologica*, vol. 94, no. 4, pp. 536–541, 2009.

[18] A. Rosenmayr, M. Pointner-Prager, M. Winkler, A. Mitterschiffthaler, B. Pelzmann, and L. Bozic, "The austrian bone marrow donor registry: providing patients in Austria with unrelated donors for transplant—a worldwide cooperation," *Transfusion Medicine and Hemotherapy*, vol. 38, pp. 292–299, 2012.

[19] J. Dehn, M. Arora, S. Spellman et al., "Unrelated donor hematopoietic cell transplantation: factors associated with a better HLA match," *Biology of Blood and Marrow Transplantation*, vol. 14, no. 12, pp. 1334–1340, 2008.

[20] J. Pidala, J. Kim, M. Schell, S. J. Lee, R. Hillgruber, and V. Nye, "Race/ethnicity affects the probability of finding an HLA-A, -B, -C and -DRB1 allele-matched unrelated donor and likelihood of subsequent transplant utilization," *Bone Marrow Transplantation*. In press.

[21] A. Rosenmayr, M. Pointner-Prager, A. Mitterschiffthaler et al., "What are a patient's current chances of finding a matched unrelated donor? Twenty years' central search experience in a small country," *Bone Marrow Transplantation*, vol. 47, pp. 172–180, 2011.

[22] Y. Chalandon, J. M. Tiercy, U. Schanz et al., "Impact of high-resolution matching in allogeneic unrelated donor stem cell transplantation in Switzerland," *Bone Marrow Transplantation*, vol. 37, no. 10, pp. 909–916, 2006.

[23] A. Woolfrey, J. P. Klein, M. Haagenson et al., "HLA-C antigen mismatch is associated with worse outcome in unrelated donor peripheral blood stem cell transplantation," *Biology of Blood and Marrow Transplantation*, vol. 17, no. 6, pp. 885–892, 2011.

[24] Y. Morishima, T. Sasazuki, H. Inoko et al., "The clinical significance of human leukocyte antigen (HLA) allele compatibility in patients receiving a marrow transplant from serologically HLA-A, HLA-B, and HLA-DR matched unrelated donors," *Blood*, vol. 99, no. 11, pp. 4200–4206, 2002.

[25] E. W. Petersdorf, C. Anasetti, P. J. Martin et al., "Limits of HLA mismatching in unrelated hematopoietic cell transplantation," *Blood*, vol. 104, no. 9, pp. 2976–2980, 2004.

[26] S. Spellman, M. Eapen, B. R. Logan, C. Mueller, P. Rubinstein, and M. I. Setterholm, "A perspective on the selection of unrelated donors and cord blood units for transplantation," *Blood*, vol. 120, pp. 259–265, 2012.

[27] A. Gratwohl, M. Stern, R. Brand et al., "Risk score for outcome after allogeneic hematopoietic stem cell transplantation: a retrospective analysis," *Cancer*, vol. 115, no. 20, pp. 4715–4726, 2009.

[28] T. Lodewyck, M. Oudshoorn, B. van der Holt et al., "Predictive impact of allele-matching and EBMT risk score for outcome after T-cell depleted unrelated donor transplantation in poor-risk acute leukemia and myelodysplasia," *Leukemia*, vol. 25, pp. 1548–1554, 2011.

[29] L. A. Baxter-Lowe, M. Maiers, S. R. Spellman et al., "HLA-A disparities illustrate challenges for ranking the impact of HLA mismatches on bone marrow transplant outcome in the United States," *Biology of Blood and Marrow Transplantation*, vol. 15, no. 8, pp. 971–981, 2009.

[30] E. Roosnek and J. M. Tiercy, "Search for an unrelated HLA-compatible stem cell donor," *Current Opinion in Hematology*, vol. 6, no. 6, pp. 365–370, 1999.

[31] M. Oudshoorn, I. I. N. Doxiadis, P. M. Van Den Berg-Loonen, C. E. M. Voorter, W. Verduyn, and F. H. J. Claas, "Functional versus structural matching: can the CTLp test be replaced by HLA allele typing?" *Human Immunology*, vol. 63, no. 3, pp. 176–184, 2002.

[32] S. Spellman, J. Klein, M. Haagenson, M. Askar, L. A. Baxter-Lowe, and J. He, "Scoring HLA class I mismatches by HistoCheck does not predict clinical outcome in unrelated hematopoietic stem cell transplantation," *Biology of Blood and Marrow Transplantation*, vol. 18, pp. 739–746, 2012.

[33] T. Kawase, Y. Morishima, K. Matsuo et al., "High-risk HLA allele mismatch combinations responsible for severe acute

graft-versus-host disease and implication for its molecular mechanism," *Blood*, vol. 110, no. 7, pp. 2235–2241, 2007.

[34] S. R. Marino, S. Lin, M. Maiers et al., "Identification by random forest method of HLA class I amino acid substitutions associated with lower survival at day 100 in unrelated donor hematopoietic cell transplantation," *Bone Marrow Transplantation*, vol. 47, pp. 217–226, 2012.

[35] M. M. Jöris, J. J. van Rood, D. L. Roelen, M. Oudshoorn, and F. H. J. Claas, "A proposed algorithm predictive for cytotoxic T cell alloreactivity," *Journal of Immunology*, vol. 188, pp. 1868–1873, 2012.

[36] N. A. Mifsud, A. W. Purcell, W. Chen, R. Holdsworth, B. D. Tait, and J. McCluskey, "Immunodominance hierarchies and gender bias in direct TCD8-cell alloreactivity," *American Journal of Transplantation*, vol. 8, no. 1, pp. 121–132, 2008.

[37] S. Morishima, S. Ogawa, A. Matsubara et al., "Impact of highly conserved HLA haplotype on acute graft-versus-host disease," *Blood*, vol. 115, no. 23, pp. 4664–4670, 2010.

[38] E. W. Petersdorf, M. Malkki, T. A. Gooley, S. R. Spellman, M. D. Haagenson, and M. M. Horowitz, "MHC-resident variation affects risks after unrelated donor hematopoietic cell transplantation," *Science Translational Medicine*, vol. 4, Article ID 144ra101, 2012.

23

Autologous Hematopoietic Stem Cell Transplantation for Multiple Myeloma without Cryopreservation

Khalid Ahmed Al-Anazi

Section of Adult Hematology and Hematopoietic Stem Cell Transplantation, Oncology Center, King Fahad Specialist Hospital, P.O. Box 15215, Dammam 31444, Saudi Arabia

Correspondence should be addressed to Khalid Ahmed Al-Anazi, kaa_alanazi@yahoo.com

Academic Editor: Ignazio Majolino

High-dose chemotherapy followed by autologous hematopoietic stem cell transplantation is considered the standard of care for multiple myeloma patients who are eligible for transplantation. The process of autografting comprises the following steps: control of the primary disease by using a certain induction therapeutic protocol, mobilization of stem cells, collection of mobilized stem cells by apheresis, cryopreservation of the apheresis product, administration of high-dose pretransplant conditioning therapy, and finally infusion of the cryopreserved stem cells after thawing. However, in cancer centers that treat patients with multiple myeloma and have transplantation capabilities but lack or are in the process of acquiring cryopreservation facilities, alternatively noncryopreserved autologous stem cell therapy has been performed with remarkable success as the pretransplant conditioning therapy is usually brief.

1. Introduction

Multiple myeloma (MM) accounts for 1% of all cancers and about 10% of all hematologic malignancies [1]. It is characterized by neoplastic proliferation of a clone of plasma cells producing a monoclonal immunoglobulin and can present as a single lesion (plasmacytoma) or multiple lesions (MM). Clonal plasma cells proliferate in the bone marrow and can cause extensive lytic bony lesions, osteopenia, and pathological fractures [2]. MM is a heterogenous disease rather than a single disease entity, as some patients progress rapidly despite therapy, whilst others may not require active therapy for a number of years [2].

Once the diagnosis of MM is made, the patient undergoes staging evaluation in order to start an appropriate line of therapy. The international staging system (ISS) divides patients into 3 categories according to serum albumin and beta-2-microglobulin levels. Conventional cytogenetics, fluorescence *in situ* hybridization (FISH), and molecular studies help to stratify patients into standard-risk, high-risk, and ultra-high-risk groups to determine prognosis and to refine management of patients. Gene expression profiling and plasma cell labeling index can identify high-risk groups and select the most appropriate novel therapies to be used [1–6].

2. Use of Novel Agents

The availability of novel agents has expanded treatment options and has improved outcomes of myeloma patients. A number of phase III clinical trials have demonstrated the efficacy of novel agent combinations and their superiority to VAD (vincristine, doxorubicin, and dexamethasone) regimen [7, 8]. Some novel agents appear to be active in high-risk patients, for example, those with adverse cytogenetics and molecular markers or certain comorbidities such as renal failure. Characterization of molecular events at cellular and marrow microenvironment levels has provided a platform for the development of various novel drugs in MM including proteasome inhibitors, immunomodulatory drugs, and HDAC (histone deacetylase) inhibitors [7, 8].

Bortezomib (velcade), the first-in-class proteasome inhibitor, was initially approved for the treatment of relapsed/refractory MM as a single agent [9, 10]. However, the great beneficial role it had exhibited in several clinical studies allowed the expansion of its role to become not only an integral part of induction therapy for newly diagnosed MM, but also a valuable element of consolidation and maintenance therapies in the pre- and posttransplant settings [9–15]. Bortezomib and dexamethasone combination has become an important part of standard induction therapy for newly diagnosed myeloma. This combination can be given twice or once weekly. The once-weekly schedule has proven to be equally effective and safer than the twice-weekly regimen specifically for patients more than 65 years of age. Bortezomib can also be safely given in various combinations with other agents including melphalan, cyclophosphamide, thalidomide, doxorubicin, and lenalidomide [7, 9, 11, 13–16]. Despite its safety profile, which allowed use in patients with renal failure and elderly individuals, the following adverse events have been reported: peripheral neuropathy, extramedullary plasmacytomas, gastrointestinal upset, myelotoxicity, and severe pulmonary complications [9, 12, 13, 15–17].

3. Autologous Stem Cell Transplantation

Since the mid-1990s, high-dose chemotherapy followed by autologous hematopoietic stem cell transplantation (auto-HSCT) has been considered the standard of care for frontline therapy in MM patients who are eligible for transplantation [18]. The choice of induction therapy has moved from conventional chemotherapy, for example VAD protocol, to newer regimens that incorporate novel agents like thalidomide, lenalidomide, and bortezomib. Upfront use of these agents, with 3-drug combinations in particular, has produced unprecedented rates of complete response (CR) that were never seen with old conventional chemotherapy and subsequent auto-HSCT [19]. Auto-HSCT offered after novel-agent-based induction therapies provides further improvement in the depth of response which is translated into longer progression-free survival, and potentially overall survival [18, 19]. Therefore, novel agents and auto-HSCT are complementary therapeutic strategies in patients with MM [19]. Improving the outcomes of HSCT in the future will require the exploration of novel strategies aimed at addressing the following issues: reduction of morbidity attributed to high-dose therapy, improving the efficacy of conditioning therapies, and the use of novel agents in the post-HSCT period [20].

For transplant-eligible patients, a bortezomib-based induction therapy is associated with improved disease control after HSCT and should, therefore, be considered the standard of care [20]. Moreover, a number of studies incorporating bortezomib as part of induction therapy have shown no adverse impact of bortezomib therapy on the yield of stem cell harvest and engraftment in patients with MM proceeding to transplant [21]. Auto-HSCT is safe and effective, but the outcome is independent of age, time from diagnosis, previous treatment, and conditioning therapy. However, achievement of CR and low international prognostic index at transplant is essential prognostically

[22, 23]. High CD34+ stem cell dose correlates well with early hematopoietic reconstitution and improvement of overall survival [22, 24]. Auto-HSCT for patients with MM can be entirely performed at the outpatient department in cancer centers that are fully equipped and can handle any evolving crisis or emergency. Outpatient auto-HSCT can result in shorter hospital stays and low transplant-related mortality and costs [25]. Studies have also shown that the use of certain conditioning therapies for HSCT can result in significant reduction or even abolition of transfusion of blood products, for example, packed red cells and platelets [26].

4. Stem Cell Mobilization

Mobilization of stem cells prior to stem cell collection and auto-HSCT in patients with MM is generally composed of 2 parts: the first part comprises the use of certain chemotherapeutic agents that include a single agent like cyclophosphamide or multiple agents in various combinations, with different dose schedules such as VAD, CD (cyclophosphamide and dexamethasone), CAD (cyclophosphamide, adriamycin, and dexamethasone), IVE (ifosfamide, etoposide, and epirubicin), EDAP (etoposide, dexamethasone, cytosine arabinoside, and cisplatin), CDVP (cyclophosphamide, doxorubicin, vincristine and prednisone), and VTD-PACE (bortezomib, thalidomide, dexamethasone, cisplatin, doxorubicin, cyclophosphamide, and etoposide), and the second part is composed of administration of growth factors such as granulocyte colony-stimulating factor (filgrastim; G-CSF), pegylated G-CSF, and plerixafor (Mozobil) in case of poor mobilization [27–40]. Various dose schedules were used in both single- or multiple-agent chemotherapeutic protocols, for example, doses of cyclophosphamide ranged from 1.0 to 7.0 gram/m^2 [34–38, 40–42]. However, recent studies have shown that adequate numbers of peripheral blood stem cells can be collected using growth factors alone, without prior chemotherapy, and that the use of cyclophosphamide for stem cell mobilization can overcome the suppressive effect of drugs, used in the treatment of MM, like lenalidomide on stem cell collection [41, 42].

Although filgrastim can be used alone for stem cell mobilization, studies have shown that the yield of stem cells was higher in patients mobilized with cyclophosphamide and G-CSF rather than with G-CSF alone, and that under certain circumstances, some regimens may be preferred to others, for example, VAD chemotherapy protocol followed by standard doses of G-CSF has been shown to be as effective as high-dose cyclophosphamide, in addition to being less toxic and allowing outpatient management with reduced cost [28, 31, 34, 35, 41, 42]. G-CSF and pegylated G-CSF may cause severe pain syndromes, and splenic rupture and may even precipitate veno-occlusive crises in patients with sickle cell anemia. However, in patients with sickle cell trait, stem cell mobilization using G-CSF is generally safe. Due to concerns of more serious adverse effects of G-CSF in patients with sickle cell trait, close monitoring of such patients should be maintained [43–47]. Plerixafor, a novel CXCR4 inhibitor, is effective in mobilization of peripheral blood stem cells in myeloma patients who fail conventional mobilization techniques. It has shown good tolerance and high success rates in patients who are labeled as poor mobilizers [29, 30, 32, 33].

5. Stem Cell Collection

Once the CD34+ cell count in peripheral blood exceeds 10.0 to 20.0 × 10^6/kg body weight, stem cell collection by leukapheresis is usually commenced. Most transplant centers make plans to obtain a target of 3.0 to 4.0 × 10^6 CD34+ cells/kg in case a single auto-HSCT is desired and a target of 6.0 to 8.0 × 10^6 CD34+ cells/kg in case a tandem transplant is planned [48–50]. The optimal count of CD34+ cells necessary for hematologic reconstitution is not well characterized, but the minimal count of 2.0 to 3.0 × 10^6 CD34+ cells/kg is generally accepted as the limit required to ensure short- as well as long-term hematologic reconstitution in the majority of patients [31, 40, 42, 48–50]. The yield of stem cell collection depends on a number of factors including age and performance status of the patient, presence of comorbidities, the previous lines of therapy given to the patient, the bone marrow reserve, upfront versus delayed auto-HSCT, the mobilization protocol used, and the technology applied in stem cell collection [42, 49].

6. Cryopreservation of Stem Cells

Cryopreservation of hematopoietic stem cells (HSCs) is routinely employed in auto-HSCT setting and is critical for cord blood transplantation. A variety of cryopreservatives have been used with different freezing and thawing techniques used in various transplantation centers. The standard and the most commonly used cryopreservative is DMSO (dimethylsulfoxide) which prevents freezing damage to living cells. DMSO is usually used at concentrations of 10% combined with normal saline and serum albumin. It is generally safe and nontoxic, but clinically it is associated with significant side effects that include nausea, vomiting, and abdominal cramps in addition to cardiovascular, neurological, respiratory, renal, hepatic, and hemolytic adverse effects. Standardization of stem cell processing using cryopreservation or mechanical freezing is of vital importance [51–53]. After cryopreservation and thawing of stem cells, a significant proportion of collected stem cells (20–30%) becomes nonviable due to early irreversible apoptosis. Therefore, systemic control for the viability of CD34+ cells immediately before reinfusion is recommended [54].

7. Autologous Transplantation without Cryopreservation

Studies have shown that peripheral blood stem cells (PBSCs) can be stored safely at 4°C for at least 5 days, while the patient receives high-dose chemotherapy. Viability of stem cells decreases progressively from day 5 onwards [55]. Liquid storage of harvested HSCs, either at room temperature or in standard blood refrigerators, is an alternative to cryopreservation. Preclinical data supporting the use of non-cryopreserved HSCs are available since 1957. Studies on mice reported successful rescue after administration of lethal doses of total body irradiation and reinfusion of bone marrow cells that had been stored for 11 days at 25°C. Subsequent *in vitro* and clinical studies on humans showed that bone marrow cells can be preserved in liquid state for 2 to 9 days without significant loss of granulocyte/macrophage-committed progenitor cells providing hematologic reconstitution to patients receiving myeloablative therapy [56]. The technique may be of value in 2 scenarios: (1) use in medical institutions from areas with limited economic resources, that is, having infrastructure to treat hematologic malignancies but not cryopreservation facilities and (2) use in medical institutions treating hematologic malignancies and in the process of establishing an HSCT program that will eventually have cryopreservation capabilities [56–59].

The use of noncryopreserved stem cells in transplantation has the following advantages: (1) simplicity of implementation and allowing auto-HSCT to be done entirely as outpatient, (2) reduction of transplant costs, (3) expansion of the number of medical institutions that offer stem cell therapy, (4) prevention of DMSO toxicity, (5) saving time between the last induction therapy and high-dose therapy, and (6) no significant reduction in viability of collected stem cells provided infusion is done within 5 days of collection. On the other hand, noncryopreserved HSCT has the following disadvantages: (1) limitation of the use of standard high-dose schedules employed in auto-HSCT, (2) plenty of coordination between various teams is required regarding timing of stem cell mobilization, apheresis, administration of high-dose therapy, and stem cell transfusion, and (3) inability to store part of the collection and reserving it for second transplant or other purposes in case a rich product is obtained [56–62].

Melphalan, which is the standard chemotherapeutic agent used in conditioning therapy prior to auto-HSCT in MM, becomes undetectable in plasma and urine 1 and 6 hours, respectively, following intravenous infusion of a high dose. Noncryopreserved stem cells can be reinfused as early as 8 hours after high-dose melphalan. Stem cell transfusion 8 to 24 hours following IV administration of melphalan has been reported to be associated with successful grafts. The dose of melphalan can range between 140 and 220 mg/m^2 [56, 59]. In a systemic review of the published studies on noncryopreserved autologous PBSCT in a variety of malignant hematological disorders including MM, the following results were obtained: (1) median time to neutrophil recovery ranged between 9 and 14 days, (2) median time to platelet recovery ranged between 13.5 and 25 days, and (3) hematopoietic reconstitution was universal in all the studies that included 560 patients. Only 1 graft failure was reported, and it was attributed to an inadequate stem cell dose [56]. Other studies reported neutrophil recovery as late as 27 days and platelet recovery as late as 37 days [57]. Treatment-related mortality was reported to range from 0.0 to 13.0%. The deaths reported were due to infections, heart failure, interstitial pneumonitis, and hepatic veno-occlusive disease [56–59, 61]. As stem cells can be stored without cryopreservation for a limited period of time, conditioning therapies for malignant hematological disorders that require administration over 6 days or more should either be excluded or these conditioning therapies should be changed altogether to be administered over 1 to 3 days. The rule of the sooner the better should therefore be applied so that harvested stem cells should be reinfused within 5 days of collection [56]. Studies comparing overnight storage of autologous stem cell apheresis products at 4°C with immediately cryopreserved products showed no statistically significant difference between the two groups regarding viability of collected stem cells, neutrophil and platelet engraftment days, safety, and even long-term outcome of the primary disease. Additional benefits of overnight storage of harvested products were reduction in costs and processing time [63–65].

8. Simplified Cryopreservation Techniques

Simplified methods of cryopreservation, that is, storage of harvested stem cells in mechanical freezers at −80°C using cryoprotective solutions that contain DMSO, have been successfully utilized in various parts of the world. Results of these simplified and less expensive cryopreservation procedures with regard to hematopoietic recovery after myeloablative therapy are comparable to standard cryopreservation techniques [66–70]. For short-term (less than 168 hours) storage of stem cells, the use of a storage medium composed of combination of super cooling, and University of Wisconsin solution was successfully used. Preservation of stem cells beyond 168 hours was associated with reduced viability of stored stem cells [71].

9. Tandem Transplantation in Myeloma

In selected subgroups of patients, tandem or second transplants may be more effective than single rounds of high-dose therapy and auto-HSCT. The timely application of a tandem transplant has extended event-free and overall survival independent of the cytogenetics and beta-2-microglobulin in some patients [72]. In most instances, a second auto-HSCT is performed using cryopreserved stem cells collected prior to the first auto-HSCT [49]. The indications for a tandem transplant in myeloma patients include relapse after first auto-HSCT or following prolonged remission and not achieving CR or near CR with the first auto-HSCT. However, in patients who are in CR or near CR, the second auto-HSCT could be performed as a salvage therapy in the future rather than an elective tandem procedure [49, 50, 72, 73].

10. Engraftment Syndrome and/or Autologous GVHD

During neutrophilic recovery following HSCT, a constellation of clinical manifestations that include fever, erythematous skin rash, nausea, vomiting, diarrhea, and noncardiogenic pulmonary edema may occur [74]. These clinical features are usually referred to as engraftment syndrome which may be a manifestation of graft versus host reaction.

This syndrome reflects cellular and cytokine interactions and may be associated with significant transplant-related mortality and morbidity due to pulmonary leak syndrome and multiorgan failure [74–77]. It has been well reported in autologous HSCT setting, and the extreme form is usually referred to as an autologous form of graft versus host disease (GVHD). The predisposing factors for auto-GVHD include MM as the primary disease, second auto-HSCT, heavily pretreated patients, high CD34+ cells infused, and achievement of high levels of absolute lymphocyte counts after HSCT [74–79]. Early recognition of this syndrome is vital in order to administer appropriate GVHD therapy which includes high-dose corticosteroids, alemtuzumab, infliximab, daclizumab, and etanercept [74–78].

11. Conclusion

Auto-HSCT without cryopreservation is feasible and can be performed successfully in cancer centers that have specific skills as well as standardized CD34+ cytometry technique in order to obtain accurate counting of progenitor cells but lack or are in the process of having cryopreservation facilities. It is simple, safe, and cost-effective. However, proper planning and coordination between various teams is vital for efficient mobilization and collection of hematopoietic progenitor cells, administration of the high-dose chemotherapy, and infusion of fresh stem cell products in a timely manner for optimal transplant outcome.

Managing teams should cautiously use filgrastim in patients with sickle cell disorders and should take into consideration the possible evolution of an engraftment syndrome after a successful autograft.

References

[1] S. V. Rajkumar, "Multiple myeloma: 2011 update on diagnosis, risk-stratification, and management," *American Journal of Hematology*, vol. 86, no. 1, pp. 57–65, 2011.

[2] S. V. Rajkumar, "Staging and prognostic studies in multiple mycloma," *UpToDate*, vol. 19.3, pp. 1–20, 2011.

[3] P. Kapoor, R. Fonseca, S. V. Rajkumar et al., "Evidence for cytogenetic and fluorescence in situ hybridization risk stratification of newly diagnosed multiple myeloma in the era of novel therapies," *Mayo Clinic Proceedings*, vol. 85, no. 6, pp. 532–537, 2010.

[4] H. Avet-Loiseau, "Ultra high-risk myeloma," *Hematology/the Education Program of the American Society of Hematology*, vol. 2010, pp. 489–493, 2010.

[5] D. Hose, T. Reme, T. Hielscher et al., "Proliferation is a central independent prognostic factor and target for personalized and risk-adapted treatment in multiple myeloma," *Haematologica*, vol. 96, no. 1, pp. 87–95, 2011.

[6] P. Segges and E. Braggio, "Genetic markers used for risk stratification in multiple myeloma," *Genetic Research International*, Article ID 798089, pp. 1–4, 2011.

[7] H. Ludwig, M. Beksac, J. Blade et al., "Current multiple myeloma treatment strategies with novel agents: a European perspective," *The Oncologist*, vol. 15, no. 1, pp. 6–25, 2010.

[8] J. P. Laubach, A. Mahindra, C. S. Mitsiades et al., "The use of novel agents in the treatment of relapsed and refractory

multiple myeloma," *Leukemia*, vol. 23, no. 12, pp. 2222–2232, 2009.

[9] J.-L. Harousseau, M. Attal, H. Avet-Loiseau et al., "Bortezomib plus dexamethasone is superior to vincristine plus doxorubicin plus dexamethasone as induction treatment prior to autologous stem-cell transplantation in newly diagnosed multiple myeloma: results of the IFM 2005-01 phase III trial," *Journal of Clinical Oncology*, vol. 28, no. 30, pp. 4621–4629, 2010.

[10] J. J. Shah and R. Z. Orlowski, "Proteasome inhibitors in the treatment of multiple myeloma," *Leukemia*, vol. 23, no. 11, pp. 1964–1979, 2009.

[11] A. Palumbo, F. Gay, P. Falco et al., "Bortezomib as induction before autologous transplantation, followed by lenalidomide as consolidation-maintenance in untreated multiple myeloma patients," *Journal of Clinical Oncology*, vol. 28, no. 5, pp. 800–807, 2010.

[12] H. Ludwig, D. Khayat, G. Giaccone, and T. Facon, "Proteasome inhibition and its clinical prospects in the treatment of hematologic and solid malignancies," *Cancer*, vol. 104, no. 9, pp. 1794–1807, 2005.

[13] S. Bringhen, A. Larocca, D. Rossi et al., "Efficacy and safety of once-weekly bortezomib in multiple myeloma patients," *Blood*, vol. 116, no. 23, pp. 4745–4753, 2010.

[14] A. Palumbo and S. V. Rajkumar, "Treatment of newly diagnosed myeloma," *Leukemia*, vol. 23, no. 3, pp. 449–456, 2009.

[15] J. J. Shah, R. Z. Orlowski, and S. K. Thomas, "Role of combination bortezomib and pegylated liposomal doxorubicin in the management of relapsed and/or refractory multiple myeloma," *Therapeutics and Clinical Risk Management*, vol. 5, no. 1, pp. 151–159, 2009.

[16] M.-V. Mateos, J. M. Hernandez, M. T. Hernandez et al., "Bortezomib plus melphalan and prednisone in elderly untreated patients with multiple myeloma: updated time-to-events results and prognostic factors for time to progression," *Haematologica*, vol. 93, no. 4, pp. 560–565, 2008.

[17] S. Miyakoshi, M. Kami, K. Yuji et al., "Severe pulmonary complications in Japanese patients after bortezomib treatment for refractory multiple myeloma," *Blood*, vol. 107, no. 9, pp. 3492–3494, 2006.

[18] P. Moreau, H. Avet-Loiseau, J.-L. Harousseau, and M. Attal, "Current trends in autologous stem-cell transplantation for myeloma in the era of novel therapies," *Journal of Clinical Oncology*, vol. 29, no. 14, pp. 1898–1906, 2011.

[19] M. Cavo, S. V. Rajkumar, A. Palumbo et al., "International myeloma working group consensus approach to the treatment of multiple myeloma patients who are candidates for autologous stem cell transplantation," *Blood*, vol. 117, no. 23, pp. 6063–6073, 2011.

[20] S. Girlat, "Stem cell transplantation for multiple myeloma: current and future status," *Hematology*, pp. 191–196, 2011.

[21] R. Manochakian, K. C. Miller, and A. A. Chanan-Khan, "Clinical impact of bortezomib in frontline regimens for patients with multiple myeloma," *The Oncologist*, vol. 12, no. 8, pp. 978–990, 2007.

[22] D. O'Shea, C. Giles, E. Terpos et al., "Predictive factors for survival in myeloma patients who undergo autologous stem cell transplantation: a single-centre experience in 211 patients," *Bone Marrow Transplantation*, vol. 37, no. 8, pp. 731–737, 2006.

[23] J. Martinez-Lopez, J. Blade, M.-V. Mateos et al., "Long-term prognostic significance of response in multiple myeloma after stem cell transplantation," *Blood*, vol. 118, pp. 529–534, 2011.

[24] N. Ketterer, G. Salles, M. Raba et al., "High CD34+ cell counts decrease hematologic toxicity of autologous peripheral blood progenitor cell transplantation," *Blood*, vol. 91, no. 9, pp. 3148–3155, 1998.

[25] M. A. Gertz, S. A. Ansell, D. Dingli et al., "Autologous stem cell transplant in 716 patients with multiple myeloma: low treatment-related mortality, feasibility of outpatient transplant, and effect of a multidisciplinary quality initiative," *Mayo Clinic Proceedings*, vol. 83, no. 10, pp. 1131–1135, 2008.

[26] G. J. Ruiz-Arguelles, A. Morales-Toquero, B. Lopez-Martinez, L. D. C. Tarin-Arzaga, and C. Manzano, "Bloodless (transfusion-free) hematopoietic stem cell transplants: the Mexican experience," *Bone Marrow Transplantation*, vol. 36, no. 8, pp. 715–720, 2005.

[27] G. Tricot, B. Barlogie, M. Zangari et al., "Mobilization of peripheral blood stem cells in myeloma with either pegfilgrastim or filgrastim following chemotherapy," *Haematologica*, vol. 93, no. 11, pp. 1739–1742, 2008.

[28] A. Nazha, R. Cook, D. T. Vogl et al., "Stem cell collection in patients with multiple myeloma: impact of induction therapy and mobilization regimen," *Bone Marrow Transplantation*, vol. 46, no. 1, pp. 59–63, 2011.

[29] G. Tricot, M. H. Cottler-Fox, and G. Calandra, "Safety and efficacy assessment of plerixafor in patients with multiple myeloma proven or predicted to be poor mobilizers, including assessment of tumor cell mobilization," *Bone Marrow Transplantation*, vol. 45, no. 1, pp. 63–68, 2010.

[30] R. F. Duarte, B. E. Shaw, P. Marin et al., "Plerixafor plus granulocyte CSF can mobilize hematopoietic stem cells from multiple myeloma and lymphoma patients failing previous mobilization attempts: EU compassionate use data," *Bone Marrow Transplantation*, vol. 46, no. 1, pp. 52–58, 2011.

[31] F. Lefrere, S. Zohar, D. Ghez et al., "The VAD chemotherapy regimen plus a G-CSF dose of $10\,\mu g/kg$ is as effective and less toxic than high-dose cyclophosphamide plus a G-CSF dose of $5\,\mu g/kg$ for progenitor cell mobilization: results from a monocentric study of 82 patients," *Bone Marrow Transplantation*, vol. 37, no. 8, pp. 725–729, 2006.

[32] J. F. DiPersio, E. A. Stadtmauer, A. Nademanee et al., "Plerixafor and G-CSF versus placebo and G-CSF to mobilize hematopoietic stem cells for autologous stem cell transplantation in patients with multiple myeloma," *Blood*, vol. 113, no. 23, pp. 5720–5726, 2009.

[33] M. J. Dugan, R. T. Maziarz, W. I. Bensinger et al., "Safety and preliminary efficacy of plerixafor (mozobil) in combination with chemotherapy and G-CSF: an open-label, multicenter, exploratory trial in patients with multiple myeloma and non-Hodgkin's lymphoma undergoing stem cell mobilization," *Bone Marrow Transplantation*, vol. 45, no. 1, pp. 39–47, 2010.

[34] J. Koren, I. Spicka, J. Straub et al., "Retrospective analysis of the results of high-dose chemotherapy with the support of autologous blood stem cells in patients with multiple myeloma. The experience of a single centre," *Prague Medical Report*, vol. 111, no. 3, pp. 207–218, 2010.

[35] K. A. Lerro, E. Medoff, Y. Wu et al., "A simplified approach to stem cell mobilization in multiple myeloma patients not previously treated with alkylating agents," *Bone Marrow Transplantation*, vol. 32, no. 12, pp. 1113–1117, 2003.

[36] U. Steidl, R. Fenk, I. Bruns et al., "Successful transplantation of peripheral blood stem cells mobilized by chemotherapy and a single dose of pegylated G-CSF in patients with multiple myeloma," *Bone Marrow Transplantation*, vol. 35, no. 1, pp. 33–36, 2005.

[37] J.-P. Fermand, S. Katsahian, M. Divine et al., "High-dose therapy and autologous blood stem-cell transplantation compared with conventional treatment in myeloma patients aged 55 to 65 years: long-term results of a randomized control trial from the group myelome-autogreffe," *Journal of Clinical Oncology*, vol. 23, no. 36, pp. 9227–9233, 2005.

[38] S. Fruehauf, J. Klaus, J. Huesing et al., "Efficient mobilization of peripheral blood stem cells following CAD chemotherapy and a single dose of pegylated G-CSF in patients with multiple myeloma," *Bone Marrow Transplantation*, vol. 39, no. 12, pp. 743–750, 2007.

[39] G. Kobbe, I. Bruns, R. Fenk, A. Czibere, and R. Haas, "Pegfilgrastim for PBSC mobilization and autologous haematopoietic SCT," *Bone Marrow Transplantation*, vol. 43, no. 9, pp. 669–677, 2009.

[40] S. Kumar, S. Giralt, E. A. Stadtmauer et al., "Mobilization in myeloma revisited: IMWG consensus perspectives on stem cell collection following initial therapy with thalidomide-, lenalidomide-, or bortezomib-containing regimens," *Blood*, vol. 114, no. 9, pp. 1729–1735, 2009.

[41] T. Mark, J. Stern, J. R. Furst et al., "Stem cell mobilization with cyclophosphamide overcomes the suppressive effect of lenalidomide therapy on stem cell collection in multiple myeloma," *Biology of Blood and Marrow Transplantation*, vol. 14, no. 7, pp. 795–798, 2008.

[42] T. Demirer, C. D. Buckner, and W. I. Bensinger, "Optimization of peripheral blood stem cell mobilization," *Stem Cells*, vol. 14, no. 1, pp. 106–116, 1996.

[43] P. Niscola, C. Romani, L. Scaramucci et al., "Pain syndromes in the setting of haematopoietic stem cell transplantation for haematological malignancies," *Bone Marrow Transplantation*, vol. 41, no. 9, pp. 757–764, 2008.

[44] A. Kuendgen, R. Fenk, I. Bruns et al., "Splenic rupture following administration of pegfilgrastim in a patient with multiple myeloma undergoing autologous peripheral blood stem cell transplantation," *Bone Marrow Transplantation*, vol. 38, no. 1, pp. 69–70, 2006.

[45] R. Veerappan, M. Morrison, S. Williams, and D. Variakojis, "Splenic rupture in a patient with plasma cell myeloma following G-CSF/ GM-CSF administration for stem cell transplantation and review of the literature," *Bone Marrow Transplantation*, vol. 40, no. 4, pp. 361–364, 2007.

[46] E. M. Kang, E. M. Areman, V. David-Ocampo et al., "Mobilization, collection, and processing of peripheral blood stem cells in individuals with sickle cell trait," *Blood*, vol. 99, no. 3, pp. 850–855, 2002.

[47] C. D. Fitzhugh, M. M. Hsieh, C. D. Bolan, C. Saenz, and J. F. Tisdale, "Granulocyte colony-stimulating factor (G-CSF) administration in individuals with sickle cell disease: time for a moratorium?" *Cytotherapy*, vol. 11, no. 4, pp. 464–471, 2009.

[48] R. M. Lemoli, G. Martinelli, E. Zamagni et al., "Engraftment, clinical, and molecular follow-up of patients with multiple myeloma who were reinfused with highly purified CD34+ cells to support single or tandem high-dose chemotherapy," *Blood*, vol. 95, no. 7, pp. 2234–2239, 2000.

[49] S. V. Rajkumar, "Autologous hematopoietic stem cell transplantation in multiple myeloma," *UpToDate*, vol. 19.3, pp. 1–24, 2011.

[50] G. Barosi, M. Boccadoro, M. Cavo et al., "Management of multiple myeloma and related-disorders: guidelines from the Italian Society of Hematology (SIE), Italian Society of Experimental Hematology (SIES) and Italian Group for Bone Marrow Transplantation (GITMO)," *Haematologica*, vol. 89, no. 6, pp. 717–741, 2004.

[51] D. Berz, E. M. McCormack, E. S. Winer, G. A. Colvin, and P. J. Quesenberry, "Cryopreservation of hematopoietic stem cells," *American Journal of Hematology*, vol. 82, no. 6, pp. 463–472, 2007.

[52] A. M. Bakken, "Cryopreserving human peripheral blood progenitor cells," *Current stem cell research & therapy*, vol. 1, no. 1, pp. 47–54, 2006.

[53] K. K. Fleming and A. Hubel, "Cryopreservation of hematopoietic and non-hematopoietic stem cells," *Transfusion and Apheresis Science*, vol. 34, no. 3, pp. 309–315, 2006.

[54] F. de Boer, A. M. Dräger, H. M. Pinedo et al., "Extensive early apoptosis in frozen-thawed CD34-positive stem cells decreases threshold doses for haematological recovery after autologous peripheral blood progenitor cell transplantation," *Bone Marrow Transplantation*, vol. 29, no. 3, pp. 249–255, 2002.

[55] G. Hechler, R. Weide, J. Heymanns, H. Köppler, and K. Havemann, "Storage of noncryopreserved periphered blood stem cells for transplantation," *Annals of Hematology*, vol. 72, no. 5, pp. 303–306, 1996.

[56] L. Wannesson, T. Panzarella, J. Mikhael, and A. Keating, "Feasibility and safety of autotransplants with noncryopreserved marrow or peripheral blood stem cells: a systematic review," *Annals of Oncology*, vol. 18, no. 4, pp. 623–632, 2007.

[57] A. Lopez-Otero, G. J. Ruiz-Delgado, and G. J. Ruiz-Arguelles, "A simplified method for stem cell autografting in multiple myeloma: a single institution experience," *Bone Marrow Transplantation*, vol. 44, no. 11, pp. 715–719, 2009.

[58] S. K. Jasuja, N. Kukar (jasuja), R. Jain, A. Bhateja, A. Jasuja, and R. Jain, "A simplified method at lowest cost for autologous, non-cryopreserved, unmanipulated, peripheral hematopoietic stem cell transplant in multiple myeloma and non-Hodgkin's lymphoma: Asian scenario," *Journal of Clinical Oncology, ASCO Annual Meeting Proceedings*, vol. 28, no. 15, Article ID è18545, 2010.

[59] M. Ramzi, M. Zakerinia, H. Nourani, M. Dehghani, R. Vojdani, and H. Haghighinejad, "Non-cryopreserved hematopoietic stem cell transplantation in multiple myeloma, a single center experience," *Clinical Transplantation*, vol. 26, no. 1, pp. 117–122, 2012.

[60] W. R. Bezwoda, R. Dansey, L. Seymour, and D. Glencross, "Non-cryopreserved, limited number (1 or 2) peripheral blood progenitor cell (PBPC) collections following GCSF administration provide adequate hematologic support for high dose chemotherapy," *Hematological Oncology*, vol. 12, no. 3, pp. 101–110, 1994.

[61] G. J. Ruiz-Arguelles, E. Lobato-Mendizabal, A. Ruiz-Arguelles, B. Perez-Romano, D. Arizpe-Bravo, and A. Marin-López, "Non-cryopreserved unmanipulated hematopoietic peripheral blood stem cell autotransplant program: long-term results," *Archives of Medical Research*, vol. 30, no. 5, pp. 380–384, 1999.

[62] G. J. Ruiz-Argüelles, A. Ruiz-Argüelles, B. Pèrvez-Romano, A. Marin-Lopez, and J. L. Delgado-Lamas, "Non-cryopreserved peripheral blood stem cells autotransplants for hematological malignancies can be performed entirely on an outpatient basis," *American Journal of Hematology*, vol. 58, no. 3, pp. 161–164, 1998.

[63] H. M. Lazarus, A. L. Pecora, T. C. Shea et al., "CD34+ selection of hematopoietic blood cell collections and autotransplantation in lymphoma: overnight storage of cells at 4 °C does not affect outcome," *Bone Marrow Transplantation*, vol. 25, no. 5, pp. 559–566, 2000.

[64] M. D. Parkins, N. Bahlis, C. Brown et al., "Overnight storage of autologous stem cell apheresis products before cryopreservation does not adversely impact early or long-term engraftment following transplantation," *Bone Marrow Transplantation*, vol. 38, no. 9, pp. 609–614, 2006.

[65] A. Donmez, S. Cagirgan, G. Saydam, and M. Tombuloglu, "Overnight refrigerator storage of autologous peripheral progenitor stem cells without cryopreservation," *Transfusion and Apheresis Science*, vol. 36, no. 3, pp. 313–319, 2007.

[66] A. Galmes, A. Gutièrrez, A. Sampol et al., "Long-term hematologic reconstitution and clinical evaluation of autologous peripheral blood stem cell transplantation after cryopreservation of cells with 5% and 10% dimethylsulfoxide at -80 °C in a mechanical freezer," *Haematologica*, vol. 92, no. 7, pp. 986–989, 2007.

[67] P. Halle, O. Tournilhac, W. Knopinska-Posluszny et al., "Uncontrolled-rate freezing and storage at-80∘C, with only 3.5-percent DMSO in cryoprotective solution for 109 autologous peripheral blood progenitor cell transplantations," *Transfusion*, vol. 41, no. 5, pp. 667–673, 2001.

[68] F. Hernandez-Navarro, E. Ojeda, R. Arrieta et al., "Hematopoietic cell transplantation using plasma and DMSO without HES, with non-programmed freezing by immersion in a methanol bath: results in 213 cases," *Bone Marrow Transplantation*, vol. 21, no. 5, pp. 511–517, 1998.

[69] C. Almici, P. Ferremi, A. Lanfranchi et al., "Uncontrolled-rate freezing of peripheral blood progenitor cells allows successful engraftment by sparing primitive and committed hematopoietic progenitors," *Haematologica*, vol. 88, no. 12, pp. 1390–1395, 2003.

[70] Y. Kudo, M. Minegishi, T. Itoh et al., "Evaluation of hematological reconstitution potential of autologous peripheral blood progenitor cells cryopreserved by a simple controlled-rate freezing method," *Tohoku Journal of Experimental Medicine*, vol. 205, no. 1, pp. 37–43, 2005.

[71] N. Matsumoto, H. Yoshizawa, H. Kagamu et al., "Successful liquid storage of peripheral blood stem cells at subzero non-freezing temperature," *Bone Marrow Transplantation*, vol. 30, no. 11, pp. 777–784, 2002.

[72] C. Gasparetto, "Stem cell transplantation for multiple myeloma," *Cancer Control*, vol. 11, no. 2, pp. 119–129, 2004.

[73] J. Mehta and S. Singhal, "Current status of autologous hematopoietic stem cell transplantation in myeloma," *Bone Marrow Transplantation*, vol. 42, no. 1, pp. S28–S34, 2008.

[74] T. R. Spitzer, "Engraftment syndrome following hematopoietic stem cell transplantation," *Bone Marrow Transplantation*, vol. 27, no. 9, pp. 893–898, 2001.

[75] C. H. Cogbill, W. R. Drobyski, and R. A. Komorowski, "Gastrointestinal pathology of autologous graft-versus-host disease following hematopoietic stem cell transplantation: a clinicopathological study of 17 cases," *Modern Pathology*, vol. 24, no. 1, pp. 117–125, 2011.

[76] R. G. L. Nellen, A. M. W. Van Marion, J. Frank, P. Poblete-Gutierrez, and P. M. Steijlen, "Eruption of lymphocyte recovery or autologous graft-versus-host disease?" *International Journal of Dermatology*, vol. 47, supplement 1, pp. 32–34, 2008.

[77] W. R. Drobyski, P. Hari, C. Keever-Taylor, R. Komorowski, and W. Grossman, "Severe autologous GVHD after hematopoietic progenitor cell transplantation for multiple myeloma," *Bone Marrow Transplantation*, vol. 43, no. 2, pp. 169–177, 2009.

[78] L. F. Porrata, "Clinical evidence of autologous graft versus tumor effect," *American Journal of Immunology*, vol. 5, no. 1, pp. 1–7, 2009.

[79] S. M. Kunisaki, G. W. Haller, A. Shimizu, H. Kitamura, R. B. Colvin, and D. H. Sachs, "Autologous graft-versus-host disease in a porcine bone marrow transplant model," *Transplantation*, vol. 74, no. 4, pp. 465–471, 2002.

24

Improving Safety of Preemptive Therapy with Oral Valganciclovir for Cytomegalovirus Infection after Allogeneic Hematopoietic Stem Cell Transplantation

Corinna Barkam, Haytham Kamal, Elke Dammann, Helmut Diedrich, Stefanie Buchholz, Matthias Eder, Jürgen Krauter, Arnold Ganser, and Michael Stadler

Department of Hematology, Hemostasis, Oncology, and Stem Cell Transplantation, Hannover Medical School, 30625 Hannover, Germany

Correspondence should be addressed to Michael Stadler, stadler.michael@mh-hannover.de

Academic Editor: David A. Rizzieri

Valganciclovir (VGC), an oral prodrug of ganciclovir (GCV), has been shown to clear cytomegalovirus (CMV) viremia in preemptive treatment of patients after allogeneic hematopoietic stem cell transplantation (alloHSCT), apparently without significant toxicity. Since VGC obviates hospitalization, it is increasingly being adopted, although not approved, in alloHSCT. When we retrospectively evaluated preemptive treatment with VGC versus GCV, foscarnet or cidofovir, in all 312 consecutive CMV viremias of 169 patients allotransplanted at our institution between 1996 and 2006, we found VGC more efficacious (79%) than non-VGC therapies (69%). The advantage of outpatient VGC, however, was outbalanced by more profound neutropenias (including two cases of agranulocytosis, one with graft loss) requiring subsequent prolonged rehospitalization. Thus, in a second, prospective cohort from 2007 to 2011 (all 202 consecutive CMV viremias of 118 yet older and sicker patients), we implemented twice weekly neutrophil monitoring during outpatient VGC treatment and avoided VGC maintenance therapy. While conserving efficacy (VGC 71%, non-VGC 72%), we could now demonstrate a reduced mean duration of hospitalization with VGC (9 days (0–66)) compared to non-VGC (25 days (0–115)), without any agranulocytosis episodes. We conclude that safe outpatient VGC therapy is possible in alloHSCT recipients, but requires frequent monitoring to prevent severe myelotoxicity.

1. Introduction

Although mortality from cytomegalovirus (CMV) infection after allogeneic hematopoietic stem cell transplantation (alloHSCT) has largely decreased with modern preemptive treatment, CMV viremias still contribute to significant morbidity and a considerable hospitalization burden for intravenous therapy with the standard first-line CMV drugs ganciclovir (GCV) and foscarnet (FCN).

Valganciclovir (VGC), an orally available prodrug hydrolyzed to GCV, with a tenfold bioavailability compared to oral GCV [1], has been licensed for therapy of CMV retinitis in HIV disease and for CMV prophylaxis after solid organ transplantation, but not after alloHSCT, due to concern about its myelotoxicity, especially in long-term

application. However, VGC has enjoyed widespread off-label use thanks to its outpatient applicability and its excellent bioavailability even in patients with impaired resorption due to intestinal graft-versus-host disease [2–4]. Several smaller trials and one large study found high efficacy (73%–100%) of VGC in the preemptive setting after alloHSCT ([5–14]; see Table 1), comparing favourably with standard CMV drugs. However, these mostly retrospective studies with short follow up may have underestimated toxicity, although some of them reported up to 27% severe hematotoxicity, especially neutropenia.

Here, we present the largest single-center study to date on VGC in preemptive treatment of CMV viremias after alloHSCT, assessing the neutropenia risk of VGC in a well-sized retrospective cohort and evaluating a prospective

TABLE 1: Studies on VGC in the preemptive setting after alloHSCT.

Author year [ref.]	Design	N patients	VGC dose	VGC efficacy	Toxicity reported
van der Heiden et al. 2006 [5]	Retrospective VGC/GCV	34	1800 mg/d	80%	None
Ayala et al. 2006 [6]	Retrospective VGC mono	18	1800 mg/d × 14, → 900 mg/d × ≥7	93%	None
Busca et al. 2007 [7]	Retrospective VGC mono	15	1800 mg/d × 14, → 900 mg/d × 14	73%	27% severe hematotoxicity
Candoni et al. 2008 [8]	Retrospective VGC mono	30	1800 mg/d versus 900 mg/d	93% 87%	≤WHO °II
de la Cruz-Vicente et al. 2008 [9]	Prospective VGC/GCV	11	1800 mg/d × 14, → 900 mg/d × 14	100%	None
Wang et al. 2008 [10]	Retrospective VGC mono	19	1800 mg/d × 14, → 900 mg/d × 14	95%	None
Takenaka et al. 2009 [11]	Retrospective VGC mono	10	1800 mg/d × 21	90%	10% severe neutropenias
Saleh et al. 2010 [12]	Retrospective VGC mono	47	1800 mg/d × ≥7, → 900 mg/d × ≥7	97%	17% severe neutropenias
Palladino et al. 2010 [13]	Retrospective VGC mono	34	1800 mg/d versus 900 mg/d	100% 83%	None
Liu et al. 2010 [14]	Prospective VGC mono	54	1800 mg/d × 14, → 900 mg/d × 14	89%	None
Ruiz-Camps et al. 2011 [15]	Prospective VGC/GCV	166		91%	5% adverse events

surveillance strategy to improve safety in outpatient VGC therapy.

2. Patients and Methods

2.1. Study Design. This is a combined retrospective and prospective comparative cohort study, analyzing all consecutive CMV viremias after alloHSCT treated preemptively at our institution during the years 1996 through 2006 (retrospective cohort 1: 169 patients; 312 CMV viremias) as well as 2007 through 2011 (prospective cohort 2: 118 patients; 202 CMV viremias). Excluded were patients originally not allotransplanted at our institution and patients without details on CMV treatment at other hospitals. Data are as of July 1st, 2012, thus allowing for at least six months of follow up. Patient data evaluation was in complete concordance with the declaration of Helsinki. All patients had given written informed consent prior to transplantation; prior to preemptive CMV therapy, informed consent was again obtained.

2.2. Diagnosis and Preemptive Treatment of CMV Viremias. According to our institutional standard operating procedures, every patient after alloHSCT was followed weekly until immune reconstitution by CMV pp65 antigen testing or, during neutropenia, by CMV DNA PCR. Preemptive therapy

was started when a significant increase of CMV pp65 antigen was noted (generally more than 5 per 400.000 leukocytes positive or CMV DNA PCR exceeding 10.000 copies per mL whole blood). Preemptive therapy of CMV viremias was selected according to the patients' toxicity profile: GCV in case of renal impairment, FCN if hematopoietic reconstitution was yet insufficient. Patients without hematopoietic or renal compromise were given the choice between intravenous GCV and oral VGC, after counseling about side effects of both drugs as well as about the off-label status of VGC. Standard doses of VGC (900 mg every 12 hours), GCV (5 mg per kg body weight every 12 hours), FCN (90 mg per kg body weight every 12 hours), or cidofovir (CDF; 5 mg per kg body weight once a week, but not as first-line therapy) were used with appropriate hydration and supportive measures and tailored according to renal function, as detailed in the manufacturers' descriptions. Initial preemptive therapy was given for at least two weeks (or changed to a second-line drug if viremia progressed); it was stopped after three consecutive negative CMV tests.

Patients were documented in the "VGC group" if they had received VGC at any time during a CMV viremia episode, if not, they belonged to the "non-VGC group."

In cohort 1, maintenance therapy was used, mostly at half the initial dose, in patients with unfavourable CMV constellation (recipient positive/donor negative; R+/D−) and in patients with repeated CMV viremias. In cohort 2,

TABLE 2: Patient cohorts of preemptive therapy for CMV viremias.

| | Cohort 1 (1996–2006) | | | Cohort 2 (2007–2011) | | |
	VGC	Non-VGC	P	VGC	Non-VGC	P
N patients	79	90	—	48	70	—
N viremias	165	147	—	67	135	—
Gender						
Female	.44	.44	n.s.	.50	.47	n.s.
Male	.56	.56		.50	.53	
Age						
Median	50	43	<0.001	53	56	n.s.
Range	18–68	18–65		20–67	19–72	
Diagnosis						
Nonmalignant	.03	.00		.03	.04	
Chronic malignancy	.24	.26	n.s.	.17	.32	n.s.
Acute malignancy	.73	.74		.80	.64	
Disease risk						
Standard	.29	.47	<0.05	.11	.23	n.s.
Advanced	.71	.53		.89	.77	
Donor						
Matched related	.28	.43		.25	.21	
Matched unrelated	.68	.52	n.s.	.44	.53	n.s.
Mismatched	.04	.05		.31	.26	
CMV						
R−/D−, R−/D+, R+/D+	.51	.67	<0.05	.69	.70	n.s.
R+/D−	.49	.33		.31	.30	
Conditioning						
Reduced intensity	.65	.30	<0.001	.83	.79	n.s.
Myeloablative	.35	.70		.17	.21	
T cell depletion						
None	.11	.40		.06	.08	
In vivo (ATG)	.84	.44	<0.001	.94	.92	n.s.
In vitro	.05	.16		.00	.00	

maintenance treatment was avoided, whenever possible, in order to prevent profound neutropenias. Patients in cohort 2 who opted for outpatient VGC were instructed to have complete blood counts controlled twice a week for early detection of neutropenia.

2.3. Patient Cohorts.
Both cohorts are described in detail in Table 2. In cohort 1, despite the retrospective study design, both the VGC and the non-VGC group were comparable for demographic, disease- and transplant-related aspects such as gender, diagnosis, and donor type. However, VGC patients of cohort 1 were generally older, had more advanced disease, showed more often the unfavourable CMV constellation R+/D−, and more of them had received reduced intensity conditioning and *in vivo* T cell depletion with antithymocyte globulin (ATG). In contrast, the VGC and the non-VGC groups of cohort 2 were much better balanced with respect to all demographic, disease- and transplant-related characteristics, even conditioning and *in vivo* T cell depletion, but especially age and disease status which were considerably less favourable in both groups of cohort 2 compared to cohort

1. Thus, a historical trend is evident towards alloHSCT in patients of ever increasing age and morbidity.

2.4. Statistics.
Due to the retrospective design of cohort 1, statistics were primarily descriptive. Statistical comparisons were calculated from cross-tables employing two-sided Chi-square tests.

3. Results and Discussion

3.1. Efficacy of VGC in Preemptive Therapy of CMV Viremias.
In cohort 1, the rate of CMV clearance was better for patients preemptively treated with VGC (79%) than with non-VGC therapies (69%), $P = 0.04$. In cohort 2, efficacy was similar in both groups: VGC cleared CMV viremia in 71%, non-VGC treatments in 72% (not significant). These results are in concordance with and confirm published studies (see Table 1).

3.2. Hospitalization Requirements for VGC versus Non-VGC Preemptive Therapies.
As expected, hospitalization for

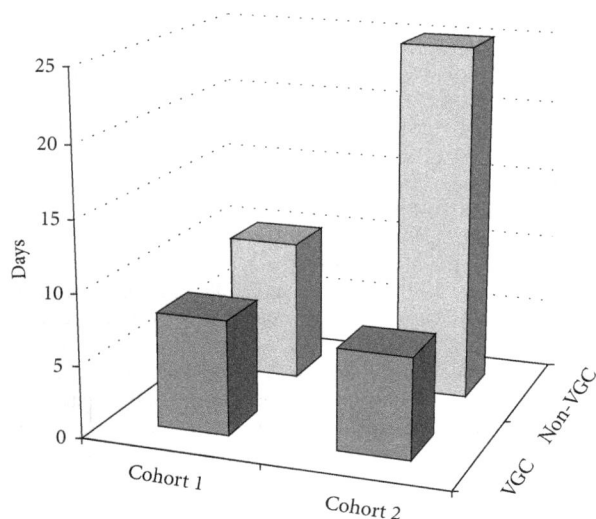

FIGURE 1: Mean total hospitalization for treatment of CMV viremia plus complications.

preemptive therapy was lower in VGC-treated patients. However, in cohort 1, severe neutropenias in the VGC group accounted for prolonged subsequent rehospitalizations. Thus, when considering both initial preemptive therapy and later treatment of complications, there was no difference between the groups in mean total hospitalisation (cohort 1: VGC 8 days (0–257); non-VGC 10 days (0–89); not significant). Of course, as suggested by the wide range of hospitalization duration in the VGC group of cohort 1, few outliers with excessive subsequent rehospitalizations (see Section 3.3) were responsible for this statistical effect which, however, highlights well the potential danger from VGC treatment in terms of profound and prolonged myelotoxicity.

This observation led us to implement frequent neutrophil monitoring during outpatient VGC treatment in cohort 2. Here, likely as a consequence of our change in surveillance strategy, we were able to demonstrate a reduced mean duration of total hospitalization after VGC (9 days (0–66)) as compared to non-VGC therapies (25 days (0–115)), with a much narrower range in the VGC group (Figure 1).

Surprisingly, mean hospitalization in the non-VGC groups differed substantially between cohorts 1 and 2. A potential explanation for this may derive from the significant differences between both cohorts, especially regarding patient age, disease risk, and mismatched donors. Compared to cohort 1, where the non-VGC group enjoyed greatly favourable characteristics with respect to the VGC group, in cohort 2, both groups were strongly disadvantaged; thus, patients may have suffered more toxicities from non-VGC therapies, too. Other possible factors for differences between the cohorts include toxicities from concomitant medications which might have been unequally distributed in consecutive cohorts. Finally, the possibility should be considered that prevalent CMV strains were becoming increasingly resistant

over time; thus, more patients might have required additional CMV therapies.

3.3. Myelotoxicity of VGC in Preemptive CMV Treatment after AlloHSCT. In cohort 1, although numerically comparable (11% in both the VGC and the non-VGC group), severe neutropenias were of greater clinical importance in the VGC group, compatible with a more profound and/or prolonged suppressive effect of VGC on granulopoiesis [2]. Especially, two cases of agranulocytosis occurred, which were confirmed by bone marrow biopsy. Whereas one patient recovered with granulocyte-colony stimulating factor after more than one month of hospitalization, the other patient additionally experienced a complete loss of his graft, eventually requiring retransplantation 6 months after preemptive VGC therapy; unfortunately, he died 4.5 months after the second transplant from infectious complications.

In cohort 2, neutropenias occurred in significant less patients of the VGC group ($n = 9$) than in patients of the non-VGC group ($n = 37$), $P = 0.004$. Conversely, the duration of neutropenias was not different (VGC: median 8 days, range 1–14; non-VGC: median 7 days, range 1–34; not significant). No cases of agranulocytosis or graft loss were observed in cohort 2.

Suppression of granulopoiesis was the most clinically relevant myelotoxicity of VGC encountered in our cohorts. When we compared frequencies of anemia, thrombocytopenia, red blood cell transfusion, and platelet substitution, we could not detect any significant differences in either cohort (data not shown).

3.4. Strengths and Limitations of the Study. The main limitations of this study are the retrospective design of cohort 1 and the difficulty to directly compare both cohorts due to the differences between them; however, the comparisons within each cohort still remain unchallenged. Another shortcoming is the nonrandomized treatment allocation, introducing a patient's bias with the patient's choice; however, this may better reflect real clinical practice in preemptive therapy of CMV viremias after alloHSCT.

Strengths of this study are its well-sized cohorts, making it the currently largest study with the longest follow up on VGC in the preemptive setting after alloHSCT. It is thus suited for the detection of rare, but severe, events and appropriate for assessment of a surveillance strategy to improve the safety of treatment with this widely used, but narrowly evaluated, yet unlicensed drug.

4. Conclusions

The present study combines adequately sized retrospective and prospective cohorts to examine the significant neutropenia risk of VGC for CMV viremia in the preemptive setting after alloHSCT. We show that outpatient VGC therapy can be safely applied in these patients, following a simple surveillance strategy with frequent neutrophil monitoring and using VGC maintenance therapy with utmost caution.

Further large, prospective studies on the use of VGC after alloHSCT are welcome.

Conflict of Interests

The authors declare that there is no potential conflict of interests.

Authors' Contribution

C. Barkam and H. Kamal are equal first coauthors.

Acknowledgments

The authors would like to thank Dr. Ludwig Hoy, Department of Biometry, Hannover Medical School, for expert statistical advice. This work has been presented in part (cohort 1) at the 2007 annual meeting of the European Group for Blood and Marrow Transplantation (EBMT).

References

[1] P. Reusser, "Oral valganciclovir: a new option for treatment of cytomegalovirus infection and disease in immunocompromised hosts," *Expert Opinion on Investigational Drugs*, vol. 10, no. 9, pp. 1745–1753, 2001.

[2] H. Einsele, P. Reusser, M. Bornhäuser et al., "Oral valganciclovir leads to higher exposure to ganciclovir than intravenous ganciclovir in patients following allogeneic stem cell transplantation," *Blood*, vol. 107, no. 7, pp. 3002–3008, 2006.

[3] D. J. Winston, L. R. Baden, D. A. Gabriel et al., "Pharmacokinetics of ganciclovir after oral valganciclovir versus intravenous ganciclovir in allogeneic stem cell transplant patients with graft-versus-host disease of the gastrointestinal tract," *Biology of Blood and Marrow Transplantation*, vol. 12, no. 6, pp. 635–640, 2006.

[4] Z. Y. Lim, G. Cook, P. R. Johnson et al., "Results of a phase I/II british society of bone marrow transplantation study on PCR-based pre-emptive therapy with valganciclovir or ganciclovir for active CMV infection following alemtuzumab-based reduced intensity allogeneic stem cell transplantation," *Leukemia Research*, vol. 33, no. 2, pp. 244–249, 2009.

[5] P. L. J. van der Heiden, J. S. Kalpoe, R. M. Barge, R. Willemze, A. C. M. Kroes, and E. F. Schippers, "Oral valganciclovir as pre-emptive therapy has similar efficacy on cytomegalovirus DNA load reduction as intravenous ganciclovir in allogeneic stem cell transplantation recipients," *Bone Marrow Transplantation*, vol. 37, no. 7, pp. 693–698, 2006.

[6] E. Ayala, J. Greene, R. Sandin et al., "Valganciclovir is safe and effective as pre-emptive therapy for CMV infection in allogeneic hematopoietic stem cell transplantation," *Bone Marrow Transplantation*, vol. 37, no. 9, pp. 851–856, 2006.

[7] A. Busca, P. de Fabritiis, V. Ghisetti et al., "Oral valganciclovir as preemptive therapy for cytomegalovirus infection post allogeneic stem cell transplantation," *Transplant Infectious Disease*, vol. 9, no. 2, pp. 102–107, 2007.

[8] A. Candoni, E. Simeone, M. Tiribelli, C. Pipan, and R. Fanin, "What is the optimal dosage of valganciclovir as preemptive therapy for CMV infection in allogeneic hematopoietic SCT?" *Bone Marrow Transplantation*, vol. 42, no. 3, pp. 207–208, 2008.

[9] F. de la Cruz-Vicente, P. Cerezuela Martinez, E. Gil-Espárraga et al., "Preemptive therapy for cytomegalovirus disease in allogeneic stem cell transplant recipients," *Transplantation Proceedings*, vol. 40, no. 9, pp. 3102–3103, 2008.

[10] Y. Wang, X. J. Huang, L. P. Xu et al., "Valganciclovir for treatment of cytomegalovirus viremia in patients following allogeneic hematopoietic stem cell transplantation," *Zhonghua yi Xue za Zhi*, vol. 88, no. 46, pp. 3265–3267, 2008.

[11] K. Takenaka, T. Eto, K. Nagafuji et al., "Oral valganciclovir as preemptive therapy is effective for cytomegalovirus infection in allogeneic hematopoietic stem cell transplant recipients," *International Journal of Hematology*, vol. 89, no. 2, pp. 231–237, 2009.

[12] A. J. M. Saleh, F. Al-Mohareb, F. Al-Rabiah et al., "High efficacy and low toxicity of short-course oral valganciclovir as pre-emptive therapy for hematopoietic stem cell transplant cytomegalovirus infection," *Hematology/ Oncology and Stem Cell Therapy*, vol. 3, no. 3, pp. 116–120, 2010.

[13] M. Palladino, L. Laurenti, P. Chiusolo et al., "Low-dose valganciclovir as preemptive therapy for cytomegalovirus infection occurring in allogeneic stem cell transplant recipients," *Acta Haematologica*, vol. 123, no. 4, pp. 230–234, 2010.

[14] K. Y. Liu, Y. Wang, M. Z. Han et al., "Valganciclovir for pre-emptive therapy of cytomegalovirus viraemia after hematopoietic stem cell transplantation: a prospective multicenter trial," *Chinese Medical Journal*, vol. 123, no. 16, pp. 2199–2205, 2010.

[15] I. Ruiz-Camps, O. Len, R. de la Cámara et al., "Valganciclovir as pre-emptive therapy for cytomegalovirus infection in allogeneic haematopoietic stem cell transplant recipients," *Antiviral Therapy*, vol. 16, no. 7, pp. 951–957, 2011.

25

Th17 Mediated Alloreactivity Is Facilitated by the Pre-Transplant Microbial Burden of the Recipient

Aleksandra Klimczak[1] and Andrzej Lange[1,2]

[1] Department of Clinical Immunology, L. Hirszfeld Institute of Immunology and Experimental Therapy, Polish Academy of Sciences, 12 Rudolfa Weigla Street, 53-114 Wroclaw, Poland
[2] Lower Silesian Center for Cellular Transplantation, National Bone Marrow Donor Registry, Grabiszyńska 105, 53-439 Wroclaw, Poland

Correspondence should be addressed to Aleksandra Klimczak, alek.klim@yahoo.com

Academic Editor: Bronwen Shaw

Acute graft-versus-host disease (aGvHD) is a major complication after hematopoietic stem cell transplantation (HSCT) and severity of aGvHD is associated with biological and genetic factors related to donors and recipients. Studies on inflammatory pathways involved in aGVHD have shown a significant impact of the gut microflora on aGvHD development giving increasing evidence in the understanding of the response of innate and adaptive immunity to microbial products. Cytokine deregulation may increase or reduce the risk of aGvHD. Damage of tissues affected by aGvHD reflects the immunological cascade of events in this disease.

1. Introduction

Allogeneic hematopoietic stem cell transplantation (HSCT) is a clinically accepted procedure in some hematological malignances, aplastic anemia, and inborn errors. It is rather a complex procedure, associated with both the adverse effect aGvHD and with the presence of beneficial alloreactivity, as it is graft versus leukemia or versus cells with inborn error reaction [1–4]. Alloreactivity influences both hematological and immunological recovery. Both alloreactivity and recovery of blood cells take place in an environment full of microbial agents in a latent form or colonizing/invading the host. Innate and adaptive immunity competence prior to and after HSCT secure an event-free course after HSCT with respect to that.

1.1. Biology of Acute GvHD. Damage of the gastrointestinal tract during the acute phase of GvHD plays a major pathophysiological role in the amplification of this systemic disease. Several experimental and clinical observations highlight the role of effector cells of the immune system migration

into the skin and gastrointestinal tract in the pathobiology of aGvHD [5]. Mice are the most often used animal model of GvHD. Differences in age, sex, genetic matching, and also gut microbiota of the mice are found to be the main players in pathophysiology of GvHD [6].

One of the first reports describing the microbial environment of the recipient as an important cofactor of gut aGvHD development was presented by Van Bekkum et al. [7, 8]. In their studies they compared the fate of conventionally and germ-free housed mice after whole-body irradiation and MHC incompatible bone marrow cell transplantation. Enteric aGvHD was less frequent in germ-free mice and in mice receiving antibiotic prophylaxis as compared to conventionally transplanted animals. The authors concluded that antigenic epitopes of microorganisms shared with gut epithelial cells may promote alloreactivity. These observations indicated that lymphocytes sensitized against microbial antigens may cross-react with epithelial cells in the gut, promoting aGvHD. Experimental studies demonstrated that loss of integrity of the gastrointestinal tract plays a major role in experimental GvHD [9]. Intestinal microflora, their

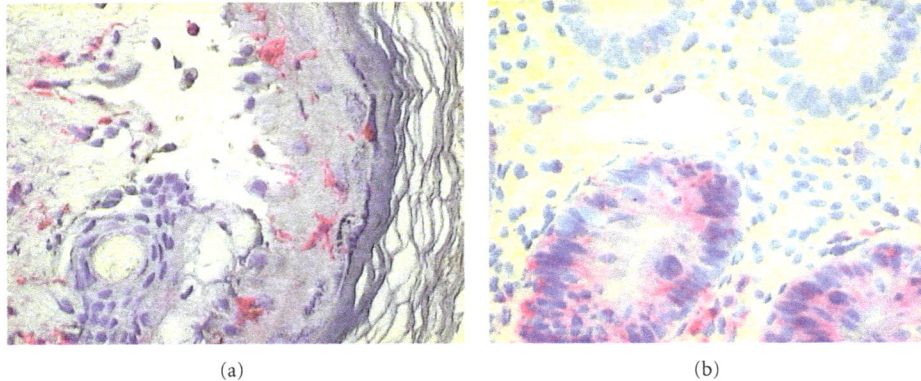

(a)   (b)

FIGURE 1: (a) HLA-DR expression on antigen presenting cells in the epidermis of the skin (+60 days after HSCT) and (b) HLA-DR expression on colon epithelial cells (+33 days after HSCT) affected by aGvHD (red staining with Permanent Red, magnifications 400x).

antigenic challenge, and released endotoxins constitute part of the microenvironment and can serve as potent triggers of inflammation in GvHD [9].

1.2. Innate Immunity and aGvHD. The studies on the role of gut microflora in initiation of aGvHD help in understanding the role of the innate and adaptive immune response evoked by microbial products in this disease [10]. Conditioning regimen damage of the gut and concomitant release of endotoxins and lipopolysaccharides (LPS) from colonizing the gut microbes activate innate immunity via Toll-like receptors (TLRs), which starts a cascade of events leading to cytokine storm, which constitutes part of the aGvHD pathomechanism [9, 11, 12]. Ligation of intestinal TLR9 by bacterial DNA increases the risk of aGvHD. TLR9 knockout mice have aGvHD of a reduced activity and intestinal damage [11]. The impact of bacterial sensing via TLRs in gut aGvHD was analyzed in an intestinal mice model which shows that MyD88 (myeloid differentiation primary-response protein 88)-dependent TLR9 signaling of bacterial DNA is essential for induction of apoptosis and cell infiltrations in the gut during aGvHD [13]. Indeed, the use of oligonucleotide (iODN) 2088, which inhibits TLR9 activation in vitro, ameliorates the symptoms of gut aGvHD in mice [13]. In contrast, mutations in TLR4 (which encodes LPS receptor) have been shown to be a biological factor reducing the risk of GvHD in experimental studies [14].

Manipulation with gut microflora in favor of *Lactobacillus rhamnosus* GG [15] makes aGvHD less aggressive. Very recent experimental and clinical studies demonstrated that microbial chaos early after HSCT and loss of intestinal flora diversity are a potential risk factors for subsequent aGvHD development [16]. In clinical practice intestinal bacterial decontamination with metronidazole and ciprofloxacin significantly reduces the severity of gut aGvHD [17], which supports the notion that intestinal microflora play a role in the pathogenesis of aGvHD.

The NOD2/CARD15 protein, restricted to intestinal epithelial cells and monocyte/macrophage lineage [18], plays a role in the innate immune response to bacterial infections

in the gastrointestinal tract. It is at present known that NOD2/CARD15 gene mutations found in patients undergoing HSCT make them more susceptible to aGvHD [19]. The cumulative incidence of 1-year transplant-related mortality and the prevalence of severe gut aGvHD affected 49% of patients with NOD2/CARD15 gene mutation as compared to 20% incidence in those without NOD2/CARD15 gene mutation. If the mutation affects donors this proportion increases to 59% and to 83% if both recipient and donor have the gene mutated [20]. Our observations also show that NOD2/CARD15 gene mutation is associated with susceptibility to severe GvHD grade III-IV [21]. Moreover, we found that mutations in the NOD2/CARD15 gene influences the level of Th17 in blood in such a way that patients with NOD2/CARD15 mutations had lower blood values of Th17 at the time of hematological recovery in the aGvHD group [22].

2. Pathophysiology of aGvHD

The conditioning regimen causes tissue damage and as a consequence several proinflammatory cytokines including IL-1 and TNF-α, and a set of chemokines, CCL2-5 and CXCL9-11, are released, thereby increasing expression of adhesion molecules, MHC antigens and costimulatory molecules on the host antigen presenting cells (APC) [1, 23]. Host APC, which survive the conditioning regimen damage, become activated and capable of confronting the transplant material antigens (Figure 1). Activation of donor T cells after interaction with host APC leads to their proliferation, differentiation, and migration. In the subsequent effector phase mononuclear cells invade the target tissue and accumulation of these cells leads to tissue destruction (Figure 2) [23, 24].

It is known, also from our own experience, that anti-CD52 monoclonal antibody (MoAb) (Campath-1H), if used as part of the conditioning regimen, greatly decreases the risk of aGvHD (unpublished). Anti-CD52 MoAb has a unique property to destroy not only lymphocytes but also APC [25].

In afferent phase 1 of aGvHD LPS of Gram-negative bacteria are the main stimulators of proinflammatory cytokines

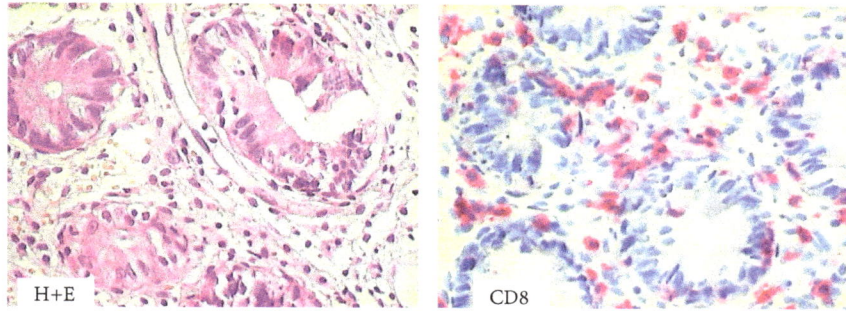

FIGURE 2: Colon biopsy specimen harvested at 33 days after HSCT from patient with clinical symptoms of aGvHD. Hematoxylin and eosin (H+E) staining documented destruction of colon crypts, and immunocytochemistry illustrate CD8+ cells invading damaged crypt epithelium (H+E magnification 200x, red staining with Permanent Red, magnifications 400x).

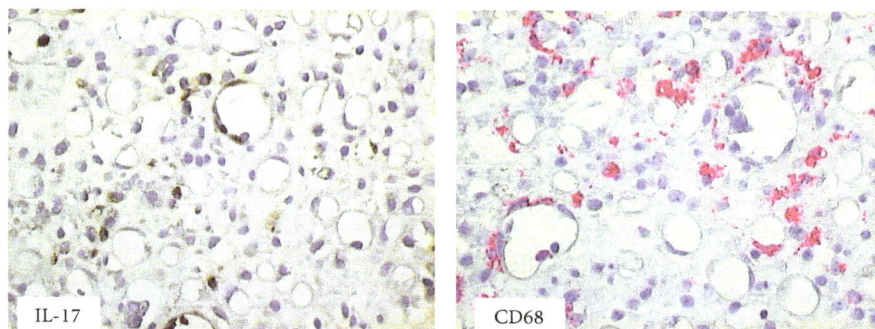

FIGURE 3: Colon biopsy specimen harvested at day 63 after HSCT from patient with clinical symptoms of aGvHD. IL-17 producing cells and macrophages CD68+ were seen within cellular infiltrates (brown staining with diaminobenzidine-tetrahydrochloride (DAB) and red staining with Permanent Red, magnifications 400x).

and chemokine receptors. The intensive conditioning regimen induces apoptosis and consequently epithelial cell damage, allowing LPS to enter the systemic circulation, activating host APC, which facilitates alloreactivity, leading to aGvHD [9, 26].

Activated T cells proliferate and secrete cytokines [1]. Th1 cells contribute to the cytokine storm associated with aGvHD, while Th2 cytokines may mitigate the impetus of alloreactivity [6]. Indeed, in our early studies we confirmed the presence of IFNγ, IP-10 as well as TNF-α and IL-6 transcripts in skin affected by aGvHD [27]. IL-2 and IFNγ prime mononuclear phagocytes to produce IL-1 and TNF-α. TNF-α, a powerful inducer of APC in the first phase, activates T cells also in the second phase of aGvHD. Again, the microbial impact plays a role in establishing a vicious circle of infection (TNFα, IL-6) and thus aggravation of aGvHD.

The role of microbial infection in aggravating aGvHD has a long history [28]. Recently we added some more information as to the role of Th17+ lymphocytes, whose differentiation is strongly supported by microbial invasion. It is a step-by-step process starting with TNF-α and IL-1 secretion in phase 1 in response to the conditioning regimen and microbial background. Among proinflammatory cytokines, IL-6 plays an important role in aggravation of aGvHD, especially when the gut is targeted [27, 29]. This cytokine is released and generated during inflammatory

processes associated with (i) the conditioning regimen, (ii) the alloreactivity associated inflammation, and (iii) bacterial and fungal infections [27]. C-reactive protein (CRP) is a reading protein of IL-6 and usually reflects microbial invasion. Notably, increase of the serum CRP level may herald gut manifestation of aGvHD [27]. Increase in serum level of IL-6 is seen early after transplant as a result of a cytokine storm described in allogeneic HSCT patients at the period of neutropenia, and then an increase may be again seen during prolonged leucopenia and at that time is usually associated with infectious complications [29]. All these events are responsible for elevation of serum CRP level during the period after HSCT [29, 30].

Following more recent observations it is known that the differentiation process of CD4+ cells into subsets depends on the cytokine milieu in their environment [31]. IL-6, if present, facilitates differentiation of CD4+ cells into Th17 cells [32, 33]. IL-17 is a cytokine of the strongest proinflammatory potential. It is known that differentiation of lymphocytes into Th17 cells may take place in the gut, where microbial products provide strong stimulation for local IL-6 production [34]. Therefore, it is not surprising that in intestinal aGvHD IL-17 producing cells are present among those infiltrating affected tissue (Figure 3) [35]. Local IL-17 production in the gut during aGvHD is seen in patients with extensive diarrhea resulting from profound damage of intestinal epithelium.

Th17 differentiation is guided by IL-6, which constitutes a primary response to bacterial and fungal infections. Th17 cells have as a hallmark receptor CCR6, which in response to their ligand CCL20 (also known as macrophage inflammatory protein-3α, MIP-3α), produced by activated macrophages in the inflammatory area of the gut, facilitates colonization of gut epithelium by IL-17 producing cells, causing severe inflammation [36, 37]. A correlation between the number of Th17 cells and the clinical course of aGvHD supports the notion that Th17 cells are involved in the active phases of aGvHD [38]. Our studies showed that IL-17 producing CD4+ lymphocytes are at a higher proportion in blood prior to aGvHD manifestation and then decrease at the time of full blown aGvHD [39]. These cells are likely marginalized in the affected tissue, exerting their strong pro-inflammatory activity.

In conclusion, the data collected since the pioneering work of Van Bekkum strongly suggest that microbial products influence the risk of aGvHD in all phases of pathobiology of this complication via activation of APC then inducing the local production of IL-6 exemplified by CRP serum level elevation to the effector phase exerted by lymphocytes of Th17 cell characteristics. Pre- and peritransplantation colonization of recipients with bacterial and fungal germs promotes alloreactivity; therefore, microbial surveillance plays an important role in securing an event-free post-transplant course. Bacterial and fungal colonization after transplant involves both Gram-positive and Gram-negative bacteria. However, up to date is not sufficiently defined which microbial populations may exert or protect aGvHD-associated damage and inflammation because both Gram-positive and Gram-negative bacteria may overgrow the intestinal flora and may worse aGvHD [16, 28]. Therefore, both Gram-positive and Gram-negative bacteria can play a role in activation of both innate and adaptive immunity with production of IL-6 with following consequences of the presence of this cytokine which may facilitate pathomechanism of aGvHD.

References

[1] S. W. Choi, J. E. Levine, and J. L. M. Ferrara, "Pathogenesis and management of graft-versus-host disease," *Immunology and Allergy Clinics of North America*, vol. 30, no. 1, pp. 75–101, 2010.

[2] A. J. Barrett, "Understanding and harnessing the graft-versus-leukaemia effect," *British Journal of Haematology*, vol. 142, no. 6, pp. 877–888, 2008.

[3] Y. Lu, C. R. Giver, and A. Sharma, "IFN-gamma and indoleamine 2,3-dioxygenase signaling between donor dendritic cells and T cells regulates graft versus host and graft versus leukemia activity," *Blood*, vol. 119, pp. 1075–1085, 2012.

[4] V. K. Prasad and J. Kurtzberg, "Cord blood and bone marrow transplantation in inherited metabolic diseases: scientific basis, current status and future directions," *British Journal of Haematology*, vol. 148, no. 3, pp. 356–372, 2010.

[5] R. Sackstein, "A revision of Billingham's tenets: the central role of lymphocyte migration in acute graft-versus-host disease," *Biology of Blood and Marrow Transplantation*, vol. 12, no. 1, pp. 2–8, 2006.

[6] J. L. Ferrara, J. E. Levine, P. Reddy, and E. Holler, "Graft-versus-host disease," *The Lancet*, vol. 373, no. 9674, pp. 1550–1561, 2009.

[7] D. W. Van Bekkum and S. Knaan, "Role of bacterial microflora in development of intestinal lesions from graft versus host reaction," *Journal of the National Cancer Institute*, vol. 58, no. 3, pp. 787–790, 1977.

[8] D. W. Van Bekkum, J. Roodenburg, P. J. Heidt, and D. Van Der Waaij, "Mitigation of secondary disease of allogeneic mouse radiation chimeras by modification of the intestinal microflora," *Journal of the National Cancer Institute*, vol. 52, no. 2, pp. 401–404, 1974.

[9] G. R. Hill and J. L. M. Ferrara, "The primacy of the gastrointestinal tract as a target organ of acute graft-versus-host disease: rationale for the use of cytokine shields in allogeneic bone marrow transplantation," *Blood*, vol. 95, no. 9, pp. 2754–2759, 2000.

[10] B. R. Blazar, W. J. Murphy, and M. Abedi, "Advances in graft-versus-host disease biology and therapy," *Nature Reviews Immunology*, vol. 12, pp. 443–458, 2012.

[11] C. Calcaterra, L. Sfondrini, A. Rossini et al., "Critical role of TLR9 in acute graft-versus-host disease," *Journal of Immunology*, vol. 181, no. 9, pp. 6132–6139, 2008.

[12] O. Penack, E. Holler, and M. R. M. Van Den Brink, "Graft-versus-host disease: regulation by microbe-associated molecules and innate immune receptors," *Blood*, vol. 115, no. 10, pp. 1865–1872, 2010.

[13] M. M. Heimesaat, A. Nogai, S. Bereswill et al., "MyD88/TLR9 mediated immunopathology and gut microbiota dynamics in a novel murine model of intestinal graft-versus-host disease," *Gut*, vol. 59, no. 8, pp. 1079–1087, 2010.

[14] T. Imado, T. Iwasaki, S. Kitano et al., "The protective role of host Toll-like receptor-4 in acute graft-versus-host disease," *Transplantation*, vol. 90, no. 10, pp. 1063–1070, 2010.

[15] A. Gerbitz, M. Schultz, A. Wilke et al., "Probiotic effects on experimental graft-versus-host disease: let them eat yogurt," *Blood*, vol. 103, no. 11, pp. 4365–4367, 2004.

[16] R. R. Jenq, C. Ubeda, and Y. Taur, "Regulation of intestinal inflammation by microbiota following allogeneic bone marrow transplantation," *Journal of Experimental Medicine*, vol. 209, pp. 903–911, 2012.

[17] D. W. Beelen, A. Elmaagacli, K. D. Müller, H. Hirche, and U. W. Schaefer, "Influence of intestinal bacterial decontamination using metronidazole and ciprofloxacin or ciprofloxacin alone on the development of acute graft- versus-host disease after marrow transplantation in patients with hematologic malignancies: final results and long-term follow-up of an open-label prospective randomized trial," *Blood*, vol. 93, no. 10, pp. 3267–3275, 1999.

[18] D. Berrebi, R. Maudinas, J. P. Hugot et al., "Card15 gene overexpression in mononuclear and epithelial cells of the inflamed Crohn's disease colon," *Gut*, vol. 52, no. 6, pp. 840–846, 2003.

[19] A. Madrigal and B. E. Shaw, "Immunogenetic factors in donors and patients that affect the outcome of hematopoietic stem cell transplantation," *Blood Cells, Molecules, and Diseases*, vol. 40, no. 1, pp. 40–43, 2008.

[20] E. Holler, G. Rogler, H. Herfarth et al., "Both donor and recipient NOD2/CARD15 mutations associate with transplant-related mortality and GvHD following allogeneic stem cell transplantation," *Blood*, vol. 104, no. 3, pp. 889–894, 2004.

[21] K. Bogunia-Kubik, E. Jaskula, D. Dłubek, A. Wójtowicz, and A. Lange, "SNP8 of the NOD2/CARD15 gene and acute GvHD contribute to CMV reactivation after allogeneic haematopoietic stem cell transplantation," *Bone Marrow Transplantation*, vol. 46, no. 1, supplement, p. S82, 2011.

[22] A. Lange, K. Suchnicki, S. Mizia, P. Czajka, A. Lach, and D. Dlubek, "Low blood levels of Th17 cells are seen in patients with aGvHD and associate with rather poor survival post HSCT," *Blood*, vol. 118, abstract 4079, 2011.

[23] P. Reddy, "Pathophysiology of acute graft-versus-host disease," *Hematological Oncology*, vol. 21, no. 4, pp. 149–161, 2003.

[24] A. Klimczak and A. Lange, "Apoptosis of keratinocytes is associated with infiltration of CD8+ lymphocytes and accumulation of Ki67 antigen," *Bone Marrow Transplantation*, vol. 26, no. 10, pp. 1077–1082, 2000.

[25] T. A. Weaver and A. D. Kirk, "Alemtuzumab," *Transplantation*, vol. 84, no. 12, pp. 1545–1547, 2007.

[26] G. R. Hill, J. M. Crawford, K. R. Cooke, Y. S. Brinson, L. Pan, and J. L. M. Ferrara, "Total body irradiation and acute graft-versus-host disease: the role of gastrointestinal damage and inflammatory cytokines," *Blood*, vol. 90, no. 8, pp. 3204–3213, 1997.

[27] A. Lange, L. Karabon, A. Klimczak et al., "Serum interferon-γ and C-reactive protein levels as predictors of acute graft-vs-host disease in allogeneic hematopoietic precursor cell (marrow or peripheral blood progenitor cells) recipients," *Transplantation Proceedings*, vol. 28, no. 6, pp. 3522–3525, 1996.

[28] S. Murphy and V. H. Nguyen, "Role of gut microbiota in graft-versus-host disease," *Leukemia & Lymphoma*, vol. 52, pp. 1844–1856, 2011.

[29] L. Karabon, A. Moniewska, A. Laba, C. Swider, and A. Lange, "IL-6 is present in sera of bone marrow-transplanted patients in aplastic period and high levels of IL-6 during acute graft-versus-host disease are associated with severe gut symptoms," *Annals of the New York Academy of Sciences*, vol. 762, pp. 439–442, 1995.

[30] S. Fuji, S. W. Kim, T. Fukuda et al., "Preengraftment serum C-reactive protein (CRP) value may predict acute graft-versus-host disease and nonrelapse mortality after allogeneic hematopoietic stem cell transplantation," *Biology of Blood and Marrow Transplantation*, vol. 14, no. 5, pp. 510–517, 2008.

[31] J. H. Niess, F. Leithäuser, G. Adler, and J. Reimann, "Commensal gut flora drives the expansion of proinflammatory CD4 T cells in the colonic lamina propria under normal and inflammatory conditions," *Journal of Immunology*, vol. 180, no. 1, pp. 559–568, 2008.

[32] J. S. Serody and G. R. Hill, "The IL-17 differentiation pathway and its role in transplant outcome," *Biology of Blood and Marrow Transplantation*, vol. 18, pp. S56–S61, 2012.

[33] E. Bettelli, Y. Carrier, W. Gao et al., "Reciprocal developmental pathways for the generation of pathogenic effector TH17 and regulatory T cells," *Nature*, vol. 441, no. 7090, pp. 235–238, 2006.

[34] H. Chung and D. L. Kasper, "Microbiota-stimulated immune mechanisms to maintain gut homeostasis," *Current Opinion in Immunology*, vol. 22, no. 4, pp. 455–460, 2010.

[35] A. Klimczak, A. Lach, E. Jaskula, and A. Lange, "IL-17 and CCR6 positive cells are present in the skin and gut with toxic lesions and even more pronounced in aGvHD," *Bone Marrow Transplantation*, vol. 46, supplement 1, p. S102, 2011.

[36] R. Varona, V. Cadenas, L. Gómez, C. Martínez-A, and G. Márquez, "CCR6 regulates CD4+ T-cell-mediated acute graft-versus-host disease responses," *Blood*, vol. 106, no. 1, pp. 18–26, 2005.

[37] C. Wang, S. G. Kang, J. Lee, Z. Sun, and C. H. Kim, "The roles of CCR6 in migration of Th17 cells and regulation of effector T-cell balance in the gut," *Mucosal Immunology*, vol. 2, no. 2, pp. 173–183, 2009.

[38] E. Dander, A. Balduzzi, G. Zappa et al., "Interleukin-17-producing t-helper cells as new potential player mediating graft-versus-host disease in patients undergoing allogeneic stem-cell transplantation," *Transplantation*, vol. 88, no. 11, pp. 1261–1272, 2009.

[39] D. Dlubek, E. Turlej, M. Sedzimirska, J. Lange, and A. Lange, "Interleukin-17-producing cells increase among CD4+ lymphocytes before overt manifestation of acute graft-versus-host disease," *Transplantation Proceedings*, vol. 42, no. 8, pp. 3277–3279, 2010.

26

What Is the Most Appropriate Source for Hematopoietic Stem Cell Transplantation? Peripheral Stem Cell/Bone Marrow/Cord Blood

Itır Sirinoglu Demiriz, Emre Tekgunduz, and Fevzi Altuntas

Hematology Clinic and Hematopotic Stem Cell Transplantation Unit, Ankara Oncology Training and Research Hospital (AOH), Yenimahalle, Demetevler, 06200 Ankara, Turkey

Correspondence should be addressed to Itır Sirinoglu Demiriz, dritir@hotmail.com

Academic Editor: Andrzej Lange

The introduction of peripheral stem cell (PSC) and cord blood (CB) as an alternative to bone marrow (BM) recently has caused important changes on hematopoietic stem cell transplantation (HSCT) practice. According to the CIBMTR data, there has been a significant decrease in the use of bone marrow and increase in the use of PSC and CB as the stem cell source for HSCT performed during 1997–2006 period for patients under the age of 20. On the other hand, the stem cell source in 70% of the HSCT procedures performed for patients over the age of 20 was PSC and the second most preferred stem cell source was bone marrow. CB usage is very limited for the adult population. Primary disease, stage, age, time and urgency of transplantation, HLA match between the patient and the donor, stem cell quantity, and the experience of the transplantation center are some of the associated factors for the selection of the appropriate stem cell source. Unfortunately, there is no prospective randomized study aimed to facilitate the selection of the correct source between CB, PSC, and BM. In this paper, we would like to emphasize the data on stem cell selection in light of the current knowledge for patient populations according to their age and primary disease.

1. Trials Comparing Bone Marrow and Peripheral Stem Cell

One of the main reasons for preferring PSC worldwide is the important advantages provided by this method to the donor. These advantages are avoidance of anesthesia, lack of the need for hospitalization or blood transfusion, and very low serious adverse event risk. The largest trial to date comparing these different stem cell sources in HLA matched sibling donor setting was the meta-analysis of IBMTR/EBMT including 536 and 288 patients, who received BM and PSC, respectively [1]. In this trial, a faster neutrophil and platelet engraftment were observed in PSC arm. However, there was no statistically significant difference for relapse and grade II–IV acute graft-versus-host disease (aGvHD) between groups. After 1 year of followup, chronic GVHD frequency was significantly higher in the PSC (65%) arm compared to BM (53%) arm.

Between 1998 and 2002, BM and PSC as a stem cell source were compared in 8 randomized trials [2–9]. Almost all of the patients included were diagnosed as leukemia. Number of patients included, remission status, conditioning regimen, GvHD prophylaxis, stem cell, and T-cell numbers were significantly different in these studies. Combined results suggest faster neutrophil and platelet engraftment with PSC compared to BM. One of the trials revealed similar grade II–IV aGVHD incidence. The largest randomized EBMT study has shown that the use of PSC significantly increased both the frequency of grade II–IV aGvHD (52%–39%; P: 0.013) and cGvHD (67%–54%; P: 0.0066) [5]. In EBMT trial omission of methotrexate on day 11 for aGVHD prophylaxis was suggested to be responsible for the increased aGVHD incidence; however, another meta-analysis was not able to verify this hypothesis [10]. Two out of four large-scale randomized trials showed increased chronic GVHD frequency (%22 and 13%) in patients treated with PSC [3, 5]. Other trials did not report statistically significant increase in chronic GVHD although an insignificant trend for increased cGvHD was observed [2, 4]. The long-term results of French [11] and EBMT [12] trials indicated a higher frequency of chronic

GVHD in the PSC compared to BM group; however, the short- and the long-term follow-up results of the North American [13] trial did not support these findings.

Graft versus tumor effect is mostly associated with the T lymphocytes. As the number of T lymphocytes is higher in PSC product compared to BM, we should expect a lower relapse rate in HSCT using PSC as stem cell source, whereas randomized trials do not report any decrease in relapse risk by using PSC.

Retrospective evaluation reveals lower transplant related mortality (TRM) in HSCT with PSC. IBMTR/EBMT results showed significant decrease in TRM with PSC in the advanced stage leukemia patients undergoing HSCT [1]. Randomized trials did not report statistically significant difference for TRM between PSC and BM. However, we cannot comment on the effect of disease subgroups, stages, and stem cell source which may have significant impact on TRM.

The most distinctive end point of HSCT is the overall survival. There are three big randomized trials reporting different results for this end point. EBMT [5] trial did not find any difference in terms of survival between BM and PSC; but another trial performed in the USA has reported a trend for increased 2-year overall survival (P: 0.06) for PBC [2]. After 30 months of followup, Canadians reported a %8 (P: 0.04) survival advantage in the PSC arm of the trial [14]. USA and Canadian trials in common indicated a survival advantage gained with PSC in advanced disease stages.

The meta-analysis of nine trials including a total of 1111 patients provides us very important data on this topic [15]. The meta-analysis confirms that the selection of PSC decreases the duration of neutrophil and platelet engraftment increases the frequency of grade III–IV aGVHD and chronic GVHD compared to BM. PSC use decreases the 3-year relapse rates in both early stage (%16–%20; P: 0.04) and advanced stage (%33–%51; P: 0.02) diseases compared to BM. On the other hand, PSC only increases the 3-year overall survival (%46–%31; P: 0.01) in the advanced stage disease group. It has been hard to generalize the results of these trials included in this meta-analysis because the majority of the patients had early stage disease such as chronic phase CML (75%) and AML in first complete remission.

Trials comparing PSC and BM as the stem cell source included almost only leukemia patients; on the other hand, very few patients diagnosed with lymphoma and myeloma have been included. Data on the stem cell source in HSCT setting for benign hematological diseases are not sufficient. EBMT has evaluated 692 severe aplastic anemia patients; over the age 20, there was no significant difference between PSC and BM in terms of cGVHD and mortality. In younger patients, cGVHD and mortality rates were higher (%27–%12) in the PSC group [16]. 5-year survival was increased %12 (%85–%73) when BM was preferred as the stem cell source in the subgroup of patients with the age $\leq$ 20. In conclusion, these data suggests that the type of the disease and the age of the patient play a role in deciding the optimal source of stem cell (Table 1).

Consequently, the randomized trials including adult patients point out that PSC increases chronic GVHD, provides overall survival advantage for advanced stage leukemia

TABLE 1: Comparison of the stem cell sources.

	Cord Blood	PB	BM
Risk for the donor	None	Yes	Yes
Duration of searching (month)	≤ 1	3–6	3–6
Factors limiting the engraftment	Cell count	HLA match	HLA match
Dominant factor affecting the outcome	Engraftment failure delayed immune recovery	GVHD	GVHD
Minimal HLA match	4/6	9/10	9/10
Risk for GVHD	Low	High	High
Acute	Low	High	High
Chronic	Low	Higher	High
DLI possibility	None	Possible	Possible
Posttransplant infection risk	Higher	High	High
Immunotheraphy possibility	None	Yes	Yes

patients, but does not significantly have an effect on survival of early stage leukemia patients. On the other hand, in none of these trials, the followup duration has exceeded 3 years and the long-term results are still not known.

The joint IBMTR/EBMT study retrospectively evaluated a large patient population for the long-term results of PSC and BM as a stem cell source [17]. Between 1995-1996 patients over the age of 20 and with different stages of AML, ALL, and CML who underwent HSCT from PSC (n: 288) and BM (n: 462) has been analyzed. Follow-up data on 413 surviving patients (BM: 272; PSC: 141) has been evaluated and a median of six years followup results has been reported. Chronic GVHD incidence was 61% in PSC group and 45% in BM group. PSC has decreased TRM in the advanced stage AML and ALL subgroup but did not increase TRM in the chronic phase CML cases. For acute leukemia patients in first complete remission, there was no significant difference on survival according to stem cell source. But in patients, who achieved second complete remission, there was a trend for increased survival with use of PBC compared to BM (%49–%42). The effectiveness of stem cell source changes according to the stage in chronic leukemia patients. In chronic phase patients, BM provided 6-year survival advantage (%64–%43), but in the accelerated phase disease PSC seems to be superior in terms of survival (%33–%25).

Another trial from IBMTR included 773 (BM: 630; PSC: 143) acute leukemia patients 8–20 of age, who underwent HSCT from HLA match sibling donor between 1995–2000. The followup period was 4 years. Chronic GVHD frequency was 33% in PSC group and 19% in BM group. PSC has increased overall survival by %10 (%58–%48). There was no significant difference between stem cell sources in aGVHD and relapse rates.

CIMBTR data was analyzed for stem cell source of unrelated donors. This trial has evaluated 911 (PSC: 331; BM: 586) patients aged 18–60 years who were diagnosed as AML, ALL, CML, and MDS between 2000 and 2003. The frequency of aGVHD on posttransplantation day 100 (%58–%45) and chronic GVHD (%56–%42) were increased in significantly higher in the PSC group. Three years TRM (%45–%44) and the overall survival (%32–%30) showed no significant difference between PSC and BM groups.

2. The Role of Cord Blood

In theory, all of the patients who are candidates for HSCT but do not have a matched sibling donor but can provide adequate cord blood are candidates for HSCT with CB. HSCT with CB can be performed with 4/6 or 3/6 match, this is why %99 of all patients belonging to all ethnic groups can find acceptable CB units [17]. Therefore, CB is a very important stem cell source alternate but in adult patients stem cell number may be inadequate and there are disadvantages such as longer duration for engraftment and accompanying infections. HSCT with CB has been increased in last two decades; for adult patients, double CB transplantations have been performed successfully but there is no prospective randomized trial head to head comparing CB, PSC, and BM as a stem cell source.

IBMTR [18] and Eurocord [19] trials have retrospectively evaluated the CB use from sibling donors for pediatric patients; under the age of 15 and 1 year survival has been reported to be above 60%. Eurocord trial compared CB (n: 113) with BM (n: 2052). CB recipients were 3 years younger ($P < 0.001$), 9 kilograms lighter ($P < 0.001$), and were treated with lower doses of methotrexate (%28–%65; $P < 0.001$) for aGVHD prophylaxis. The median cell number was 4.7×10^7 nucleated cell/kg in CB recipients. Neutrophil and platelet engraftment ratios were lower with CB compared to BM. Grade II–IV aGVHD (%14–%24; $P = 0.02$) and chronic GVHD (%6–%15; $P = 0.02$) frequency were significantly lower in patients who received CB. There was no difference between groups in terms of 3 years overall survival (CB: %64; BM: %66). These data suggests that CB from HLA matched sibling has similar outcomes as BM from HLA match sister/brother for the pediatric group.

Unrelated CB transplantation data is mostly based on retrospective analysis. Two of three New York Blood Center studies are conducted in 0–11 years old children who were diagnosed with a hematological malignancy and 87% of all grafts were one or two antigen mismatched. The most important factor for the neutrophil engraftment in this series of 861 cases has been found to be the infused cell number. Neutrophil engraftment duration was median of 5 days earlier ($P = 0.0027$) in transplantations with HLA full matched compared to the HLA mismatched CB transplants [20]. HLA mismatch increases the risk of severe GVHD. Grade III–IV aGVHD rate was 8% with HLA A, B, DRB1 matched transplantations, but in mismatched cases it has been increased to 28% ($P = 0.006$). Multivariate analysis revealed that the most important markers for relapse were

the stage of the disease and GVHD. The 3-year survival rates are predicted as 27% and 47% in hematological malignancies and genetic diseases, respectively.

In adult patients, CIBMTR/EBMT has retrospectively evaluated a total of 1525 patients who underwent unrelated HSCT for acute leukemia between 2002 and 2006 and randomized them into 3 different groups (CB: 165; BM: 472; PSC: 888) [21]. Disease-free survival ratios were similar between 8/8 and 7/8 HLA matched BM, PSC cases, and CB recipients. Considering that the 70% of CB group received two antigen mismatched transplants, this success of CB is remarkable. On the other hand, TRM was higher in the CB group when compared with 8/8 HLA matched PSC ($P = 0.003$) and BM ($P = 0.003$). Grade II–IV aGVHD ($P = 0.002$) and chronic GVHD ($P = 0.003$) frequency decreased with CB when compared to allele matched PSC; however, aGVHD ratios did not change when we compared the CB patients with 8/8 HLA matched BM recipients, but chronic GVHD frequency decreased in the CB group ($P = 0.01$).

Basic factors associated with the success of the HSCT with CB are cell number and the degree HLA match. The New York Blood Center (NYBC) has analyzed 910 CB transplantations and revealed that products with $\geq 5 \times 10^7$/kg cell count provided significantly higher 3-year survival rate [22]. The same data confirmed an absolute 3-year survival advantage of 25% with 6/6 HLA matched compared to 5/6 HLA matched CB HSCT. The joint CIBMTR/NYBC trial retrospectively evaluated 619 acute leukemia patients under age 16 during 1995–2003 period; 5-year survival ratios were higher with 6/6 HLA matched CB compared to 8/8 HLA matched BM transplantation (%63–%45). When there is one antigen mismatched CB, it is reasonable to increase the cell number ($>3 \times 10^7$/kg) with double donor to provide the same 5-year survival rate as HLA matched BM (%45) [23].

3. Conclusion

When we choose PSC instead of BM as the stem cell source, the following points should be beer in mind:

(i) chronic GvHD frequency increases,

(ii) in advanced stage leukemias TRM decreases,

(iii) in early phase CML cases TRM increases,

(iv) in advanced stage CML patients survival rate increases,

(v) survival in chronic phase CML cases decreases,

(vi) no effect can be achieved on relapse ratios,

(vii) no difference on disease-free survival and overall survival on acute leukemia,

(viii) aGVHD risk is similar with BM recipients in pediatric and adolescent acute leukemia patients, but chronic GVHD frequency is higher. Relapse ratios are similar in both BM and PSC groups. However, PSC increases TRM and overall mortality,

(ix) aGVHD frequency is similar in aplastic anemia patients. Mortality increases in the group of patients under the age of 20,

(x) acute and chronic GVHD frequency increases with unrelated transplantations. Survival rates are similar to BM recipients.

When we use CB for HSCT, the following points should be emphasized:

(i) An HSCT candidate, but who does not have HLA matched sister/brother and who can provide adequate cord blood for transplantation, can be a recipient.

(ii) The optimal graft selection procedure is still a matter of debate. The most important parameters are the number of nucleated cells and HLA match.

(iii) The success of the cord blood practice depends on the primary disease, conditioning regimen, defrosting the product and the experience of the HSCT center.

(iv) Especially when HLA mismatched unrelated and 5/6 HLA matched CB grafts are compared, CB can be a good alternative to unrelated transplantations.

References

[1] R. E. Champlin, N. Schmitz, M. M. Horowitz et al., "Blood stem cells compared with bone marrow as a source of hematopoietic cells for allogeneic transplantation," *Blood*, vol. 95, no. 12, pp. 3702–3709, 2000.

[2] W. I. Bensinger, P. J. Martin, B. Storer et al., "Transplantation of bone marrow as compared with peripheral-blood cells from HLA-identical relatives in patients with hematologic cancers," *New England Journal of Medicine*, vol. 344, no. 3, pp. 175–181, 2001.

[3] D. Blaise, M. Kuentz, C. Fortanier et al., "Randomized trial of bone marrow versus lenograstim-primed blood cell allogeneic transplantation in patients with early-stage leukemia: a report from the soeiete francaise de greffe de moelle," *Journal of Clinical Oncology*, vol. 18, no. 3, pp. 537–546, 2000.

[4] S. Couban, D. R. Simpson, M. J. Barnett et al., "A randomized multicenter comparison of bone marrow and peripheral blood in recipients of matched sibling allogeneic transplants for myeloid malignancies," *Blood*, vol. 100, no. 5, pp. 1525–1531, 2002.

[5] N. Schmitz, M. Beksac, D. Hasenclever et al., "Transplantation of mobilized peripheral blood cells to HLA-identical siblings with standard-risk leukemia," *Blood*, vol. 100, no. 3, pp. 761–767, 2002.

[6] D. Heldal, G. Tjønnfjord, L. Brinch et al., "A randomised study of allogeneic transplantation with stem cells from blood or bone marrow," *Bone Marrow Transplantation*, vol. 25, no. 11, pp. 1129–1136, 2000.

[7] H. K. Mahmoud, O. A. Fahmy, A. Kamel, M. Kamel, A. El-Haddad, and D. El-Kadi, "Peripheral blood vs bone marrow as a source for allogeneic hematopoietic stem cell transplantation," *Bone Marrow Transplantation*, vol. 24, no. 4, pp. 355–358, 1999.

[8] R. Powles, J. Mehta, S. Kulkarni et al., "Allogeneic blood and bone-marrow stem-cell transplantation in haematological malignant diseases: a randomised trial," *The Lancet*, vol. 355, no. 9211, pp. 1231–1237, 2000.

[9] A. C. Vigorito, W. M. Azevedo, J. F. C. Marques et al., "A randomised, prospective comparison of allogeneic bone marrow and peripheral blood progenitor cell transplantation in the treatment of haematological malignancies," *Bone Marrow Transplantation*, vol. 22, no. 12, pp. 1145–1151, 1998.

[10] W. I. Bensinger, M. Al-Jurf, C. Annasetti et al., "Individual patient data meta-analysis of allogeneic peripheral blood stem cell transplant vs bone marrow transplant in the management of hematological malignancies: indirect assessment of the effect of day 11 methotrexate administration," *Bone Marrow Transplantation*, vol. 38, no. 8, pp. 539–546, 2006.

[11] M. Mohty, M. Kuentz, M. Michallet et al., "Chronic graft-versus-host disease after allogeneic blood stem cell transplantation: long-term results of a randomized study," *Blood*, vol. 100, no. 9, pp. 3128–3134, 2002.

[12] N. Schmitz, M. Beksac, A. Bacigalupo et al., "Filgrastim-mobilized peripheral blood progenitor cells versus bone marrow transplantation for treating leukemia: 3-Year results from the EBMT randomized trial," *Haematologica*, vol. 90, no. 5, pp. 643–648, 2005.

[13] M. E. D. Flowers, P. M. Parker, L. J. Johnston et al., "Comparison of chronic graft-versus-host disease after transplantation of peripheral blood stem cells versus bone marrow in allogeneic recipients: long-term follow-up of a randomized trial," *Blood*, vol. 100, no. 2, pp. 415–419, 2002.

[14] Z. S. Pavletic, M. R. Bishop, S. R. Tarantolo et al., "Hematopoietic recovery after allogeneic blood stem-cell transplantation compared with bone marrow transplantation in patients with hematologic malignancies," *Journal of Clinical Oncology*, vol. 15, no. 4, pp. 1608–1616, 1997.

[15] Stem Cell Trialists' Collaborative Group, "Allogeneic peripheral blood stem-cell compared with bone marrow transplantation in the management of hematologic malignancies: an individual patient data meta-analysis of nine randomized trials," *Journal of Clinical Oncology*, vol. 23, no. 22, pp. 5074–5087, 2005.

[16] H. Schrezenmeier, J. R. Passweg, J. C. W. Marsh et al., "Worse outcome and more chronic GVHD with peripheral blood progenitor cells than bone marrow in HLA-matched sibling donor transplants for young patients with severe acquired aplastic anemia," *Blood*, vol. 110, no. 4, pp. 1397–1400, 2007.

[17] P. G. Beatty, K. M. Boucher, M. Mori, and E. L. Milford, "Probability of finding HLA-mismatched related or unrelated marrow or cord blood donors," *Human Immunology*, vol. 61, no. 8, pp. 834–840, 2000.

[18] E. Gluckman, V. Rocha, A. Boyer-Chammard et al., "Outcome of cord-blood transplantation from related and unrelated donors," *New England Journal of Medicine*, vol. 337, no. 6, pp. 373–381, 1997.

[19] V. Rocha, J. E. Wagner, K. A. Sobocinski et al., "Graft-versus-host disease in children who have received a cord blood or bone marrow transplant from an HLA-identical sibling," *New England Journal of Medicine*, vol. 342, no. 25, pp. 1846–1854, 2000.

[20] P. Rubinstein and C. E. Stevens, "Placental blood for bone marrow replacement: the New York Blood Center's program and clinical results," *Best Practice and Research*, vol. 13, no. 4, pp. 565–584, 2000.

[21] M. Eapen, V. Rocha, G. Sanz et al., "Effect of graft source on unrelated donor haemopoietic stem-cell transplantation in adults with acute leukaemia: a retrospective analysis," *The Lancet Oncology*, vol. 11, no. 7, pp. 653–660, 2010.

[22] Center for International Blood and Marrow Transplant Research (CIBMTR), Summary slides-trends and survival data, http://www.cibmtr.org/ .

[23] M. Eapen, P. Rubinstein, M. J. Zhang et al., "Outcomes of transplantation of unrelated donor umbilical cord blood and bone marrow in children with acute leukaemia: a comparison study," *The Lancet*, vol. 369, no. 9577, pp. 1947–1954, 2007.

Permissions

The contributors of this book come from diverse backgrounds, making this book a truly international effort. This book will bring forth new frontiers with its revolutionizing research information and detailed analysis of the nascent developments around the world.

We would like to thank all the contributing authors for lending their expertise to make the book truly unique. They have played a crucial role in the development of this book. Without their invaluable contributions this book wouldn't have been possible. They have made vital efforts to compile up to date information on the varied aspects of this subject to make this book a valuable addition to the collection of many professionals and students.

This book was conceptualized with the vision of imparting up-to-date information and advanced data in this field. To ensure the same, a matchless editorial board was set up. Every individual on the board went through rigorous rounds of assessment to prove their worth. After which they invested a large part of their time researching and compiling the most relevant data for our readers.

The editorial board has been involved in producing this book since its inception. They have spent rigorous hours researching and exploring the diverse topics which have resulted in the successful publishing of this book. They have passed on their knowledge of decades through this book. To expedite this challenging task, the publisher supported the team at every step. A small team of assistant editors was also appointed to further simplify the editing procedure and attain best results for the readers.

Apart from the editorial board, the designing team has also invested a significant amount of their time in understanding the subject and creating the most relevant covers. They scrutinized every image to scout for the most suitable representation of the subject and create an appropriate cover for the book.

The publishing team has been an ardent support to the editorial, designing and production team. Their endless efforts to recruit the best for this project, has resulted in the accomplishment of this book. They are a veteran in the field of academics and their pool of knowledge is as vast as their experience in printing. Their expertise and guidance has proved useful at every step. Their uncompromising quality standards have made this book an exceptional effort. Their encouragement from time to time has been an inspiration for everyone.

The publisher and the editorial board hope that this book will prove to be a valuable piece of knowledge for researchers, students, practitioners and scholars across the globe.

List of Contributors

Esteban Arrieta-Bolaños
Clinical Research Group, The Anthony Nolan Research Institute, Royal Free & University College Medical School, London NW3 2QG, UK
University College London Cancer Institute, London WC1E 6DD, UK
Centro de Investigaciones en Hematología y Trastornos Afines (CIHATA), Universidad de Costa Rica, 11501-2060 San José, Costa Rica

J. Alejandro Madrigal
Clinical Research Group, The Anthony Nolan Research Institute, Royal Free & University College Medical School, London NW3 2QG, UK
University College London Cancer Institute, London WC1E 6DD, UK

Bronwen E. Shaw
Clinical Research Group, The Anthony Nolan Research Institute, Royal Free & University College Medical School, London NW3 2QG, UK
Haemato-Oncology Research Unit, Division of Molecular Pathology, The Institute of Cancer Research, London SM2 5NG, UK

Netanel Horowitz, Noa Lavi, Noam Benyamini and Viki Held
Department of Hematology and Bone Marrow Transplantation, Rambam Health Care Campus, P.O. Box 9602, Haifa 31096, Israel

Ilana Oren
Unit of Infectious Diseases, Rambam Health Care Campus, P.O. Box 9602, Haifa 31096, Israel
Bruce Rappaport Faculty of Medicine, Technion – Israel Institute of Technology, P.O. Box 9602, Haifa 31096, Israel

Tsila Zuckerman and Irit Avivi
Department of Hematology and Bone Marrow Transplantation, Rambam Health Care Campus, P.O. Box 9602, Haifa 31096, Israel
Bruce Rappaport Faculty of Medicine, Technion – Israel Institute of Technology, P.O. Box 9602, Haifa 31096, Israel

Zipi Kra-Oz
Virology Laboratory, Rambam Health Care Campus, P.O. Box 9602, Haifa 31096, Israel

Monika Dzierzak-Mietla, M.Markiewicz, Anna Koclega, Patrycja Zielinska, Malgorzata Sobczyk-Kruszelnicka and Slawomira Kyrcz-Krzemien
Department of Hematology and Bone Marrow Transplantation, Medical University of Silesia, Dabrowskiego 25, 40-032 Katowice, Poland

Urszula Siekiera
2HLA and Immunogenetics Laboratory, Regional Blood Center, Raciborska 15, 40-074 Katowice, Poland

Sylwia Mizia
Lower Silesian Center for Cellular Transplantation with National Bone Marrow Donor Registry, Grabiszynska 105, 53-439 Wroclaw, Poland

Meral Beksaç
Department of Hematology, Ankara University Unrelated Donor Registry and Cord Blood Bank, Ankara, Turkey
Ankara Tip Fakultesi Hematoloji Bilim Dali, Cebeci Yerleskesi, Dikimevi, 06620 Ankara, Turkey

Klara Dalva
HLA Typing Laboratories, Department of Hematology, Ankara University School of Medicine, `Ibni Sina Hospital, Sihhiye, 06100 Ankara, Turkey

Emilia Jaskula
Department of Clinical Immunology, L. Hirszfeld Institute of Immunology and Experimental Therapy, Polish Academy of Sciences, 12 Rudolfa Weigla Street, 53-114 Wroclaw, Poland

Jolanta Bochenska, Edyta Kocwin and Agnieszka Tarnowska
Lower Silesian Center for Cellular Transplantation, National Bone Marrow Donor Registry, Grabiszyńska 105, 53-439 Wroclaw, Poland

Andrzej Lange
Department of Clinical Immunology, L. Hirszfeld Institute of Immunology and Experimental Therapy, Polish Academy of Sciences, 12 Rudolfa Weigla Street, 53-114 Wroclaw, Poland
Lower Silesian Center for Cellular Transplantation, National Bone Marrow Donor Registry, Grabiszyńska 105, 53-439 Wroclaw, Poland

David Steiner
Department of Cybernetics, Czech Technical University in Prague, Karlovo N´am˘est´ı 13, 121 35 Prague 2, Czech Republic

Catherine Stavropoulos-Giokas, Amalia Dinou and Andreas Papassavas
Hellenic Cord Blood Bank, Biomedical Research Foundation Academy of Athens (BRFAA), 4 Soranou Efessiou Street, 115 27 Athens, Greece

Anita Ryningen, Håkon Reikvam, Ina Nepstad, Kristin Paulsen Rye and Øystein Bruserud
Division of Hematology, Institute of Medicine, University of Bergen, N-5021 Bergen, Norway

Department of Medicine, Haukeland University Hospital, N-5021 Bergen, Norway

Natalia Daniela Escudero and Patricia Mónica Mandalunis
Histology and Embryology Department, School of Dentistry, University of Buenos Aires, Marcelo T de Alvear 2142 1° piso sector A, (C1122AAH) Ciudad Autónoma de Buenos Aires, C1122AAH Buenos Aires, Argentina

Nigel P.Murray
Hematology, Division of Medicine, Hospital de Carabineros de Chile, Simón Bolívar 2200, Ñuñoa, 7770199 Santiago, Chile
Instituto de Bio-Oncología, Avenida Salvador 95, Oficina 95, Providencia, 7500710 Santiago, Chile
Circulating Tumor Cell Unit, Faculty of Medicine, Universidad Mayor, Renato Sánchez 4369, Las Condes, 7550224 Santiago, Chile

Eduardo Reyes
Hematology, Division of Medicine, Hospital de Carabineros de Chile, Simón Bolívar 2200, Ñuñoa, 7770199 Santiago, Chile
Faculty of Medicine, Universidad Diego Portales, Manuel Rodriguez Sur 415, 8370179 Santiago, Chile

Pablo Tapia
Faculty of Medicine, Universidad Pontificia Católica de Chile, Avenida Libertador Bernardo O'Higgins 340, 8331150 Santiago, Chile

Leonardo Badínez
Radiotherapy, Fundación Arturo López Pérez, Rancagua 899, Providencia, 7500921 Santiago, Chile

Nelson Orellana
Hematology, Division of Medicine, Hospital de Carabineros de Chile, Simón Bolívar 2200, Ñuñoa, 7770199 Santiago, Chile

Jennifer L. Granick and Dori L. Borjesson
Department of Pathology, Microbiology, Immunology, University of California School of Veterinary Medicine, Davis, CA 95616, USA

Scott I. Simon
Department of Biomedical Engineering, University of California, Davis, CA 95616, USA

Anna Koclega, MiroslawMarkiewicz, Monika Dzierzak-Mietla, Patrycja Zielinska, Malgorzata Sobczyk Kruszelnicka and Slawomira Kyrcz-Krzemien
Department of Hematology and BMT, Medical University of Silesia, Dabrowskiego 25, 40-032 Katowice, Poland

Urszula Siekiera and Alicja Dobrowolska
HLA and Immunogenetics Laboratory, Regional Blood Center, Raciborska 15, 40-074 Katowice, Poland

Mizia Sylwia and Andrzej Lange
Lower Silesian Center for Cellular Transplantation with National Bone Marrow Donor Registry, Grabiszynska 105, 53-439 Wroclaw, Poland

Kamonnaree Chotinantakul and Wilairat Leeanansaksiri
Stem Cell Therapy and Transplantation Research Group, Suranaree University of Technology, Nakhon Ratchasima 30000, Thailand
School of Microbiology, Institute of Science, Suranaree University of Technology, Nakhon Ratchasima 30000, Thailand

Elisa Dorantes-Acosta
Leukemia Clinic, Mexican Children's Hospital Federico Gómez, 06720 Mexico City, DF, Mexico
Oncology Research Unit, Oncology Hospital, Mexican Institute of Social Security, 06720 Mexico City, DF, Mexico
Medical Sciences Program, National Autonomous University of Mexico, 04510 Mexico City, DF, Mexico

Rosana Pelayo
Oncology Research Unit, Oncology Hospital, Mexican Institute of Social Security, 06720 Mexico City, DF, Mexico

Vivek Roy
Division of Hematology/Oncology, Mayo Clinic, 4500 San Pablo Road, Jacksonville, FL 32224, USA

Meerim Park
Department of Pediatrics, College of Medicine, Chungbuk National University, Cheongju, Republic of Korea

Jong Jin Seo
Department of Pediatrics, Asan Medical Center Children's Hospital, University of Ulsan College of Medicine, Seoul, Republic of Korea

Raymond Alexanian, Kay Delasalle, Michael Wang, Sheeba Thomas and Donna Weber
University of Texas MD Anderson Cancer Center, Houston, TX 77030-4009, USA

Vidyasagar Devaprasad Dedeepiya, Subramani Baskar, Sadananda RaoManjunath and Rajappa Senthilkumar
Division of Translational Medicine, Nichi-In Centre for Regenerative Medicine (NCRM), C 16 & 17, Vijaya Health Centre Premises, 175 NSK Salai, Vadapalani, Chennai-600026, Tamil Nadu, India
Department of Biotechnology, Acharya Nagarjuna University, Nagarjuna Nagar, Guntur 522 510, India

Yegneswara Yellury Rao
Department of Medicine, KG Hospital, Arts College Road, Coimbatore 641018, India

Gosalakkal A. Jayakrishnan
Department of Cardiothoracic Surgery, Omega Hospital, Mangalore, Mahaveera Circle, Kankanady, Mangalore 575002, India

Jutty K. B. C. Parthiban
Division of Translational Medicine, Nichi-In Centre for Regenerative Medicine (NCRM), C 16 & 17, Vijaya Health Centre Premises, 175 NSK Salai, Vadapalani, Chennai-600026, Tamil Nadu, India

Samuel J. K. Abraham
Division of Translational Medicine, Nichi-In Centre for Regenerative Medicine (NCRM), C 16 & 17, Vijaya Health Centre Premises, 175 NSK Salai, Vadapalani, Chennai-600026, Tamil Nadu, India
Department of Surgery, Faculty of Medicine, University of Yamanashi, 1110 Shimokato, Yamanashi, Chuo 409-3898, Japan

SylwiaMizia, Dorota Dera-Joachimiak, Malgorzata Polak, Katarzyna Koscinska and
Mariola Sedzimirska
Division of the National Bone Marrow Donor Registry, Lower Silesian Center for Cellular Transplantation, Grabiszynska 105, 53-439 Wroclaw, Poland

Andrzej Lange
Division of the National Bone Marrow Donor Registry, Lower Silesian Center for Cellular Transplantation, Grabiszynska 105, 53-439 Wroclaw, Poland
Institute of Immunology and Experimental Therapy, Polish Academy of Sciences, 53-114 Wroclaw, Poland

Abraham S. Kanate
Myeloma and Lymphoma Service, Osborn Hematopoietic Malignancy and Transplantation Program, West Virginia University, Morgantown, WV 26506, USA

Mohamed A. Kharfan-Dabaja
Blood and Marrow Transplantation, Moffitt Cancer Center, Tampa, FL 33612, USA

Mehdi Hamadani
Myeloma and Lymphoma Service, Osborn Hematopoietic Malignancy and Transplantation Program, West Virginia University, Morgantown, WV 26506, USA
Division of Hematology and Oncology, West Virginia University, P.O. Box 9162, 1 Medical Center Drive, Morgantown, WV 26506, USA

J.-M. Tiercy
National Reference Laboratory for Histocompatibility, Transplantation Immunology Unit, Department of Medical Specialties and Department of Genetics and Laboratory Medicine, Geneva University Hospitals, University of Geneva, 1211 Geneva, Switzerland

Khalid Ahmed Al-Anazi
Section of Adult Hematology and Hematopoietic Stem Cell Transplantation, Oncology Center, King Fahad Specialist Hospital, P.O. Box 15215, Dammam 31444, Saudi Arabia

Corinna Barkam, Haytham Kamal, Elke Dammann, Helmut Diedrich, Stefanie Buchholz, Matthias Eder, Jürgen Krauter, Arnold Ganser and Michael Stadler
Department of Hematology, Hemostasis, Oncology, and Stem Cell Transplantation, Hannover Medical School, 30625 Hannover, Germany

Aleksandra Klimczak
Department of Clinical Immunology, L. Hirszfeld Institute of Immunology and Experimental Therapy, Polish Academy of Sciences, 12 Rudolfa Weigla Street, 53-114 Wroclaw, Poland

Andrzej Lange
Department of Clinical Immunology, L. Hirszfeld Institute of Immunology and Experimental Therapy, Polish Academy of Sciences, 12 Rudolfa Weigla Street, 53-114 Wroclaw, Poland
Lower Silesian Center for Cellular Transplantation, National Bone Marrow Donor Registry, Grabiszyńska 105, 53-439 Wroclaw, Poland

Itır Sirinoglu Demiriz, Emre Tekgunduz and Fevzi Altuntas
Hematology Clinic and Hematopotic Stem Cell Transplantation Unit, Ankara Oncology Training and Research Hospital (AOH), Yenimahalle, Demetevler, 06200 Ankara, Turkey